GLENFIELD
X-RAY

GLENFIELD GENERAL HOSPITAL
X-RAY DEPARTMENT

An Atlas of Transvaginal Sonography

GLENFIELD GENERAL HOSPITAL
X-RAY DEPARTMENT

An Atlas of Transvaginal Sonography

Jonathan Carter
M.B., B.S., Dip. R.A.C.O.G.,
F.A.C.A., M.S., F.R.A.C.O.G.
Assistant Professor
Director Ultrasound Research
Department of Obstetrics and Gynecology
Division of Gynecologic Oncology
University of Minnesota
Minneapolis, Minnesota

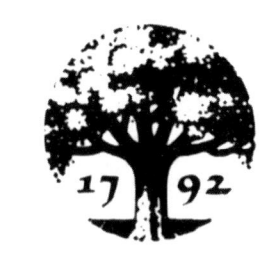

J.B. Lippincott Company
Philadelphia

Acquisitions Editor: Lisa McAllister
Sponsoring Editor: Emilie Linkins
Production Manager: Janet Greenwood
Design Coordinator: Glenn Whaley/GW Graphics
Interior Design: Angie Blackwell/GW Graphics
Cover Design: Angie Blackwell/GW Graphics
Printer/Binder: Walsworth Publishing Company

Copyright © 1994, by J. B. Lippincott Company. All rights reserved. No part of this book may be used or reproduced in any manner whatsoever without written permission except for brief quotations embodied in critical articles and reviews. Printed in the United States of America. For information write J.B. Lippincott Company, 227 East Washington Square, Philadelphia, Pennsylvania 19106.

Library of Congress Cataloging-In-Publication Data

Carter, Jonathan,
    An atlas of transvaginal sonography/Jonathan Carter.
      p. cm.
    Includes bibliographical references.
    ISBN 0-397-51460-3
1. Transvaginal ultrasonography—Atlases. I. Title. [DNLM: 1. Genital Diseases, Female—ultrasonography—atlases.
2. Ultrasonography, Prenatal—atlases. 3. Genitalia, Female—ultrasonography—atlases. WP 17 C323a 1994]
RG107. 5.T73C37-1994
618'.047543—dc20
DNLM/DLC
for Library of Congress
                                                                                        93-48347
                                                                                           CIP

The authors and publisher have exerted every effort to ensure that drug selection and dosage set forth in this text are in accord with current recommendations and practice at the time of publication. However, in view of ongoing research, changes in government regulations, and the constant flow of information relating to drug therapy and drug reactions, the reader is urged to check the package insert for each drug for any change in indications and dosage and for added warnings and precautions. This is particularly important when the recommended agent is a new or infrequently employed drug.

This book is dedicated to my family. To my parents Bob and Elizabeth who stimulated, encouraged and financed my lifelong dream to become a doctor. To my sister, Noni, who through her family consolidated us as a strong family unit through the good and bad times. To my brother Timothy who works harder than all of us, and whom we all love and cherish. And to Andrew who has grown from the baby to the leader of the family.

To my wife Janet for her devoted love and attention and our son Nicholas, to whom I dedicate the rest of my life.

Preface

Transvaginal sonography (TVS) is rapidly emerging as an extension to the normal pelvic examination. By performing a TVS after a pelvic examination, the physician can combine tactile physical impression with visual identification of pathology that literally allows "seeing into the pelvis." This information, in combination with knowledge of pelvic anatomy and understanding of gynecologic disease processes, facilitates immediate formulation of an accurate diagnosis.

Although all sonographers need to understand the physics of sound and ultrasound, the clinically oriented sonographer, like the colposcopist, recognizes patterns of images to formulate a sonographic diagnosis. For the novice, and less experienced sonographer, an atlas of representative images for education and future reference is crucial. Currently such an atlas of TVS does not exist. Available texts on sonography provide extensive dialogue on disease processes, but lack quality images. The same can be said for older texts on transabdominal sonography. The orientation and quality of the transvaginal ultrasound images are, in addition, very different from images obtained transabdominally. Many of the previous texts discussing use of ultrasound in gynecology are of limited value because of these differences.

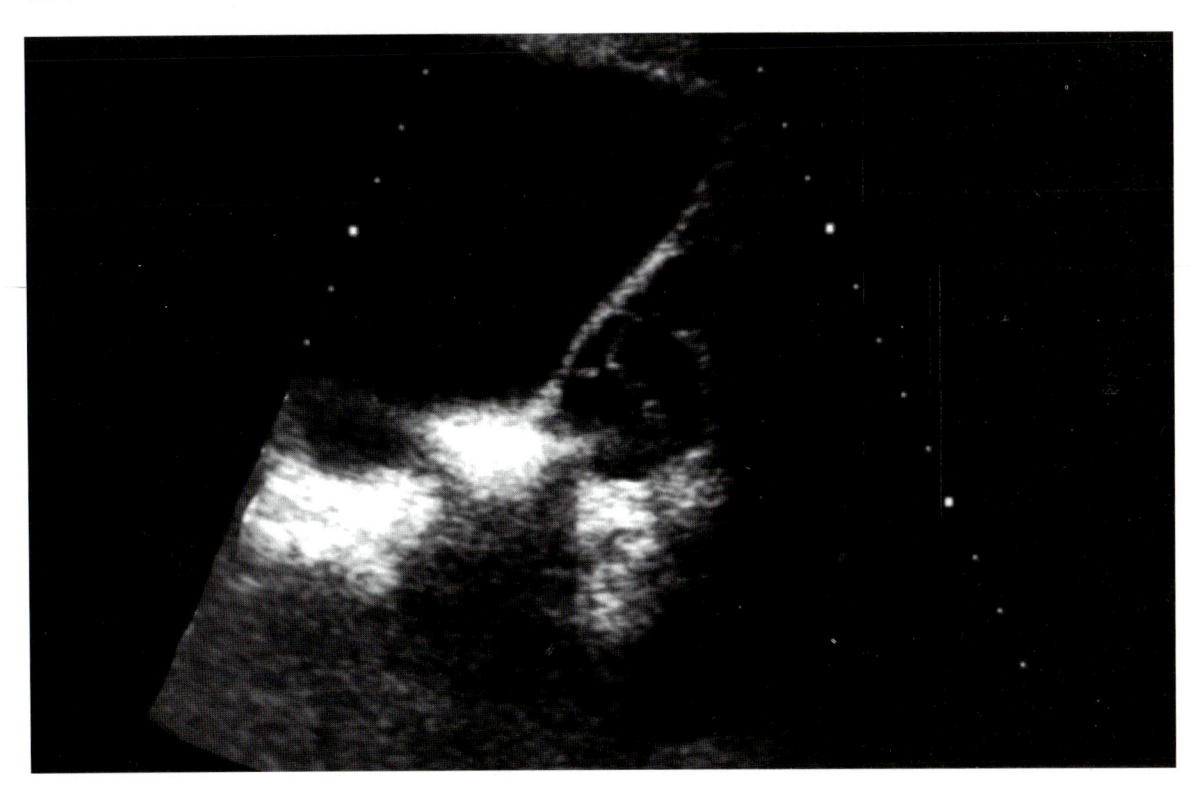

Figure I. Transabdominal sonogram, through a distended bladder, of a cystic ovarian tumor. Internal morphology is difficult to determine.

Preface

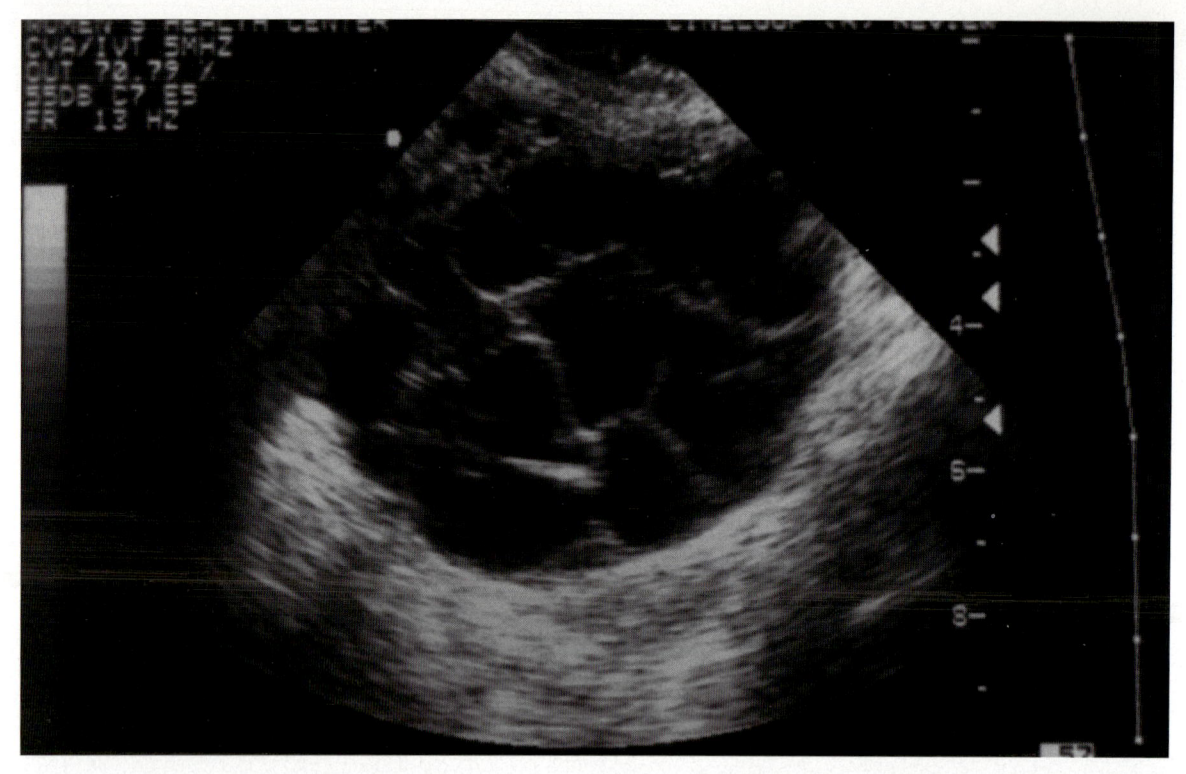

Figure II. *Superior image obtained by transvaginal sonography, clearly depicting the internal morphology of this ovarian tumor.*

This *Atlas* was compiled by a clinician for use by clinicians. The intent of this reference book is not to be a definitive text on gynecologic pathology, nor is it to be a text on transvaginal sonography. This *Atlas* is designed to provide the clinician with visual information and to educate those utilizing this fantastic imaging modality.

The author wishes to thank Selina Blatz and Dr. Jacques Stassart for some images related to reproductive endocrinology.

Jonathan Carter

Contents

Chapter 1
Color Doppler in Transvaginal Sonography 1

Chapter 2
Limitations and Artifacts 13

Chapter 3
The Examination 21

Chapter 4
Cervix 23

Chapter 5
Uterus 33

Chapter 6
Fallopian Tube 63

Chapter 7
Ovary 67

Chapter 8
Normal Early Pregnancy 101

Chapter 9
Abnormal Early Pregnancy 111

Chapter 10
Gestational Trophoblastic Disease 119

Chapter 11
Uterine Cancer 129

Chapter 12
Cervical Cancer 149

Chapter 13
Ovarian Cancer 161

Chapter 14
Recurrent Gynecologic Cancer 177

Chapter 15
Infertility 183

Chapter 16
Urinary Tract 195

Chapter 17
Bowel 201

Chapter 18
Miscellaneous Lesions 209

Bibliography 223

1 Color Doppler in Transvaginal Sonography

The use of color Doppler in TVS is helpful for the majority of diagnostic evaluations. Bursts or pulses of ultrasound are emitted from the transducer at a frequency determined by the transducer characteristics. Returning echoes have different frequencies (Doppler shifted frequencies) depending upon the object they strike and its motion. A color is assigned to each shifted frequency. Thus, in assessing blood flow, the ultrasound echoes are reflected from moving red blood cells. The frequency of the returning echo is thus altered by the velocity of the red blood cell, and the direction of its travel, either toward or away from the transducer. Blood flow velocity or blood flow indices are calculated according to the Doppler equation.

The iliac vessels serve as anatomic landmarks for transvaginal sonography, but their flow measurements are not clinically useful. Although many previous texts have stated the internal iliac vessels lie adjacent to the ovary and are used for their identification, in reality, ovarian location is variable, and can be found overlying either the common iliac vessels, the external iliac vessels or the internal iliac vessels.

The uterine artery is a branch of the internal iliac that courses along the base of the broad ligament. As it approaches the cervix, it divides into a descending vaginal and anterior uterine branch that ascends in a convoluted and tortuous fashion up the lateral edge of the uterus, within the leaves of the broad ligament. The spectral appearance of the uterine artery varies throughout the menstrual cycle. In the proliferative phase of the cycle, uterine flow velocity is typically of a high resistance pattern. From the time of ovulation and throughout the luteal phase of the cycle, resistance decreases. Postmenopausal women typically show a low velocity, high impedance pattern that increases with age.

The ovarian artery is a branch of the aorta and reaches the ovary through fascial condensation known as the infundibulopelvic ligament. The ovary is further supplied by an adnexal branch of the uterine artery. Like the uterine vessels, the ovarian blood supply is altered at different stages throughout the menstrual cycle. A low-velocity, high-impedance pattern is seen during the follicular phase. At ovulation, the velocity increases and resistance indices decrease, signifying a low-impedance vascular bed. This is more pronounced on the side of the corpus luteum and results from the neovascularization of the dominant follicle.

An Atlas of Transvaginal Sonography

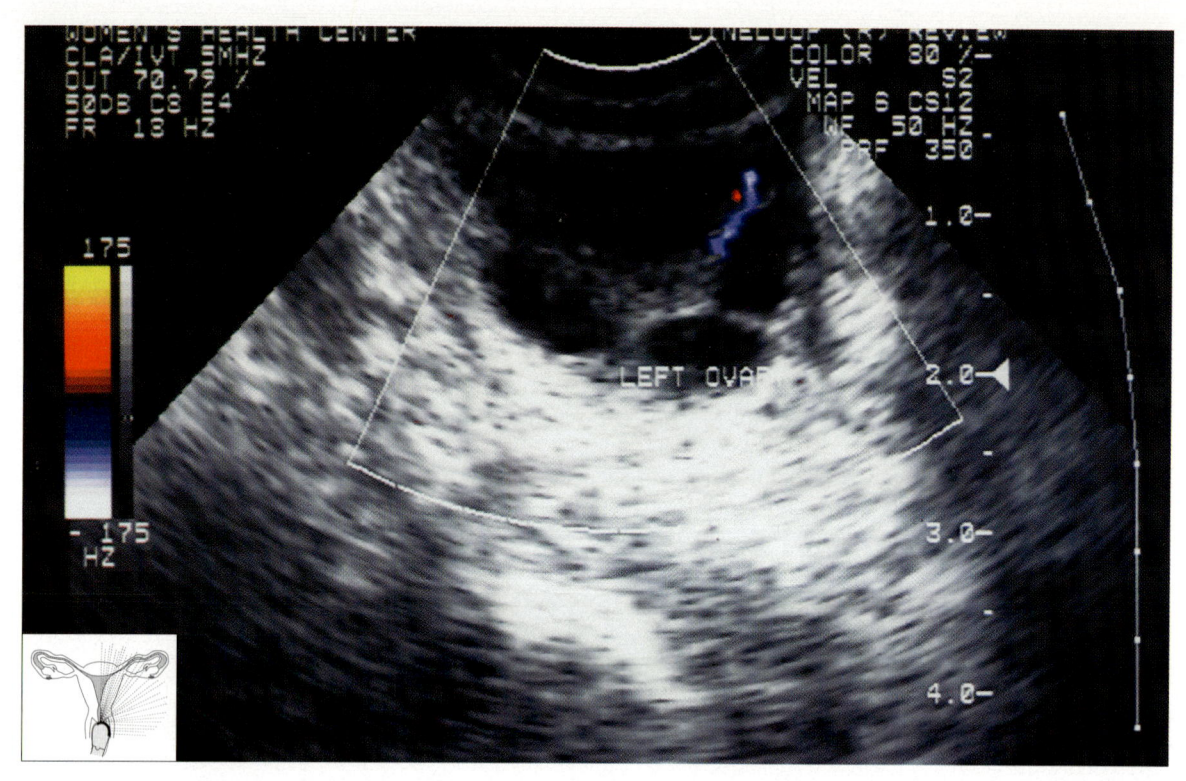

Figure 1-1. *Normal intraovarian flow. Low-velocity fine-branching tapering vessel.*

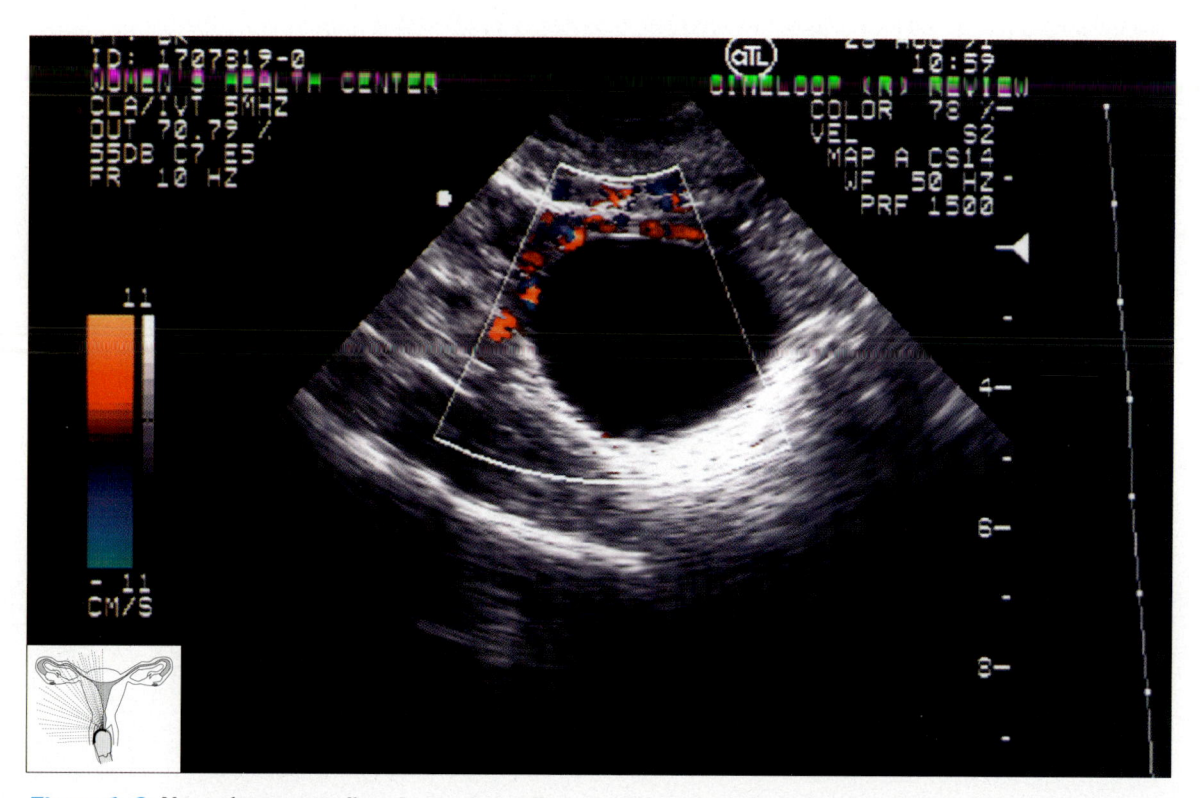

Figure 1-2. *Normal pericystic flow. Low-velocity flow around the periphery of this ovarian cyst.*

Color Doppler in Transvaginal Sonography

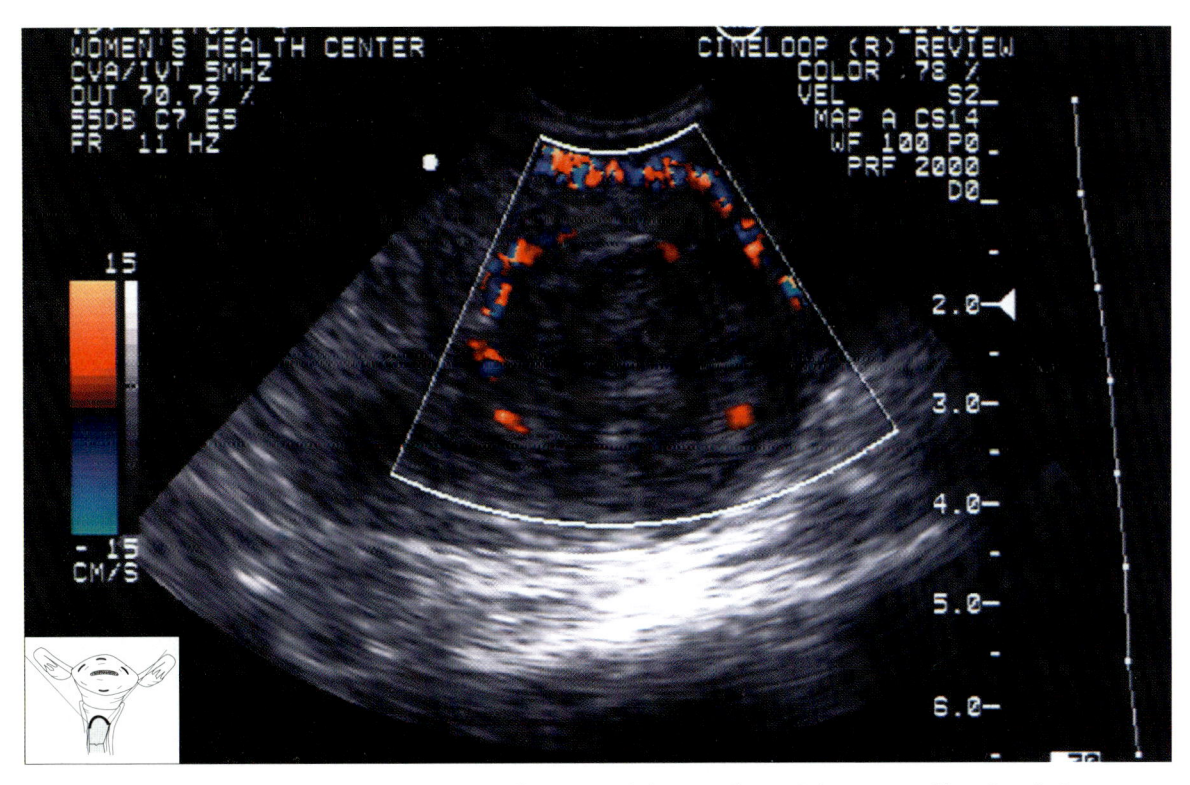

Figure 1-3. Normal uterine flow. Low-velocity flow around the periphery of this uterine fibroid and absent intratumor flow.

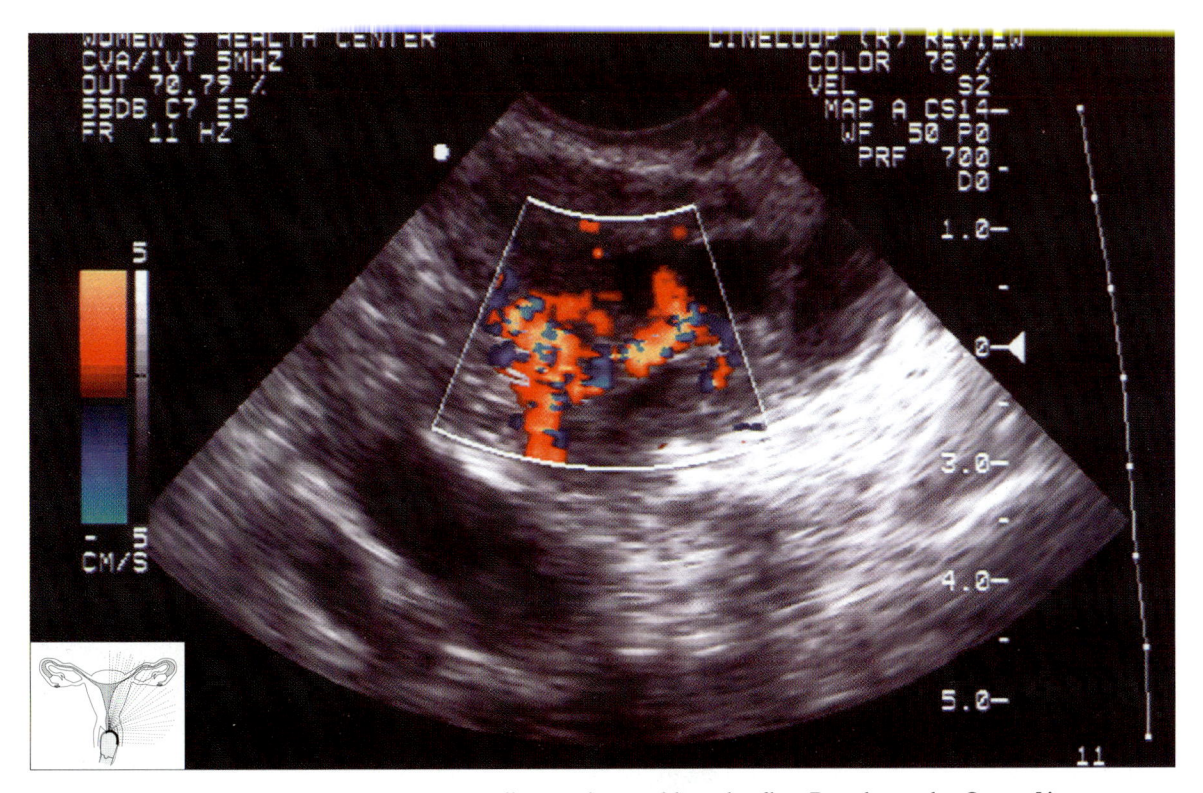

Figure 1-4. Increased and abnormal ovarian flow as depicted by color flow Doppler in this Stage IA ovarian cancer.

An Atlas of Transvaginal Sonography

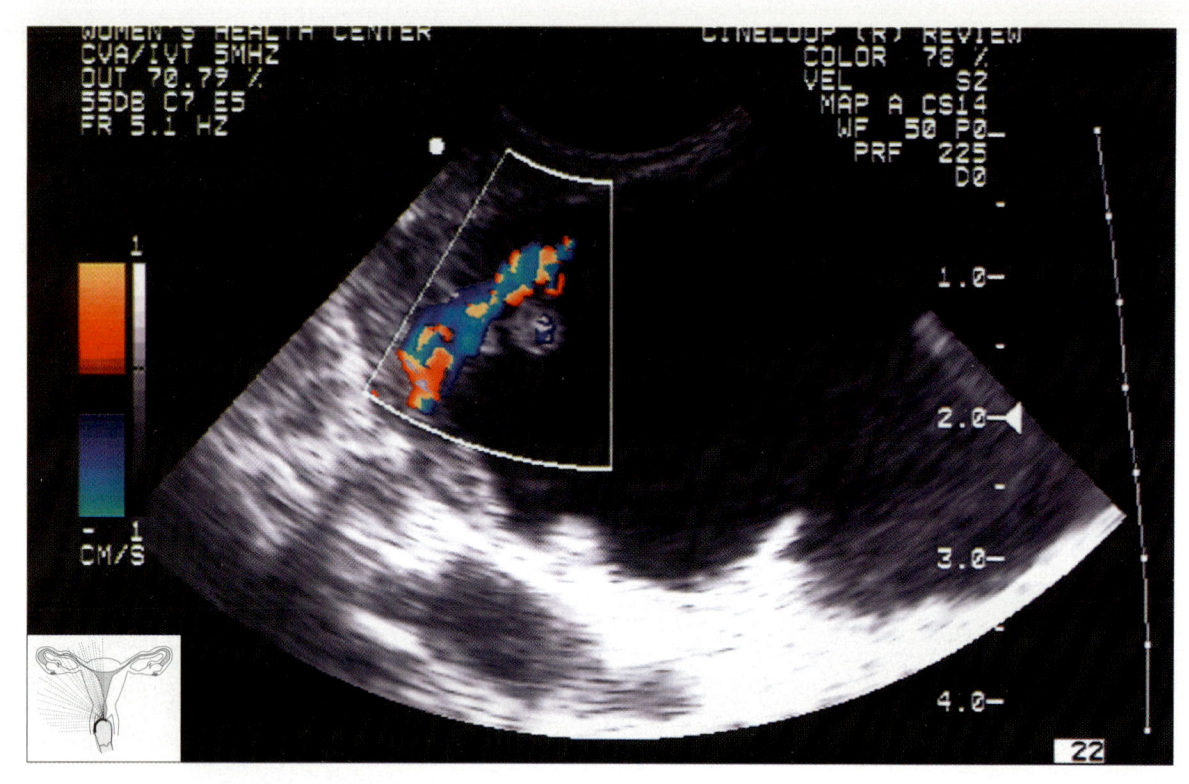

Figure 1-5. *Increased flow within the solid component of this ovarian cancer.*

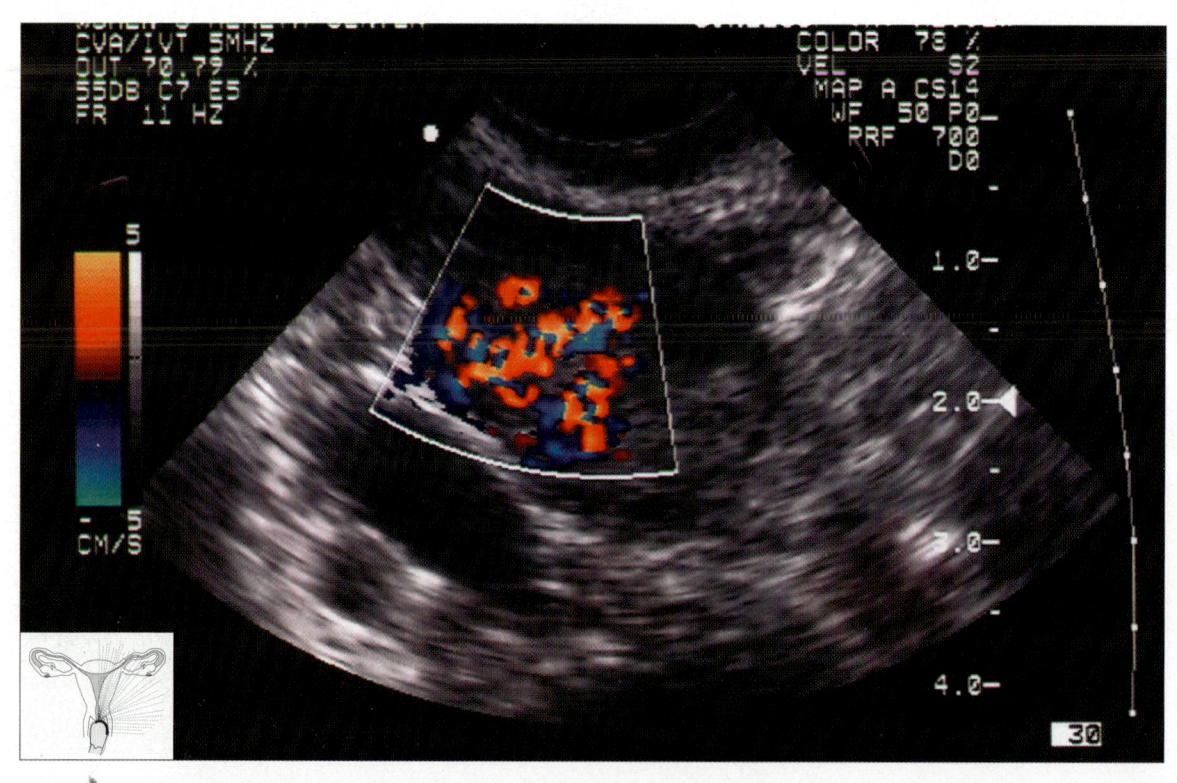

Figure 1-6. *Abnormal and increased color flow in this early ovarian cancer.*

Color Doppler in Transvaginal Sonography

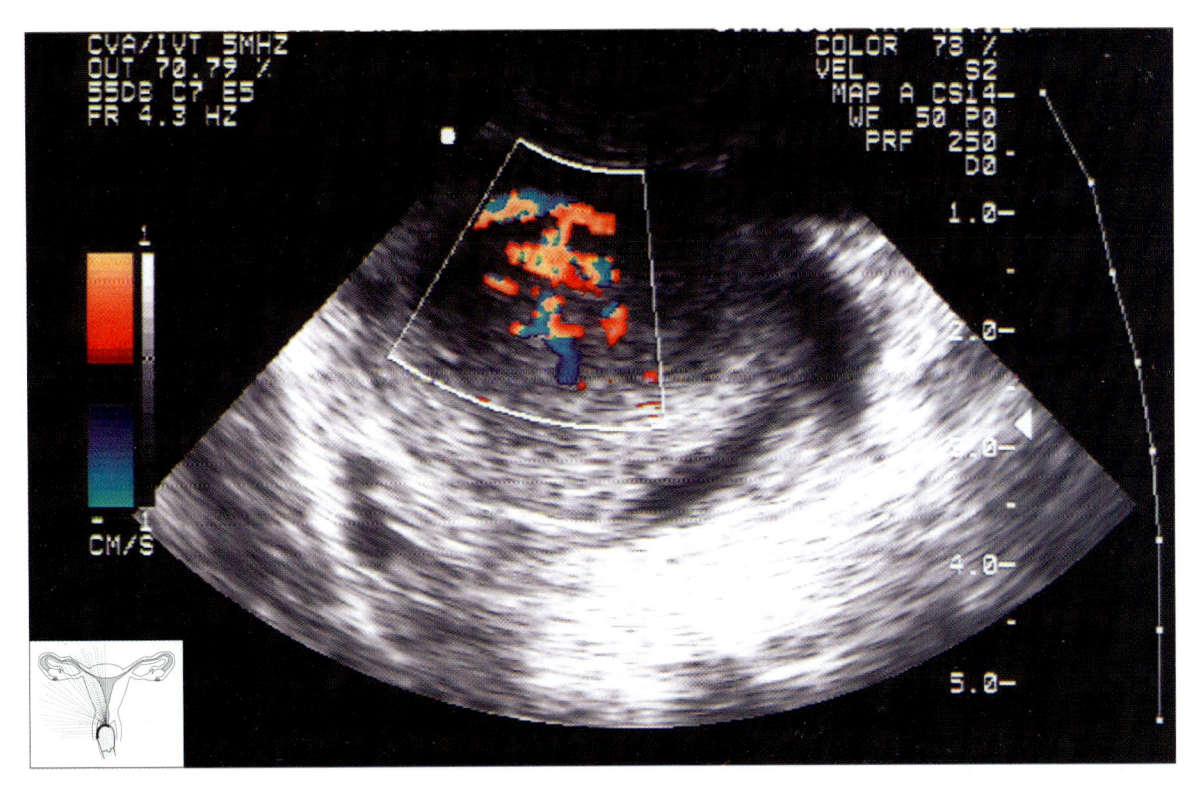

Figure 1-7. Increased central and peripheral flow in this solid ovarian tumor.

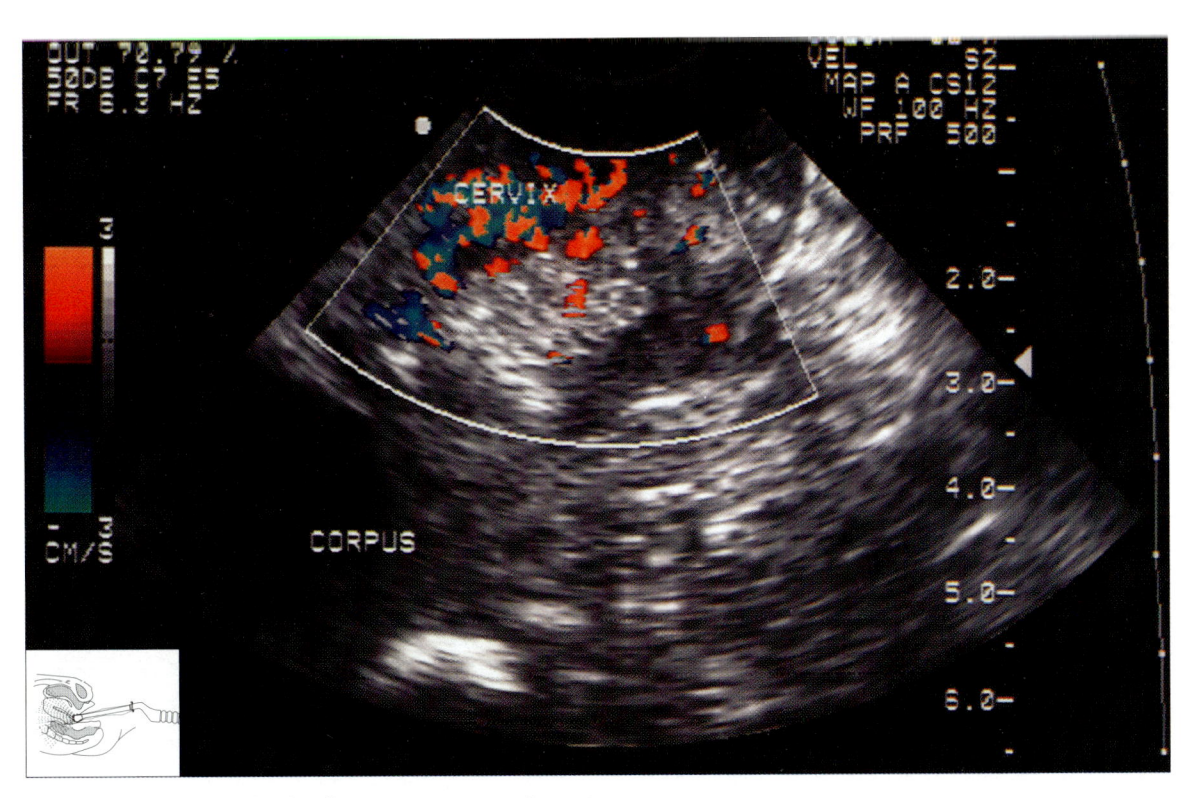

Figure 1-8. Increased color flow in a patient with cervix cancer.

An Atlas of Transvaginal Sonography

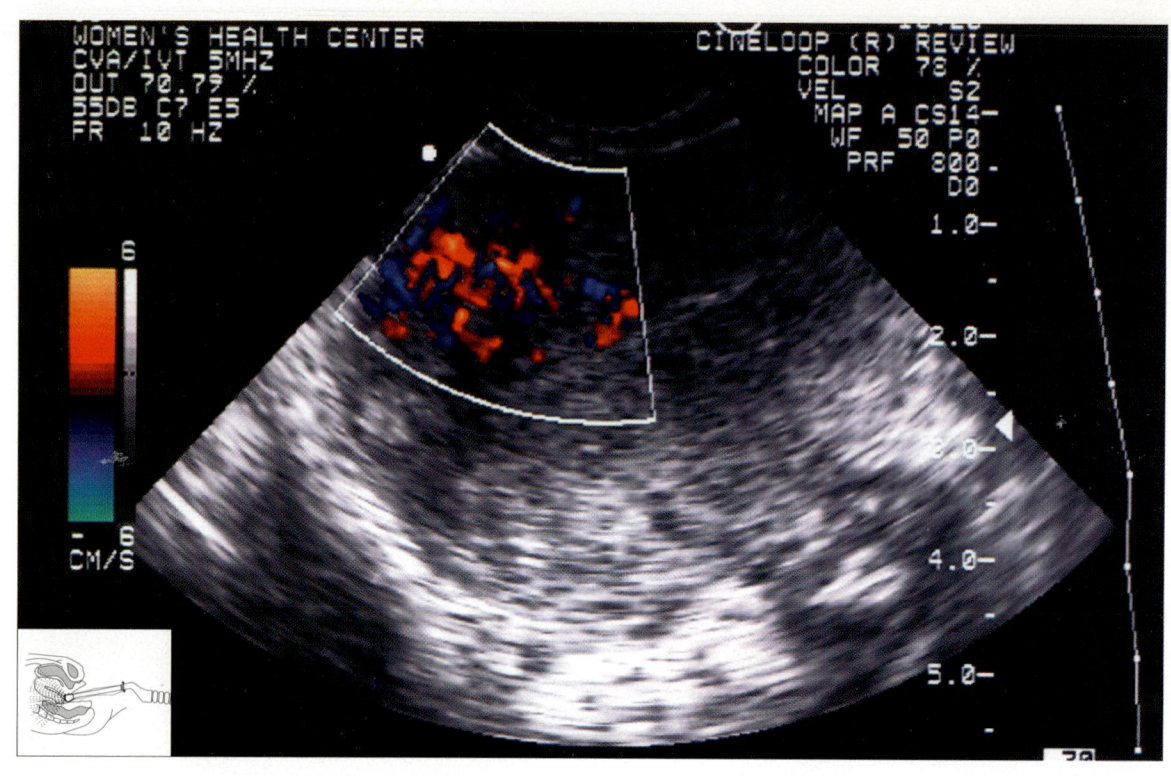

Figure 1-9. Increased color flow in a patient with an invasive hydatidiform mole.

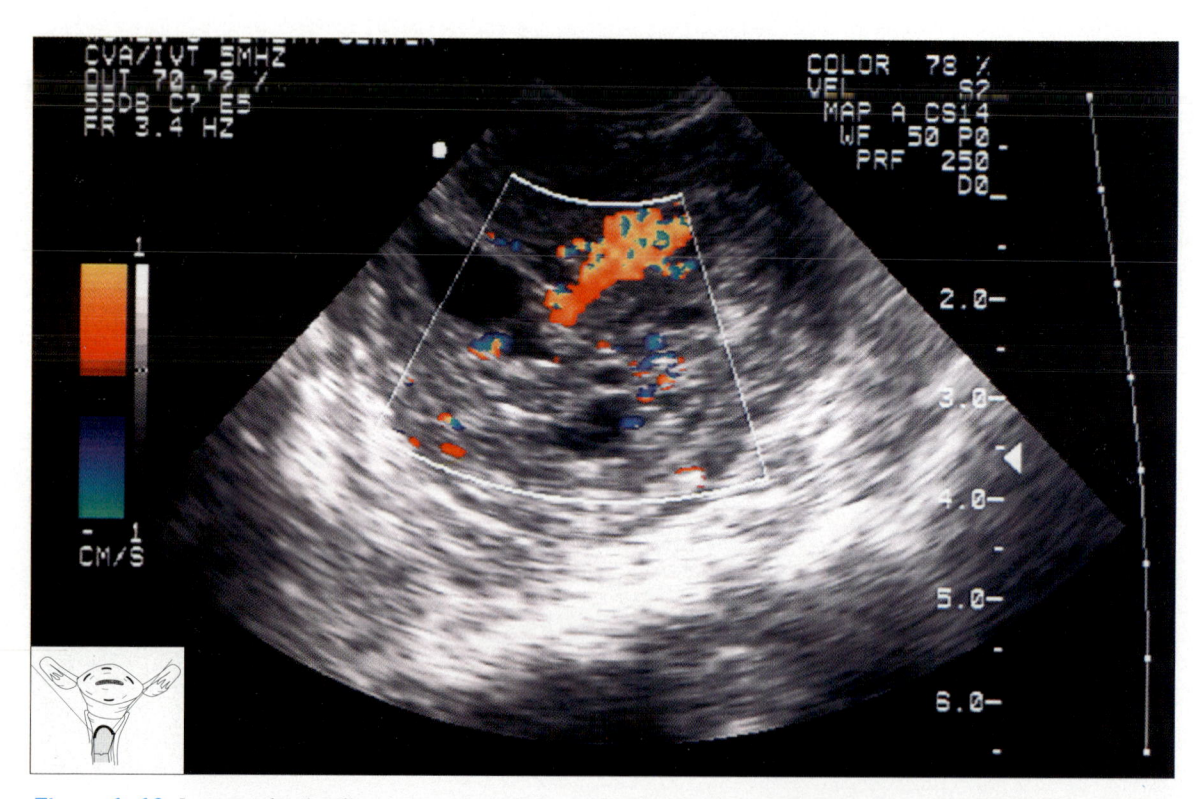

Figure 1-10. Increased color flow in a patient with a cystic-solid mixed Mullerian sarcoma of uterus.

6

Color Doppler in Transvaginal Sonography

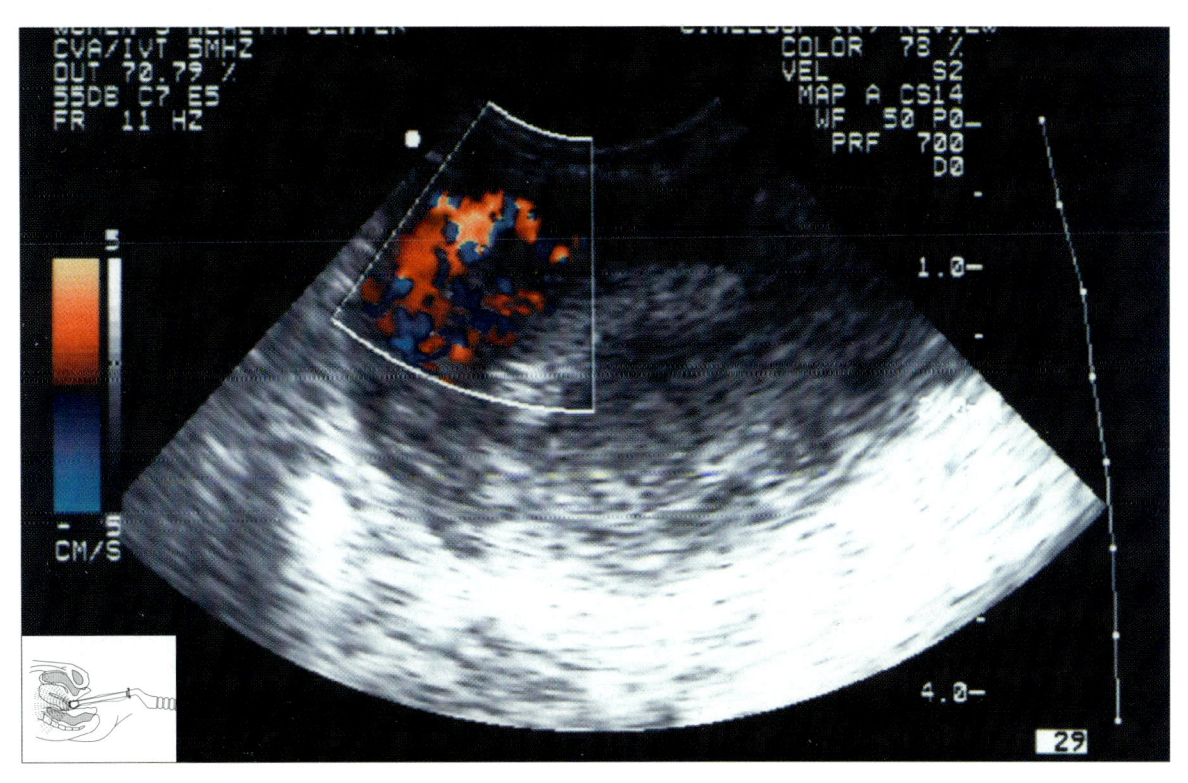

Figure 1-11. Increased color flow in a patient with invasive endometrial cancer.

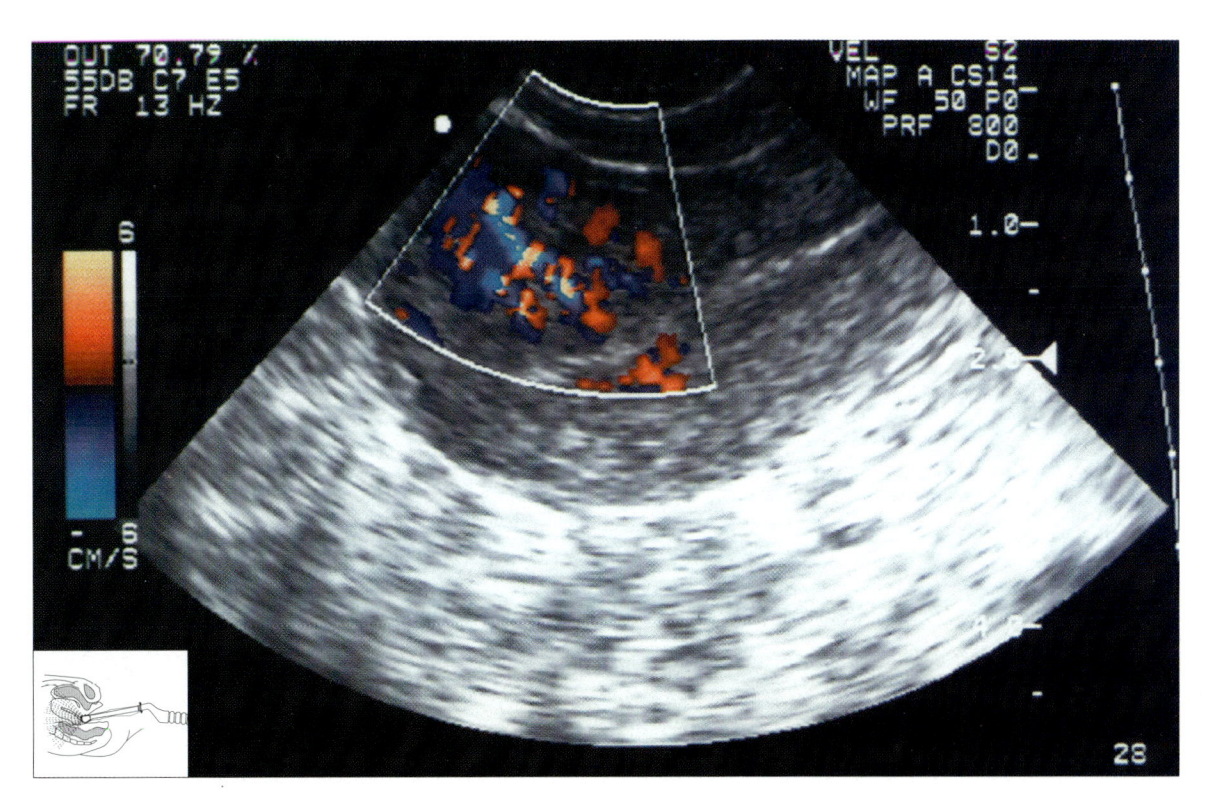

Figure 1-12. Increased color flow in a patient with an invasive mole.

An Atlas of Transvaginal Sonography

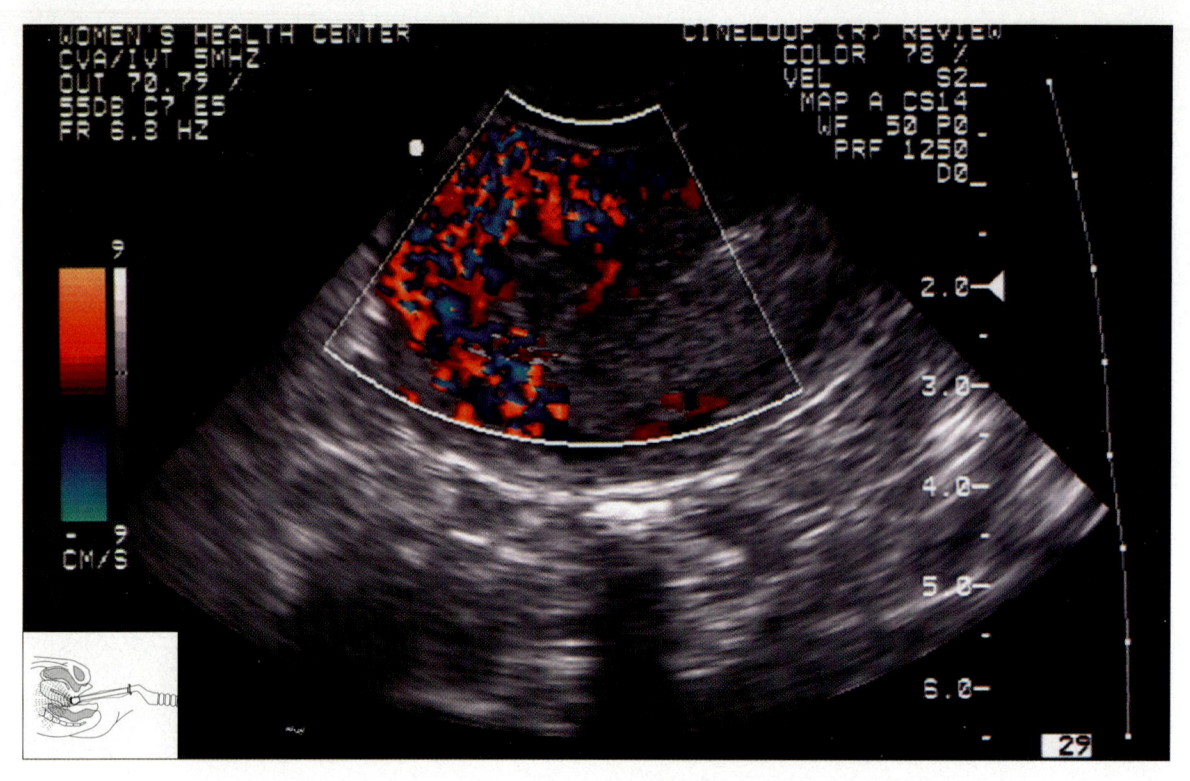

Figure 1-13. *Increased color flow in a patient with an invasive mole.*

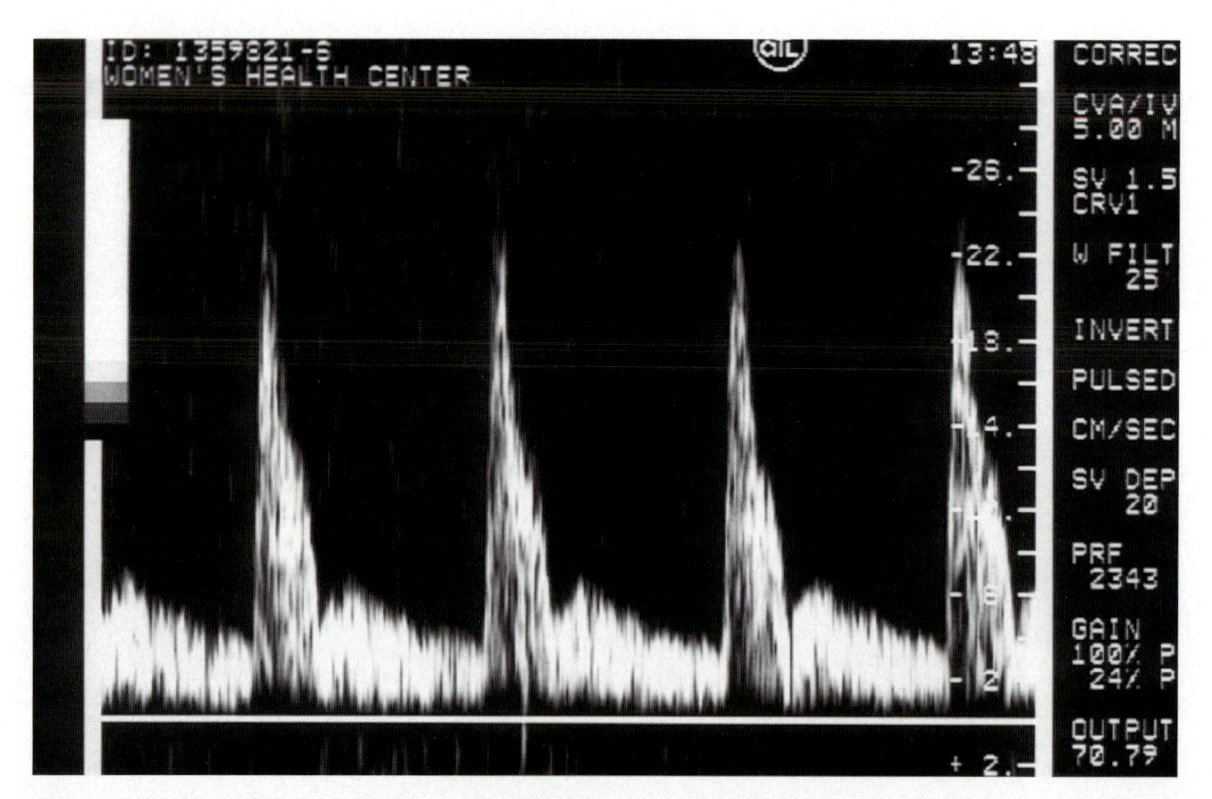

Figure 1-14. *Normal uterine artery spectral waveform.*

Color Doppler in Transvaginal Sonography

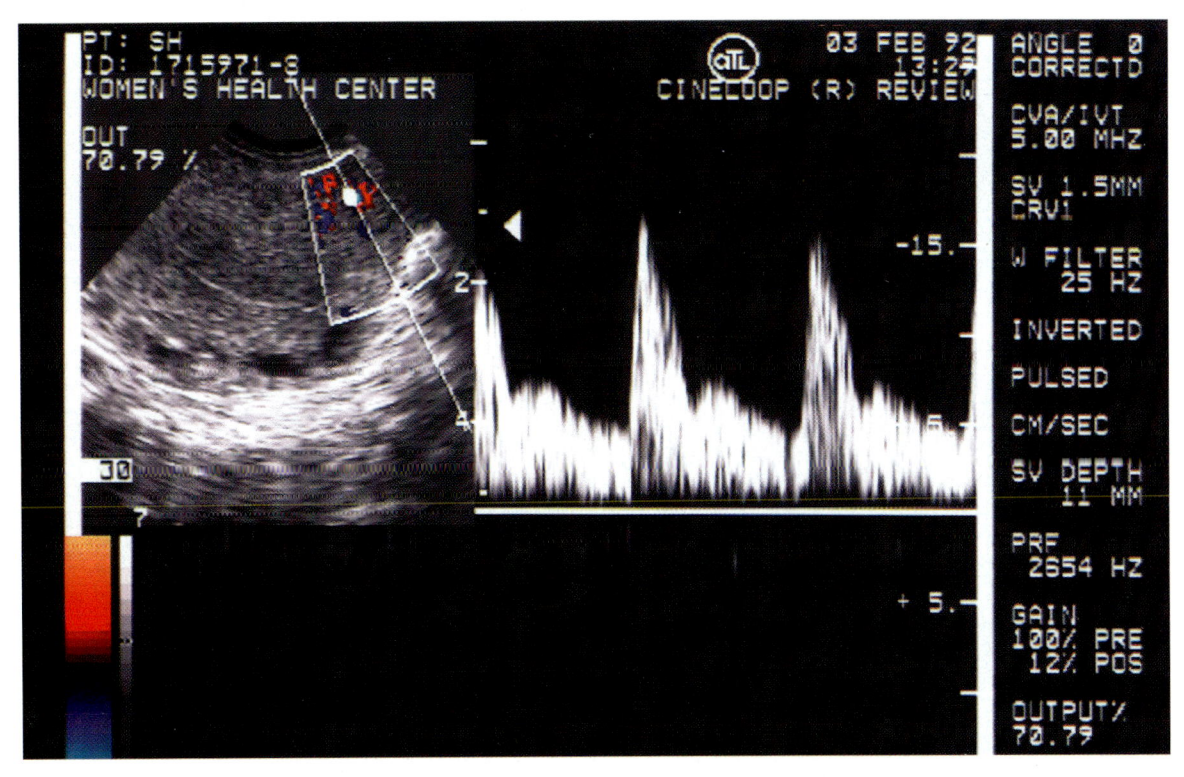

Figure 1~15. Uterine artery spectral waveform in a patient with a benign tumor.

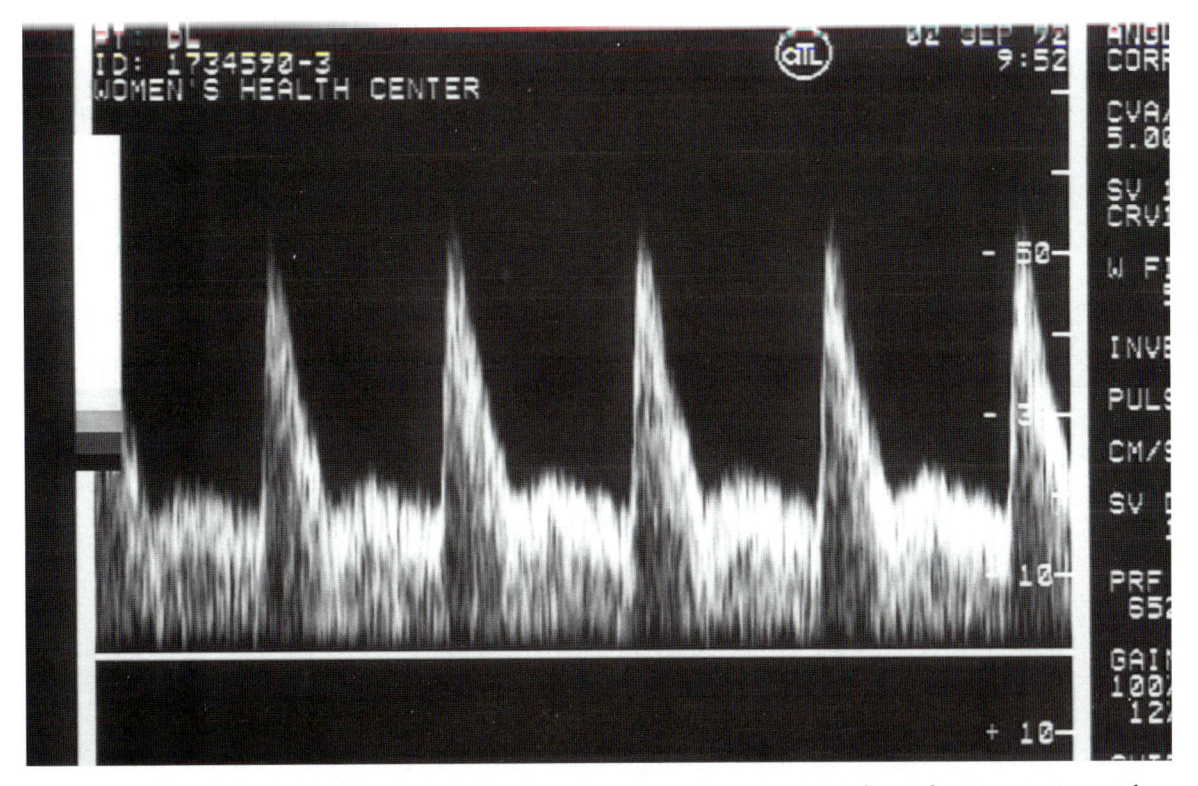

Figure 1~16. Increased diastolic flow but otherwise normal uterine artery spectral waveform in a patient with a benign uterine tumor.

9

An Atlas of Transvaginal Sonography

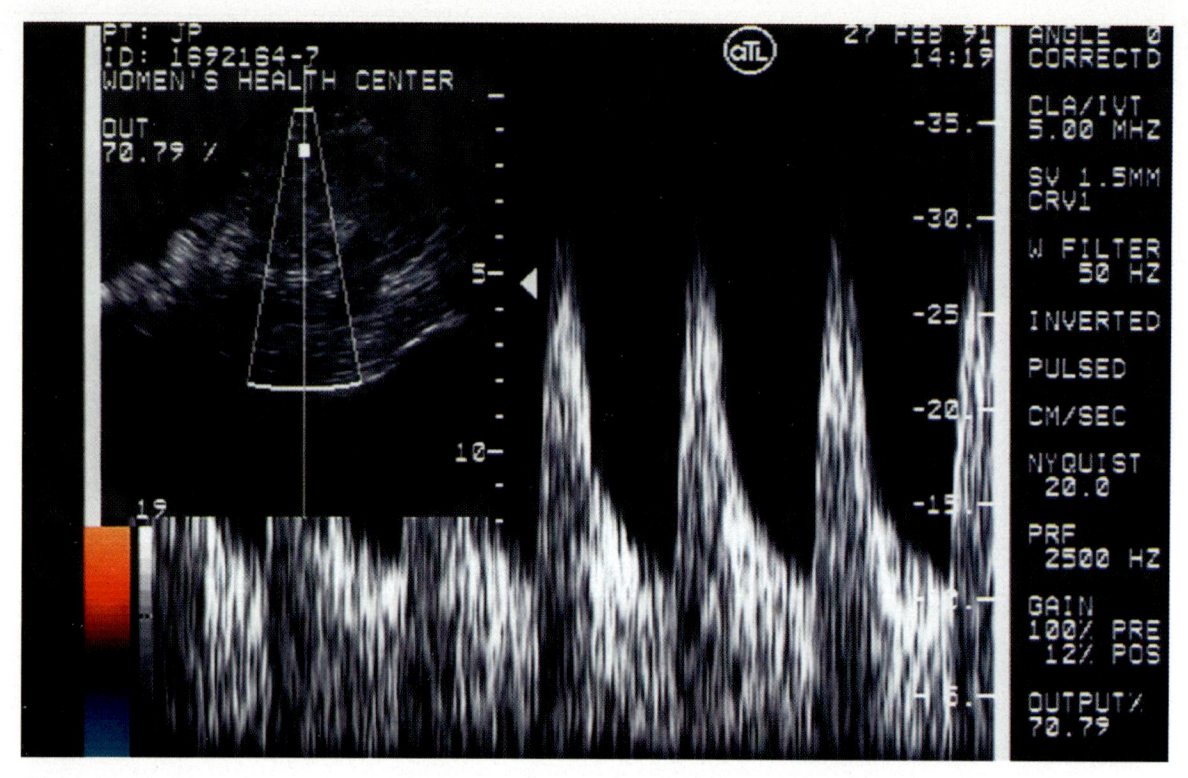

Figure 1-17. *Typical uterine artery spectral waveform in a patient with a fibroid. There is some spectral broadening in diastole, but the systolic:diastolic ratio is maintained.*

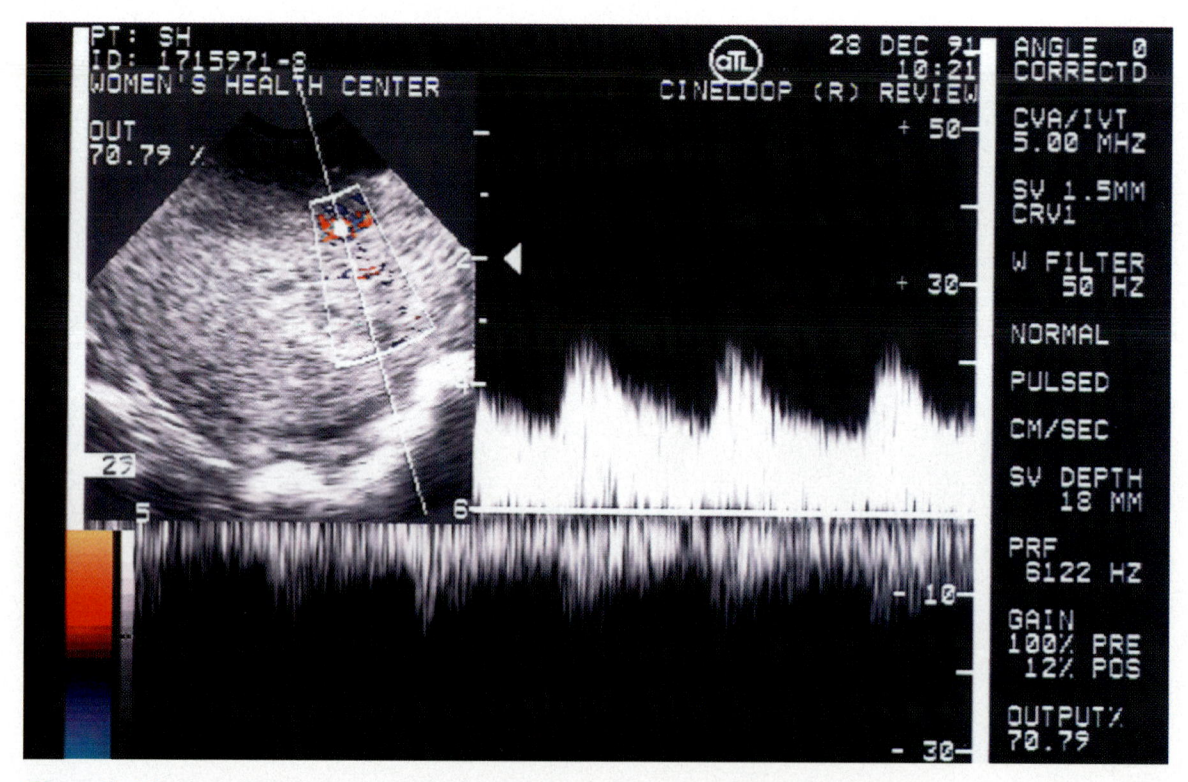

Figure 1-18. *Abnormal uterine artery flow in a patient with endometrial cancer.*

Color Doppler in Transvaginal Sonography

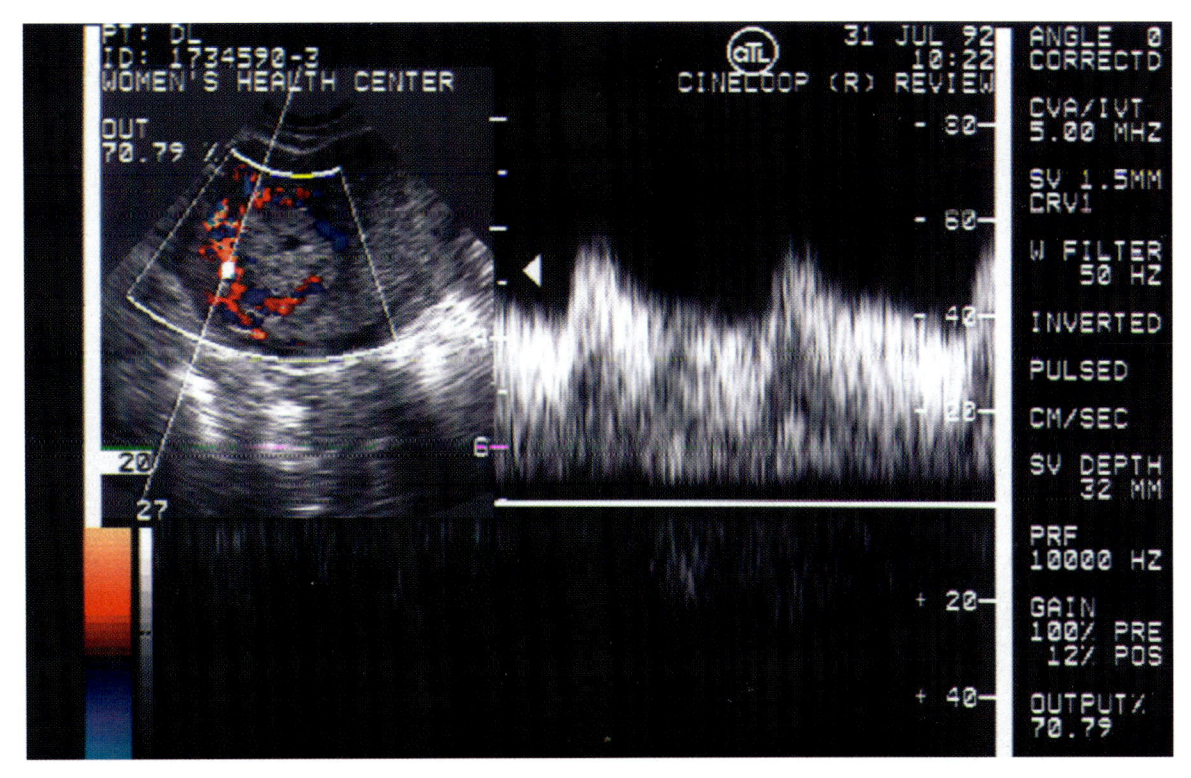

Figure 1-19. Abnormal uterine artery flow in a patient with invasive gestational trophoblastic disease. Increased diastolic flow and an abnormal PI and RI confirmed the malignant nature of this uterine tumor.

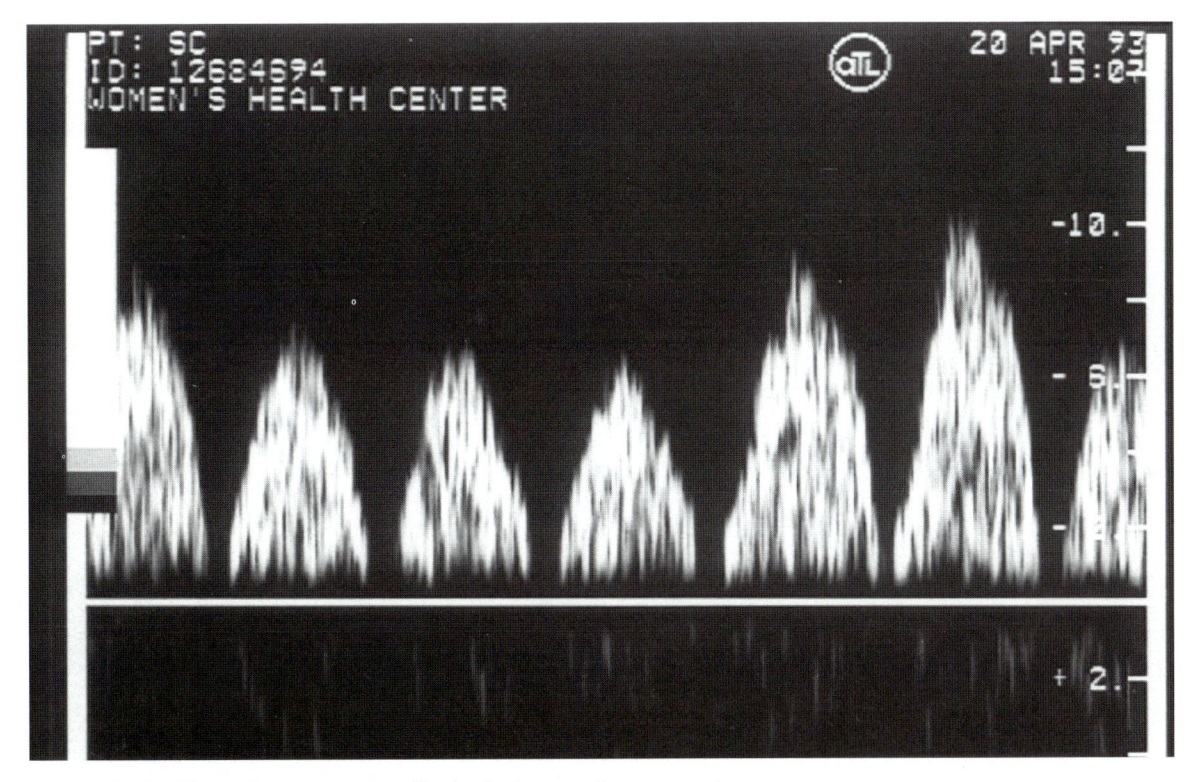

Figure 1-20. Normal ovarian artery flow velocity waveform.

An Atlas of Transvaginal Sonography

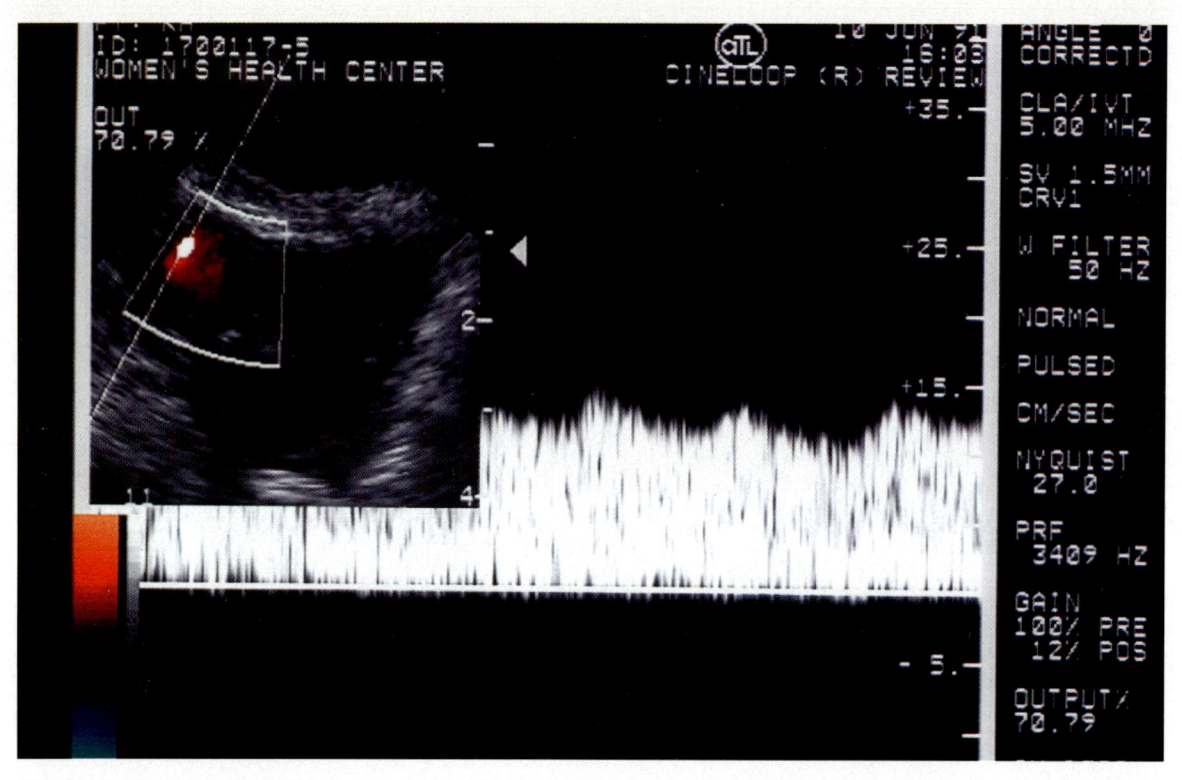

Figure 1-21. *Diastolic flow is so prominent that it almost approaches systolic flow in this highly malignant ovarian tumor.*

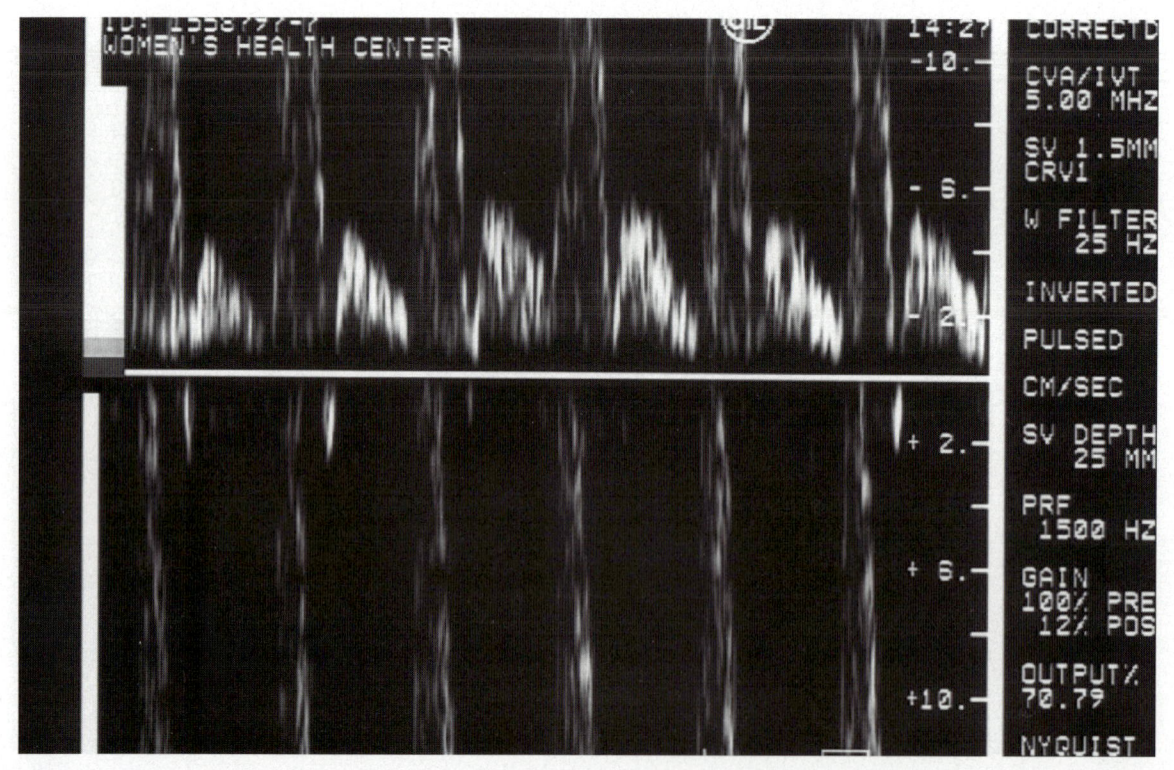

Figure 1-22. *Incorrect or "aliasing" of the spectral waveform. The Doppler shift frequency is "folding over" the spectral display. A change in the baseline and pulse repetition frequency should correct this error.*

12

2   Limitations and Artifacts

The major limitations of transvaginal scanning are limited depth of field and bowel interference resulting in an obstructed field of view. Commonly encountered artifacts include reverberation, ring-down (comet tail), mirror image, shadows, enhancement, duplication, and beam thickness and side lobe.

Artifacts

Reverberation

In reverberation artifacts, echoes are "bounced" back and forth between the transducer and tissue interface. The transducer incorrectly assigns a deeper tissue depth to the reverberating beam that is twice the distance from the transducer as true interface.

Ring-Down (Comet Tail)

Ring-down is another type of reverberation artifact produced when an ultrasound beam hits a metallic structure, such as a surgical clip, or from gas within the colon. It appears as numerous, tiny, parallel echoes in a line deep to the structure.

Mirror Image

Mirror image artifact occurs when the sound beam is deflected away from the transducer. The reflected sound may hit a strong interface, be bounced back to the "mirror," and then back to the transducer. The machine receives the echo and displays it in the direction the transducer was pointing, which is incorrect.

Shadows

Shadows may be reflective or absorptive, and can be caused by calcification, bowel gas, or inhomogeneous structures due to fat and hair within (ovarian) dermoid tumors.

Enhancement

Enhancement is the opposite of shadowing, where echoes returning from structures deep to cysts appear more intense than if the cyst were not interposed.

Duplication

Duplication artifact occurs with transabdominal sonography, not in TVS, when imaging over the linea alba in the transverse plane. The refracted beam can erroneously produce duplication of signals, thus, for example, making a singleton gestation appear to be a twin gestation.

Beam Thickness and Side Lobe

Side lobe artifact is produced when beams other than the main beam, called side lobes, strike an interface and reflect the echo back to the transducer. The transducer has no way of knowing that the echo originated from a side lobe and mistakenly displays it on the screen.

An Atlas of Transvaginal Sonography

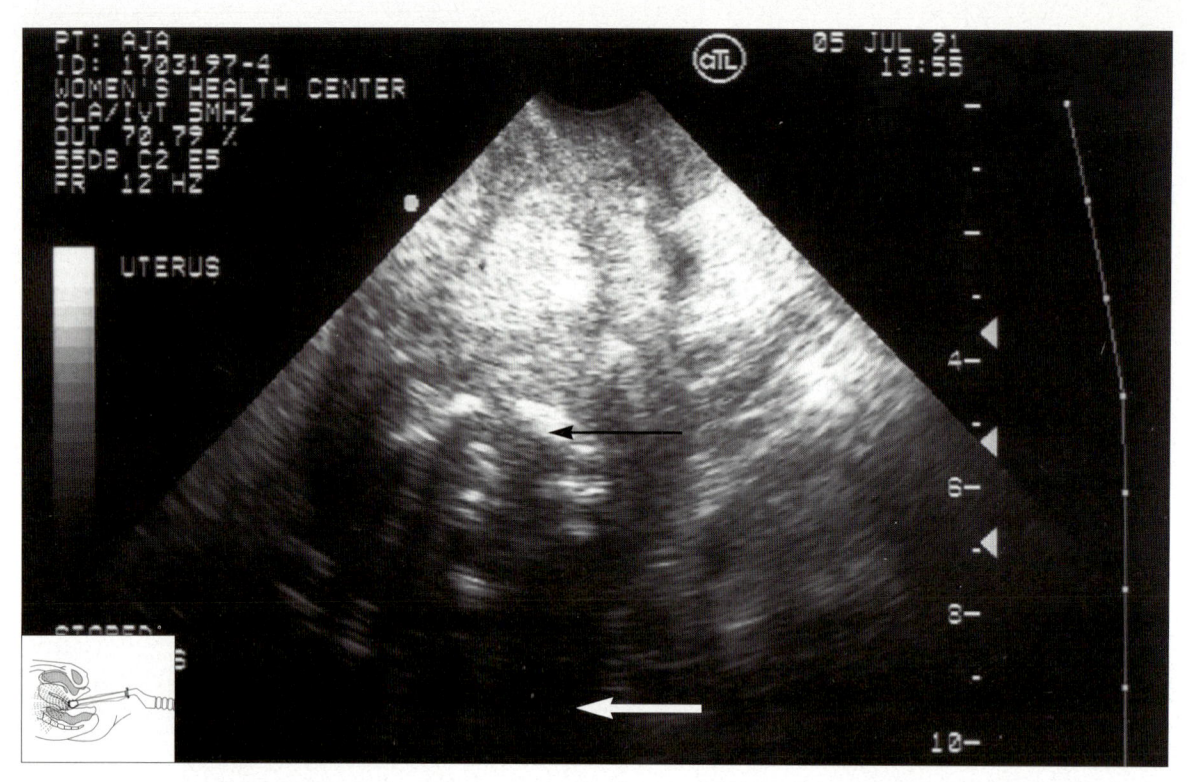

Figure 2-1. This retroverted postmenopausal uterus contains a calcified fundal fibroid (small arrow) that is producing characteristic posterior acoustical shadowing (large arrow).

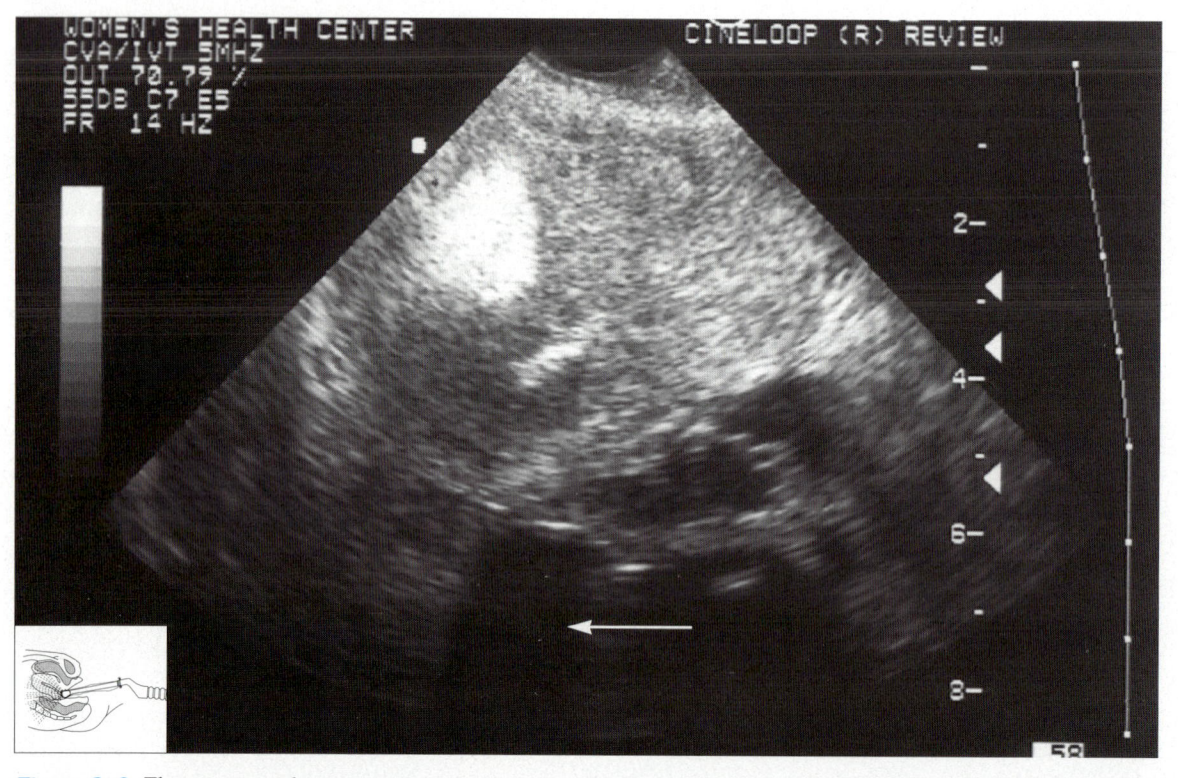

Figure 2-2. This anteverted uterus contains echogenic endometrium and a small calcified postero-fundal arcuate vessel, both producing a minor degree of posterior acoustical shadowing. More prominent are the loops of small bowel in the cul-de-sac producing dense posterior shadowing (arrow). This is related to the high impedance at the air-fluid interface in the bowel lumen.

Limitations and Artifacts

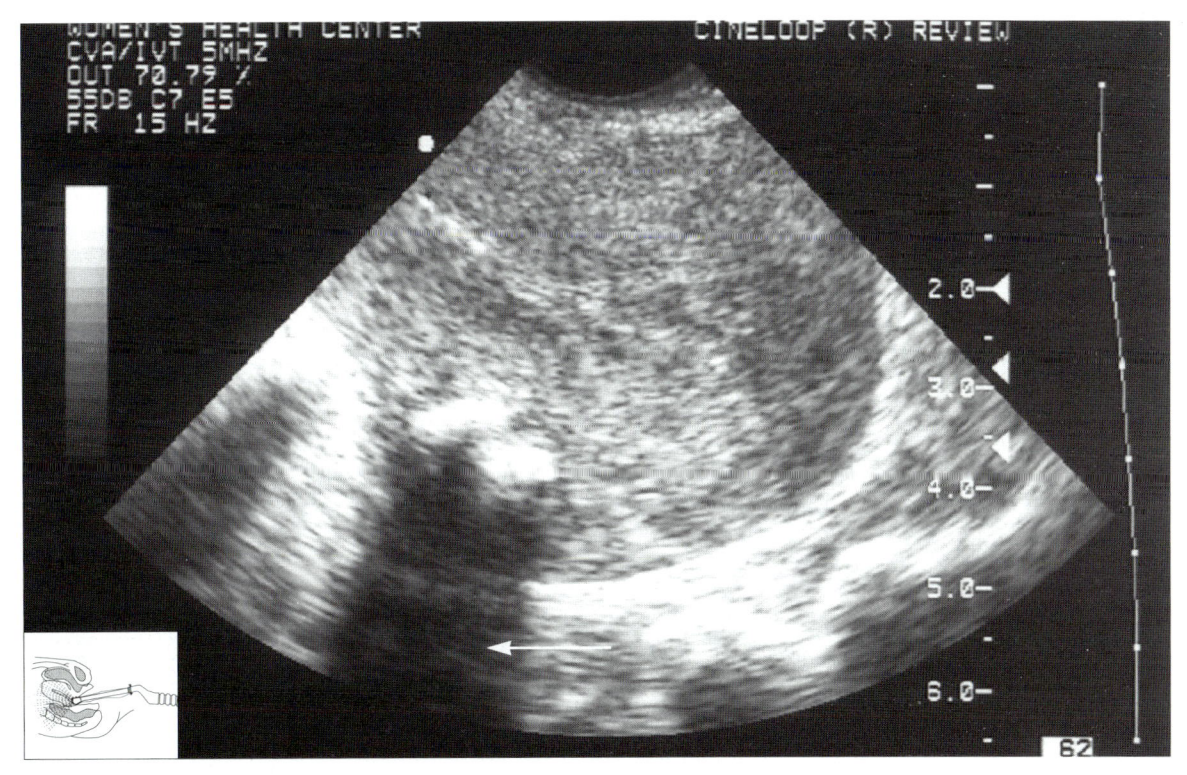

Figure 2-3. This premenopausal retroverted uterus contains two calcified arcuate vessels in the anterior wall myometrium, again producing dense posterior shadowing (arrow).

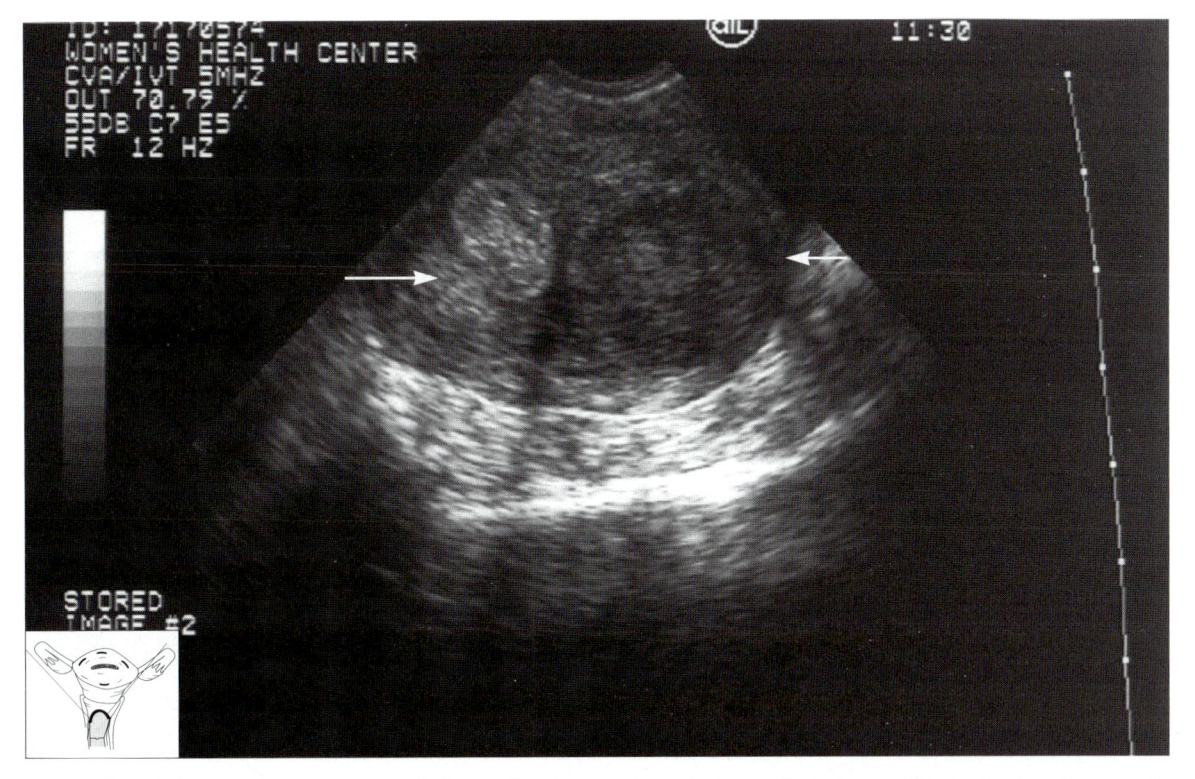

Figure 2-4. This transverse or coronal plane of a premenopausal uterus shows two artifacts. A mirror image of the endometrial cavity is produced (large arrow), while edge shadows (small arrow) are seen from the lateral borders of the fibroid due to defocusing of the sound beam at the edge of the lesion.

An Atlas of Transvaginal Sonography

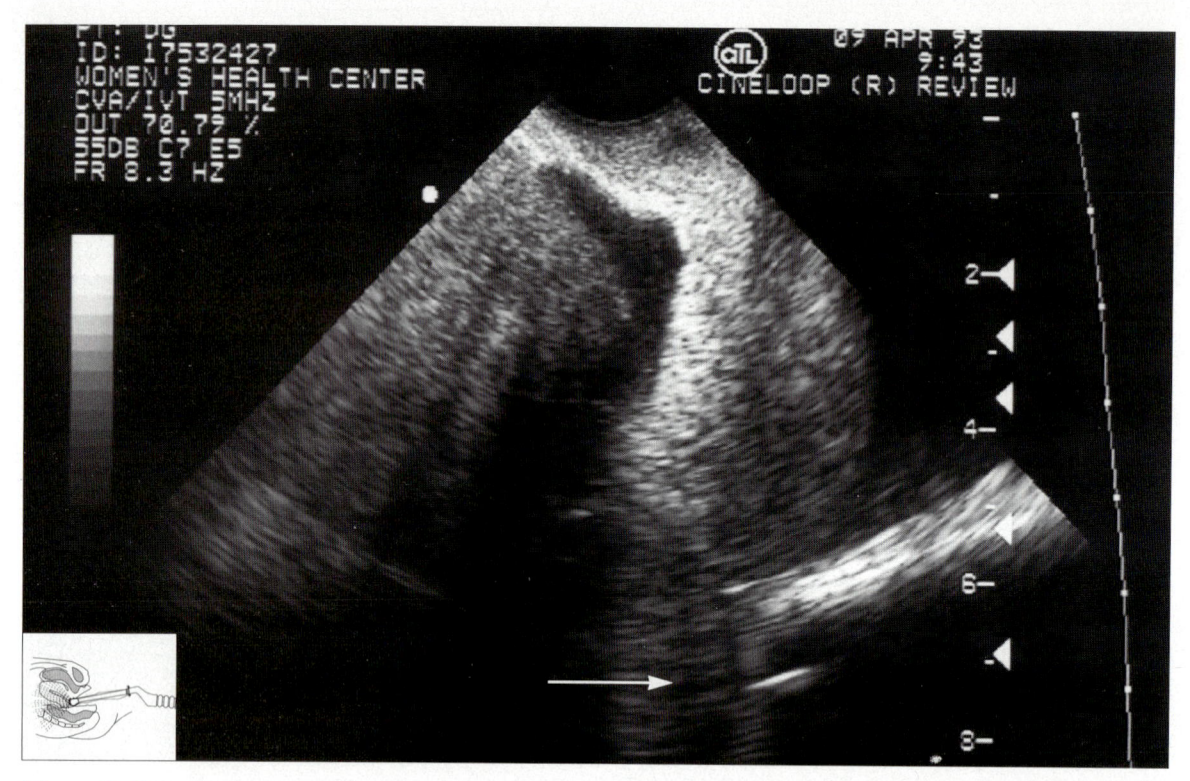

Figure 2~5. *Sagittal section of a retroverted uterus and solid adnexal mass, bathed in ascitic fluid. Inferior to the uterus is a mirror image artifact (arrow).*

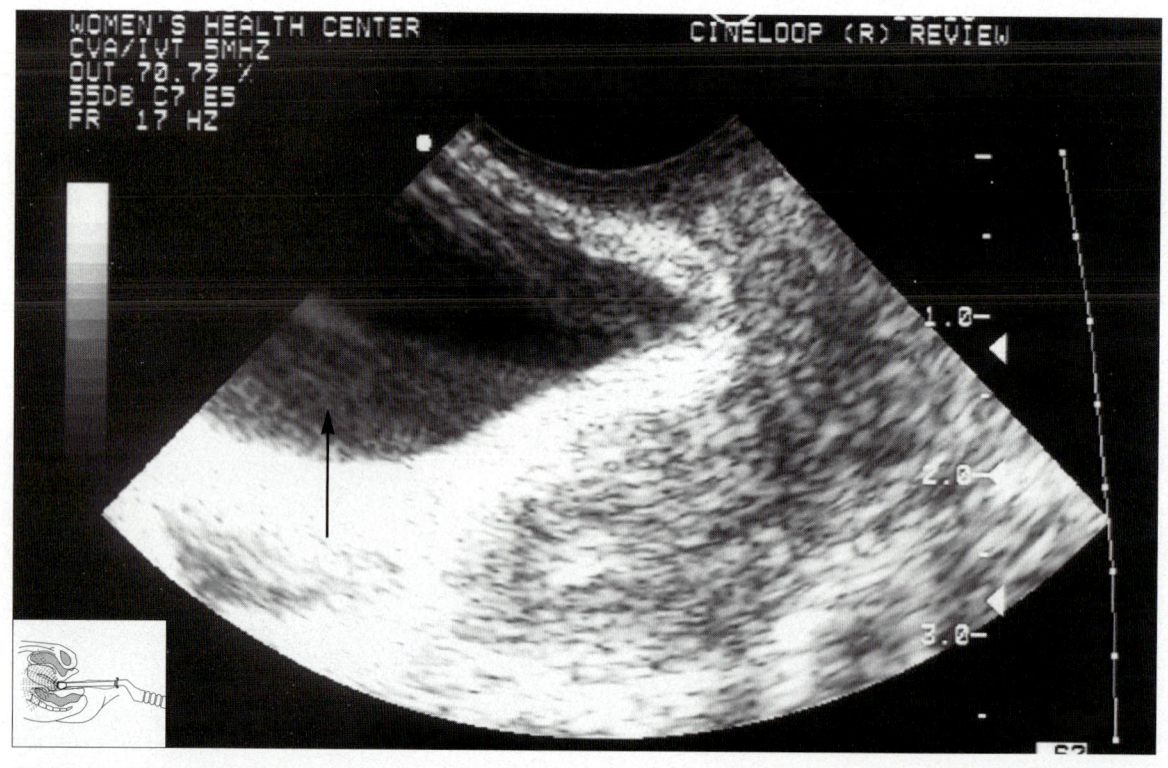

Figure 2~6. *This image of a partially distended bladder and anteverted uterus demonstrates side lobe artifact or arcs of echoes within the bladder (arrow).*

16

Limitations and Artifacts

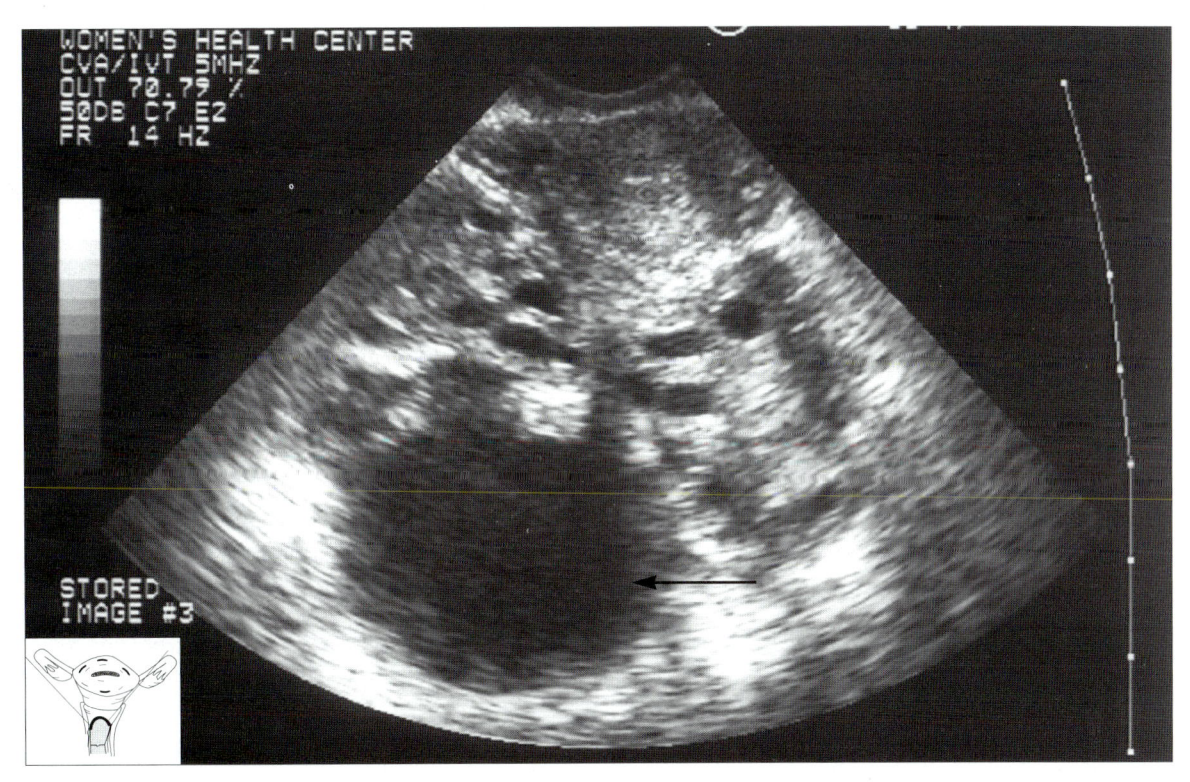

Figure 2-7. *Transverse section through the uterus and what was initially believed to be an adnexal cyst (arrow). The cyst disappeared on altering the scan angle of the transducer. Note that there is not a clear "cyst wall," giving further evidence of its artifactual nature.*

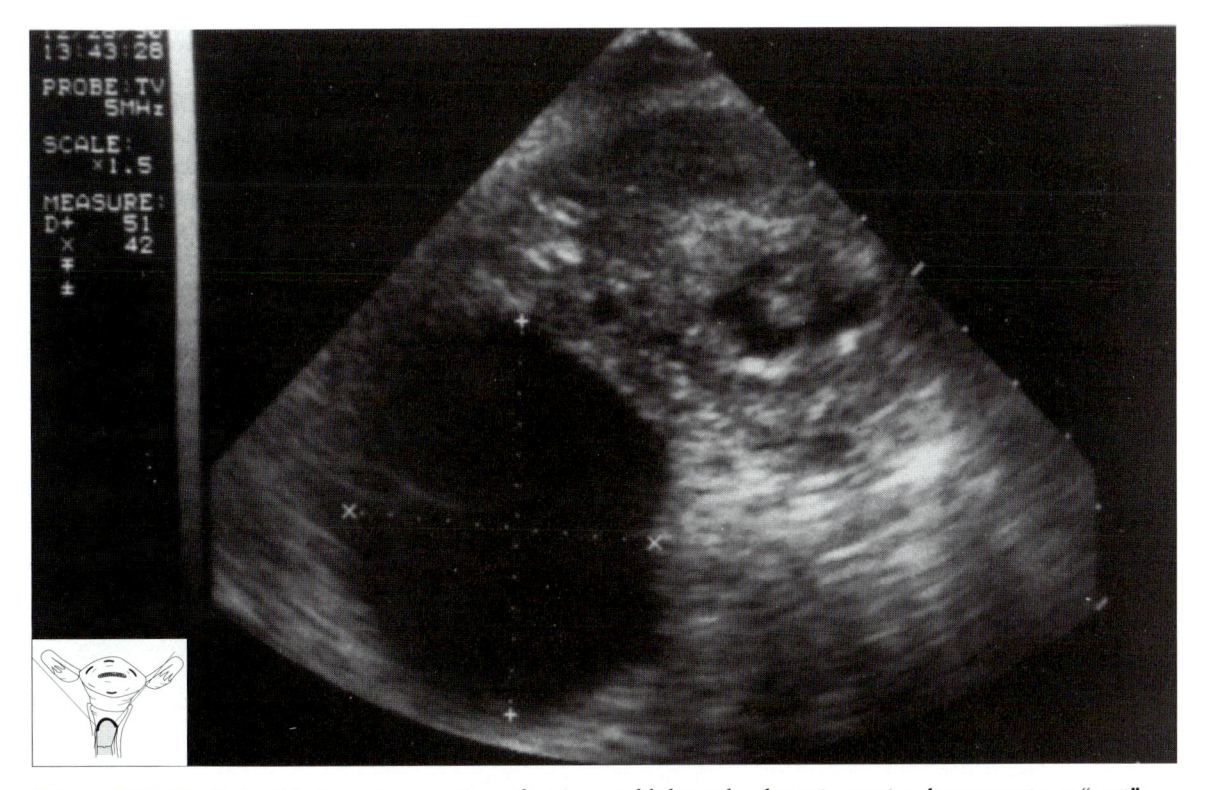

Figure 2-8. *Similarly, this transverse section of uterus and bilateral polycystic ovaries demonstrates a "cyst" deep to the ovaries and again without clear cyst walls evident. Again, a pseudo or artifactual cyst.*

17

An Atlas of Transvaginal Sonography

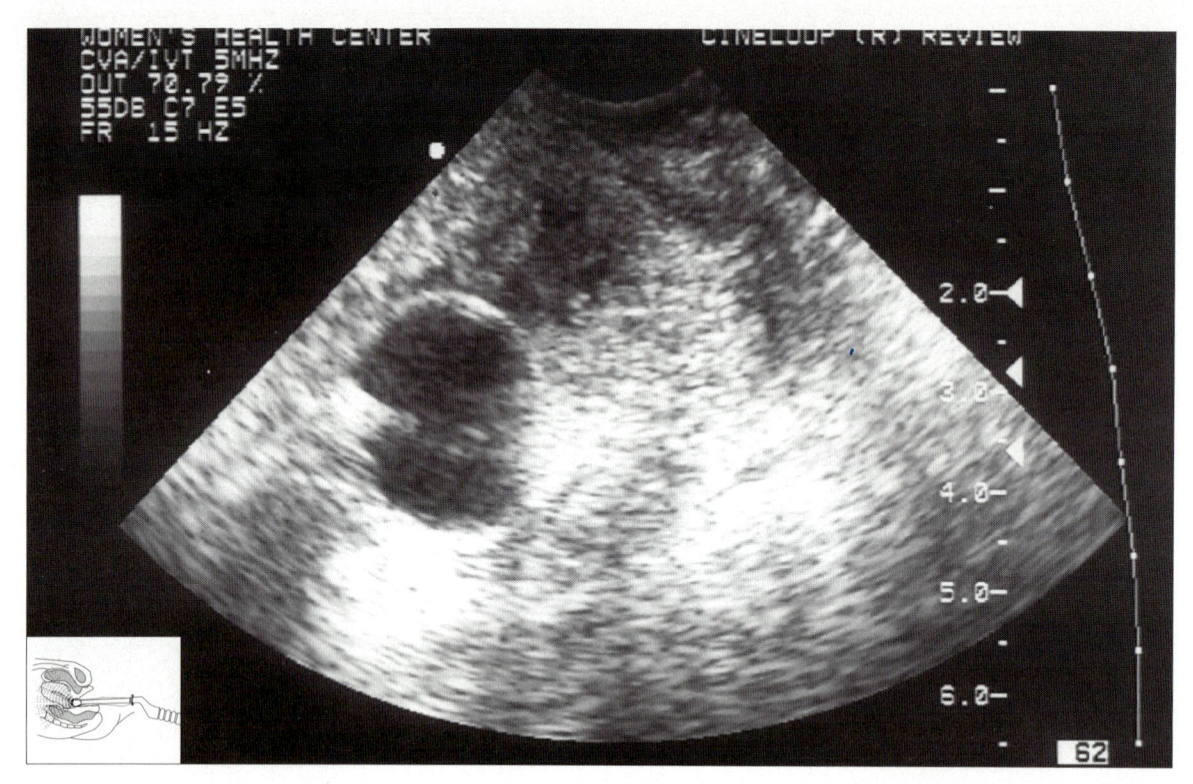

Figure 2~9. *Not an ovarian cyst, but a Foley balloon. The bladder is empty, its walls contracted and thickened.*

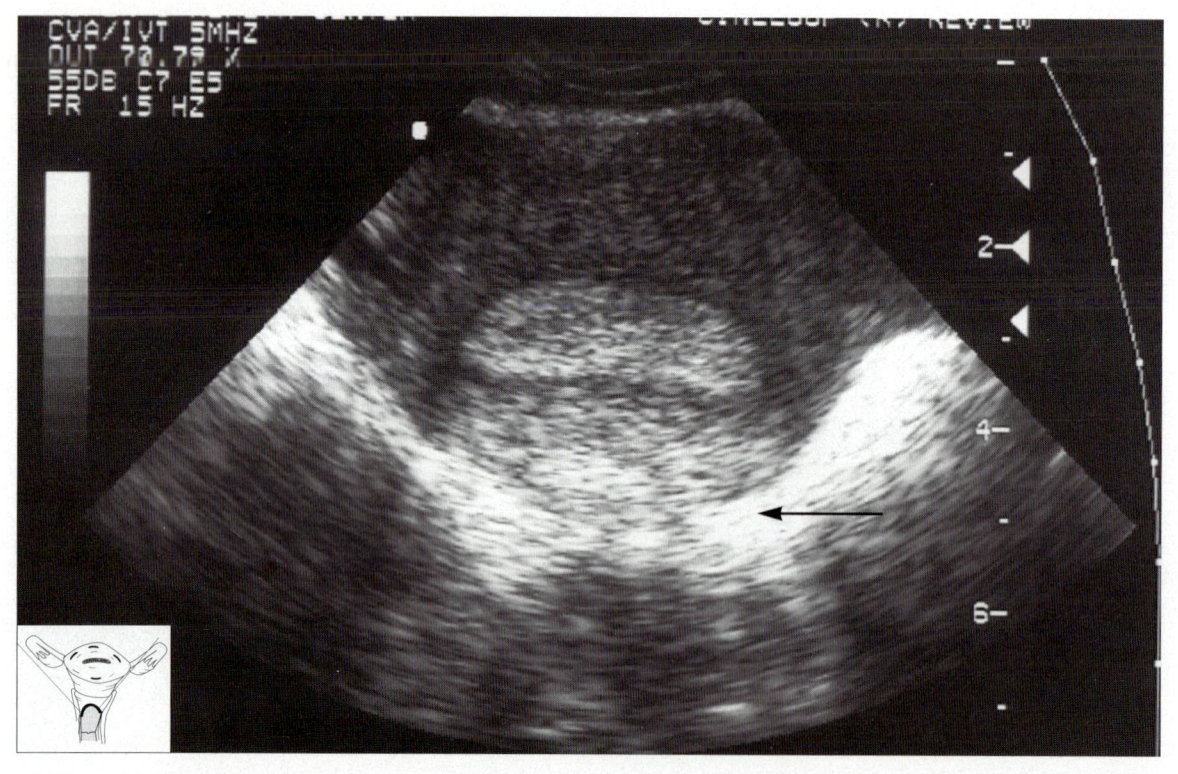

Figure 2~10. *Sagittal section through uterus demonstrating echoic luteal phase endometrium with posterior acoustic enhancement (arrow).*

Limitations and Artifacts

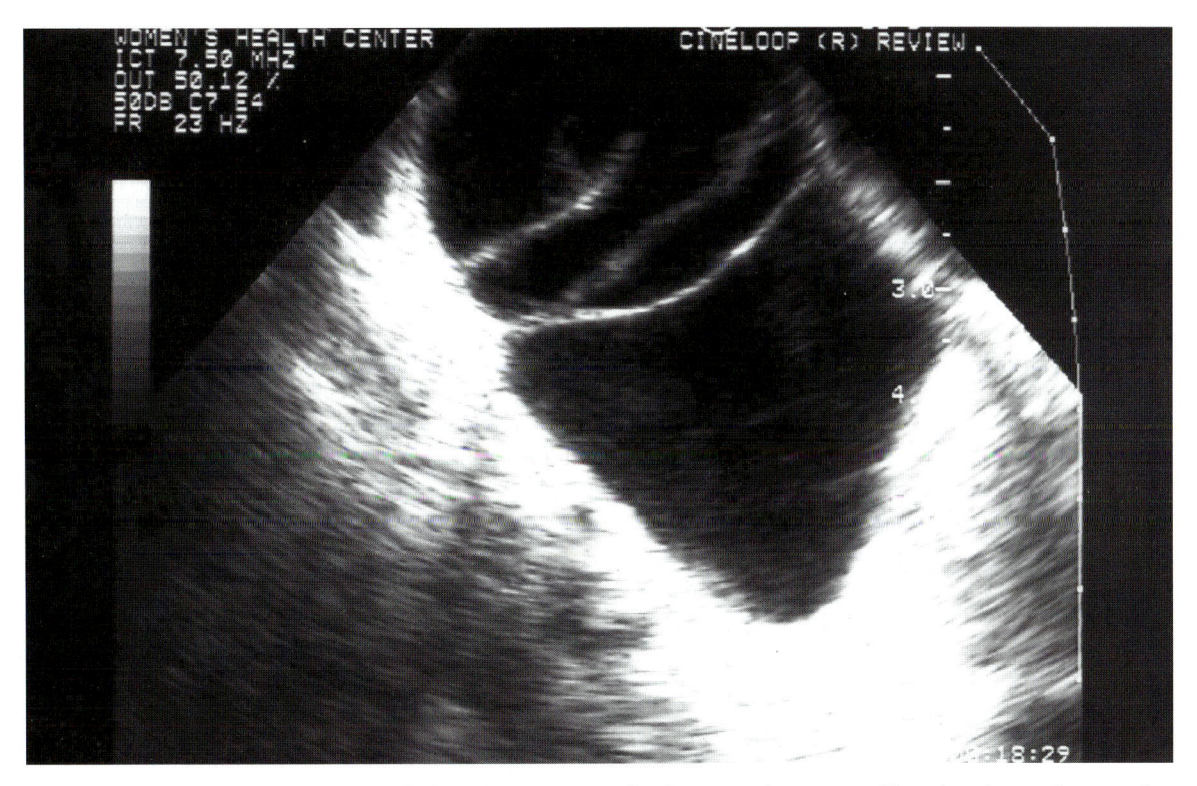

Figure 2-11. Transabdominal scan of a large cystic, septated pelvic mass that was unable to be adequately imaged by TVS.

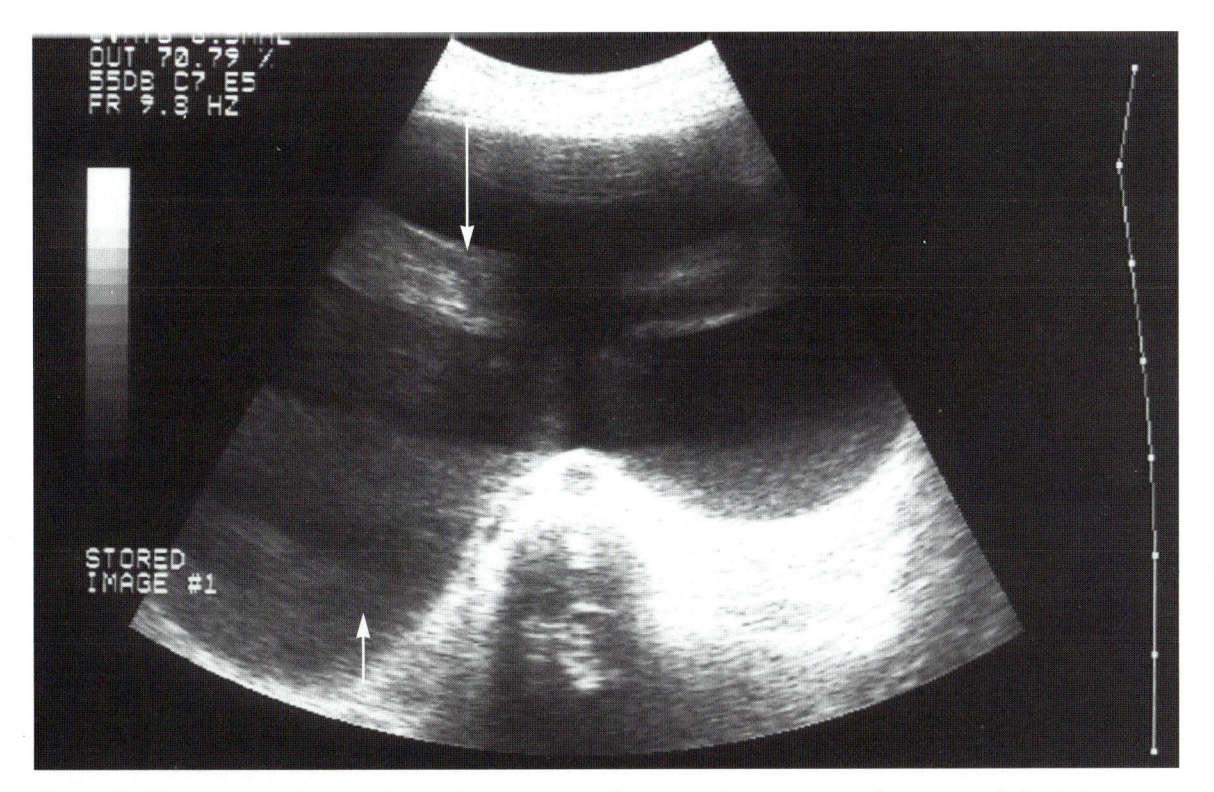

Figure 2-12. This transabdominal scan demonstrates a huge simple ovarian cyst that occupied the entire abdominal cavity. Reverberation and side lobe artifact (large arrow) are seen within the cyst while beam width artifact simulating sludge (small arrow) in the dependent portion of the cyst is seen.

An Atlas of Transvaginal Sonography

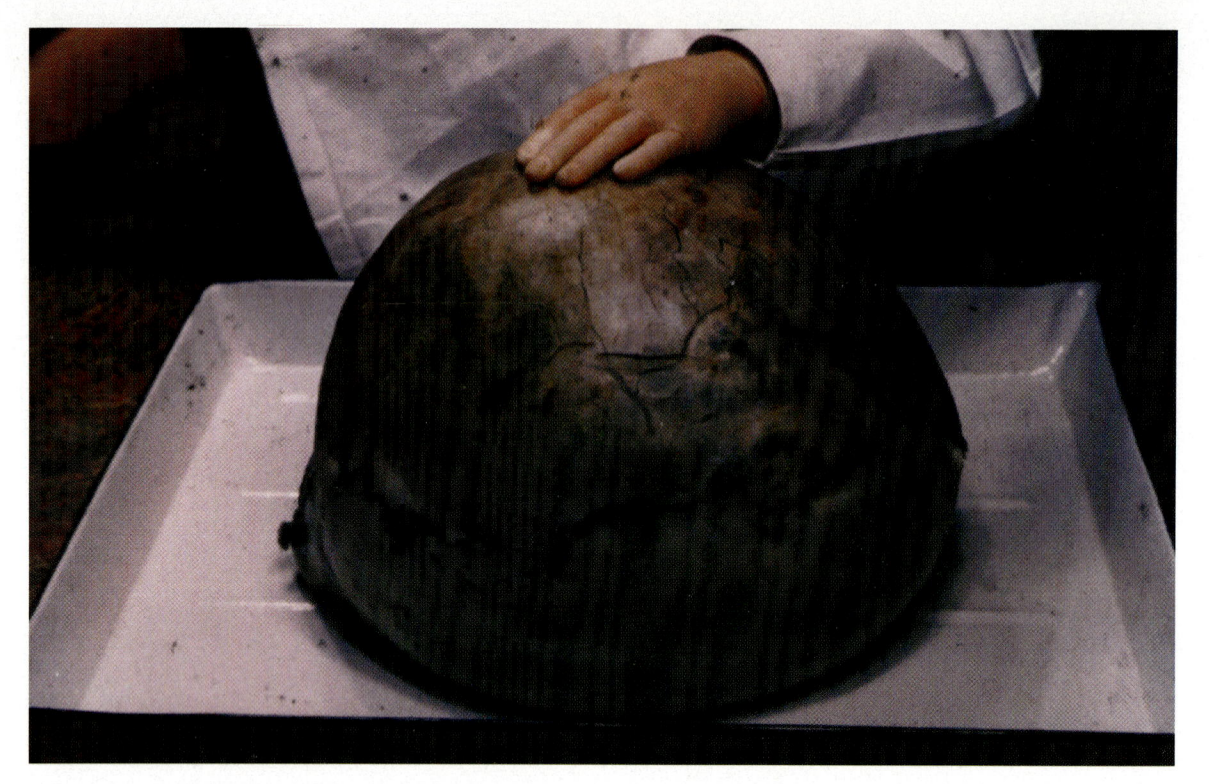

Figure 2-13. *Huge simple mucinous cystadenoma.*

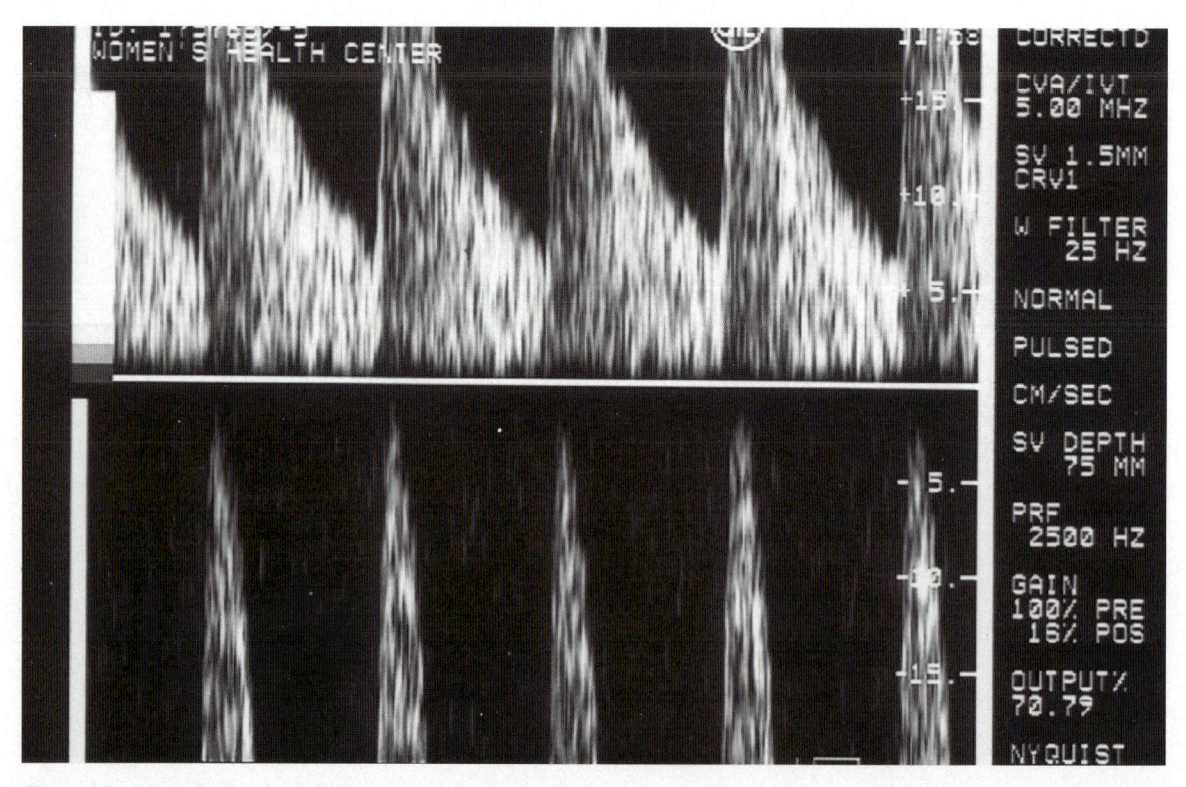

Figure 2-14. *"Aliasing" of the spectral waveform. The Doppler shift frequency is "folding over" the spectral display. A change in the baseline and pulse repetition frequency should correct this error.*

3 The Examination

A transvaginal sonogram is more comfortable for the patient than a transabdominal examination because a distended bladder is not an examination prerequisite. The transvaginal sonographic examination, like the pelvic examination, is performed respecting patient privacy and dignity.

Procedure

Most of the images in this *Atlas* have been captured using a 5.0 MHz curved array intravaginal transducer, incorporating a field of view of 90°, 0.5 mm axial resolution, and 1.5 mm lateral resolution. After the patient is placed in a lithotomy position, a disposable sheath is filled with coupling gel and the transducer inserted into the sheath. Gel is applied on the outside of the sheath for lubrication. After the sheath-covered transducer is inserted into the vagina, the pelvis is systematically scanned. The sagittal plane is scanned from pelvic side wall to side wall, and then the coronal plane is scanned by rotating the transducer 90° from cul-de-sac to anterior abdominal wall. Next, pelvic organs are scanned in the sagittal plane initially, and then in the coronal plane.

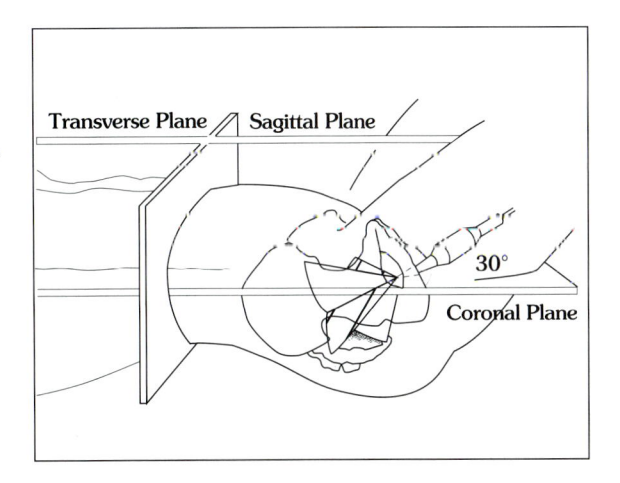

Figure 3-1. Demonstration of the transverse, sagittal, and coronal planes in a female figure in the lithotomy position. These true anatomic planes can be compared with pelvic imaging planes when the sound beam is being diverted from side to side in the pelvis (final plane in the pelvis) and when the sound beam is directed anteriorly and posteriorly in the pelvis (clear plane in the pelvis). The pelvic planes can vary considerably by manipulating the transducer. However, the pelvic plane never corresponds to a true anatomic transverse plane, and rarely are true sagittal or coronal planes imaged. (Illustration by Delilah R. Cohn, Nashville, TN.)

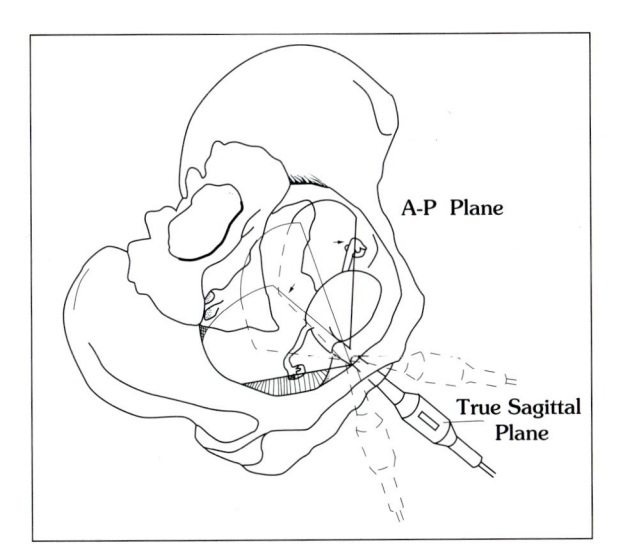

Figure 3-2. Projection of the bony pelvis showing several AP-pelvic planes obtained by moving the transducer from side to side. Only the central AP-pelvic planes correspond to the anatomic sagittal plane. (Illustration by Delilah R. Cohn, Nashville, TN.)

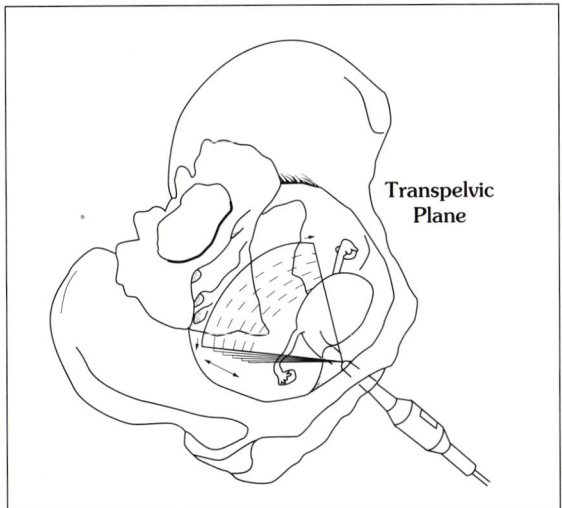

Figure 3-3. Projection showing the bony pelvis with a transducer oriented in such a way as to project the sound beam from side to side in the pelvis. Multiple different T-pelvic planes can be imaged by moving the transducer handle up or down or right or left, projecting the sound beam in different T-pelvic planes. (Illustration by Delilah R. Cohn, Nashville, TN.)

An Atlas of Transvaginal Sonography

If appropriate, color Doppler is activated. The color gate is positioned, and its size optimized to maximize frame rate. An appropriate blood vessel is identified and on-line spectral Doppler analysis performed. A spectralanalysis of the arterial wave-form is obtained. From this wave-form the peak systolic, diastolic and mean velocities are determined and the pulsatility index (PI) and resistance index (RI) calculated.

The PI and RI are angle independent estimates of flow. The PI is defined as the ratio of the difference between the peak systolic and the diastolic frequencies to the mean frequency, as obtained from the spectral analysis. The RI is defined as the ratio of the difference between the peak systolic and the diastolic frequencies to the systolic frequency.

To visualize areas with decreased blood flow, the velocity range was lowered to 1-4 cm/sec by lowering the pulse repetition frequency. The wall filter was set at its minimum (50 Hz), and the sample volume size set at 1.5 mm. The spatial peak temporal average intensity was approximately 65 mW/cm^2, which is well within the highest limit recommended by the Bioeffects Committee of the American Institute of Ultrasound in Medicine.

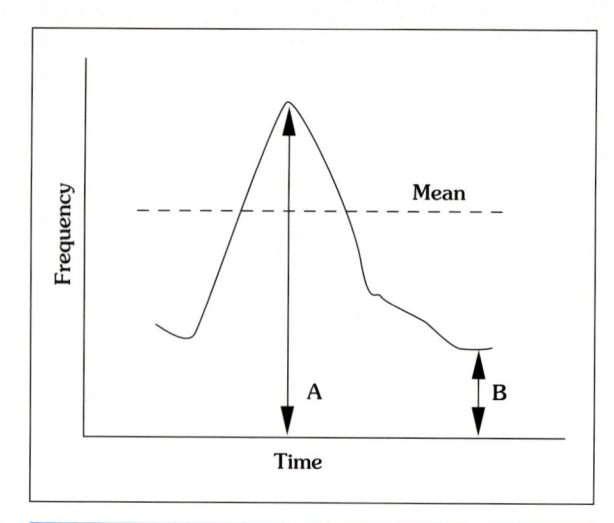

Pulsatility Index (PI)	A-B / Mean
Resistance Index (RI)	A-B / A
Systolic / Diastolic Ratio	A / B

Figure 3-4. *Derivation of resistance indices, where A = peak systolic Doppler shift frequency; B = end diastolic shift frequency; and Mean = mean maximum Doppler shift frequency over the cardiac cycle.*

The examination concludes with allowing the patient, if she desires, to review the scan and appropriate findings. The transducer is removed from the patient's vagina, and the sheath removed and wiped free of coupling gel. Excess gel is wiped from the patient and she is assisted to the sitting position. The sonographer then leaves the examination area to generate the report. This provides the patient an opportunity to toilet and dress. The transducer is then sterilized in the appropriate fashion, as recommended by the manufacturer.

4 Cervix

The cervix, depending on version of the uterus, can be visualized in most instances by slowly withdrawing and angulating the probe. It should be scanned in both sagittal and coronal planes. Relevant sonographic information includes its position, whether midline or deviated. Its size, or more correctly its volume, is measured in three planes—anterior, longitudinal, and transverse.

Scan Findings

On gray scale imaging it is uniformly isoechoic. Intratumoral, or more correctly intracervical, blood flow is not prominent. The parametria extend from the lateral cervix toward the pelvic side wall with a fine taper. With color flow the uterine vessels can be traced out to the side wall and their origin from the internal iliac artery and vein, identifying their origin.

As in the corpus, the endocervical glands and mucus formation vary throughout the menstrual cycle. Midcycle, the cervical mucus production increases, producing an echogenic interface and a clearly defined endocervical canal. Intratumoral blood is usually not prominent.

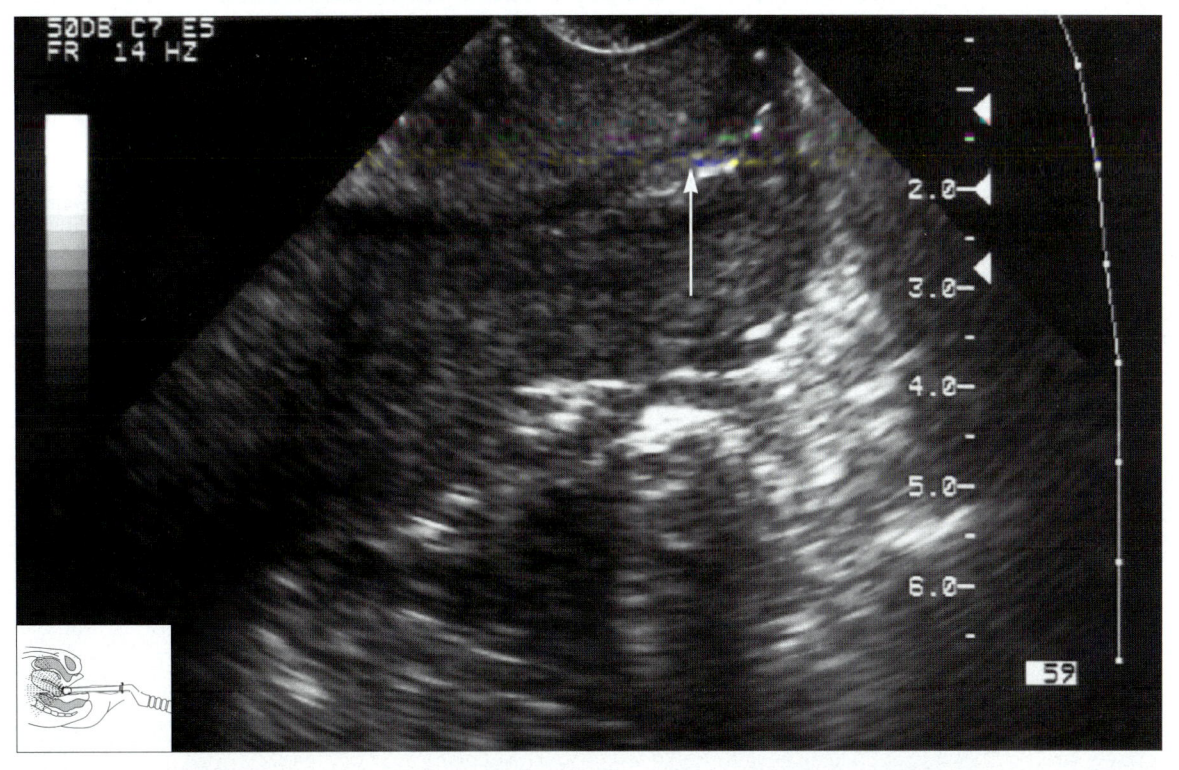

Figure 4-1. Sagittal scan through the lower uterine segment and cervix. Midcycle endocervical mucus appears as the echogenic line (arrow).

An Atlas of Transvaginal Sonography

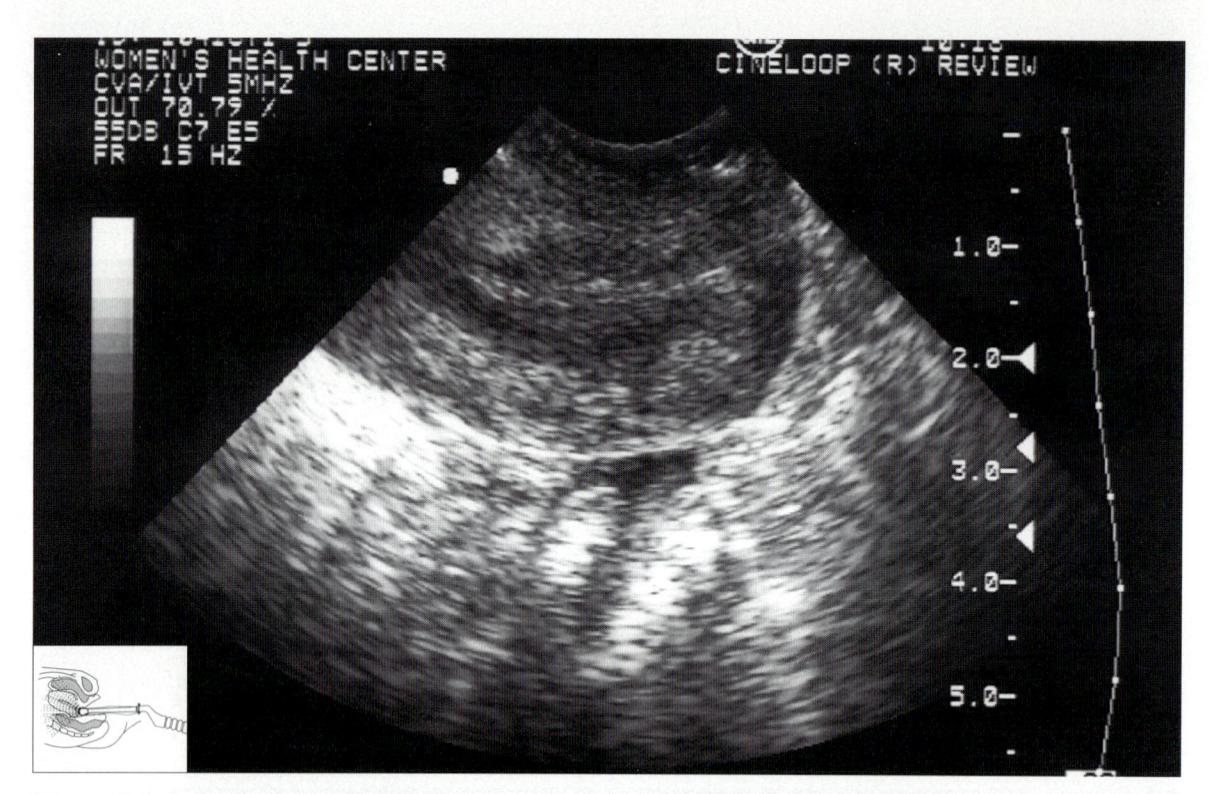

Figure 4-2. Sagittal section of a cervix.

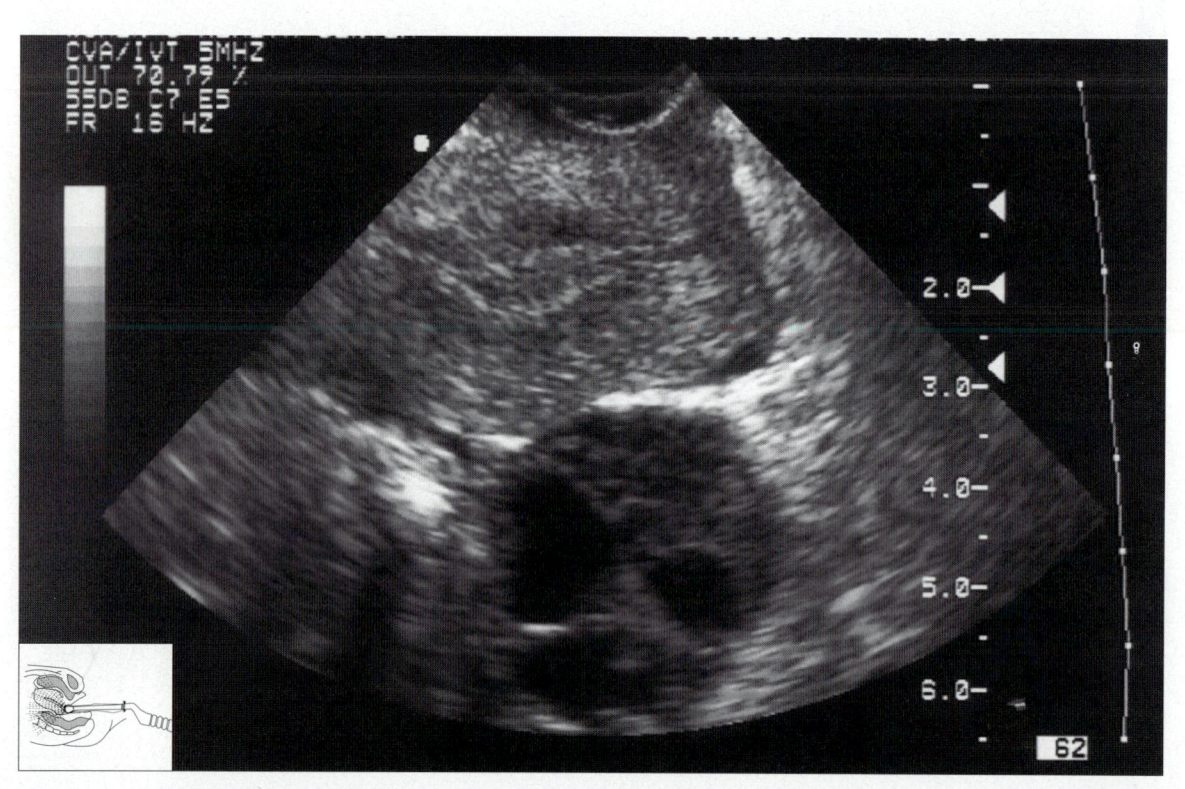

Figure 4-3. Sagittal section of cervix with distension of endocervix. A mobile cystic ovary is seen posterior to the cervix, within the cul-de-sac.

Cervix

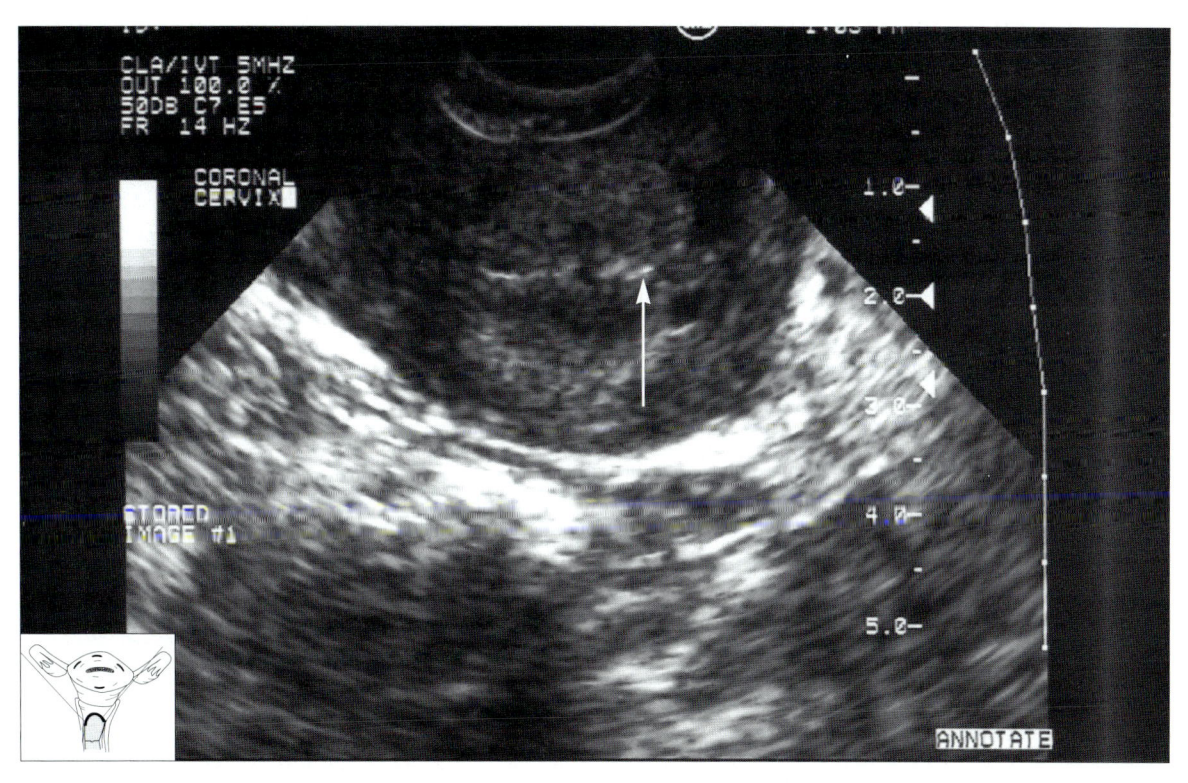

Figure 4-4. Coronal section of a normal cervix. The central portion is clearly seen. Endocervical mucus appears as an echogenic central line (arrow).

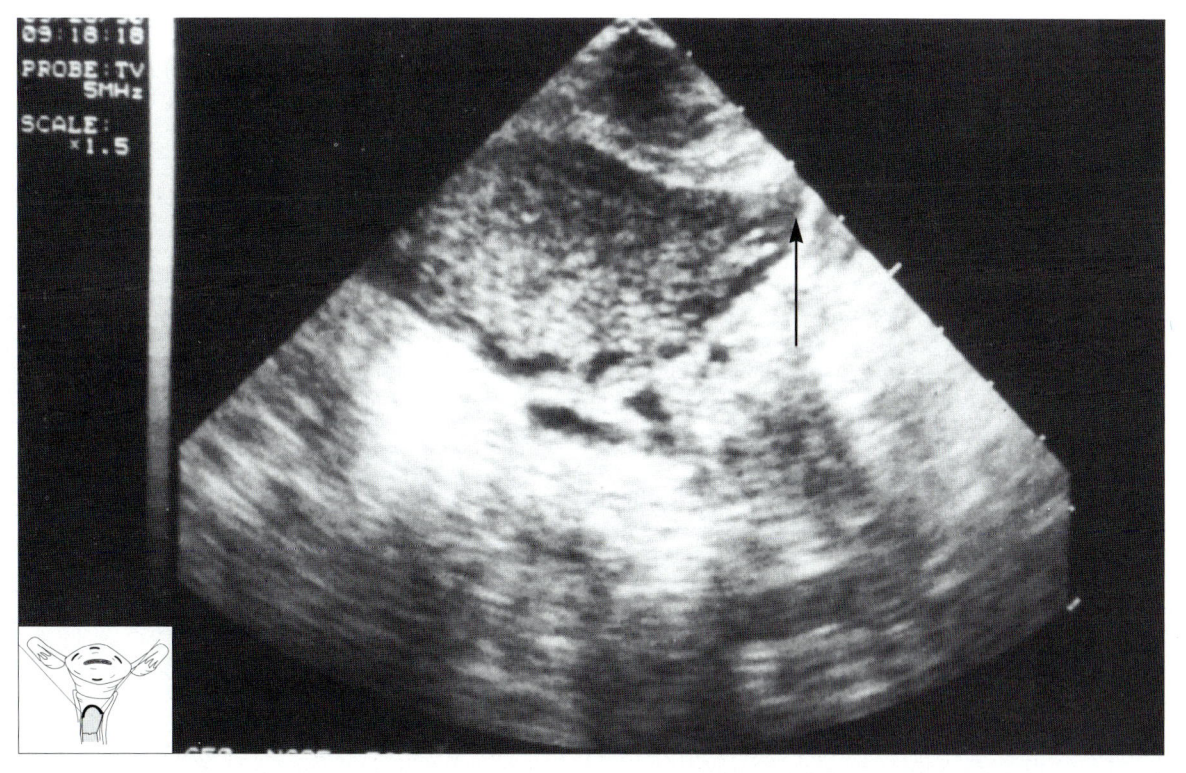

Figure 4-5. Normal cervical parametria. Coronal view through cervix demonstrating thin tapering parametria (arrow).

An Atlas of Transvaginal Sonography

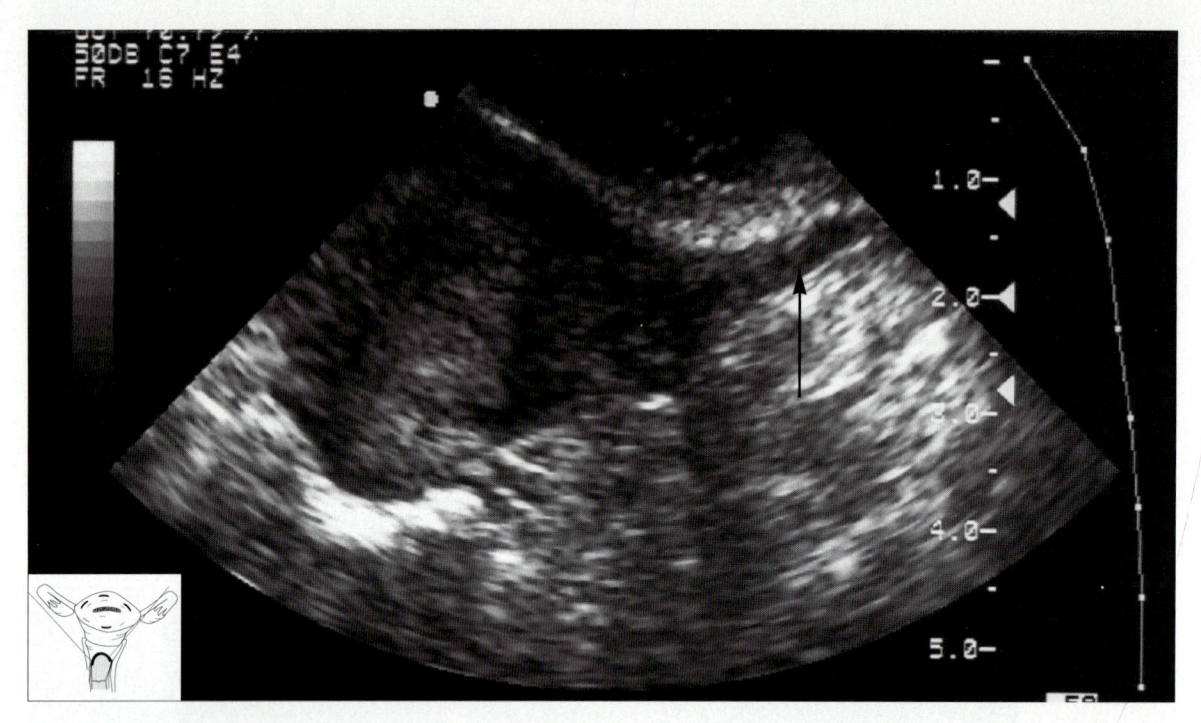

Figure 4-6. Thin, tapering, normal parametria (arrow).

Benign Cervical Pathology

Benign lesions that can be imaged include Nabothian follicles or mucus retention cysts, cervical or prolapsed uterine leiomyomas and xanthomatous fibromas, and cervical and prolapsed uterine polyps.

Nabothian Follicles (Mucus Retention Cysts)

Nabothian follicles or mucus retention cysts are often seen throughout the reproductive years. They are caused by blockage of the gland ducts with continued secretion of mucinous material. They are located near the endocervical canal and can cause irregularities of the ectocervix.

Scan Findings

They are anechoic structures and demonstrate characteristic "through transmission" related to their fluid content. They may vary in size from a few millimeters to more than a centimeter. They can be single or multiple, and may be situated in the endocervix or ectocervix.

Cervix

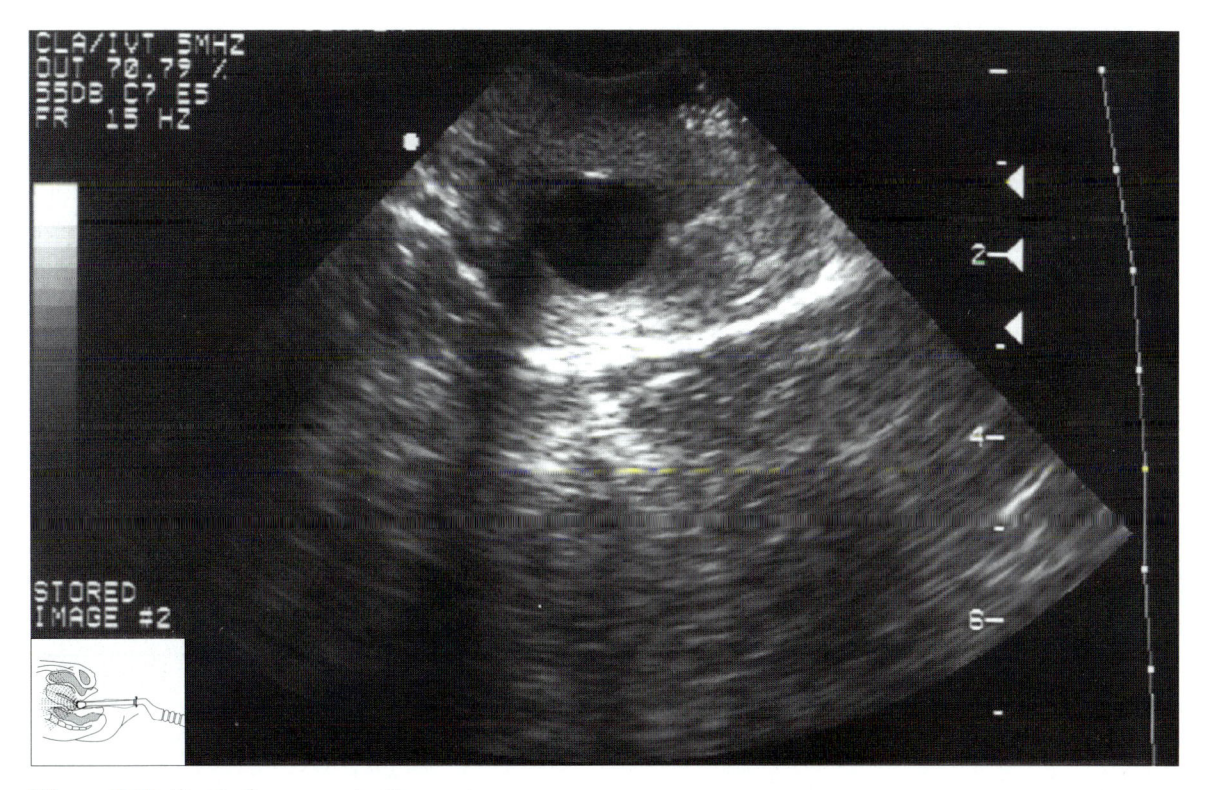

Figure 4-7. Cervical mucus retention cyst.

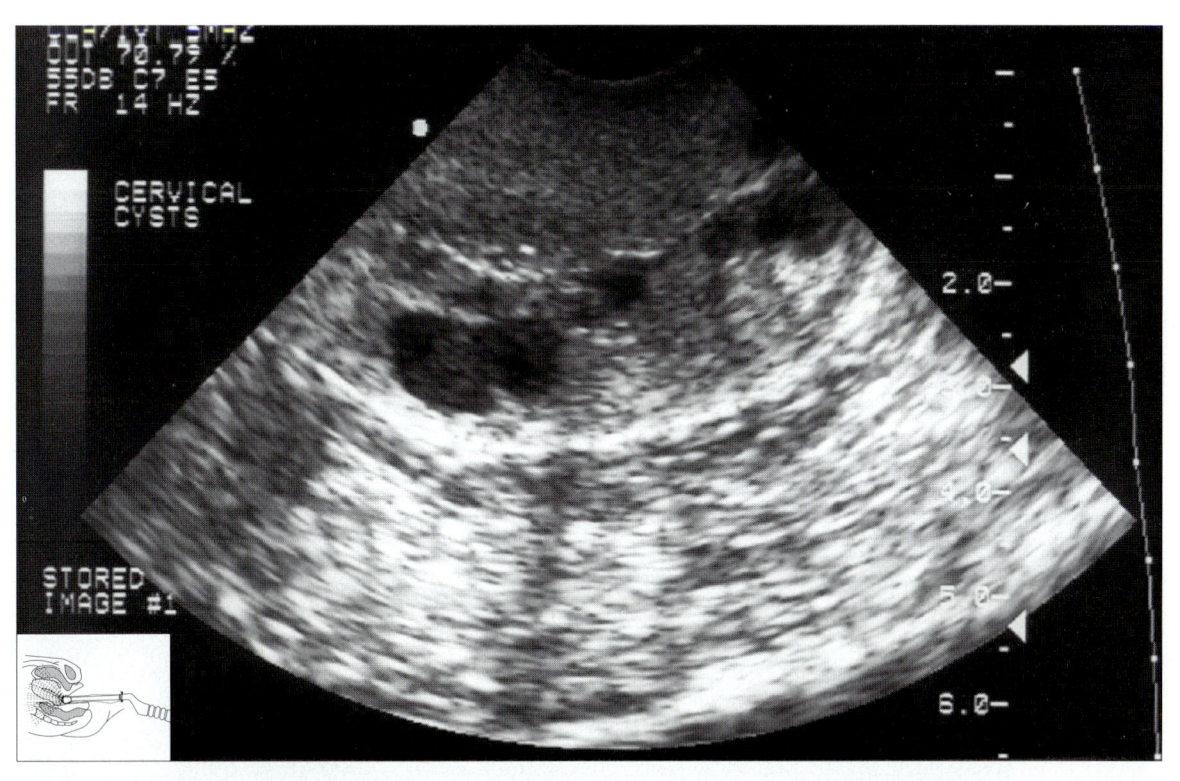

Figure 4-8. Multiple small endocervical and ectocervical mucus retention cysts (Nabothian follicles).

An Atlas of Transvaginal Sonography

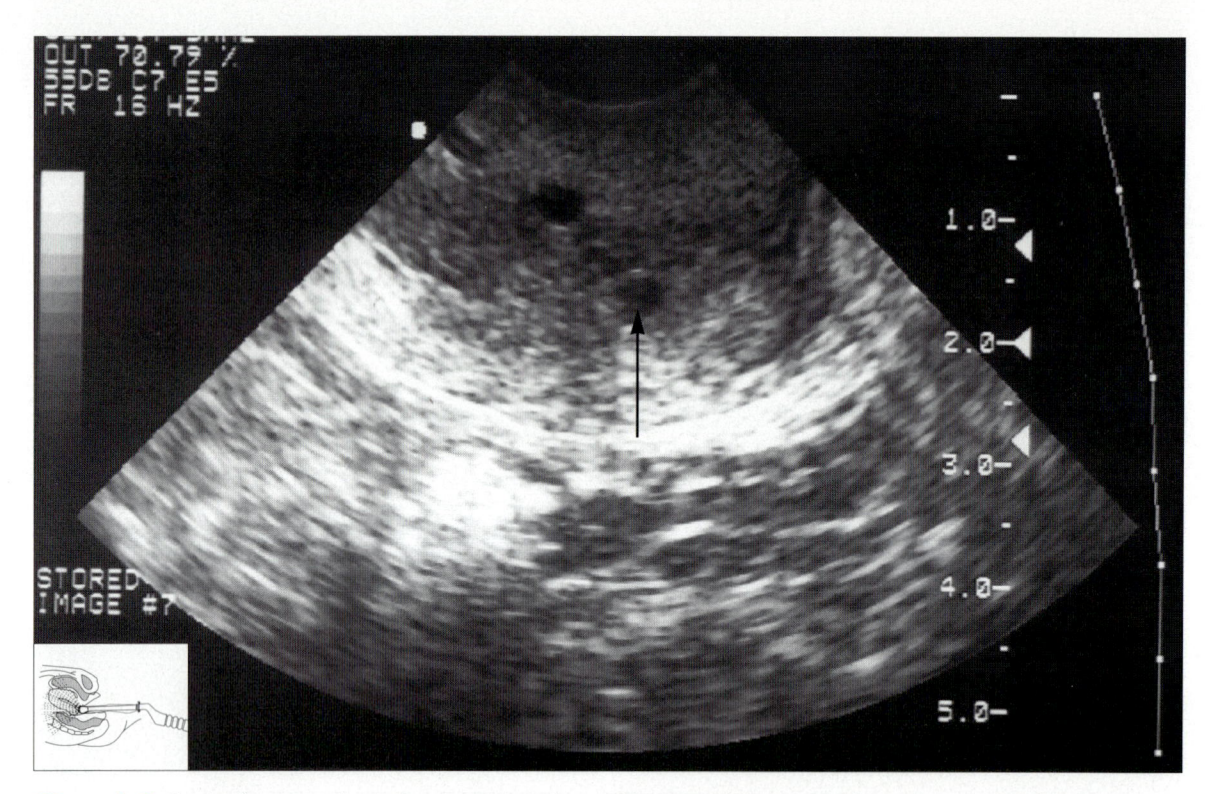

Figure 4-9. *Sagittal section through a normal, early, proliferative-phase cervix demonstrating small mucus retention cysts (arrow).*

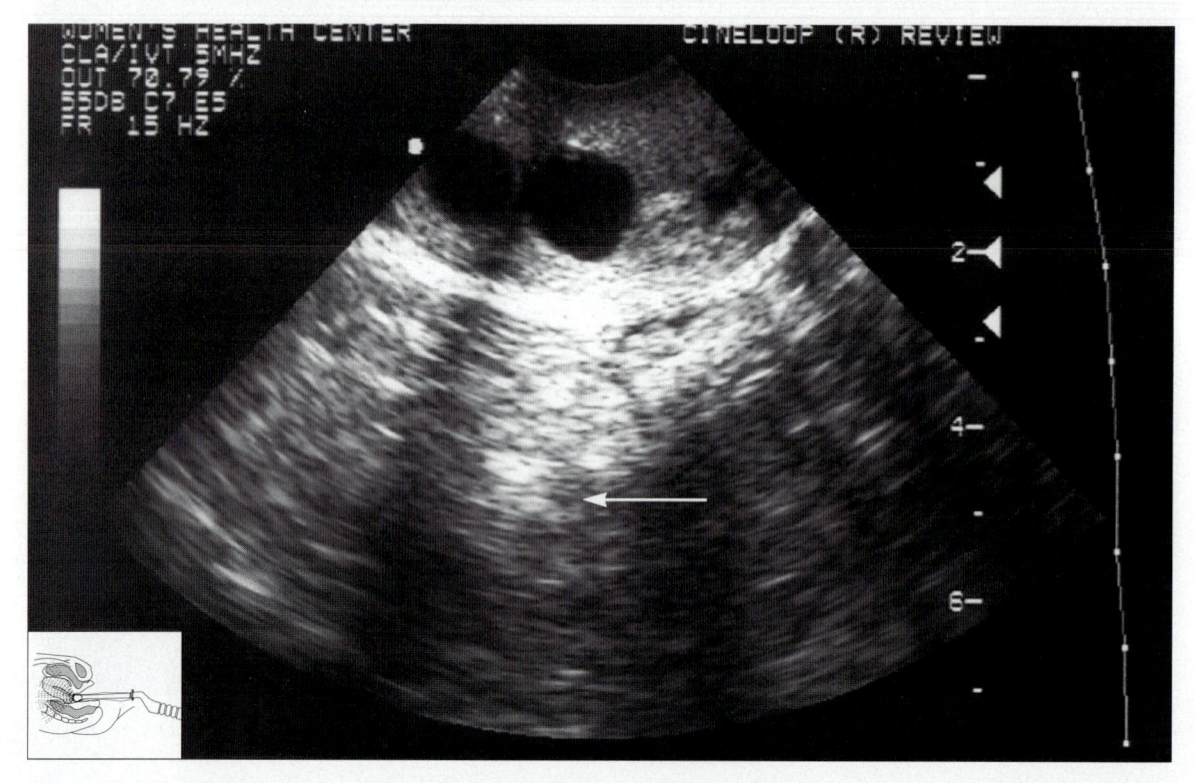

Figure 4-10. *Large, anechoic, endocervical cysts, displaying characteristic "through transmission" (arrow).*

Cervix

Cervical Leiomyomas (Fibroids)

Cervical leiomyomas or fibroids are uncommon smooth muscle tumors of the cervix. Like their uterine counterpart, they may be intramural or pedunculated.

Scan Findings

Classically, cervical fibroids have a mixed echogenic appearance on gray-scale sonography. There is often prominent acoustic shadowing, and obtaining clear images may be difficult. Intratumoral blood flow is usually not prominent but flow is seen around the periphery, within their pseudo capsule.

Even more uncommon are xanthomatous fibromas within the cervical stroma. Color flow helps differentiate this growth from a fibroid or polyp by confirming peripheral flow.

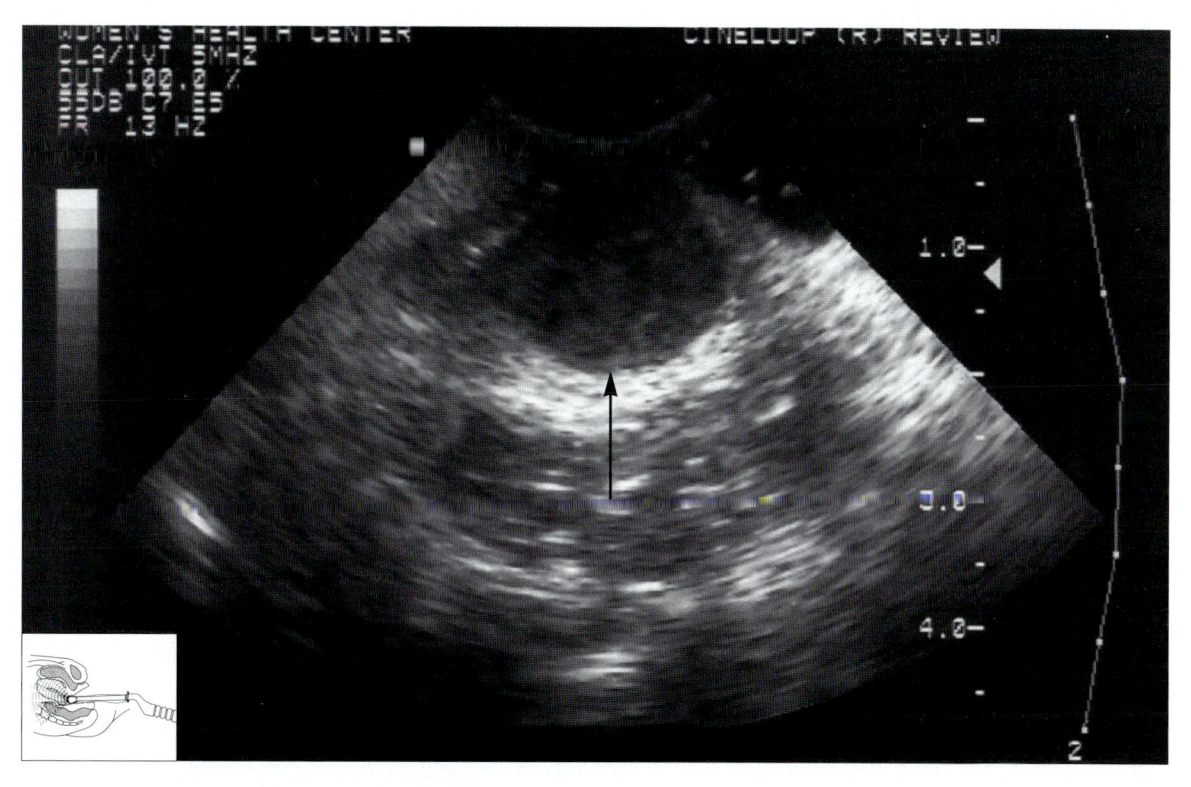

Figure 4-11. A large hypoechoic endocervical tumor (arrow). The endocervical canal contains echoic mucus. This lesion was originally thought to be a mucus cyst.

An Atlas of Transvaginal Sonography

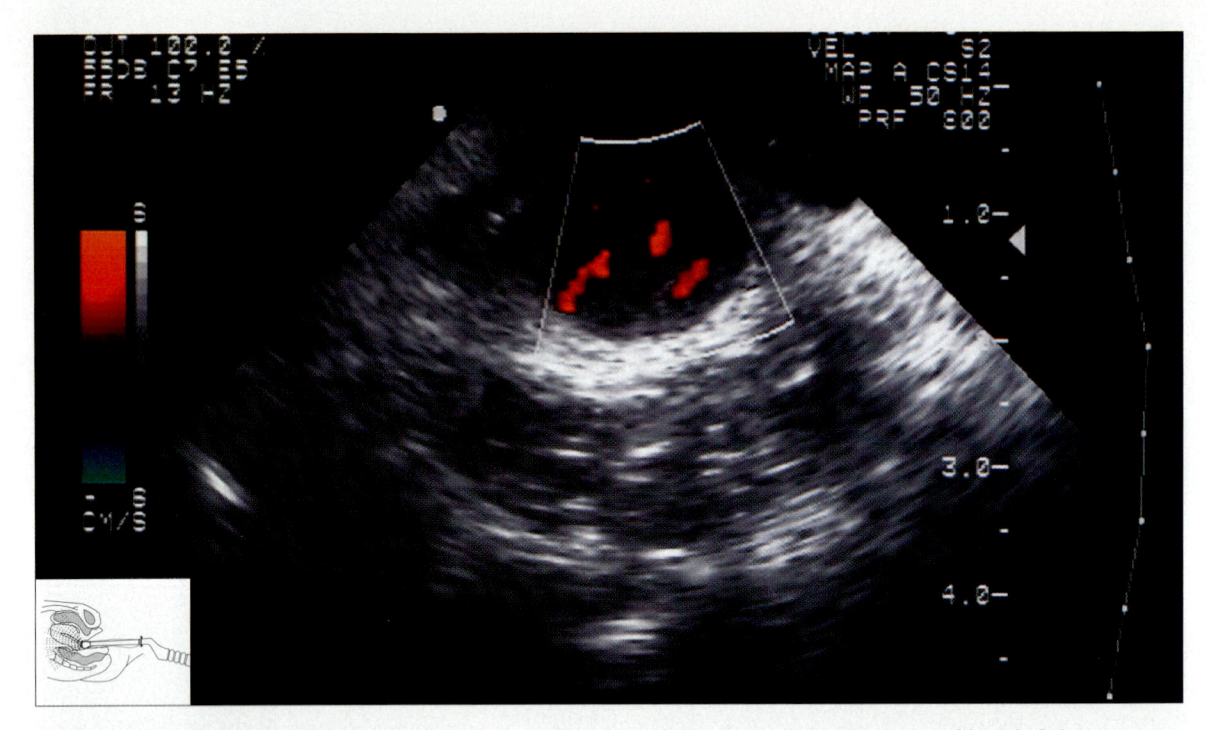

Figure 4-12. *Color flow Doppler confirms the solid nature of this cervical xanthomatous fibroid. Other characteristics that help confirm its solid nature include its lack of "through transmission" and the fact that it contains internal echoes rather than being anechoic.*

Cervical and Prolapsed Uterine Polyps

Cervical and prolapsed uterine polyps are benign overgrowths of the epithelial lining of the endocervix, resulting in an exophytic polyploid growth.

Scan Findings

Cervical and prolapsed uterine polyps can vary in appearance from iso- to hyperechoic. If these polyps are isoechoic, they can be very difficult to distinguish from the surrounding cervical stroma. These polyps can also be very difficult to distinguish from an isoechoic prolapsed uterine fibroid.

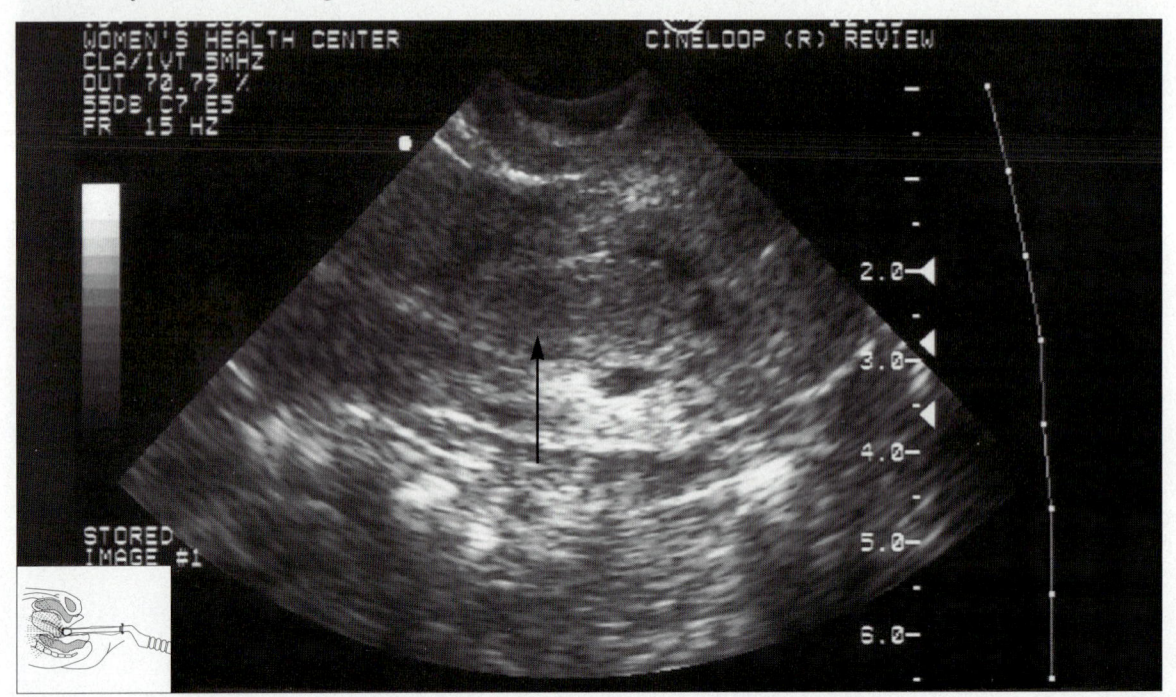

Figure 4-13. *An isoechoic endocervical polyp (arrow), which may be confused with an isoechoic fibroid.*

30

Cervical Stump

Although infrequently performed these days, a subtotal hysterectomy leaves the uterine cervix in situ. In patients claiming to have had a hysterectomy, occasionally the cervical stump may confuse the sonographer and lead him or her to diagnose a central pelvic mass.

Scan Findings

The scan findings of a cervical stump are essentially those of a normal cervix, without an attached uterine corpus. Its internal morphology is homogeneously isoechoic. Echoic mucus can be seen within the endocervix. Normal parametria extend in a tapering fashion toward the pelvic side wall.

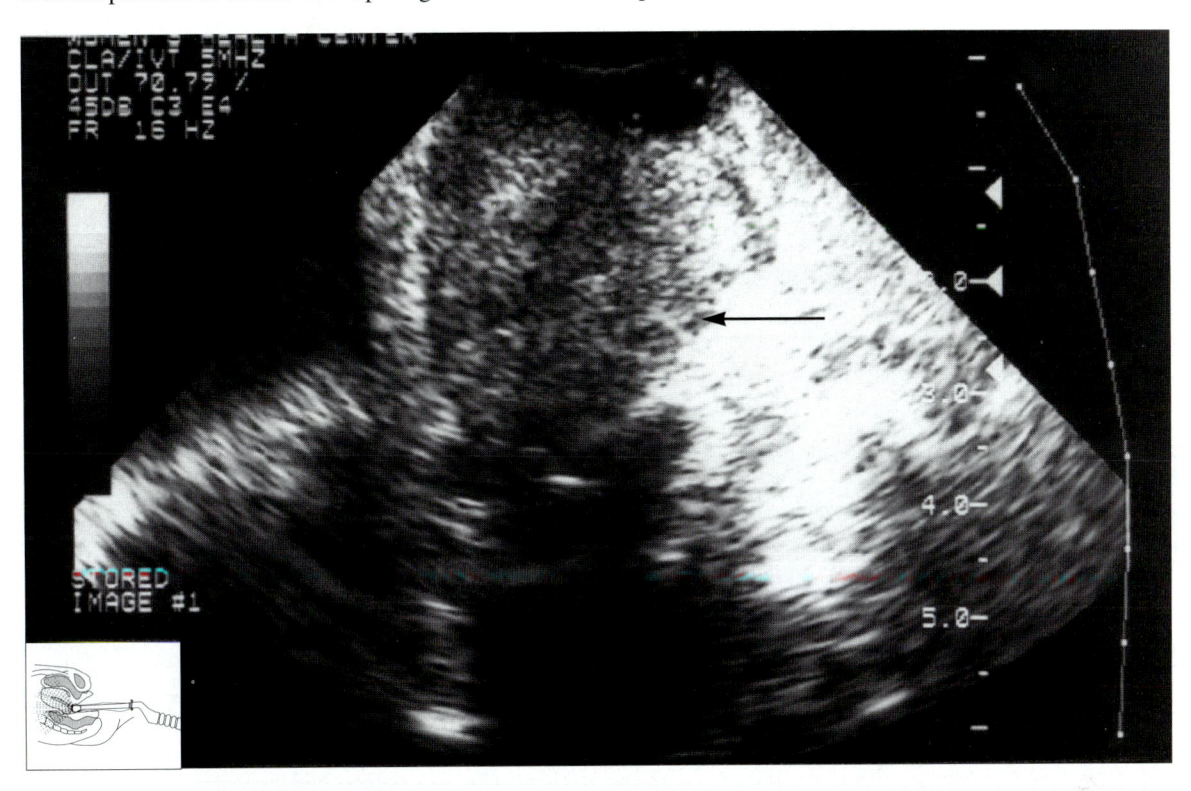

Figure 4-14. Patient with a history of a hysterectomy was referred with a central pelvic mass. TVS confirmed a remnant cervix (arrow) and no cancer. A review of the records confirms a subtotal hysterectomy was performed.

Cervical Stenosis

The ectocervix may become atrophic and stenotic in the postmenopausal years, leading to the buildup of retained uterine fluid.

Scan Findings

The scan findings of retained cervical fluid are similar to those of retained uterine fluid. Echogenic material may imply retained blood while clear fluid may imply retained mucus. The cervical stroma is ballooned or distended outward, resulting in thinning of the normal cervical parenchyma.

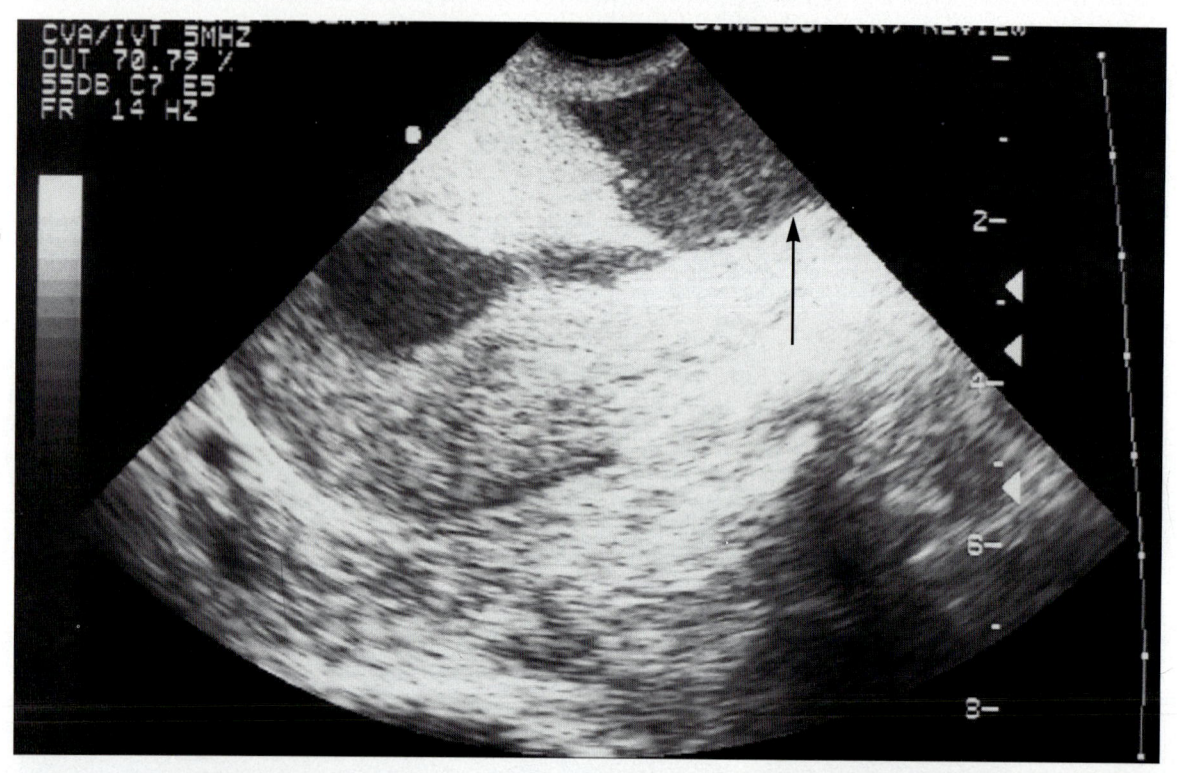

Figure 4-15. Sagittal section through corpus and endocervix demonstrating a ballooned cervix distended with echogenic fluid (arrow) and with communication with the uterine cavity. The patient had stenosis of the ectocervix and was on hormone replacement therapy resulting in hematometra and hematocervix.

5 Uterus

The uterine corpus is ideally suited to transvaginal ultrasound imaging. It lies directly within the focal zone of the transducer, without intervening bowel to potentially obscure the image. The uterus is scanned in sagittal and coronal planes to obtain a 3D impression of its size, shape and relationship to other pelvic structures.

The uterine artery, a branch of the internal iliac artery, supplies blood to the uterus. It can be visualized just lateral to the cervix, approximately at the cervical-corpus junction. The uterine artery can be traced laterally to its origin in the pelvic side wall, in the base of the broad ligament. Although not essential, color Doppler ultrasound makes its identification easier.

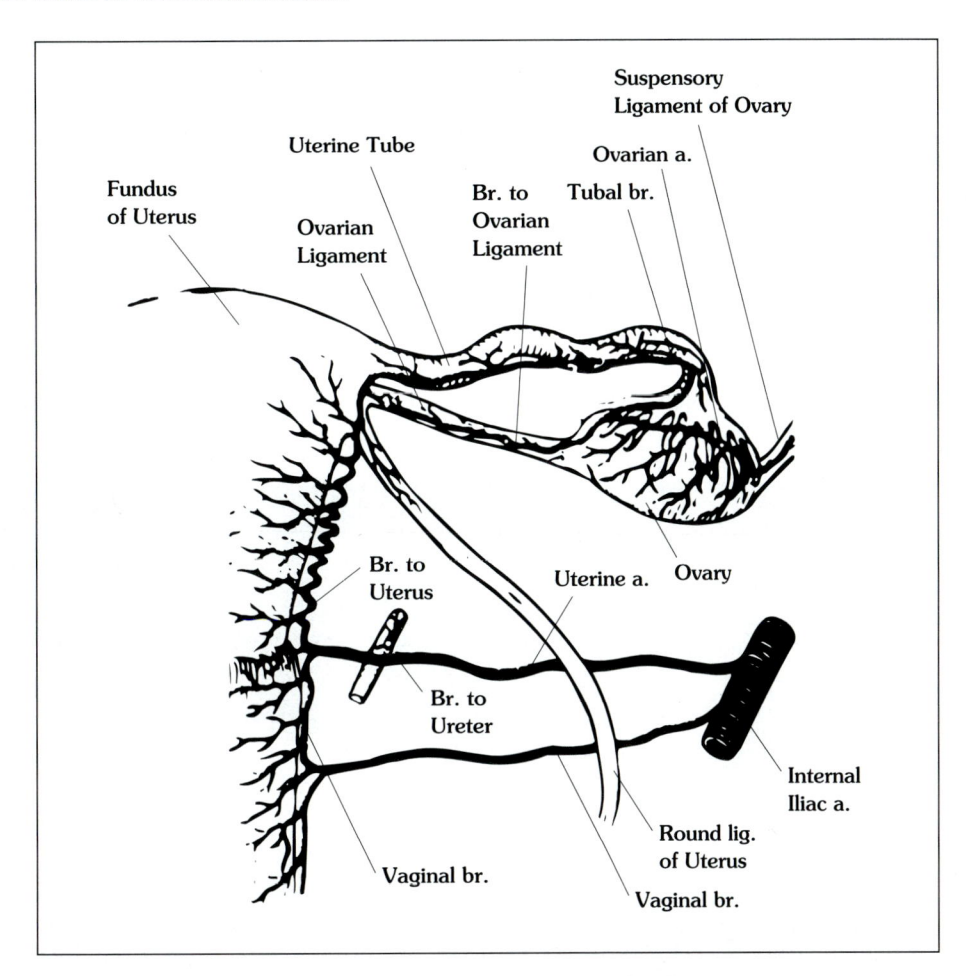

Figure 5-1. Normal uterine arterial supply. A complex network of arcuate arteries originate as branches (br.) from the uterine artery (a). A complex venous system (not shown) accompanies the arterial supply. (From Woodburne RT, Burkel WE, editors: Essentials of Human Anatomy, ed 8, New York, 1988, Oxford University, p. 541.)

An Atlas of Transvaginal Sonography

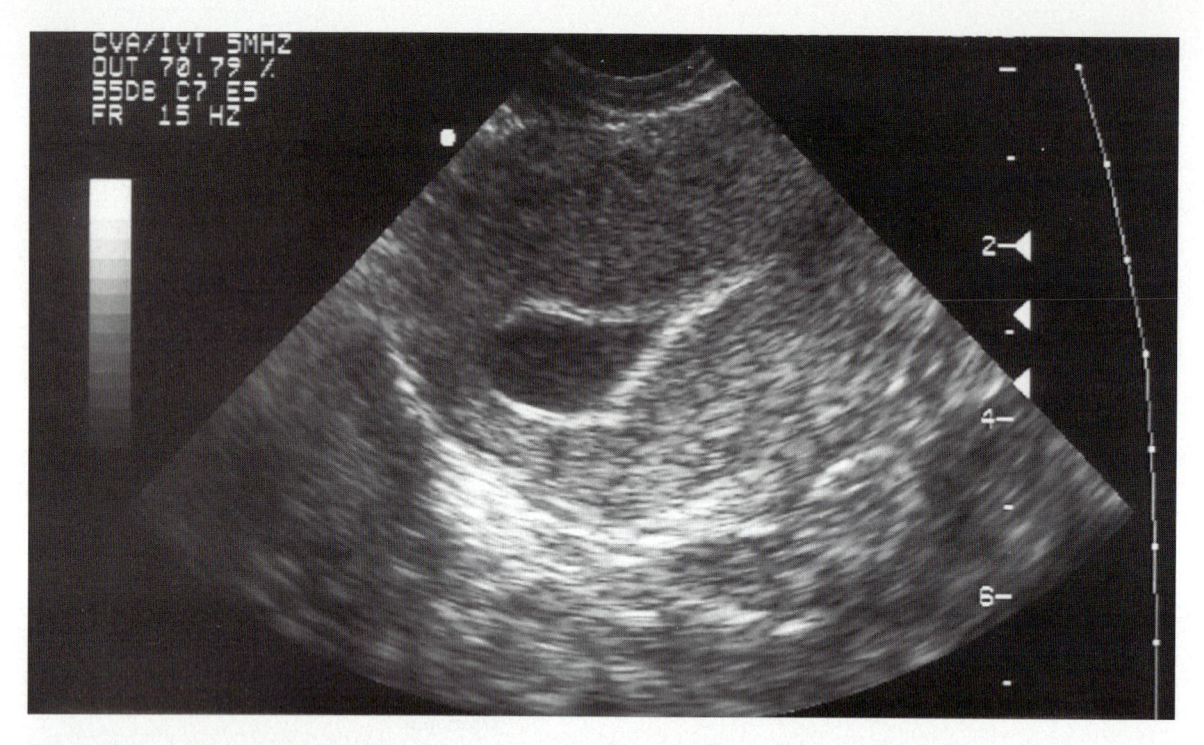

Figure 5-2. *Sagittal section through an anteverted uterus. Fluid has been instilled within the uterine cavity to demonstrate the thin, echogenic endometrium.*

Scan Findings

Sagittal and coronal imaging identifies uterine size (normal, small, enlarged), shape (regular or irregular), version (anteverted or retroverted), and position (midline or deviated). The myometrium often appears as homogenous and isoechoic. Immediately adjacent to the endometrium is a dense compact layer of myometrium, referred to as the subendometrial halo. The importance of this layer is that it becomes disrupted with invasive uterine malignancies.

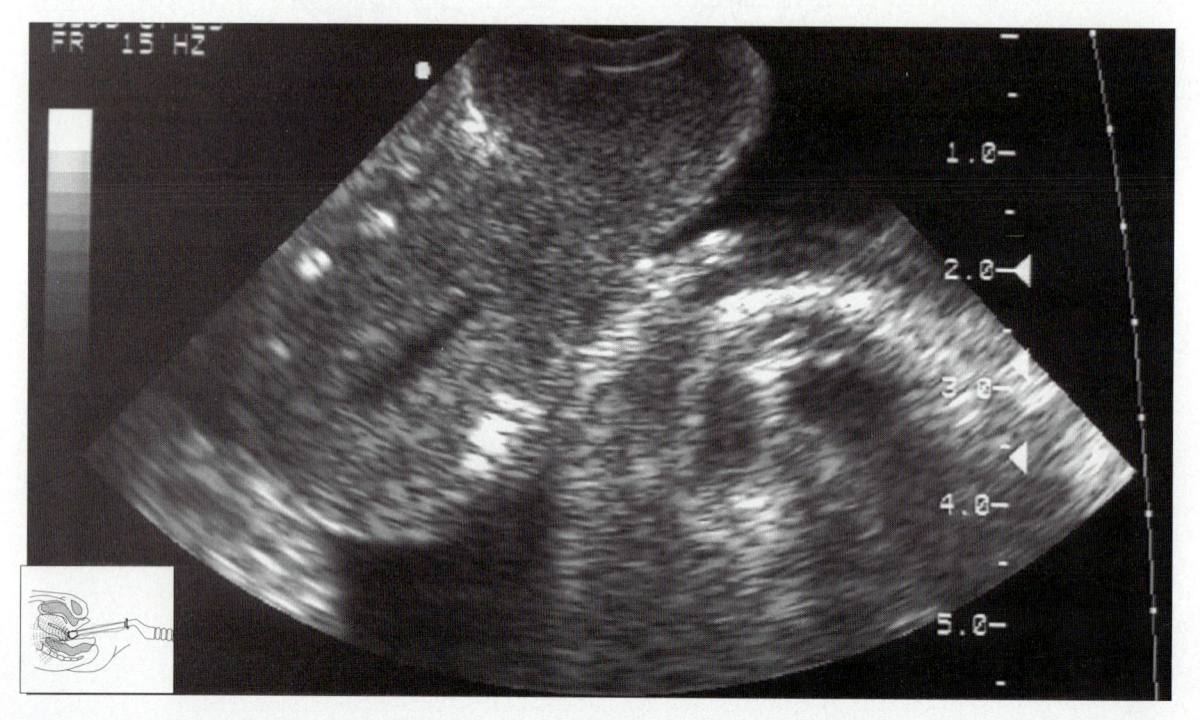

Figure 5-3. *Sagittal uterine section through an anteverted uterus, bathed in ascitic fluid. Calcified arcuate vessels (arrow) within the peripheral myometrium.*

Uterus

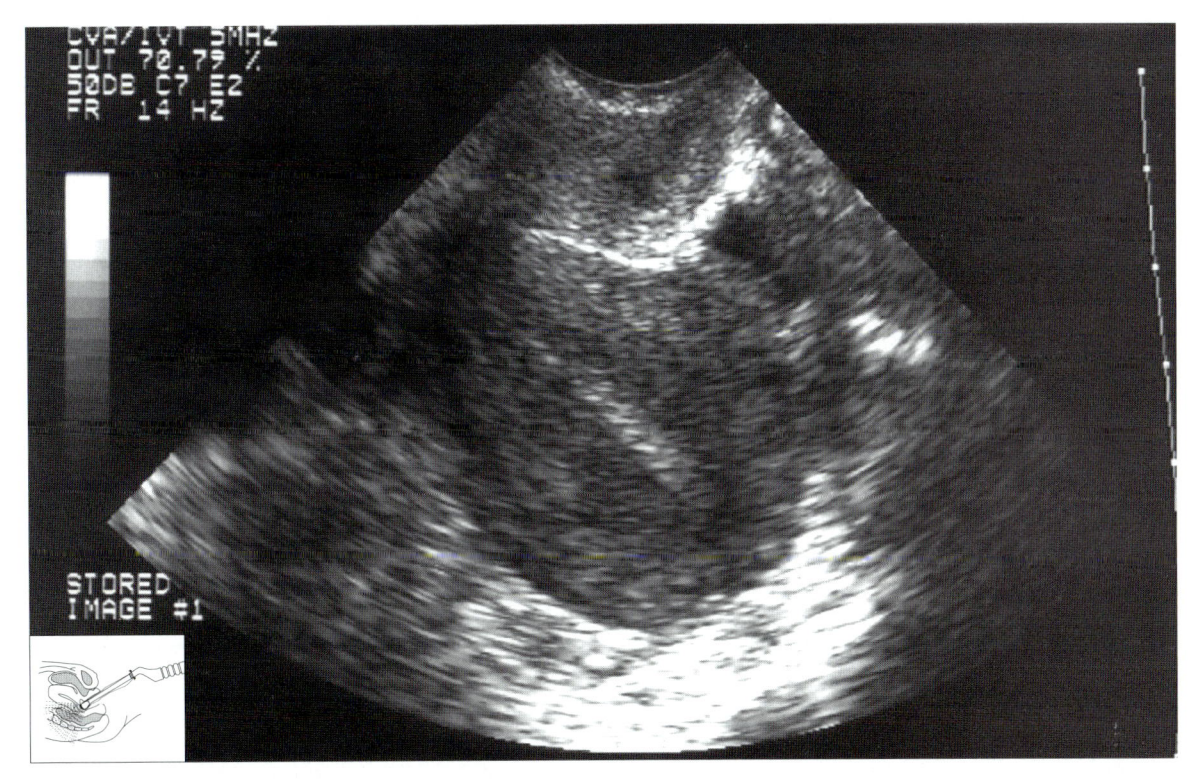

Figure 5-4. Retroverted retroflexed uterus.

An Atlas of Transvaginal Sonography

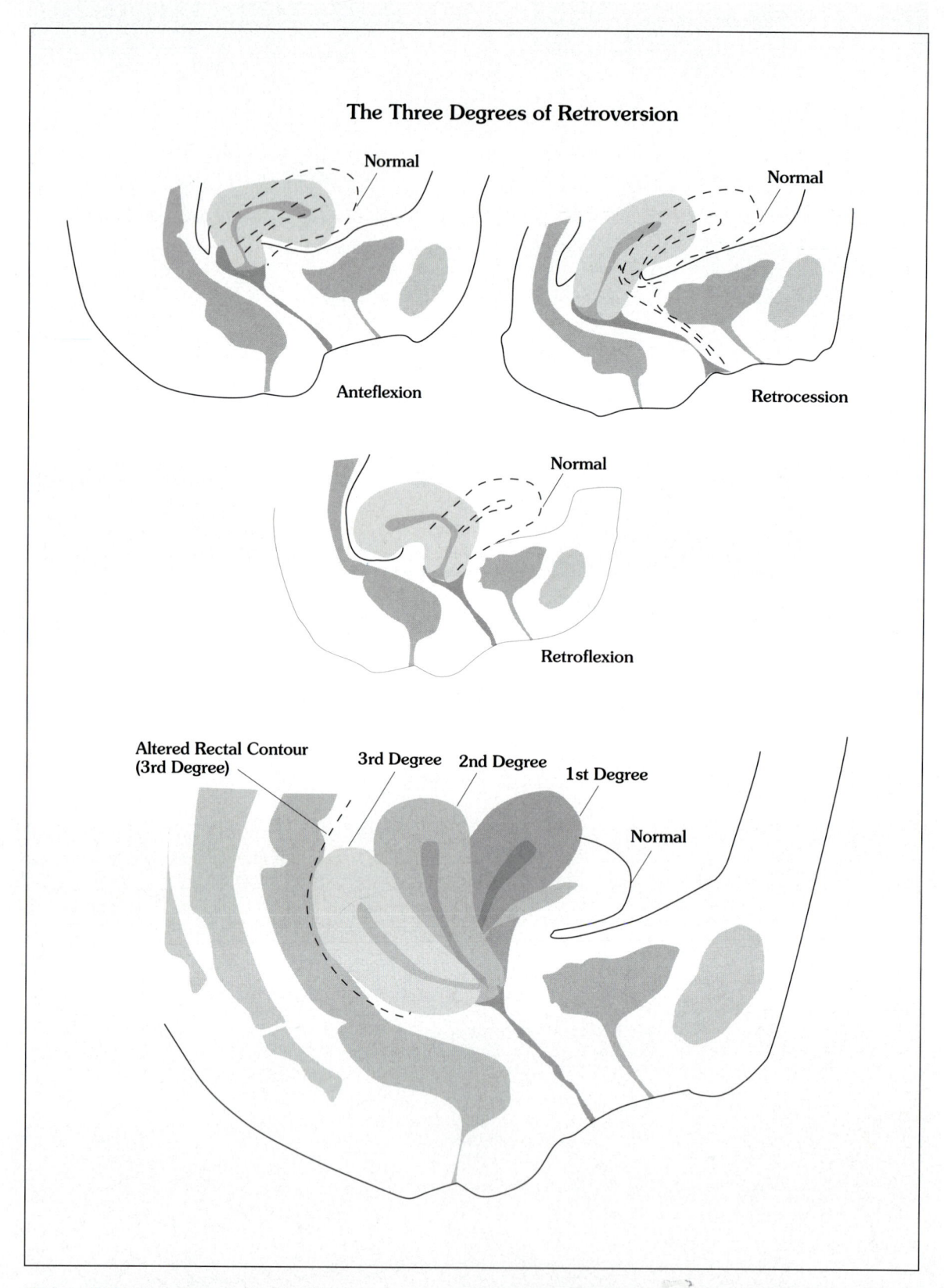

Figure 5-5. *Diagrammatic representation of uterine version, clearly demonstrating the differences between ante and retroversion and ante and retroflexion.*

Uterus

Menstrual Cycle Changes

The changes in endometrial histology occurring throughout the menstrual cycle are reflected in the sonographic images obtained. Proliferative phase endometrium is typically 3-5 mm thick and iso- or hypoechoic. The endometrial stripe is thin and intrauterine blood flow is absent. The midcycle or periovulatory period is ultrasonographically characterized by a "three line" endometrial stripe. With increasing glycogen accumulation in the luteal phase, the endometrium sonographically increases in thickness to 5-15 mm and is echoic. Uterine blood flow is increased on color flow.

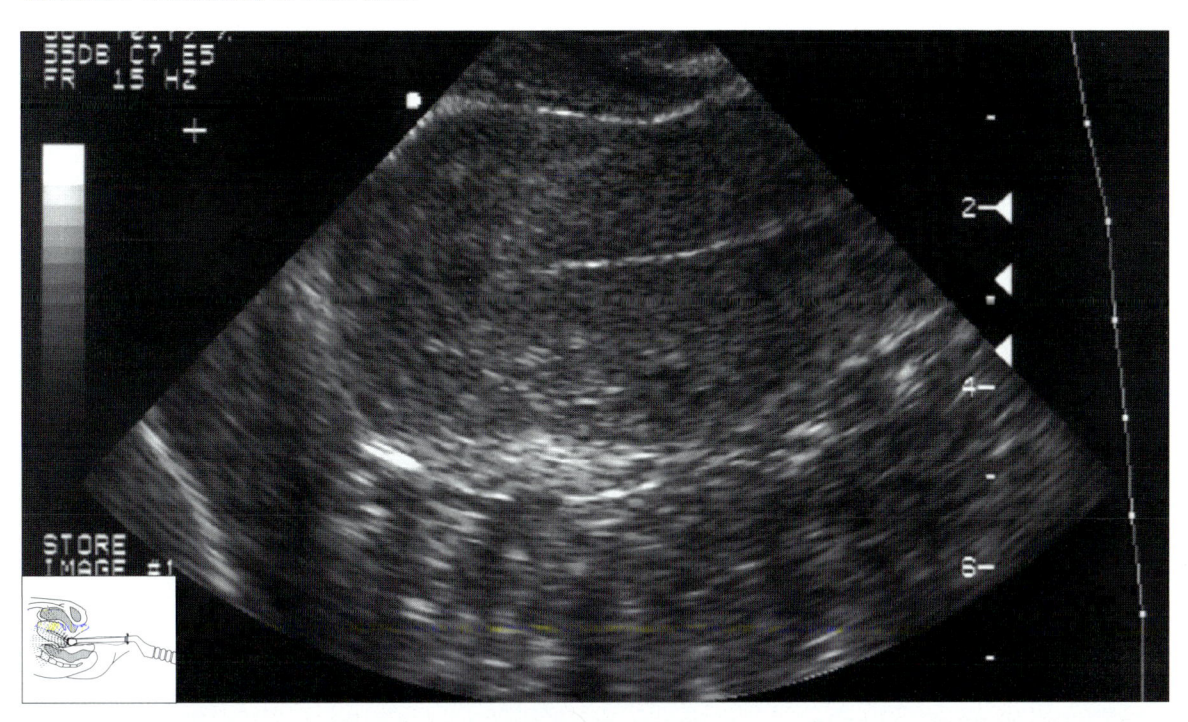

Figure 5-6. Sagittal uterine scan demonstrating early proliferative phase endometrium. The endometrial stripe is thin and isoechoic, with a small amount of echoic intrauterine fluid.

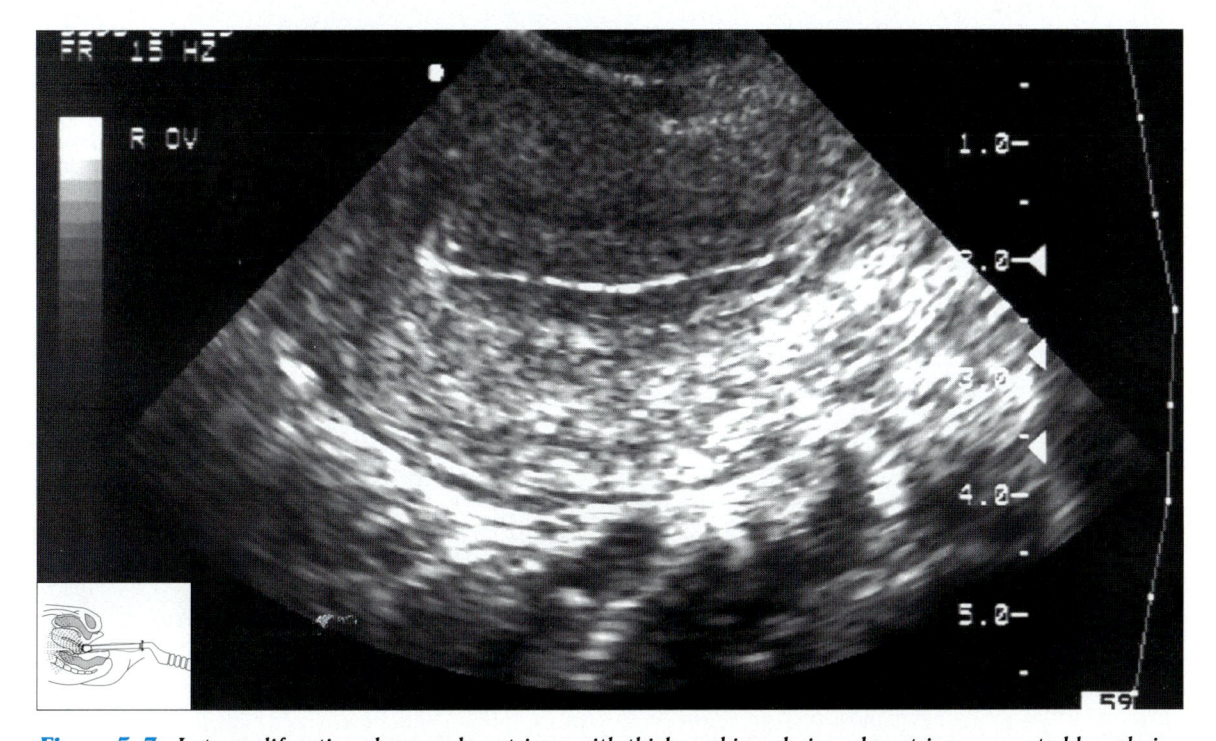

Figure 5-7. Late proliferative phase endometrium, with thickened isoechoic endometrium separated by echoic intrauterine fluid.

An Atlas of Transvaginal Sonography

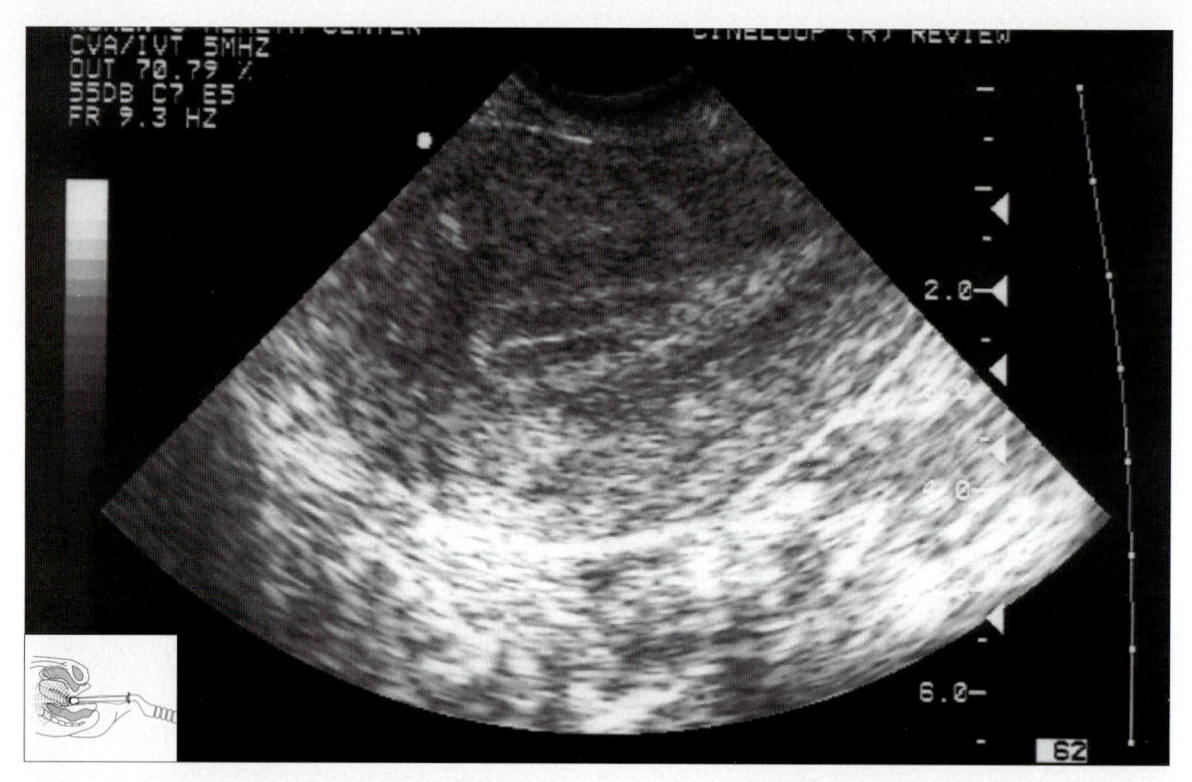

Figure 5-8. Periovulatory phase endometrium clearly demonstrating the "three line sign." The basal endometrium has developed increased echogenicity.

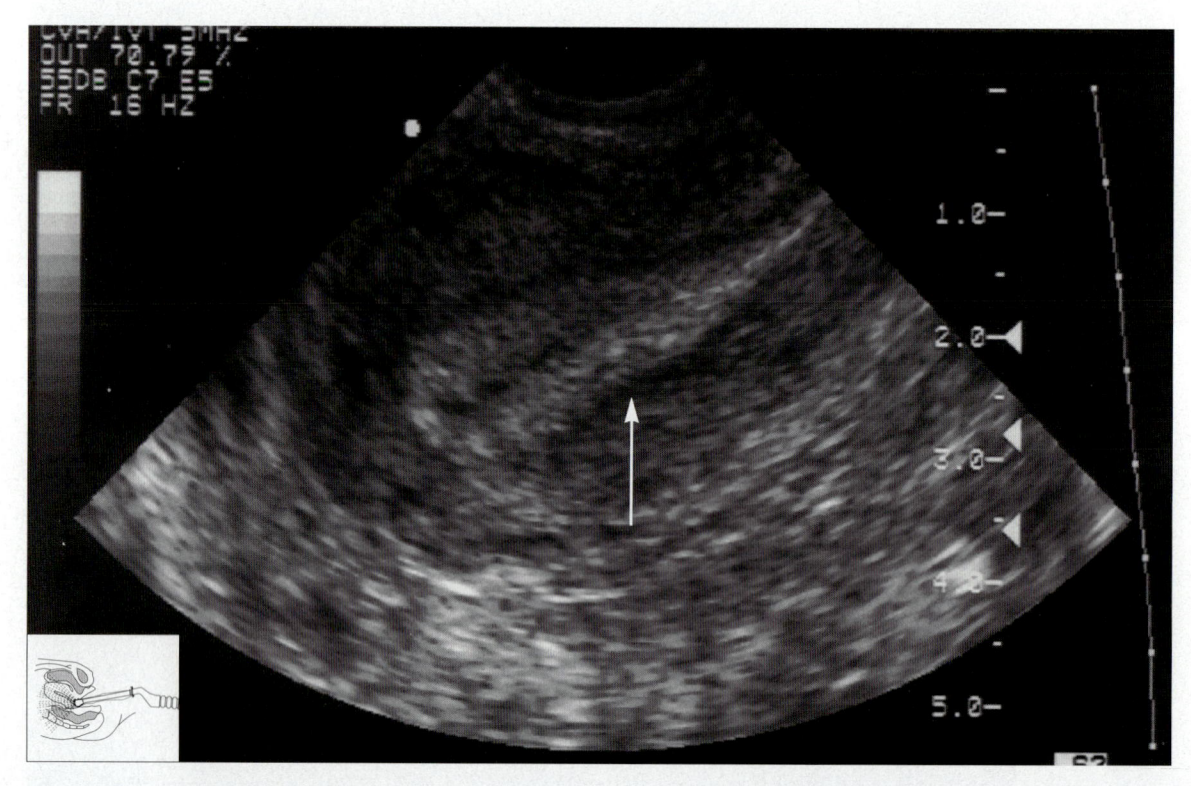

Figure 5-9. Luteal phase endometrium, demonstrating thickened, echoic endometrium, surrounded by a hypoechoic layer of compact myometrium referred to as the "subendometrial halo" (arrow).

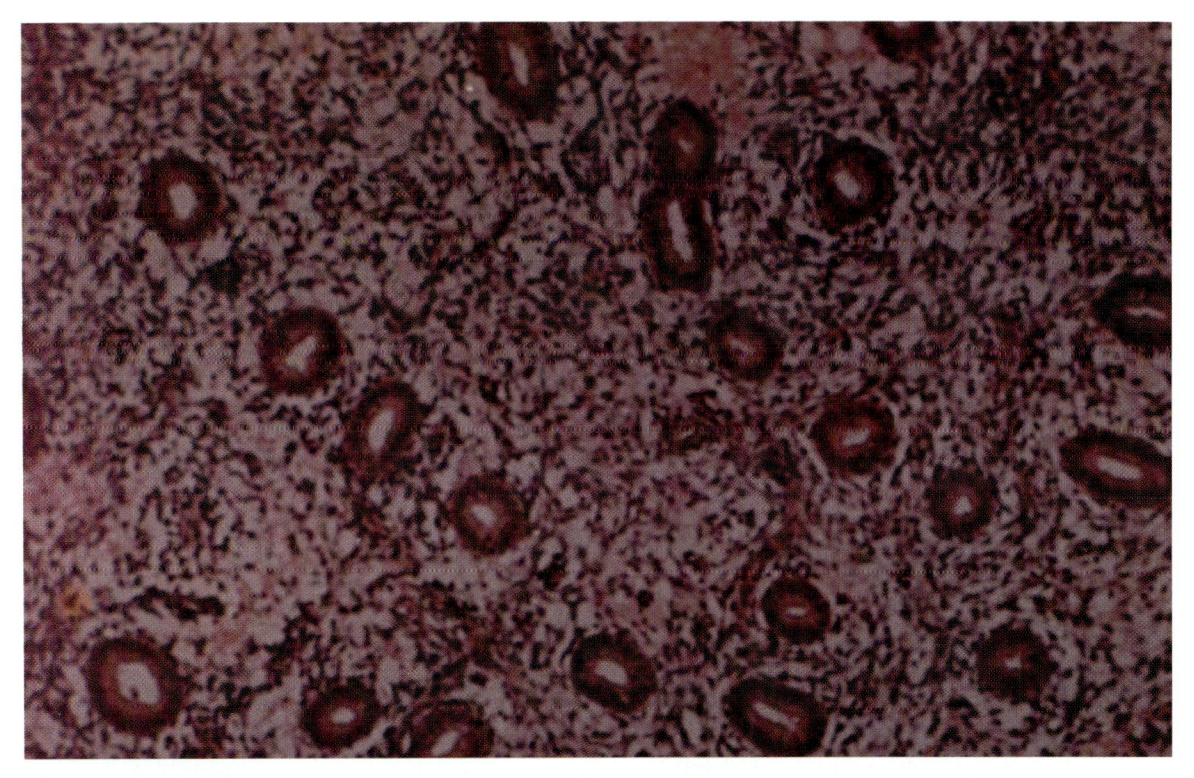

Uterus

Figure 5-10. *Proliferative phase endometrium, with small, sparsely spaced glands.*

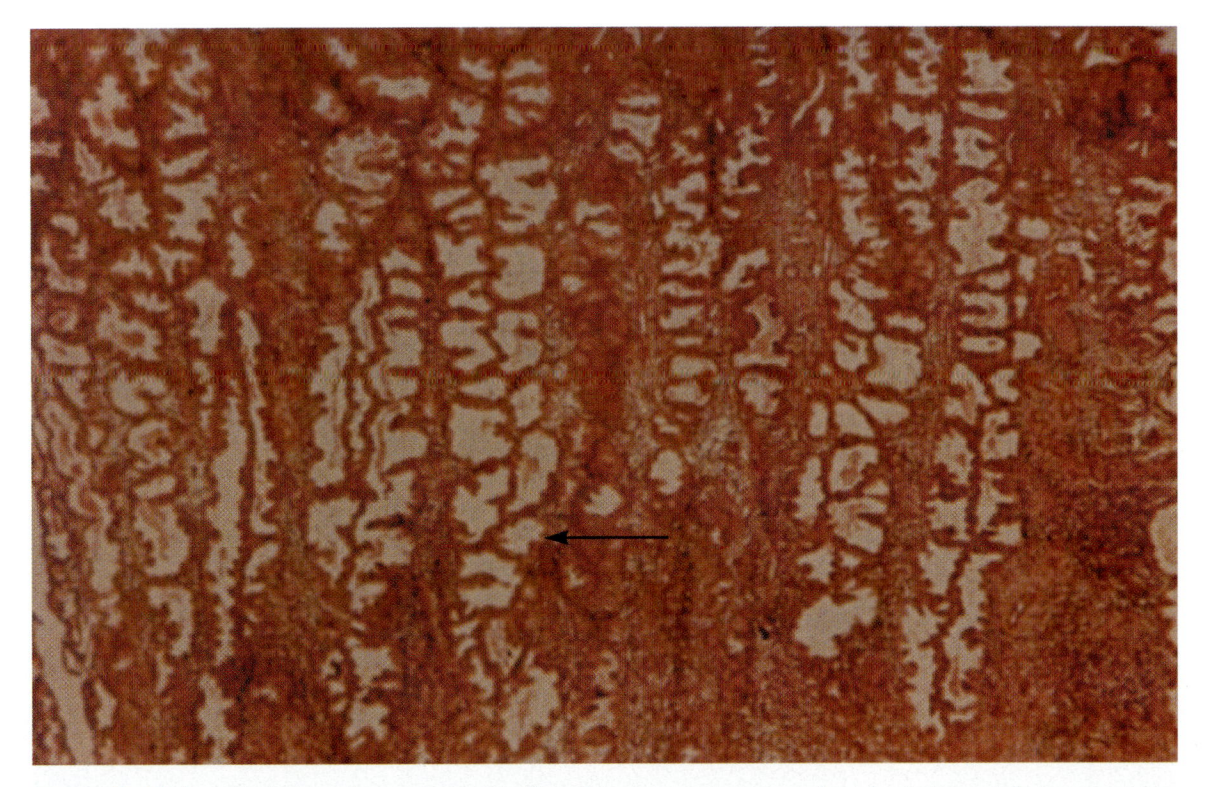

Figure 5-11. *Luteal phase endometrium, with dilated, tortuous, glycogen laden glands (arrow) that account for the hyperechoic appearance on gray-scale sonography.*

An Atlas of Transvaginal Sonography

Postmenopausal Changes

Postmenopausal endometrium is typically thin, less than 5-6 mm and is hypoechoic. Thickened, echoic postmenopausal endometrium probably warrants endometrial biopsy. Also commonly seen in postmenopausal patients are calcified arcuate vessels. They are densely echoic regions in the periphery of the myometrium with characteristic posterior acoustic shadowing.

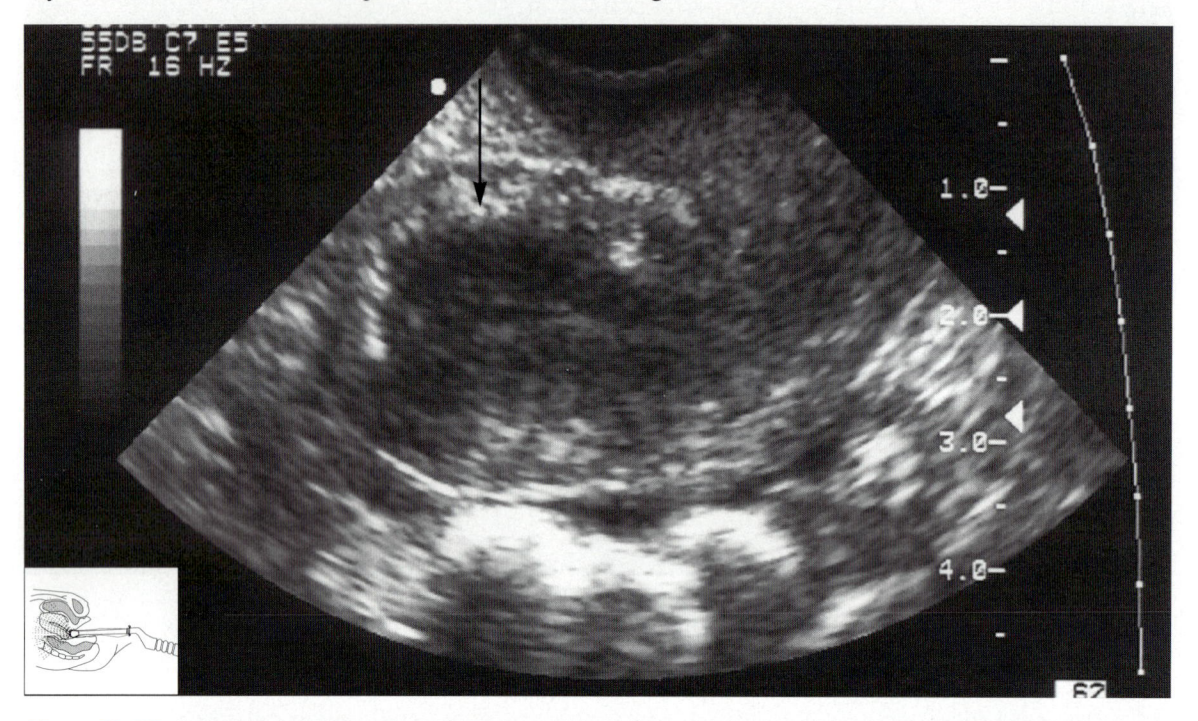

Figure 5-12. Anteverted postmenopausal uterus with atrophic, isoechoic endometrium. Calcification of the arcuate vessels is demonstrated in the peripheral myometrium (arrow).

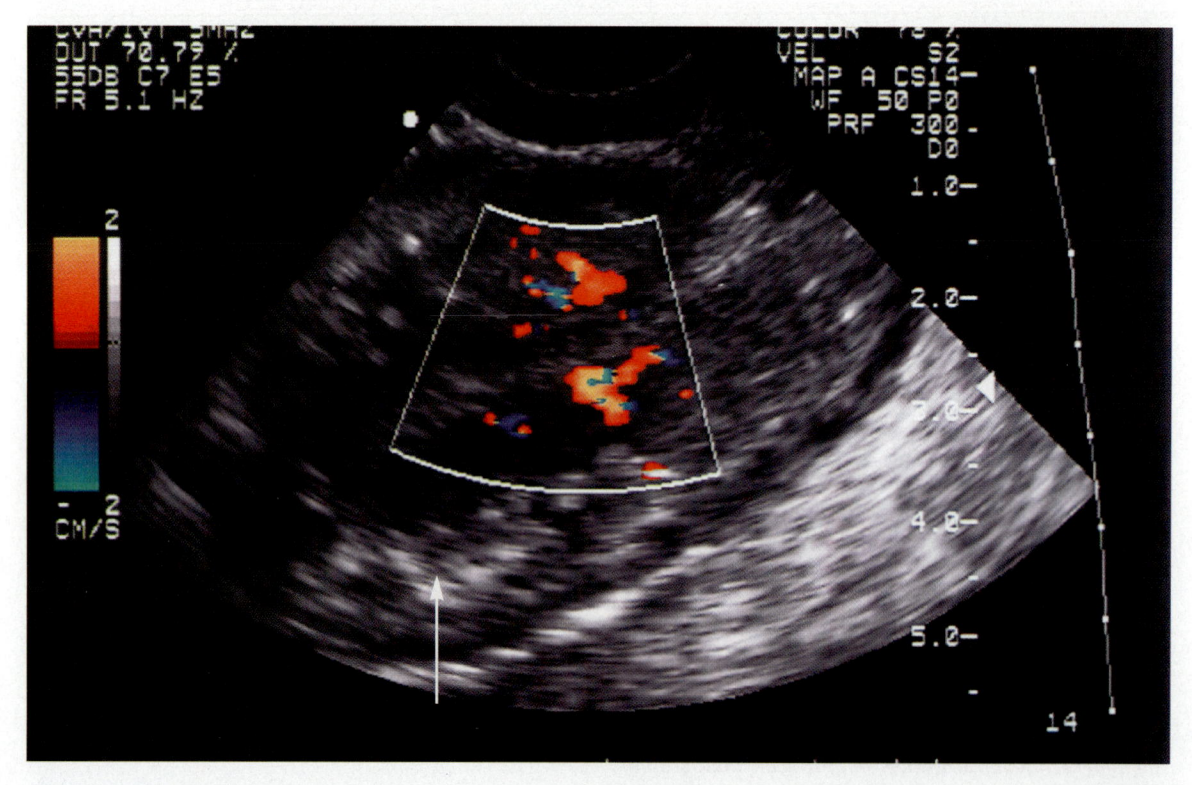

Figure 5-13. Prominent color flow in postmenopausal woman. The uterus is anteverted and contains calcified arcuate vessels (arrow). The endometrium is echoic and thickened, and the subendometrial halo appears intact.

Benign Uterine Pathology

Not only can uterine size, shape, and morphology be assessed by transvaginal sonography, but the following benign lesions can also be imaged. These include fibroids, adenomyosis, the endometrial hyperplasias, endometrial polyps, intrauterine fluid, and intrauterine contraceptive devices.

Fibroids

Fibroids, or leiomyomas, are the most common benign tumor of the uterus occurring in about 20-30% of women over age 35. They are thought to arise from totipotential primitive cells that become muscle cells, connective tissue cells and blood vessels. Since these tumors are estrogen-dependent, they appear and grow during the reproductive years, pregnancy, and under the influence of hormone replacement theory (HRT). Fibroids vary in size and shape, but tend to be well-circumscribed, demarcated, and encapsulated within a "pseudo capsule" formed by flattened uterine muscle. They are usually firm in consistency, but this will vary with degeneration. They can undergo red, hyaline, cystic or calcific degeneration. A fibroid can be situated in a submucosal, intramural or subserous location. Subserous leiomyomas can cause considerable diagnostic problems and need to be excluded from ovarian solid tumors.

Scan Findings

The sonographic appearance of this tumor also depends on the presence and type of degeneration and on the vascular supply. Sonographically, fibroids appear as mild to moderate echogenic masses that can distort the shape or cavity of the uterus. Their echogenicity depends upon the relative ratio of fibrous tissue to smooth muscle. With a predominant fibrous component, echogenicity is increased. Isoechoic leiomyomas can be difficult to distinguish from the adjacent myometrium. Interfaces between the normal myometrium and the pseudo capsule can often be identified as a clear demarcation.

Calcific degeneration is recognized as clusters of high level echoes with distal acoustical shadowing. Cystic and hyaline degeneration have irregular anechoic areas within the fibroid. Red degeneration occurs more commonly in pregnancy, and appears as a homogenous, tender mass within the myometrium. The uncommon lipoleiomyoma appears as a densely echogenic, spherical, uterine tumor.

Color flow Doppler shows normal uterine artery flow, and the PI and RI are greater than 1.0 and 0.5 respectively. Tumoral flow is dependent on presence of degeneration but is typically absent. When present, intratumoral flow is low velocity. Prominent peripheral flow, which tends to be venous in nature, is seen.

An Atlas of Transvaginal Sonography

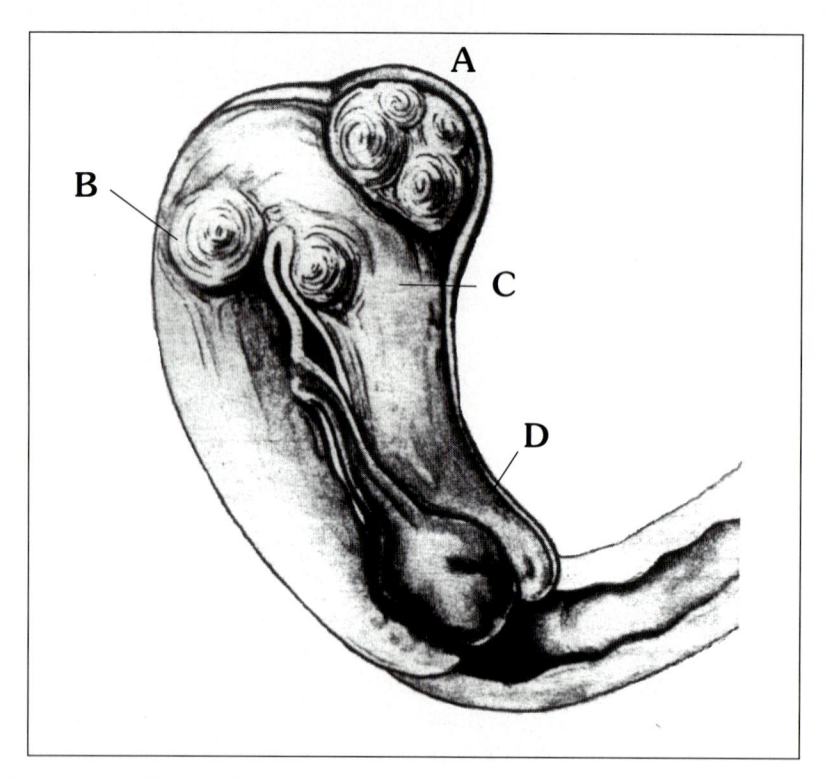

Figure 5-14. Leiomyomas. Various locations of leiomyomas include subserosal (A), intramural (B), submucosal (C), and cervical with long stalk (D).

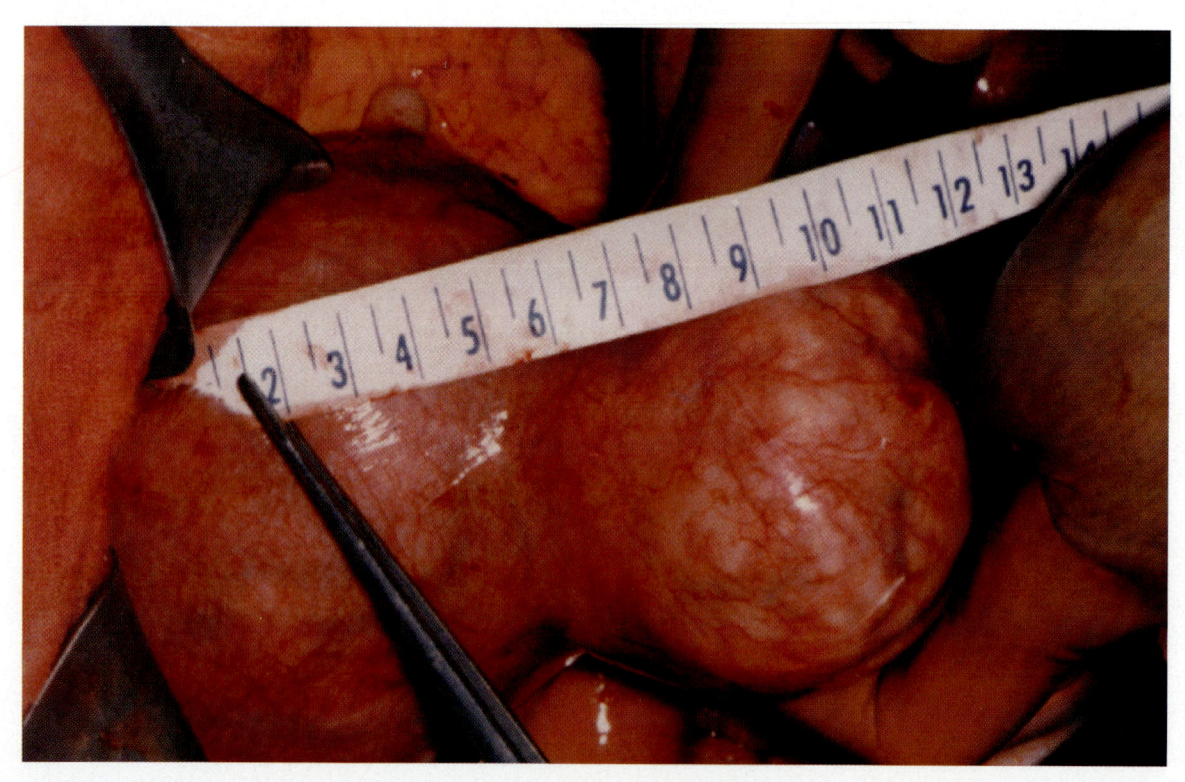

Figure 5-15. Serosal fibroid, displaying characteristic peripheral vasculature.

Uterus

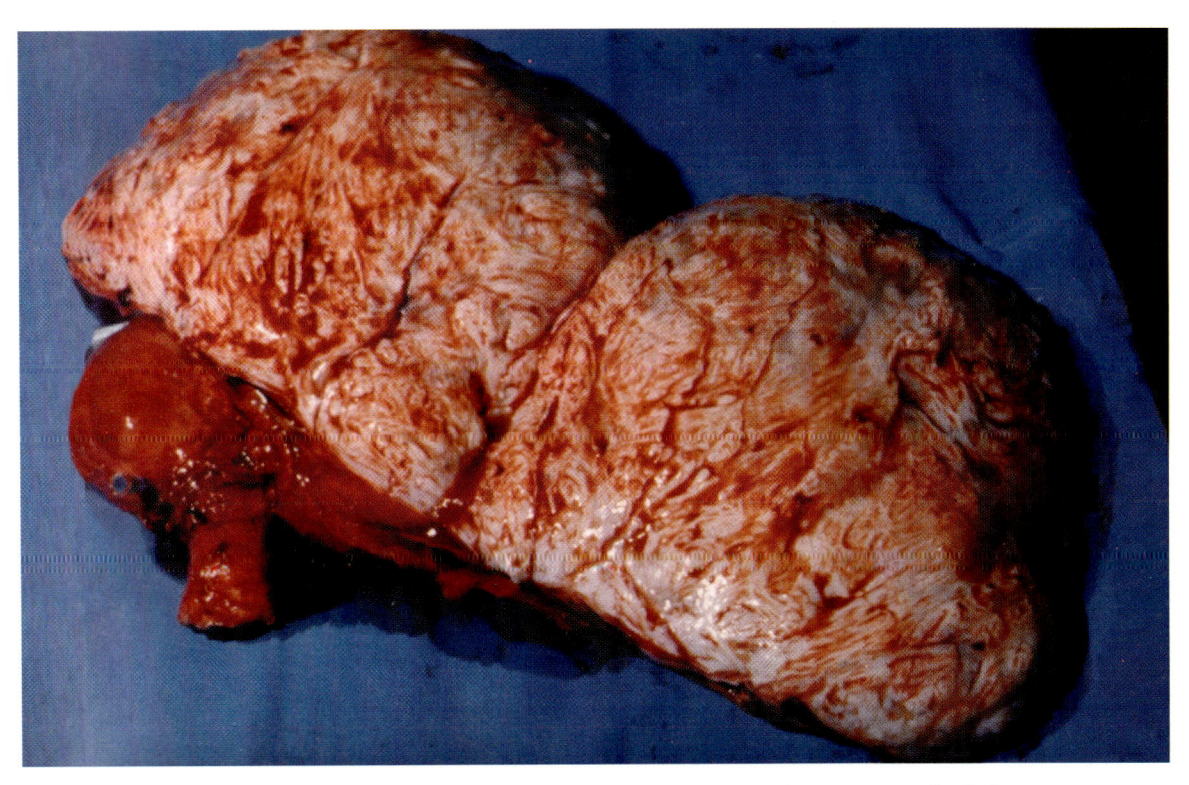

Figure 5-16. Cut surface of a large intramural fibroid demonstrating its characteristic whorled appearance.

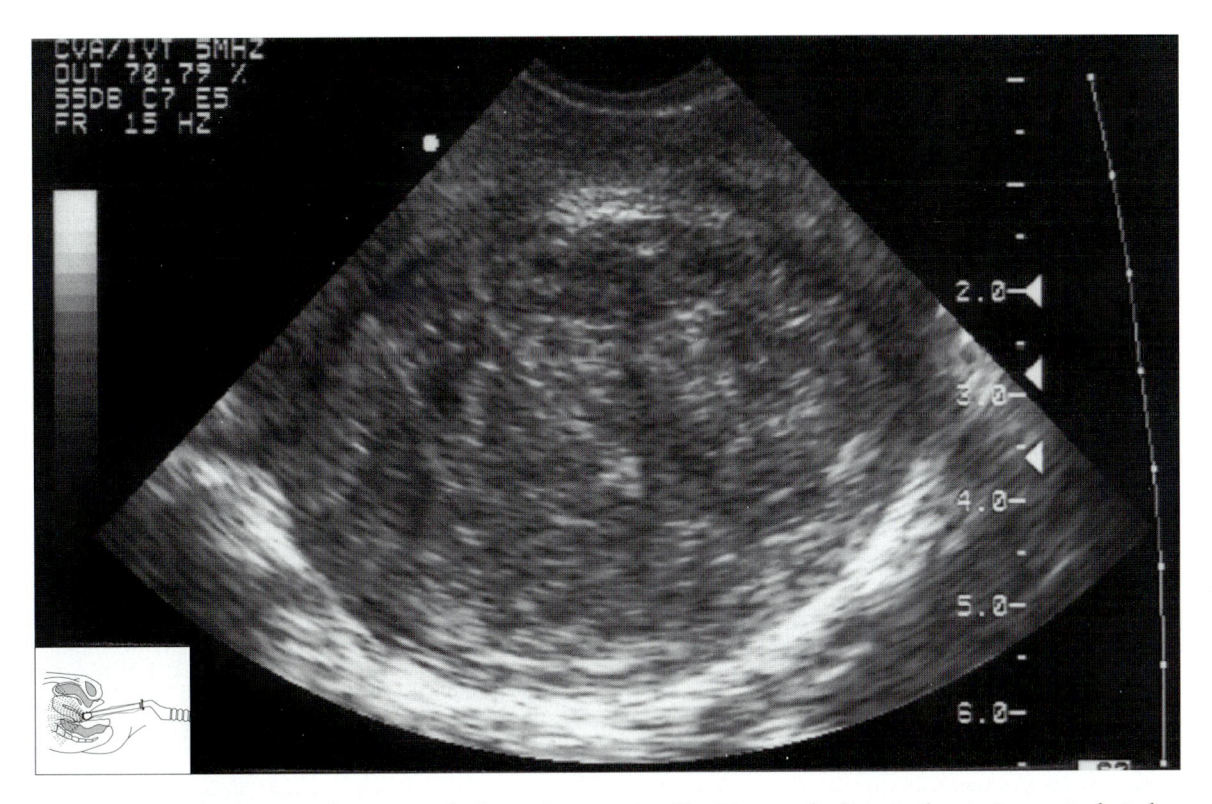

Figure 5-17. This large, well-circumscribed isoechoic uterine fibroid not only distorts the uterine cavity but also the uterine shape. Internal morphology reveals a mixed pattern.

An Atlas of Transvaginal Sonography

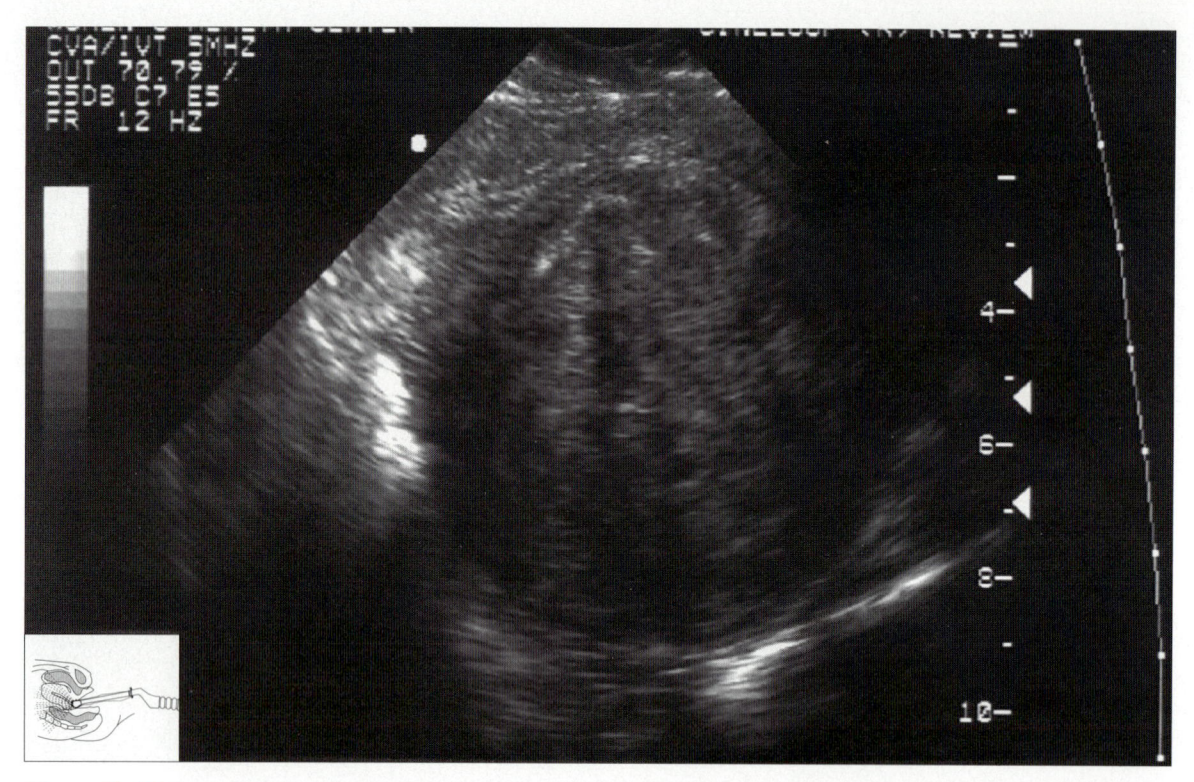

Figure 5-18. Large mixed echogenic fibroid causing distortion of uterine shape. Areas of iso- and hypoechoic areas contribute to the acoustical shadowing behind the tumor.

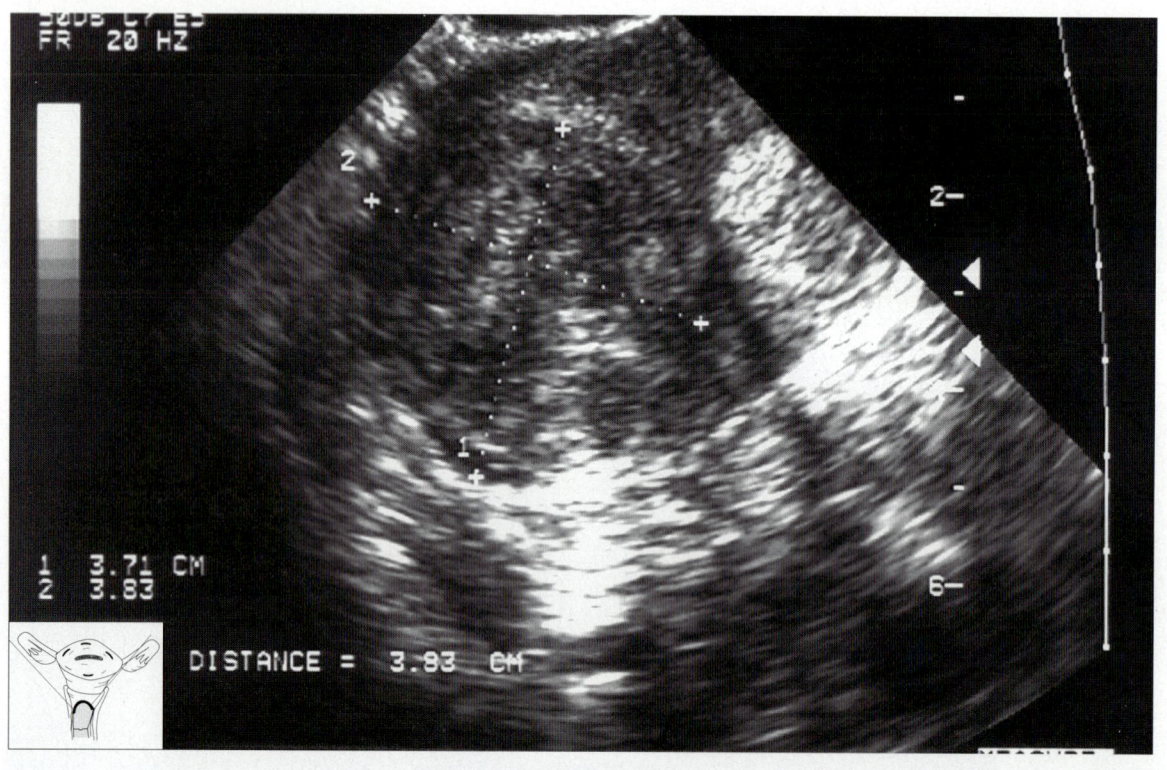

Figure 5-19. Coronal scan through the lower uterine segment with a 4-cm broad ligament fibroid. The patient was clinically thought to have an adnexal mass.

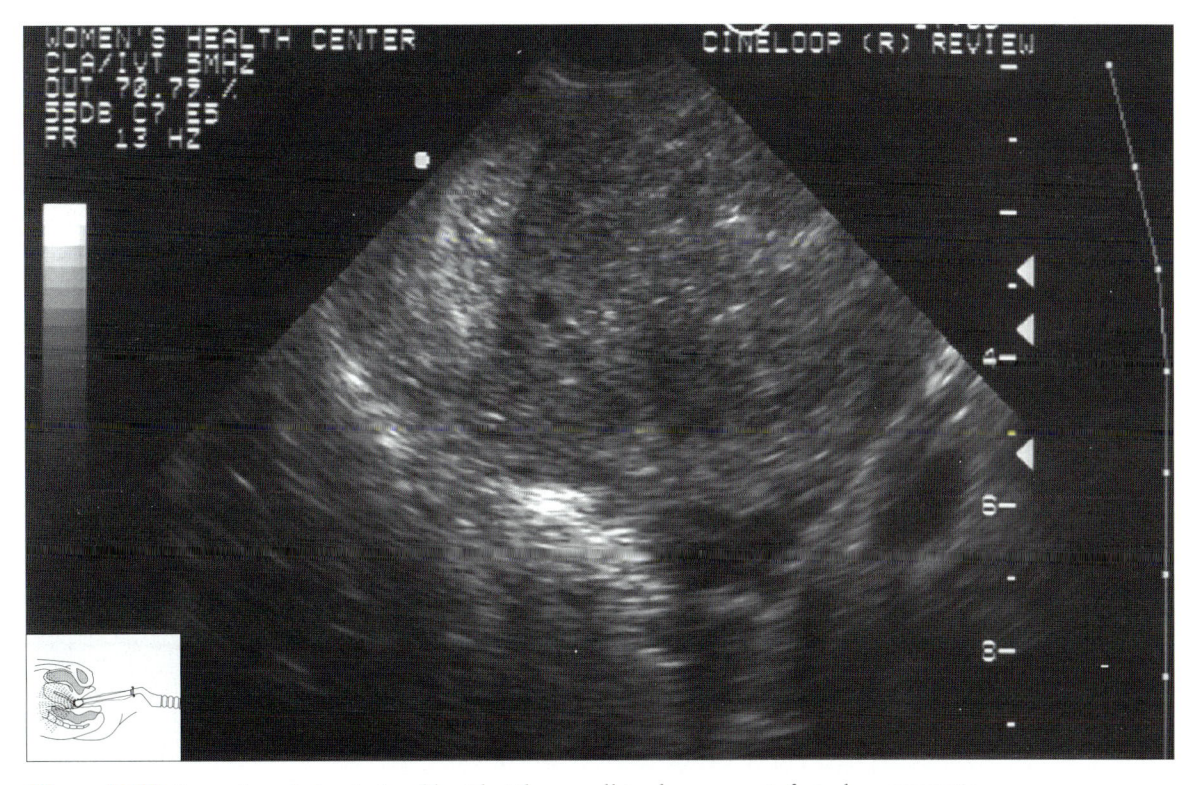

Figure 5~20. Large isoechoic uterine fibroid with a small isodense area inferiorly representing hemorrhagic necrosis.

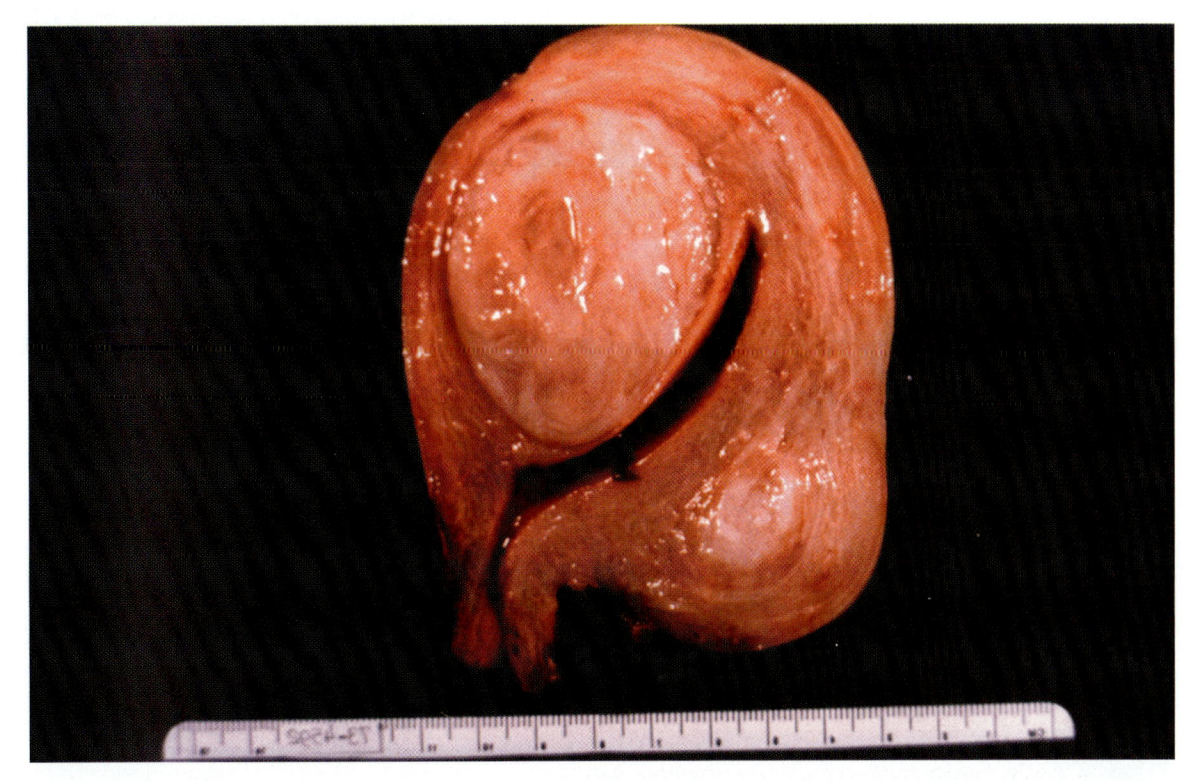

Figure 5~21. Anterior and posterior intramural fibroids, encroaching upon, but not involving, the uterine cavity.

An Atlas of Transvaginal Sonography

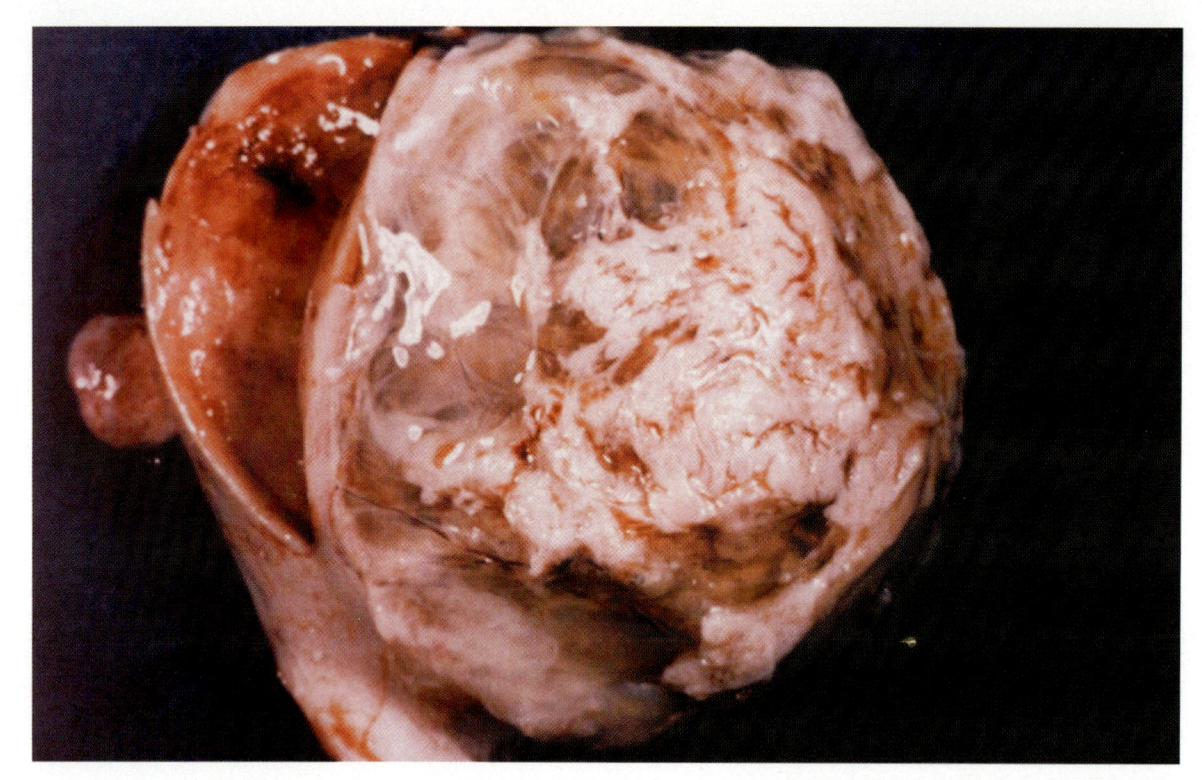

Figure 5-22. Cystic degeneration of a large uterine fibroid.

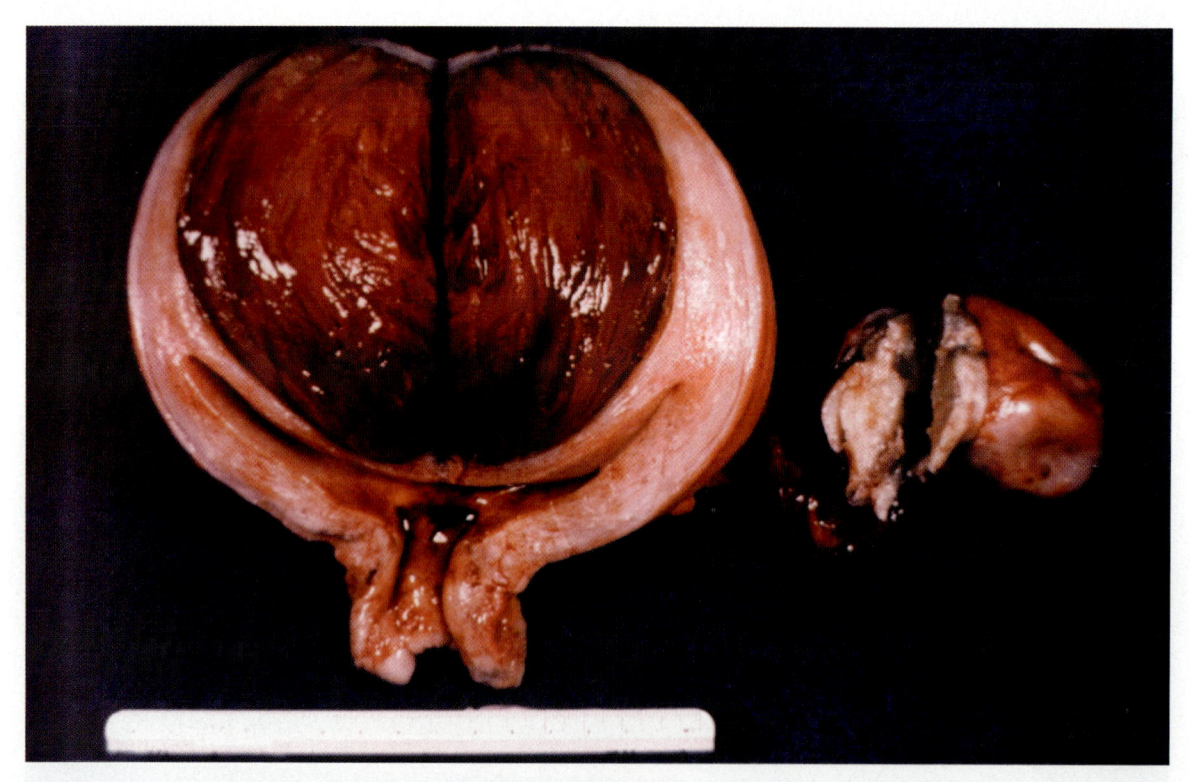

Figure 5-23. Red degeneration of a large intramural fibroid.

Uterus

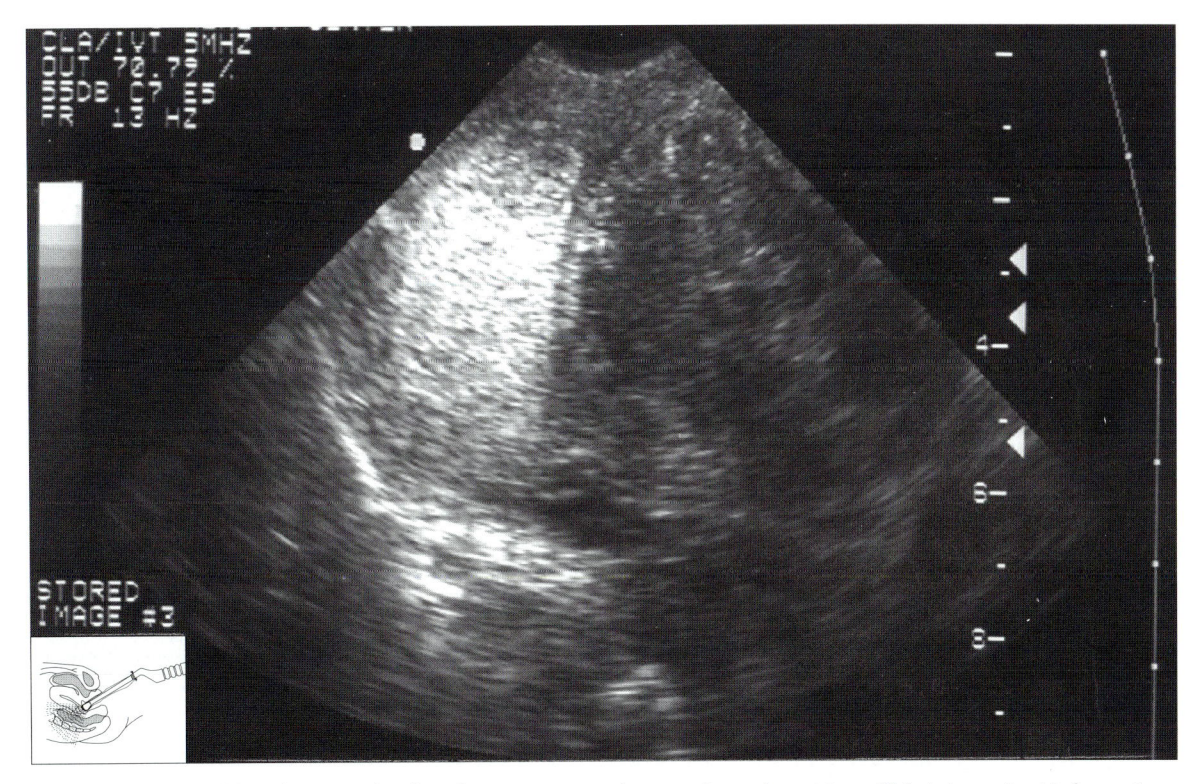

Figure 5-24. *The fibroid approaches but does not encroach upon the endometrium. This is important information if a myomectomy is being considered.*

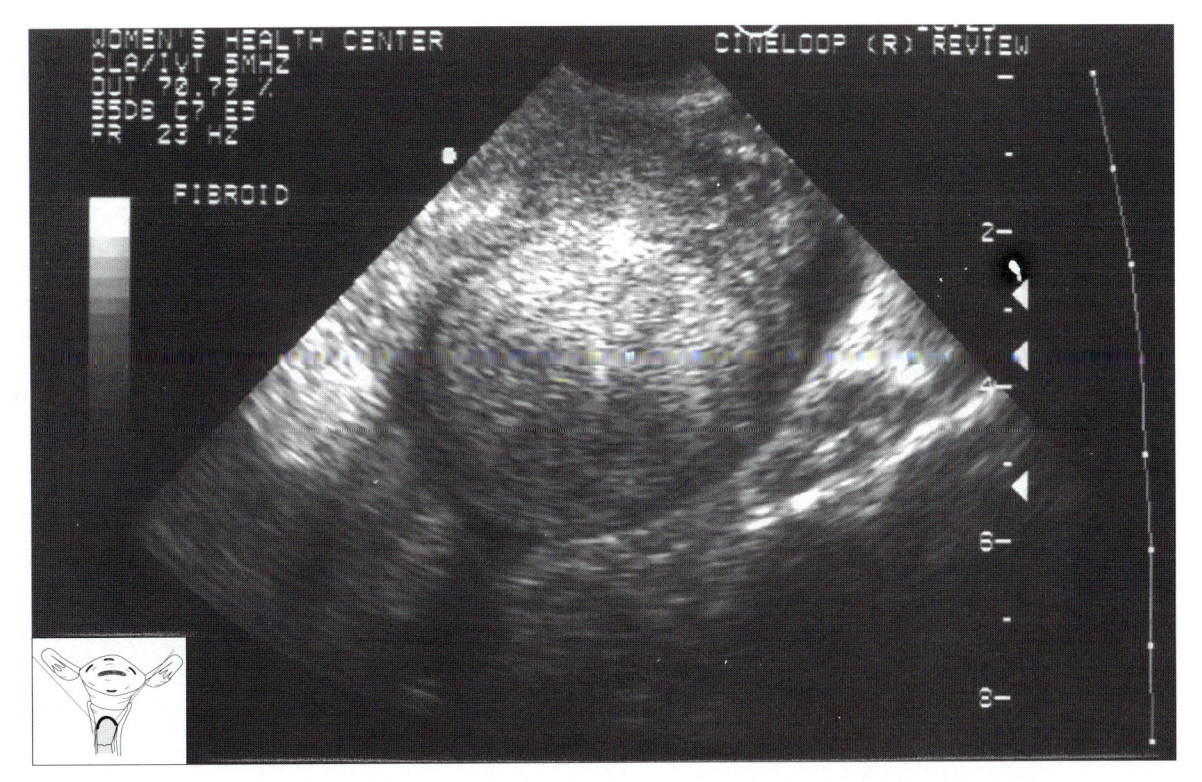

Figure 5-25. *This intramural fibroid appears slightly more echoic than the surrounding myometrium.*

An Atlas of Transvaginal Sonography

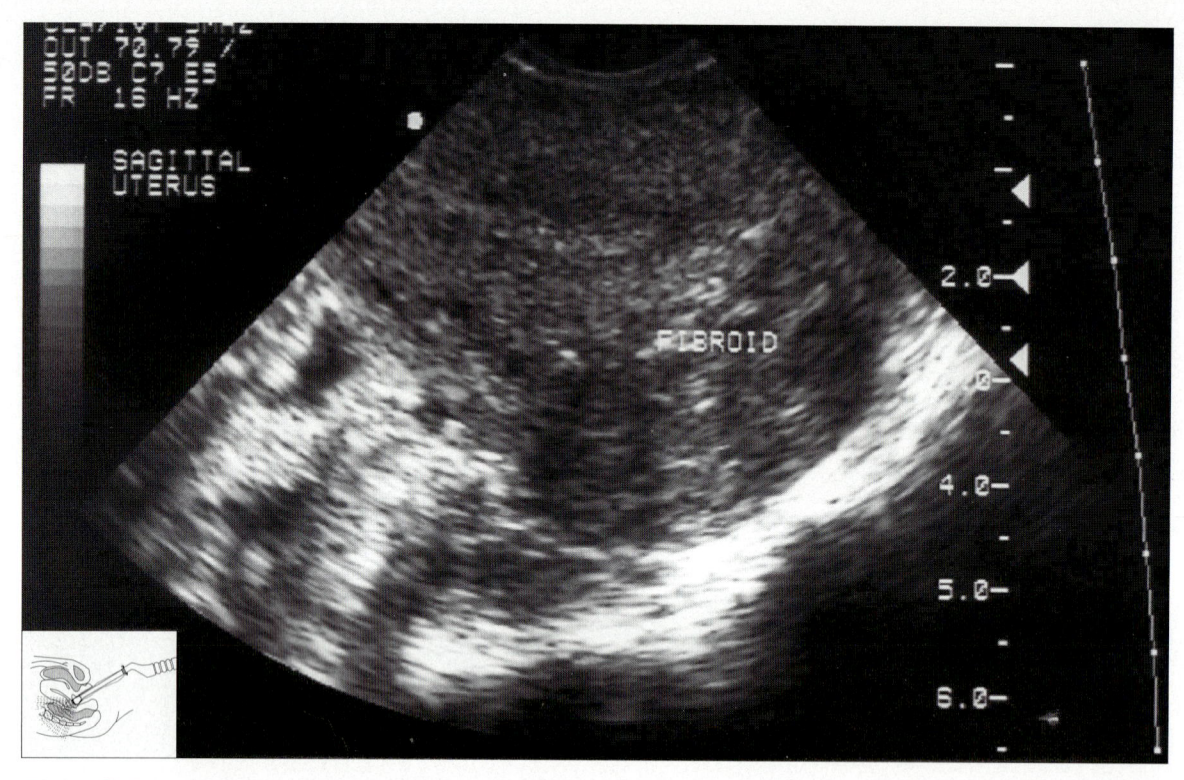

Figure 5-26. A small, clinically insignificant serosal fibroid.

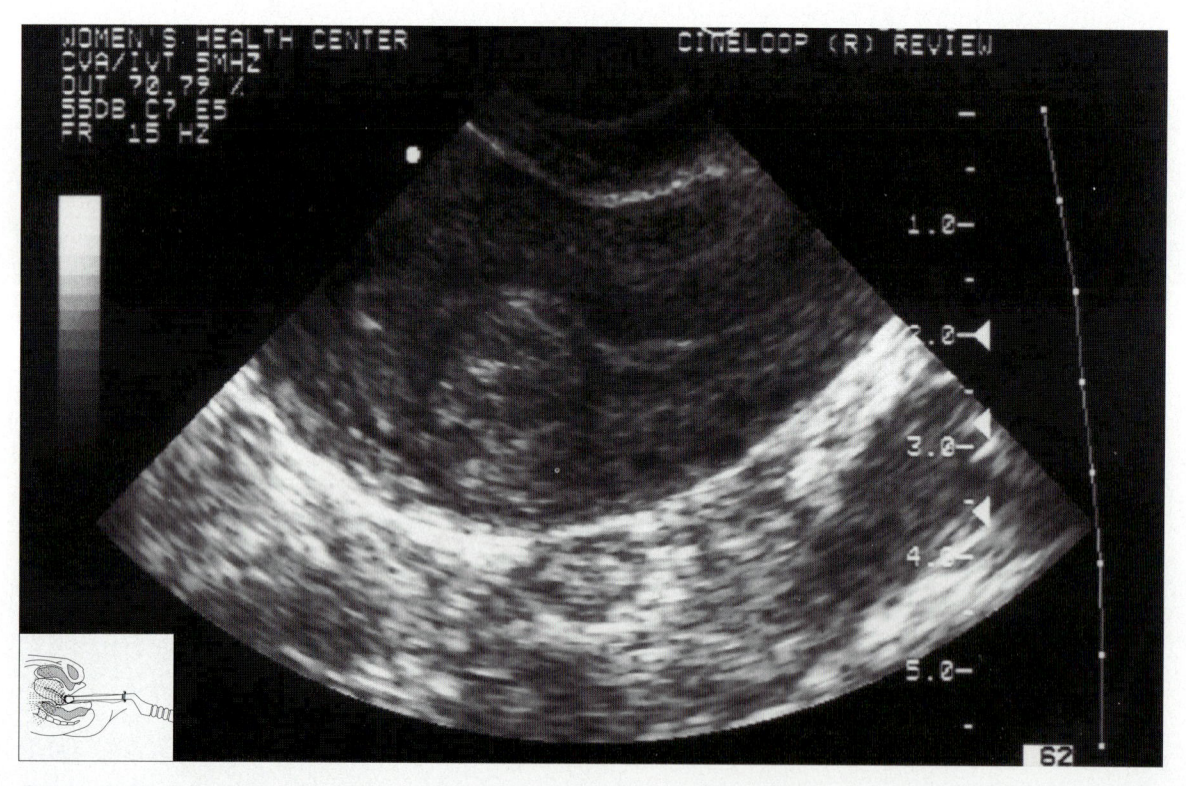

Figure 5-27. A small, but clinically significant, intramyometrial soft-tissue tumor causing gross distortion of the uterine cavity.

Uterus

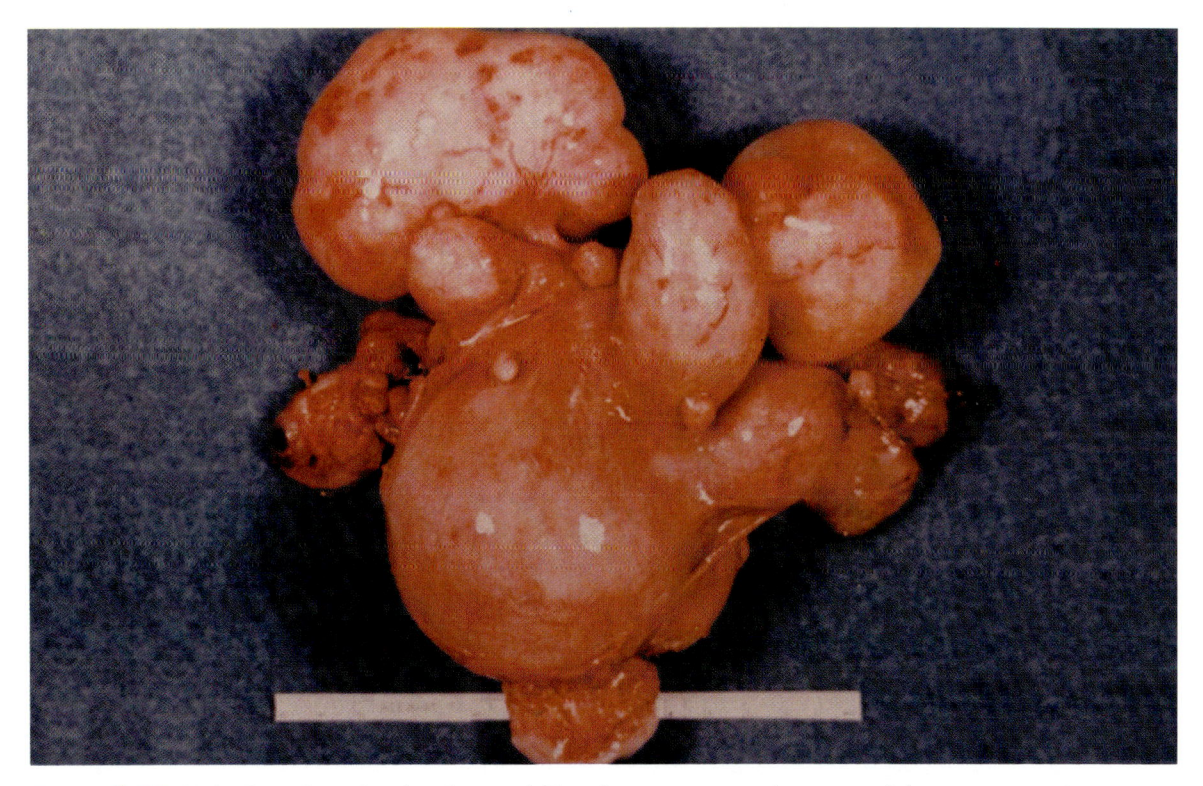

Figure 5-28. Multiple pedunculated and serosal fibroids causing gross distortion of the uterine contour.

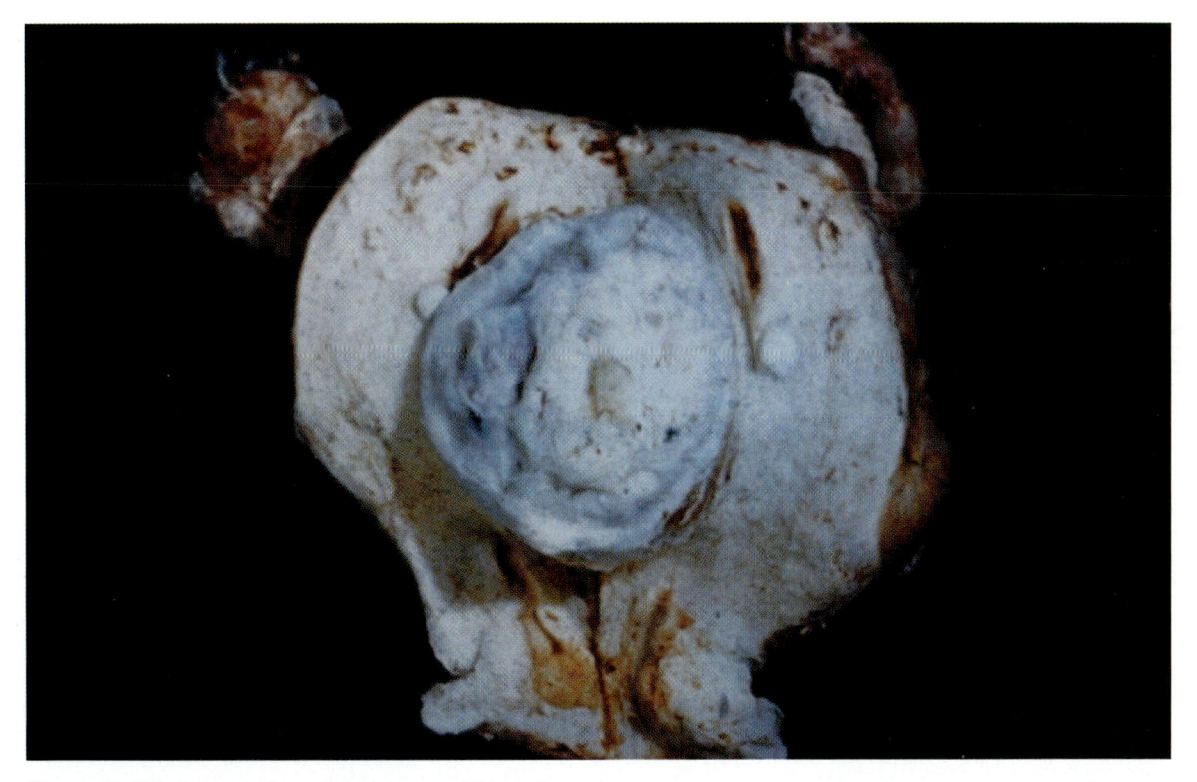

Figure 5-29. Large pedunculated mucosal fibroid.

An Atlas of Transvaginal Sonography

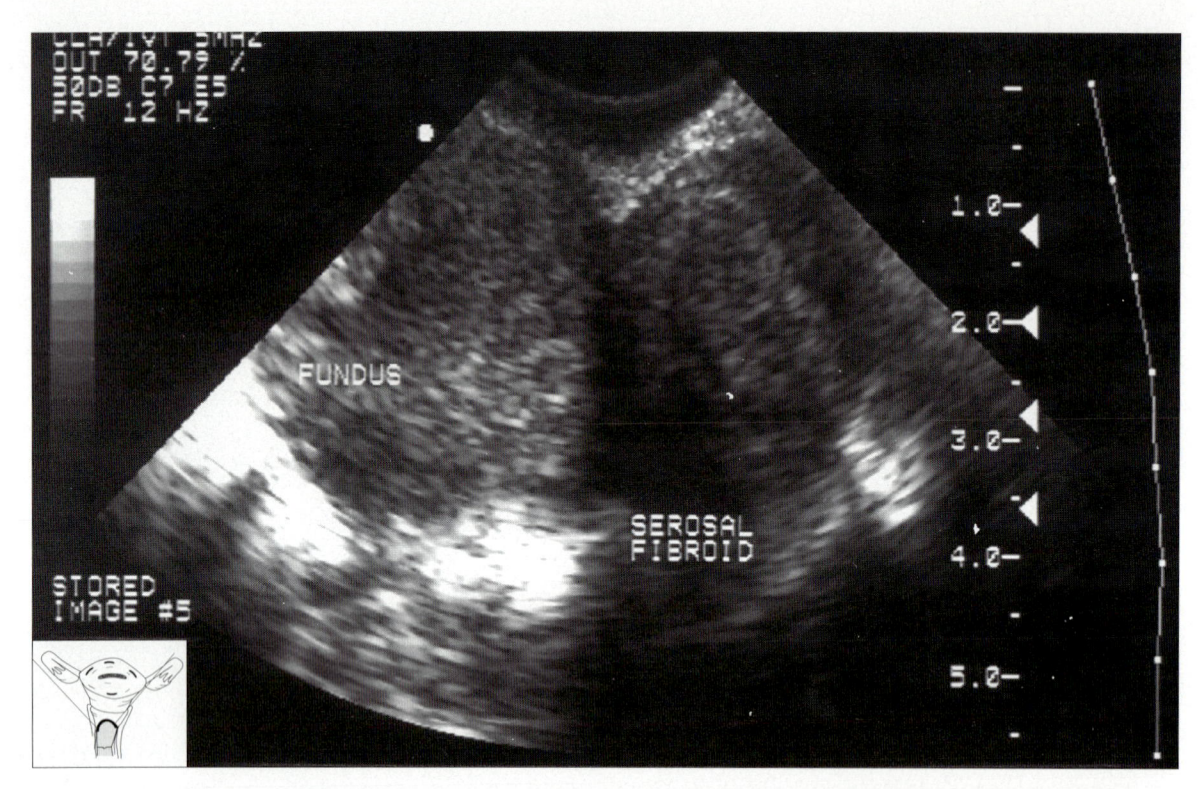

Figure 5-30. *This serosal fibroid was clinically thought to be a solid adnexal mass. Differing tissue interfaces within the fibroid contribute to the shadowing and enhancement posterior to the lesion.*

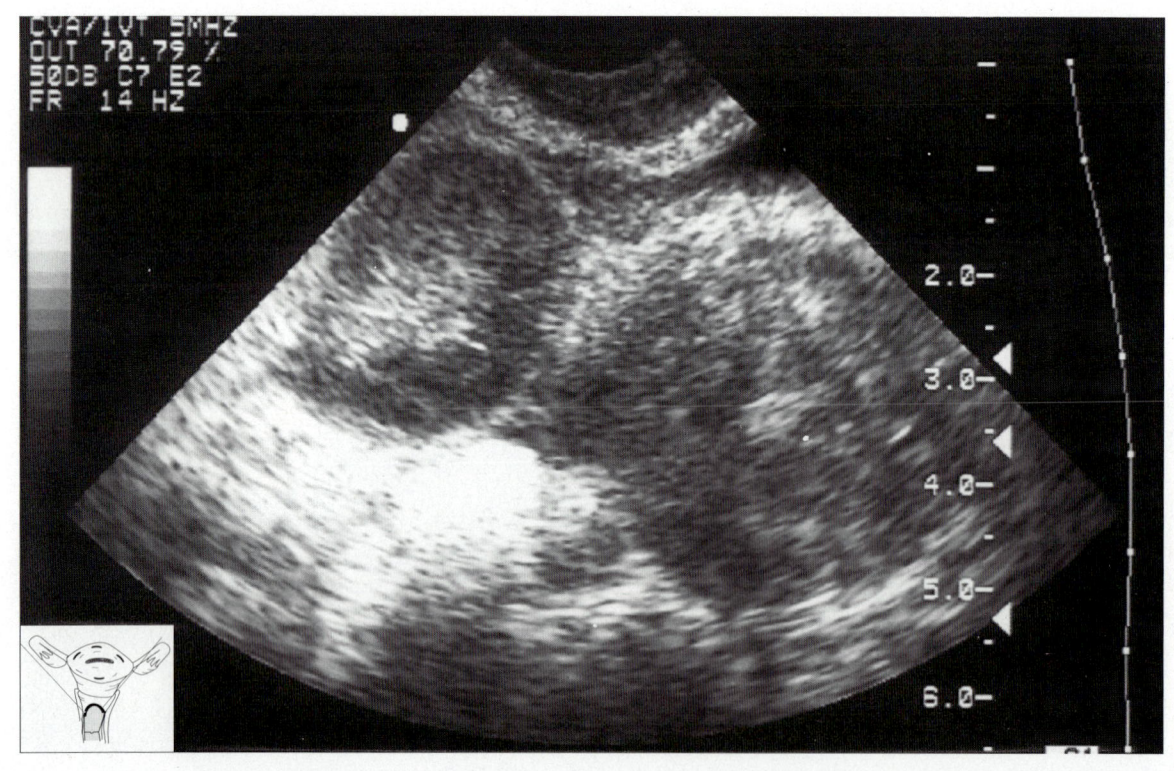

Figure 5-31. *Coronal section of an isoechoic pedunculated uterine fibroid demonstrating a central echoic region representing degeneration.*

Uterus

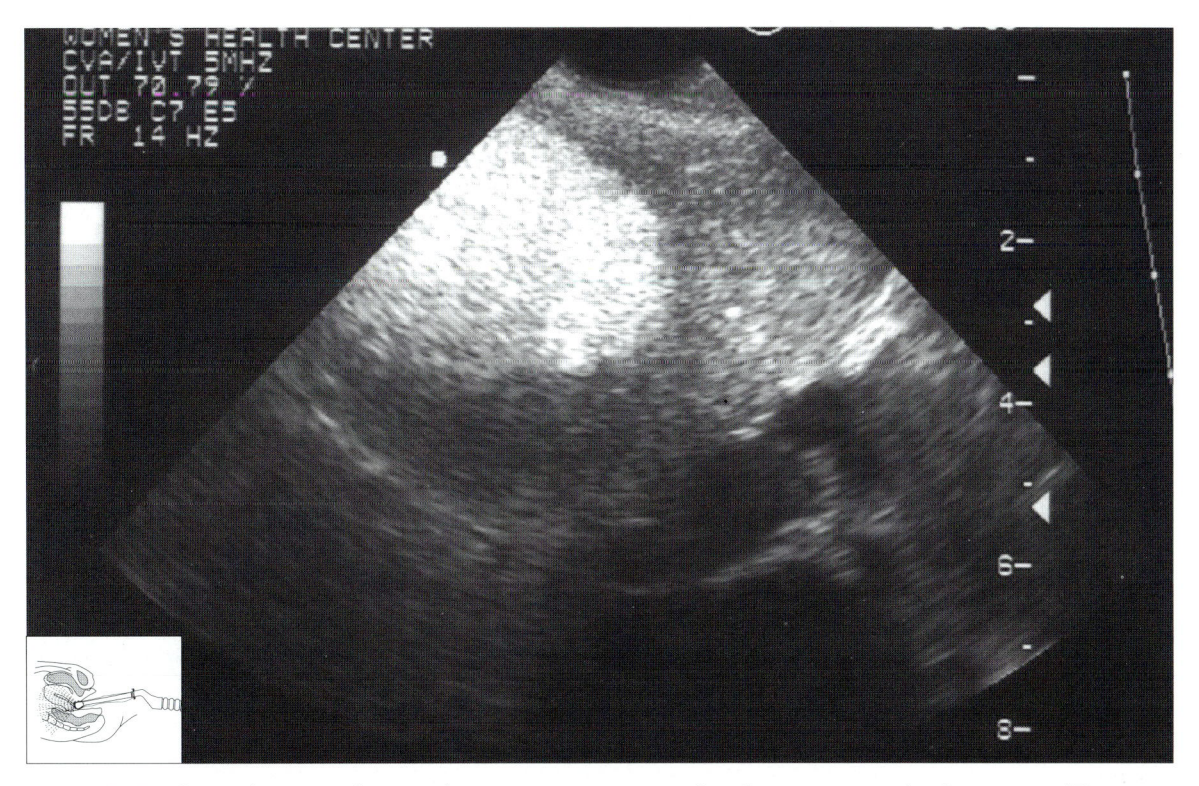

Figure 5-32. *Sagittal section of uterus demonstrating an intensely echogenic uterine lipoleiomyoma. The ultrasound appearance is classic for this tumor.*

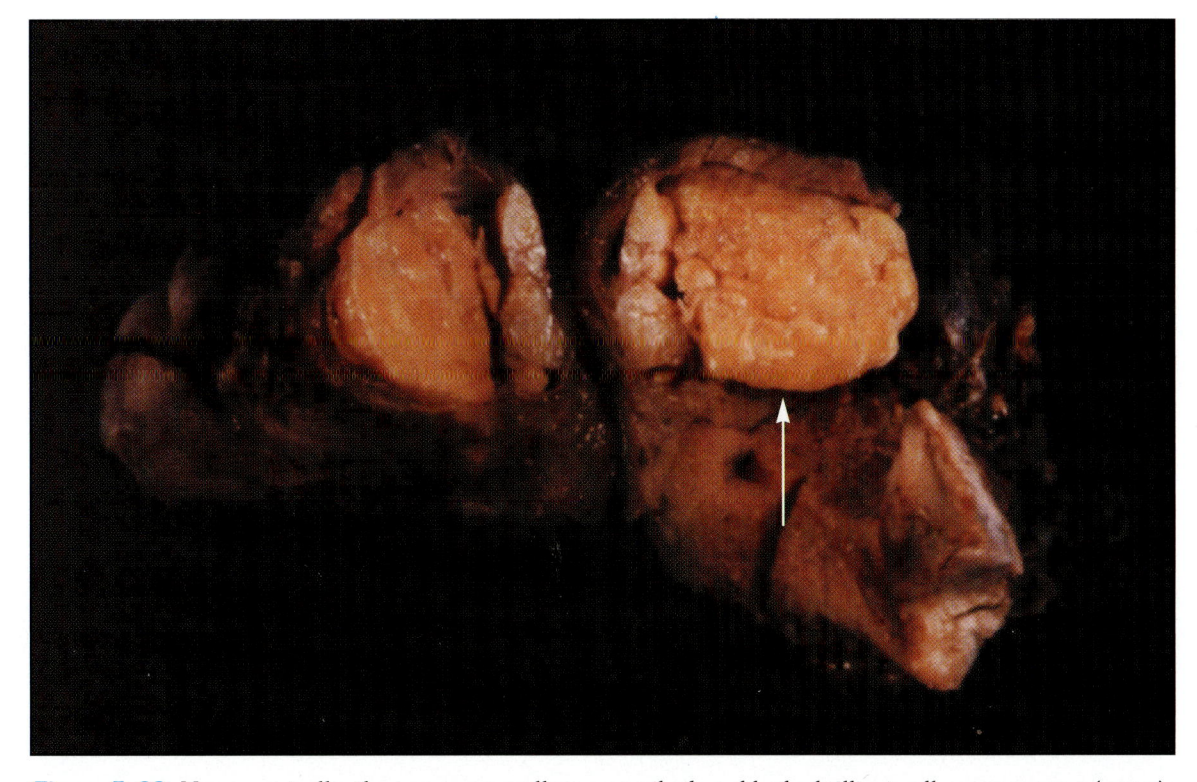

Figure 5-33. *Macroscopically, the tumor was well-circumscribed, and had a brilliant yellow appearance (arrow).*

An Atlas of Transvaginal Sonography

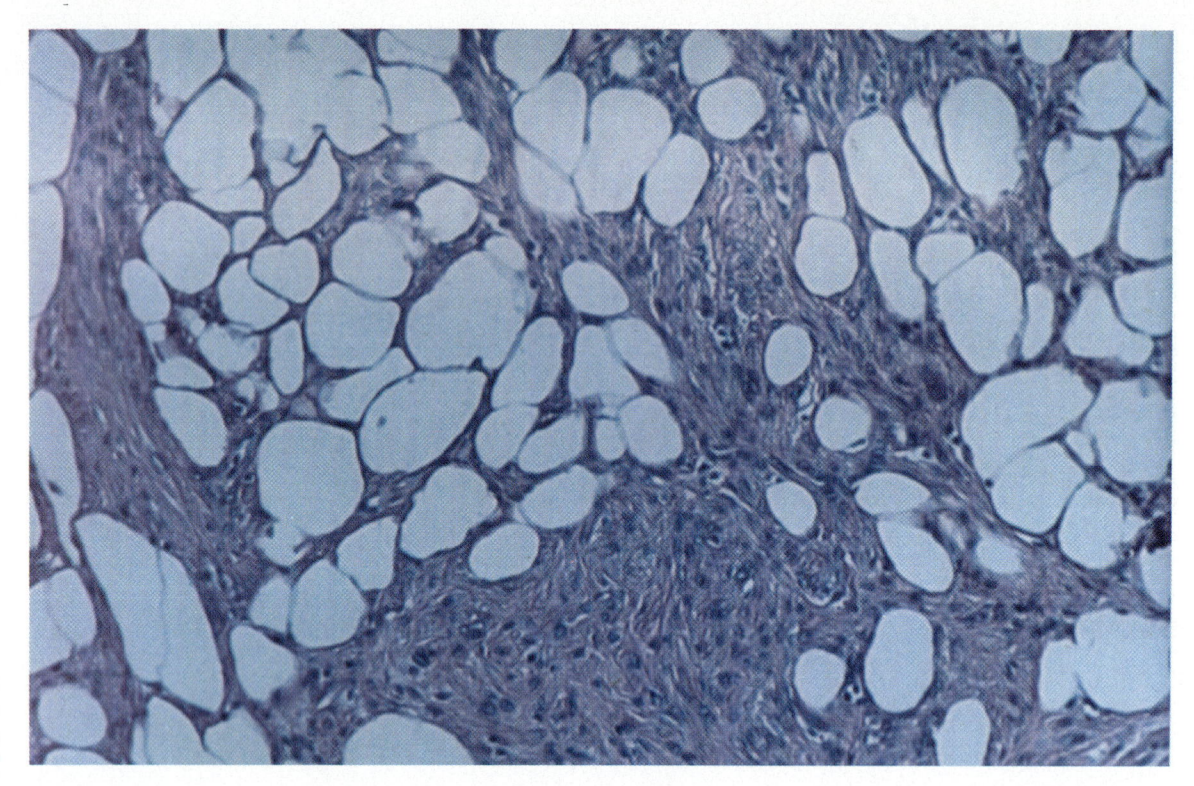

Figure 5-34. Histologically, the tumor is composed of fat cells.

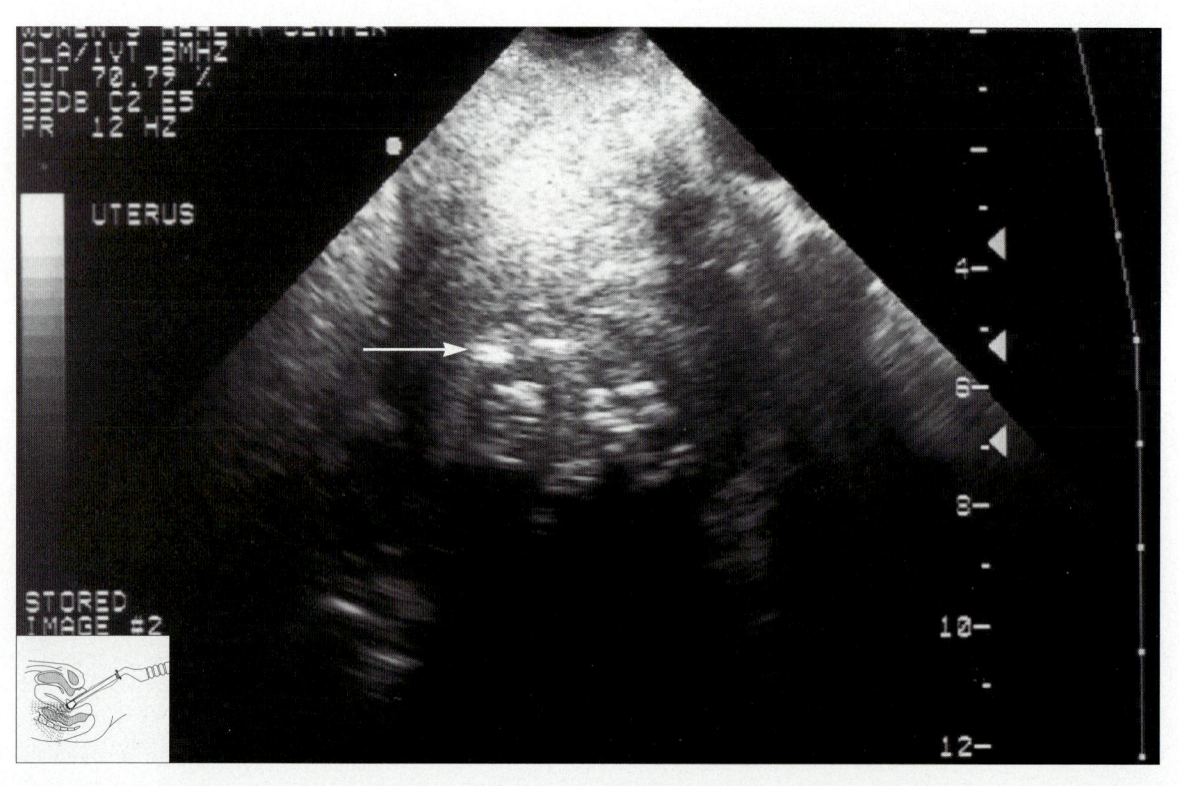

Figure 5-35. Retroverted uterus with a poorly defined echoic endometrium. Within the fundus is a calcified fibroid (arrow). The calcified areas produce the characteristic posterior acoustic shadowing.

Uterus

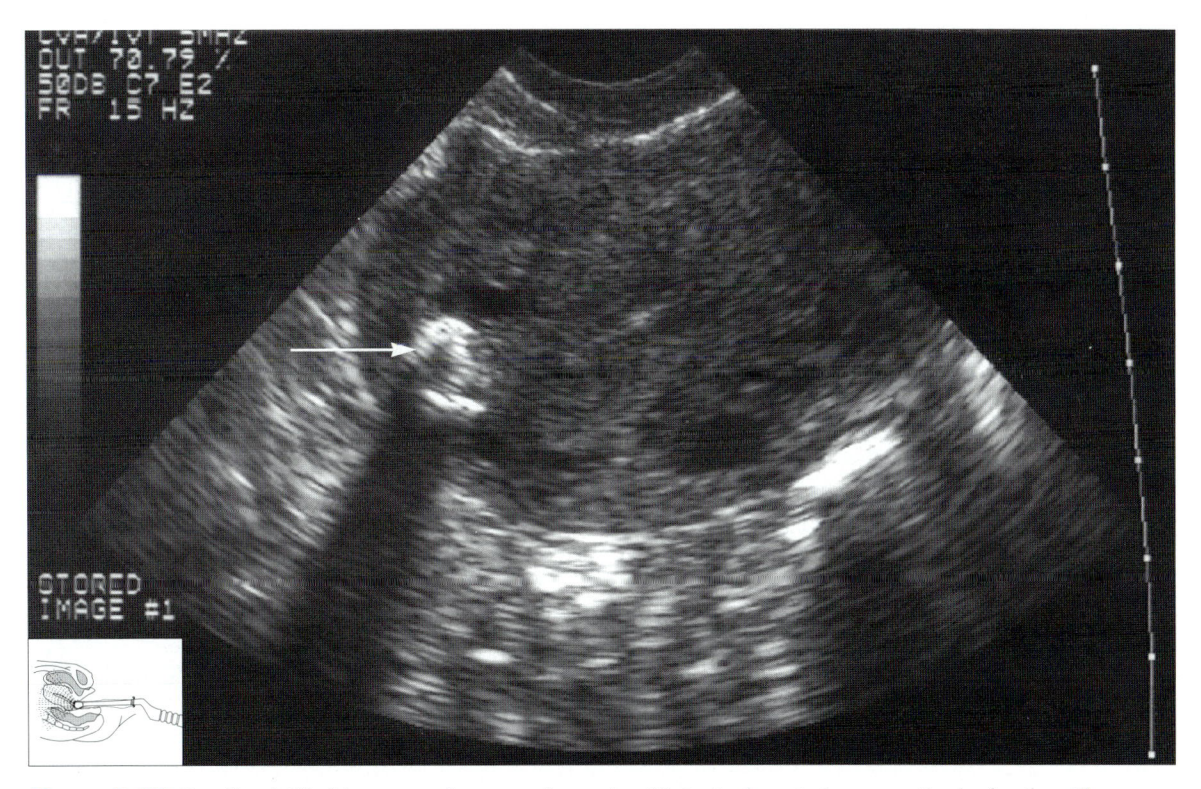

Figure 5-36. *Small calcified intramural myoma (arrow), with typical posterior acoustic shadowing. The peripheral myometrium has distended arcuate vessels.*

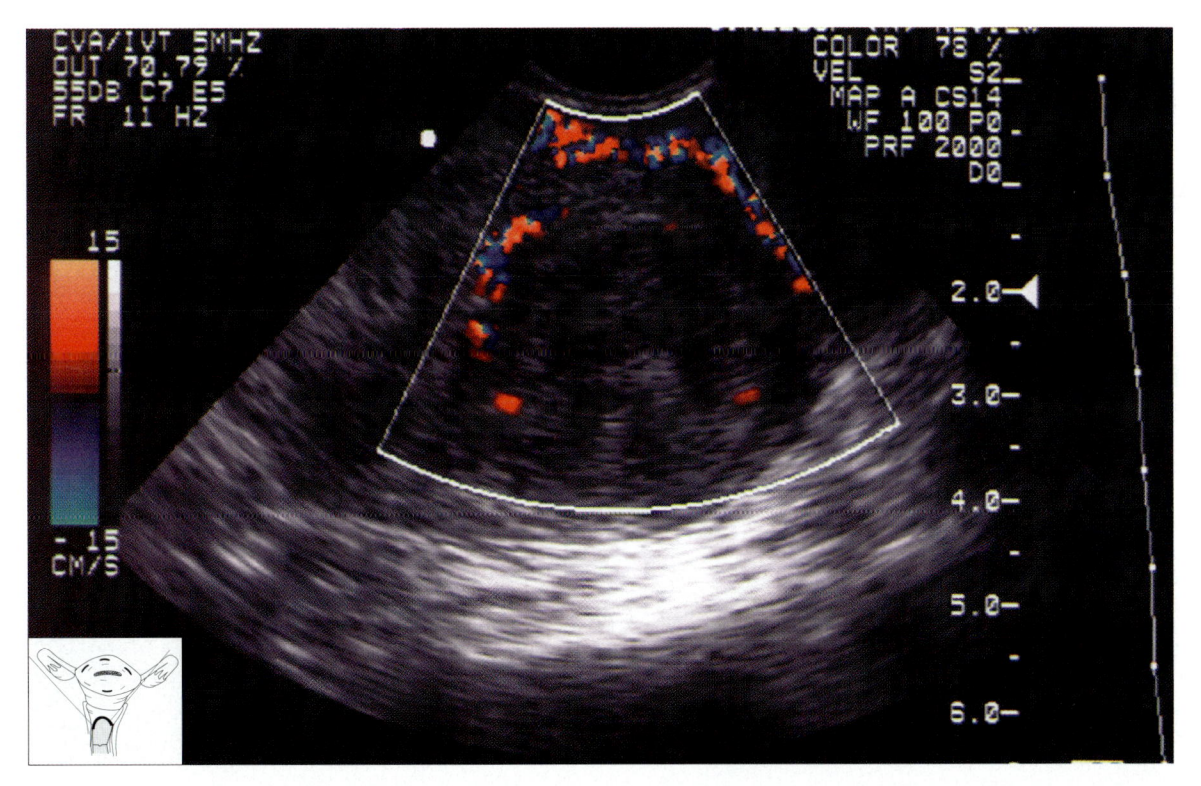

Figure 5-37. *Color flow Doppler of a broad ligament uterine fibroid. The peripheral flow around the tumor is characteristic for a benign tumor.*

An Atlas of Transvaginal Sonography

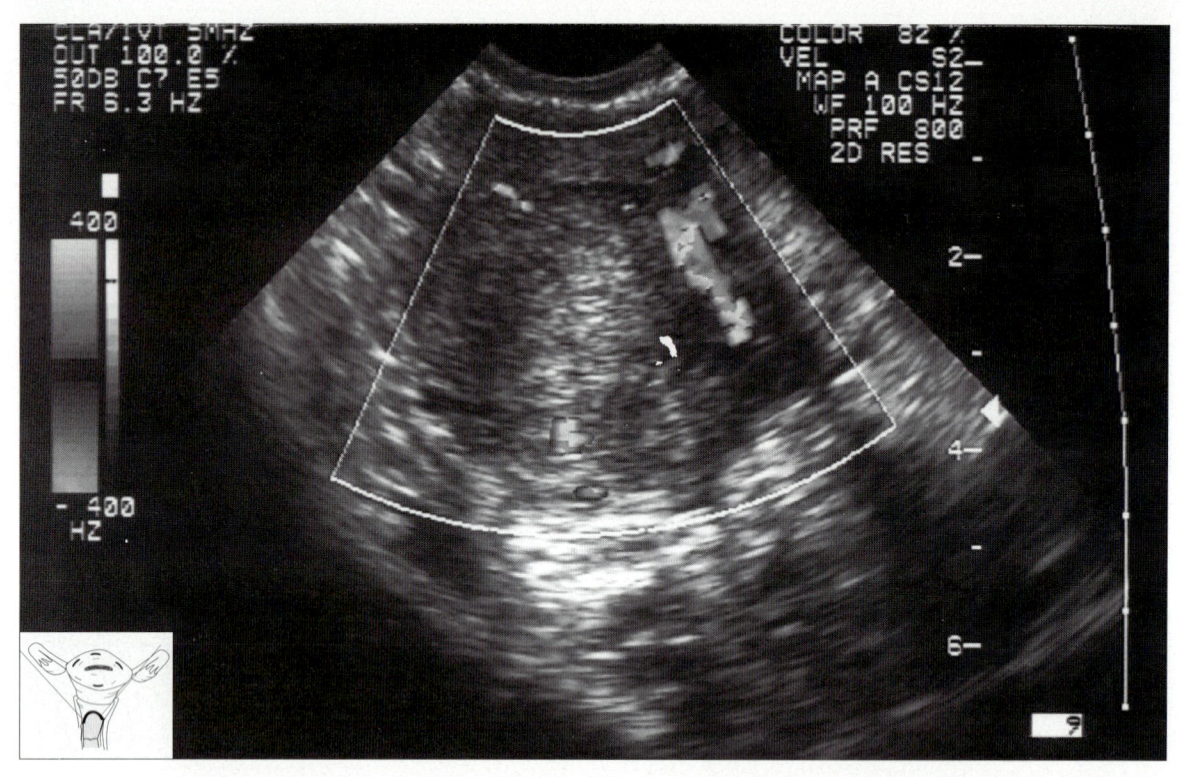

Figure 5-38. Prominent peripheral flow around the tumor and lack of intratumor flow confirm the benign nature of this presumed fibroid.

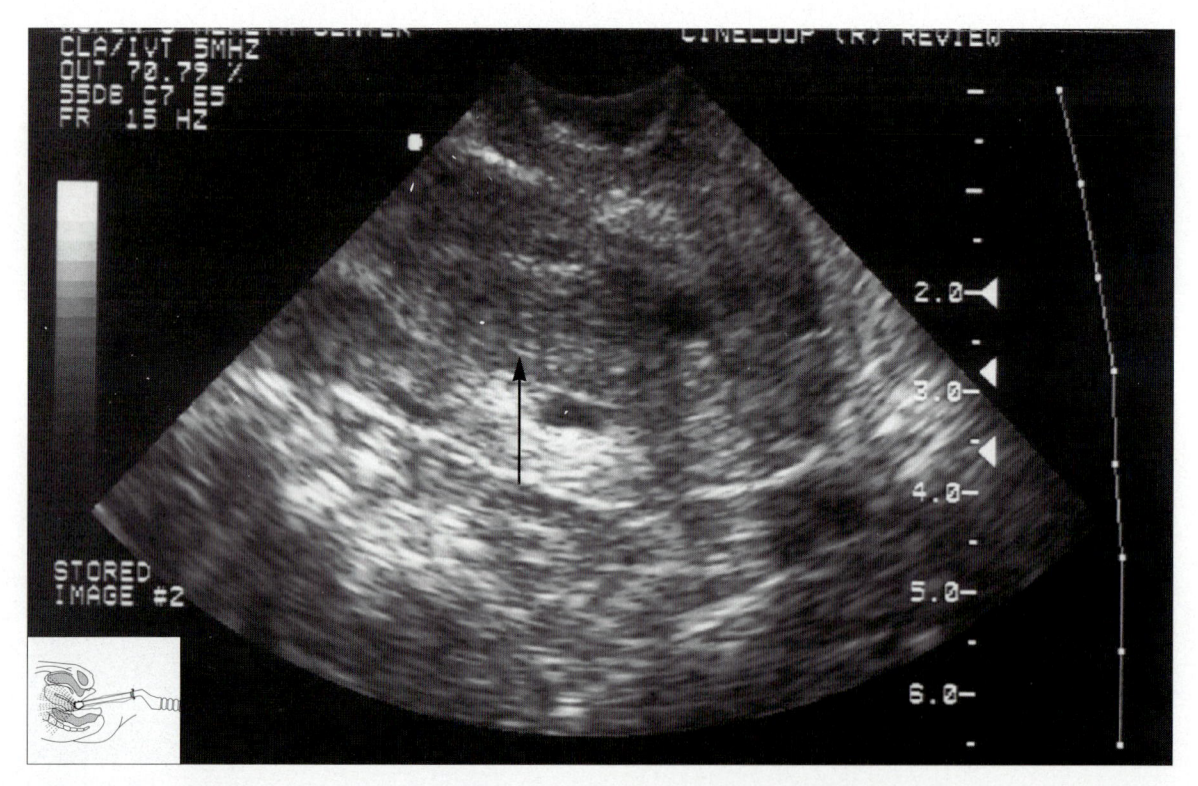

Figure 5-39. Sagittal view of the lower uterine segment and cervix demonstrating an isoechoic prolapsed submucous fibroid (arrow).

Uterus

Adenomyosis

Adenomyosis, also called internal endometriosis, is an estrogen dependent condition marked by the presence of heterotopic endometrium within the myometrium. The incidence varies between 10-20%, peaking between ages 40-50. About half are associated with fibroids and about 10-15% have endometriosis.

This condition causes the uterine corpus to be symmetrically enlarged, with the walls being markedly thickened. The posterior wall is more often involved than the anterior wall. The thickened uterine wall consists of coarsely trabeculated areas that are granular in appearance, and cystic areas that can contain serous fluid or old blood.

Scan Findings

Although adenomyosis is a pathological diagnosis, it can often be suspected sonographically by a symmetrically enlarged uterus, thickened myometrium and multiple sonolucent areas of hemorrhage and clot within the myometrium.

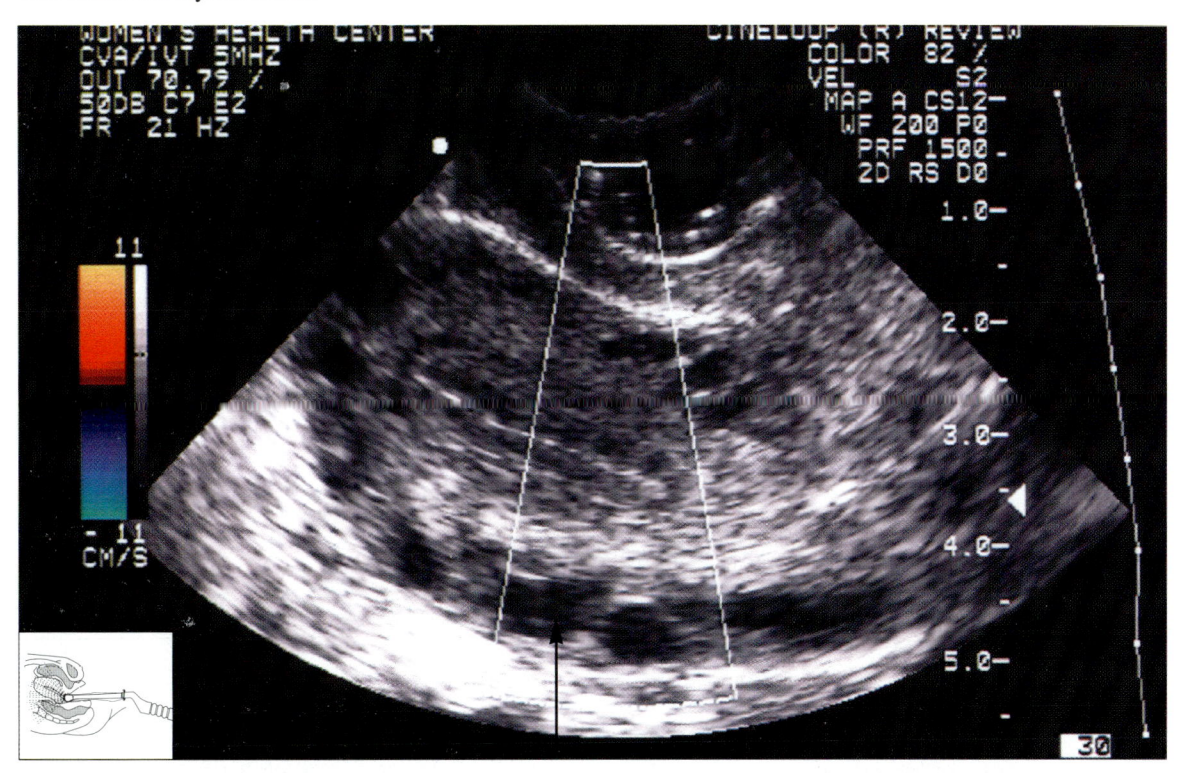

Figure 5-40. Anteverted uterus with midcycle endometrium. In the peripheral myometrium, distended, prominent, anechoic vascular spaces are seen (arrow).

Endometrial Hyperplasia

Endometrial hyperplasia comprises a group of histological patterns of the endometrium characterized by overgrowth of the glandular and stromal elements. They are secondary to persistent, unopposed estrogen stimulation. Endometrial hyperplasias are important because of their malignancy potential. They are classified as simple hyperplasias (cystic hyperplasia); complex hyperplasia (adenomatous or moderate adenomatous hyperplasia); and atypical hyperplasia (severe adenomatous hyperplasia, adenomatous hyperplasia with atypia, carcinoma in situ).

The malignant potential of cystic hyperplasia is <1% over 15 years, for complex hyperplasia is 1-4% over 13 years, and 20-25% over 11 years for atypical hyperplasia.

Scan Findings

Transvaginal sonography is unable to differentiate between the different histologic variants of the endometrial hyperplasias. The endometrium appears thickened, greater than 5-6 mm, hyperechoic, and importantly, the subendometrial halo is intact. Color Doppler is nonspecific and flow, if present, is typically not increased.

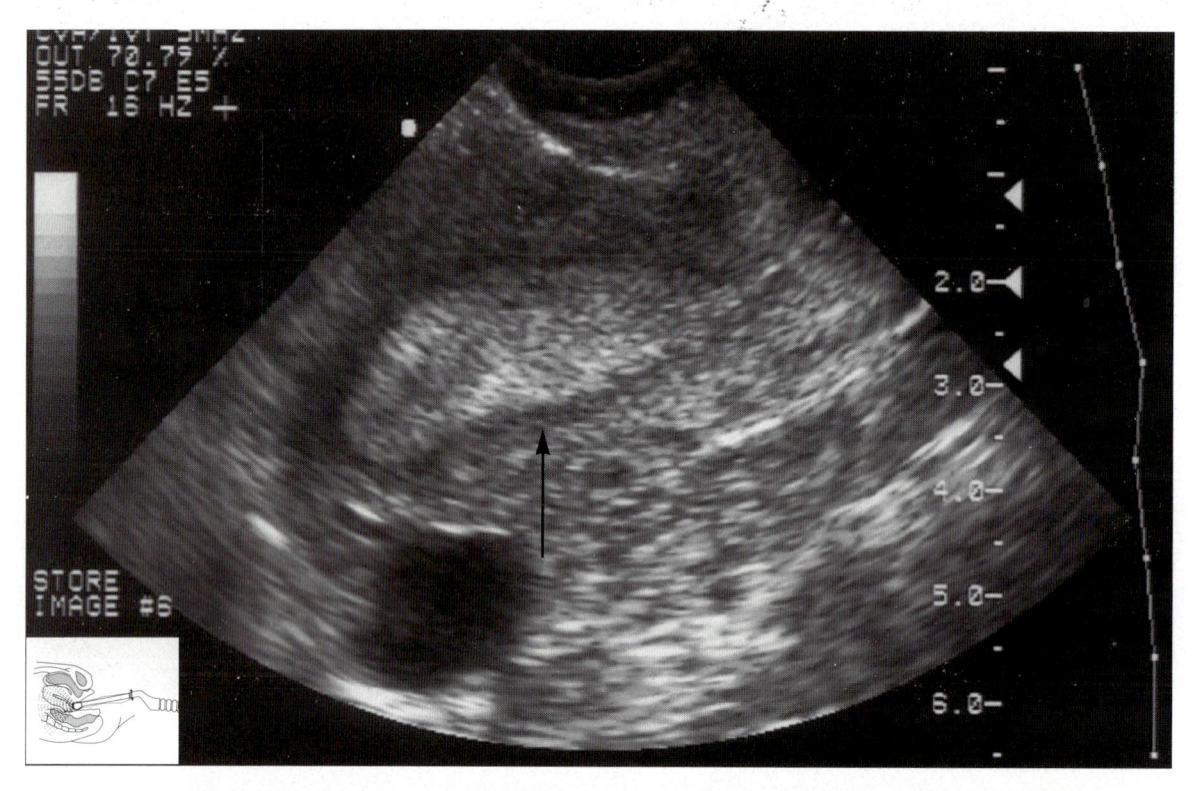

Figure 5-41. This perimenopausal patient complained of increasing uterine bleeding. The endometrium is markedly thickened and intensely echoic. Pathology revealed endometrial hyperplasia. Note that the subendometrial halo is intact (arrow).

Uterus

Endometrial Polyps

Endometrial polyps are the result of focal overgrowth of endometrial glands and stroma. Histologically, they are composed of weakly proliferative glands but rarely show active proliferative or secretory changes. They are usually secondary to unopposed estrogen therapy. These polyps are usually present during the fifth decade and can cause abnormal uterine or postmenopausal bleeding. Benign polyps are only rarely (< 0.5%) associated with endometrial cancer. Their malignant potential is zero.

Scan Findings

Endometrial polyps are easily seen on transvaginal sonography. They can be iso-, hypo- or hyperechoic depending upon the background hormonal milieu, degree of proliferation, and amount of fluid and glycogen accumulation. Isoechoic endometrial polyps can be confused with, and thus must be distinguished from, adjacent myometrium and submucous or pedunculated fibroids.

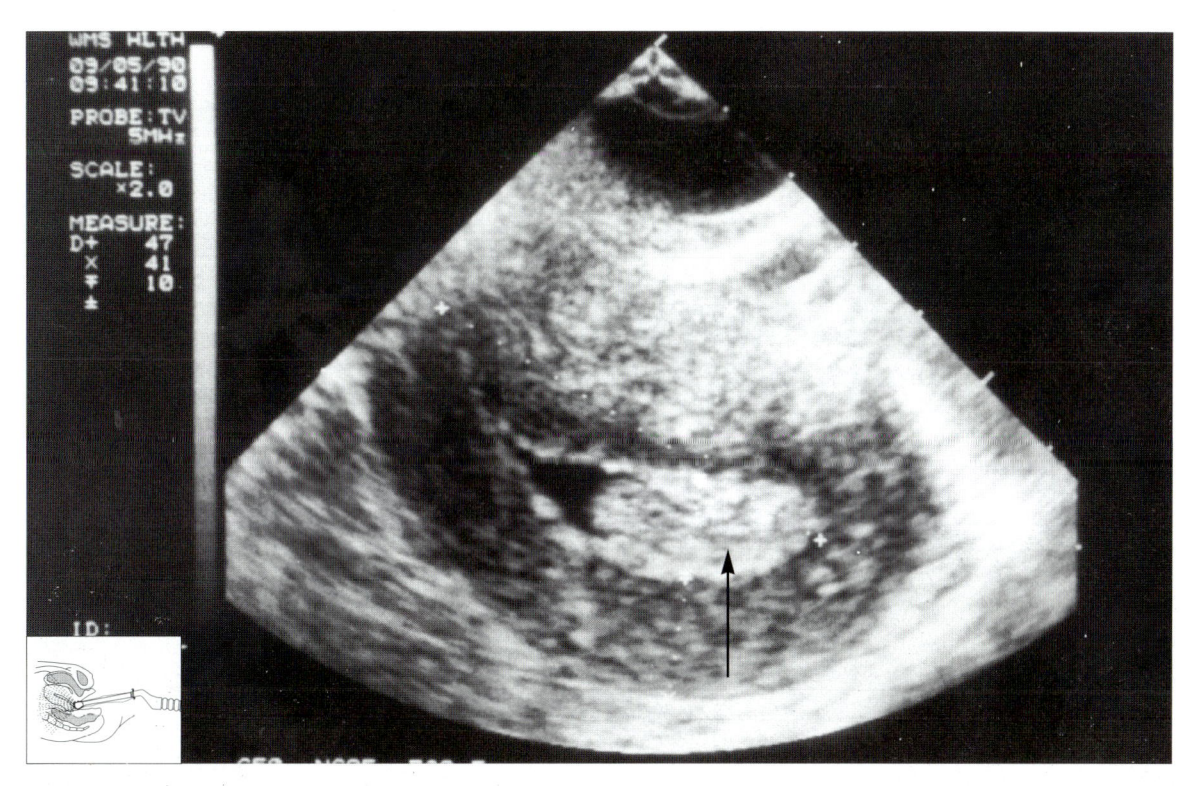

Figure 5-42. This postmenopausal woman presented with uterine bleeding. TVS reveals a retroverted uterus with an echoic endometrial polyp (arrow).

An Atlas of Transvaginal Sonography

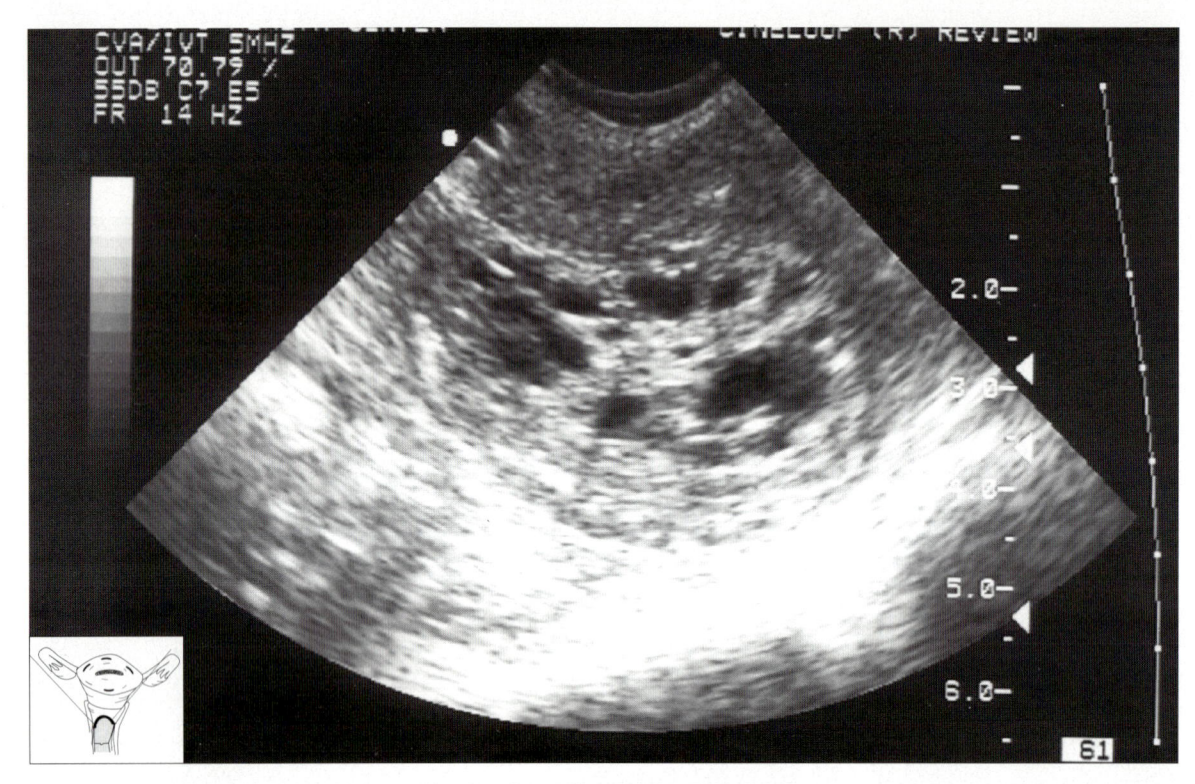

Figure 5-43. Echoic cystic endometrial polyp distending the uterine cavity.

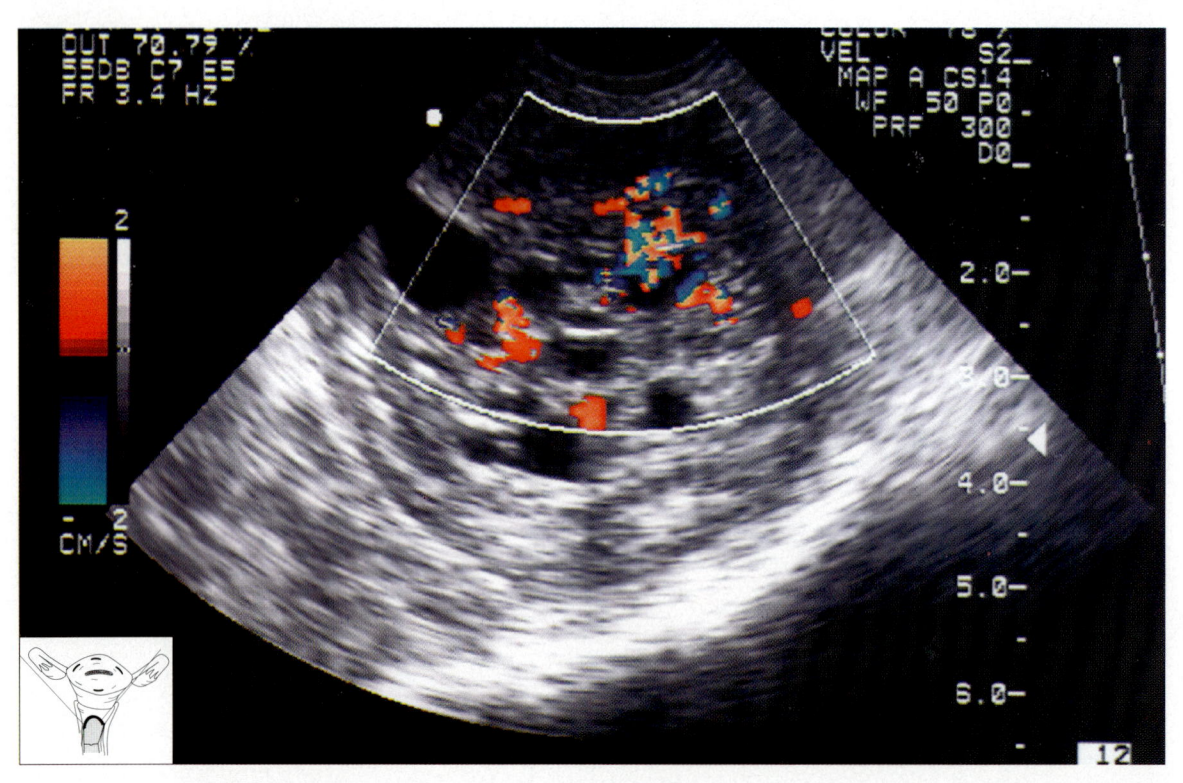

Figure 5-44. Color flow Doppler reveals essentially peripheral flow.

Uterus

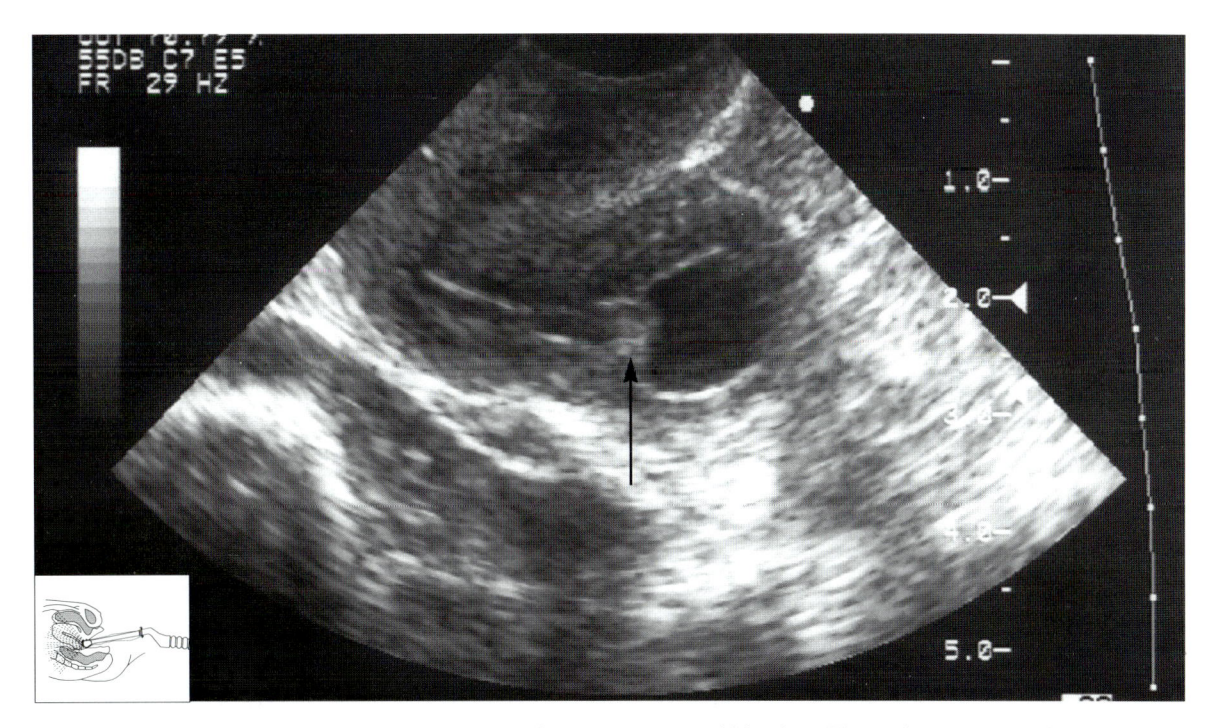

Figure 5-45. *Retroverted uterus in a patient with postmenopausal bleeding. The endometrium is thin and atrophic, and the uterine cavity distended by mucus (hydrometra). An echoic endometrial polyp in seen in the lower uterine segment (arrow).*

Intrauterine Fluid

Intrauterine fluid can be mucus (hydrometra), pus (pyometra) or blood (hematometra) and can be seen distending the myometrium. The etiology includes pregnancy-related conditions, pelvic inflammatory disease, congenital vaginal or cervical atresia, cervical stricture or fibrosis, or endometrial or cervical cancer.

Scan Findings

Sonographically, the distending media is clear if mucinous or echogenic if pus or blood. Careful attention to the endometrium and cervix is essential to avoid missing associated cancerous neoplasms.

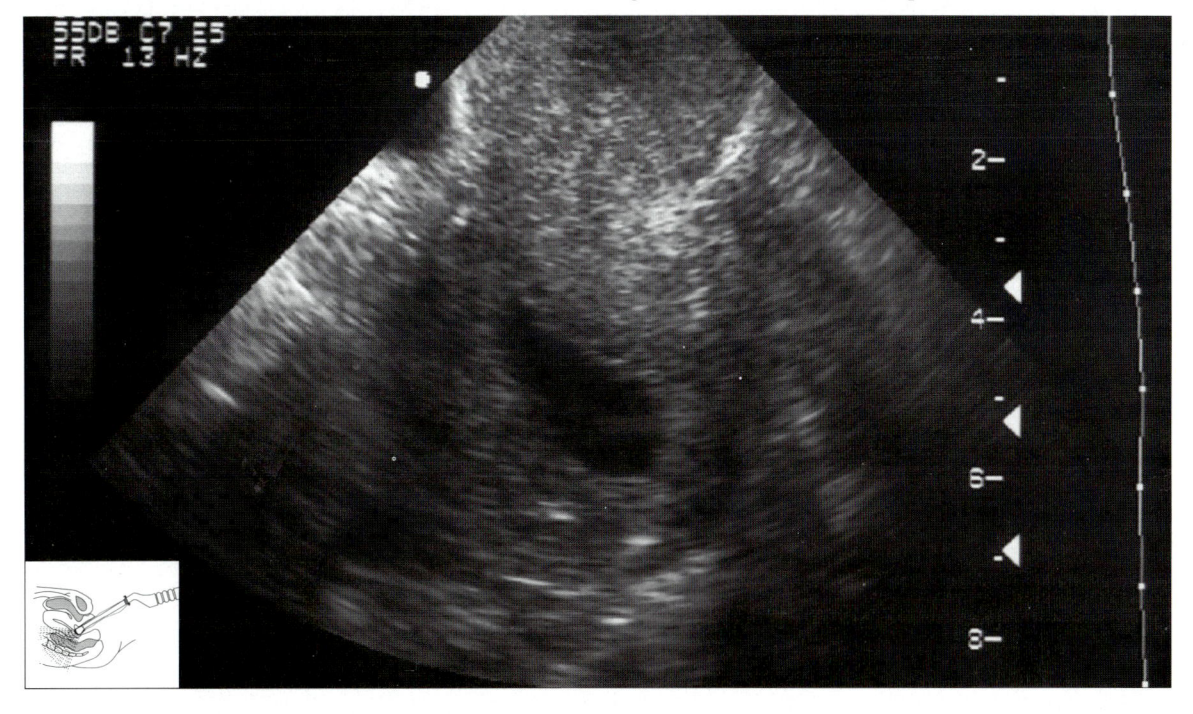

Figure 5-46. *Retroverted uterus with a tear-drop shaped uterine cavity distended by clear mucinous fluid. The endometrium is thin and isoechoic.*

An Atlas of Transvaginal Sonography

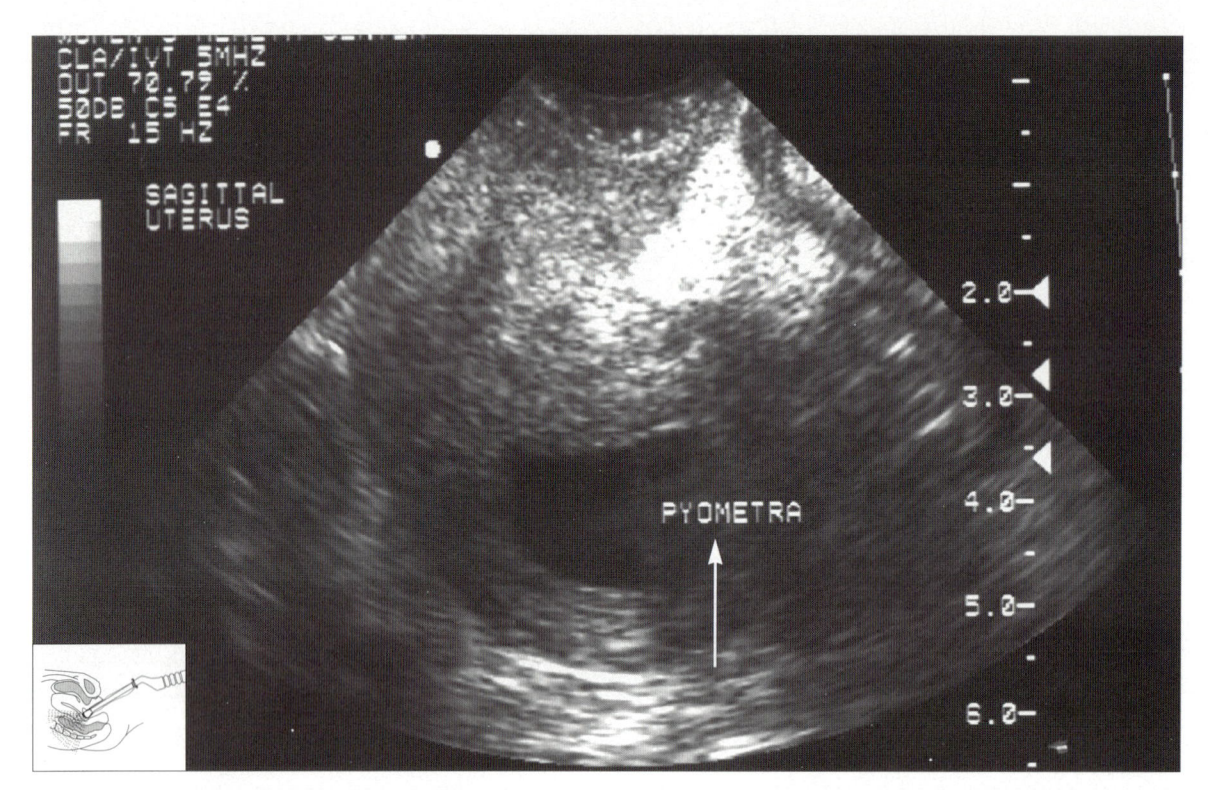

Figure 5-47. Pyometra in a patient with offensive vaginal discharge. The uterus is retroverted and the cavity is distended by fluid that demonstrates layering in the fundus (arrow).

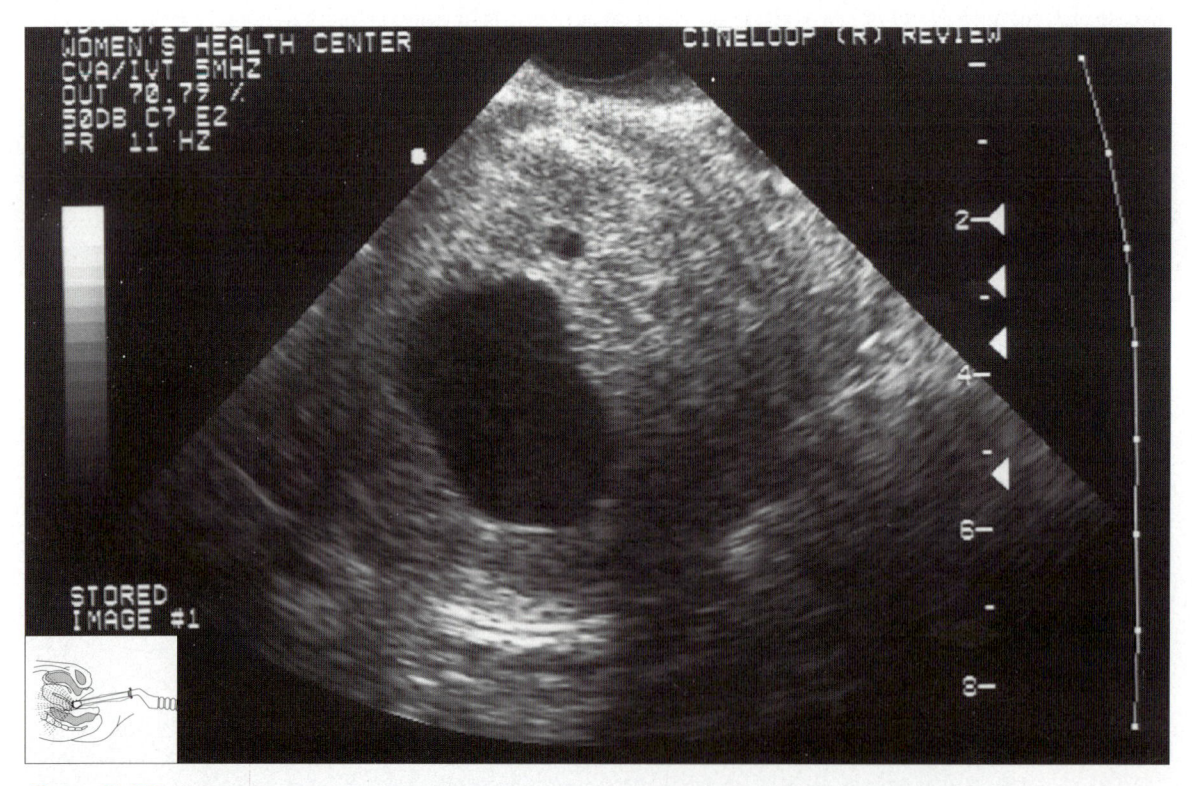

Figure 5-48. Hematometra in a premenopausal woman post cone biopsy. The uterine cavity is distended by echogenic fluid.

Uterus

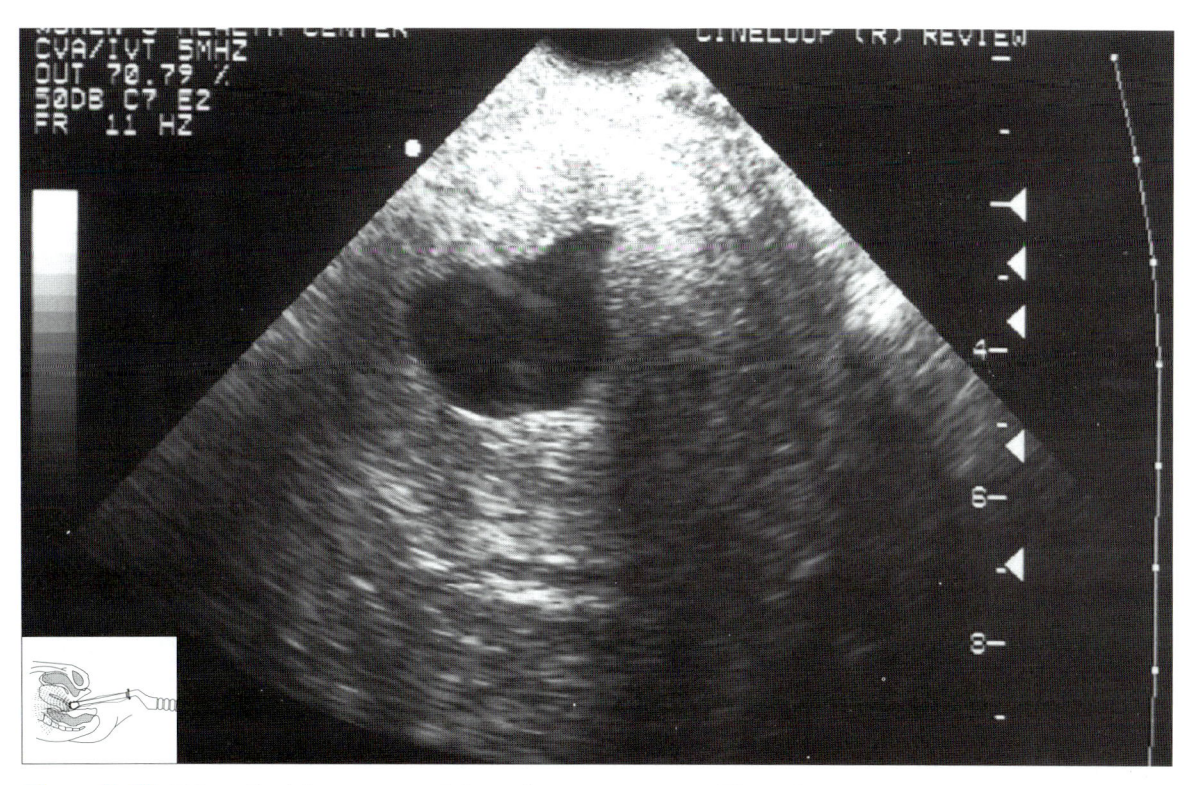

Figure 5-49. *Echoic fluid (hematometra) distending uterine cavity. The endometrium is thin and isoechoic.*

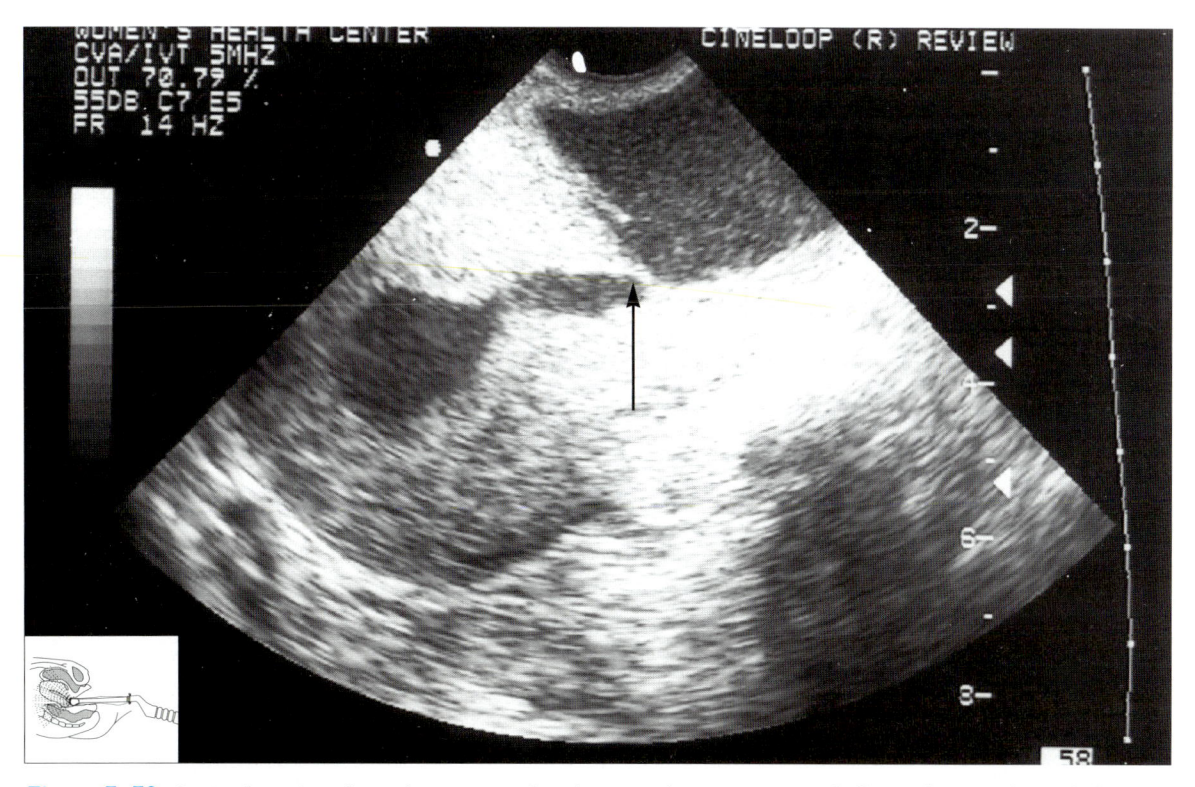

Figure 5-50. *Sagittal section through corpus and endocervix demonstrating a ballooned cervix distended with echogenic fluid (small arrow) and with communication with the uterine cavity. The patient had stenosis of the ectocervix and was on hormone replacement therapy resulting in hematometra and hematocervix. A small membrane (large arrow) acting as a valve at the upper cervix prevents massive distention of the uterine cavity as compared to the cervix.*

An Atlas of Transvaginal Sonography

Intrauterine Contraceptive Device

Intrauterine contraceptive devices (IUD) are plastic or metal-plastic devices inserted into the uterine cavity to prevent conception. To obtain their contraceptive effect, these devices must lie within the uterine cavity.

Scan Findings

Transvaginal sonography can identify a correctly placed or a misplaced IUD. They appear as a highly echogenic interface that produces characteristic posterior acoustical shadowing. Sites of inappropriately located devices include the myometrium, broad ligament, cul-de-sac or within bowel mesentery.

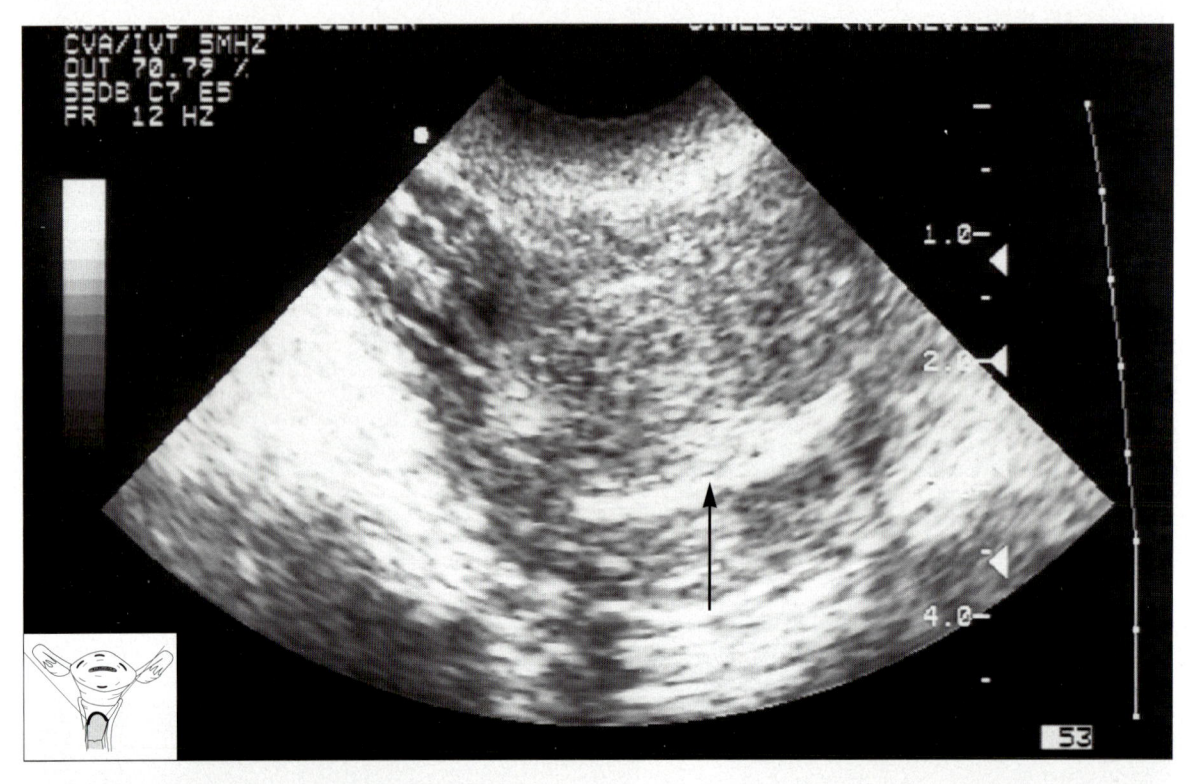

Figure 5-51. Coronal section through the mid portion of the uterus demonstrating an intrauterine contraceptive device (arrow). This was a plastic device and appears sonographically as an intensely echogenic line. Often there will be posterior acoustical shadowing or posterior reverberation artifact.

6   Fallopian Tube

The fallopian tubes are paired, Mullerian duct-derived structures whose function is to convey oocytes from the ovaries to the uterus and transmit the spermatozoa in the opposite direction. Fertilization usually occurs within the distal tube. Each tube is about 10cm long, located at the upper margin of the broad ligament, attached medially to the uterus and extends out laterally to the ovary. They are composed of smooth muscle.

Scan Findings

Normal fallopian tubes are usually not visualized by sonography, but occasionally in the luteal phase of the menstrual cycle, the echogenic endometrium can be traced out into the tubal ostia and for a variable distance along the isthmic portion of the tube. In the presence of ascites the fallopian tubes can be seen "floating" in the sea of peritoneal fluid.

Benign Tubal Pathology
Pelvic Inflammatory Disease

Pelvic inflammatory disease is an acute pelvic infection resulting from an ascending polymicrobial infection. Although the true incidence is unknown, there are probably over 250,000 new cases per year in the United States. It is caused by a variety of organisms depending on the country and area.

The infection causes the fallopian tubes to become edematous with distention of the tubal wall and destruction of the tubal epithelium. The fimbria become occluded, causing a distended pus-containing tube. The tube can be involved by this process in a focal, segmental or diffuse way and usually both tubes are affected to some degree. If the tube and ovary are involved together in this inflammatory process, without any part of the ovary being visible, then a tubo-ovarian abscess is present. Purulent exudate will also be present in the cul-de-sac.

Scan Findings

Although PID cannot be confirmed sonographically, there can be a high index of suspicion if pressure with the ultrasound probe elicits tenderness or pain, which is generated from the inflamed pelvic peritoneum, or if a distended fluid-filled fallopian tube is seen. These characteristic hydro- or pyosalpinges appear as elongated, or sausage-shaped cystic structures. Careful examination of their internal structure often reveals a thickened tubal mucosa and small mucosal folds projecting into the hydrosalpinx. Due to the nature of the underlying disease process, these tubal masses have increased flow on color flow Doppler. Loculated echogenic pus can be present within the cul-de-sac.

An Atlas of Transvaginal Sonography

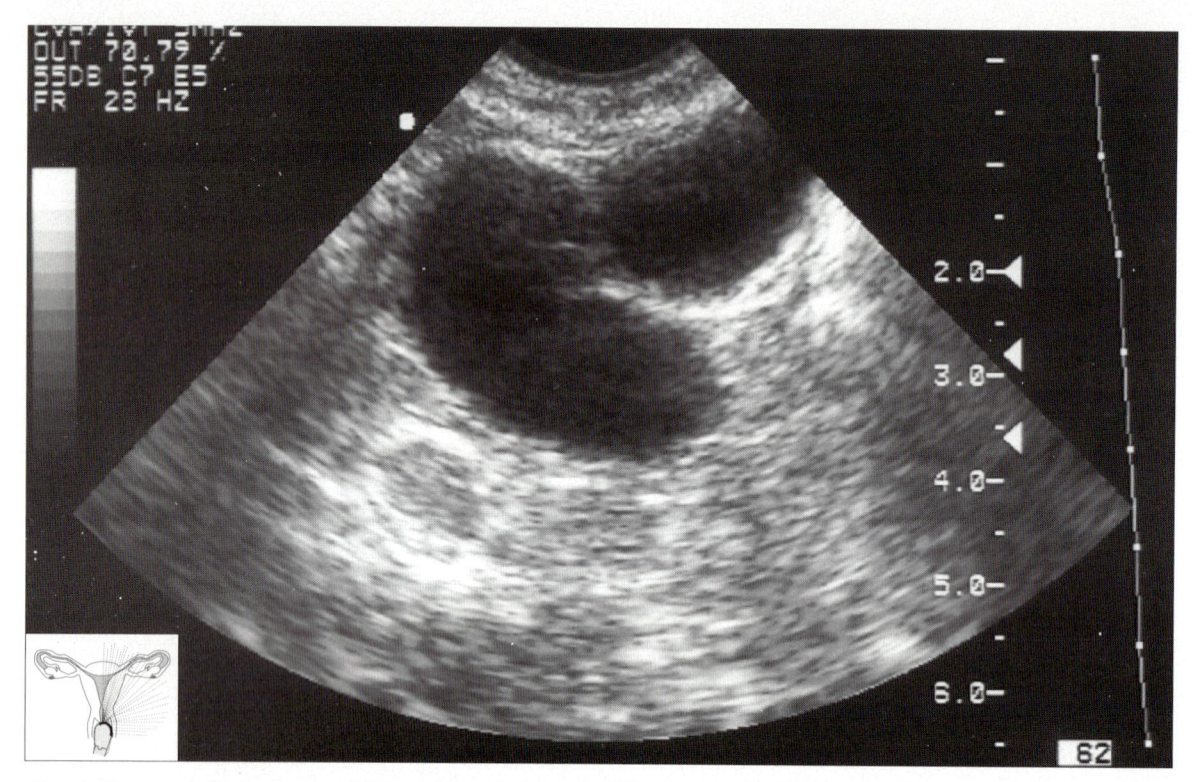

Figure 6~1. Sausage-shaped, tortuous fallopian tube, distended by serous fluid.

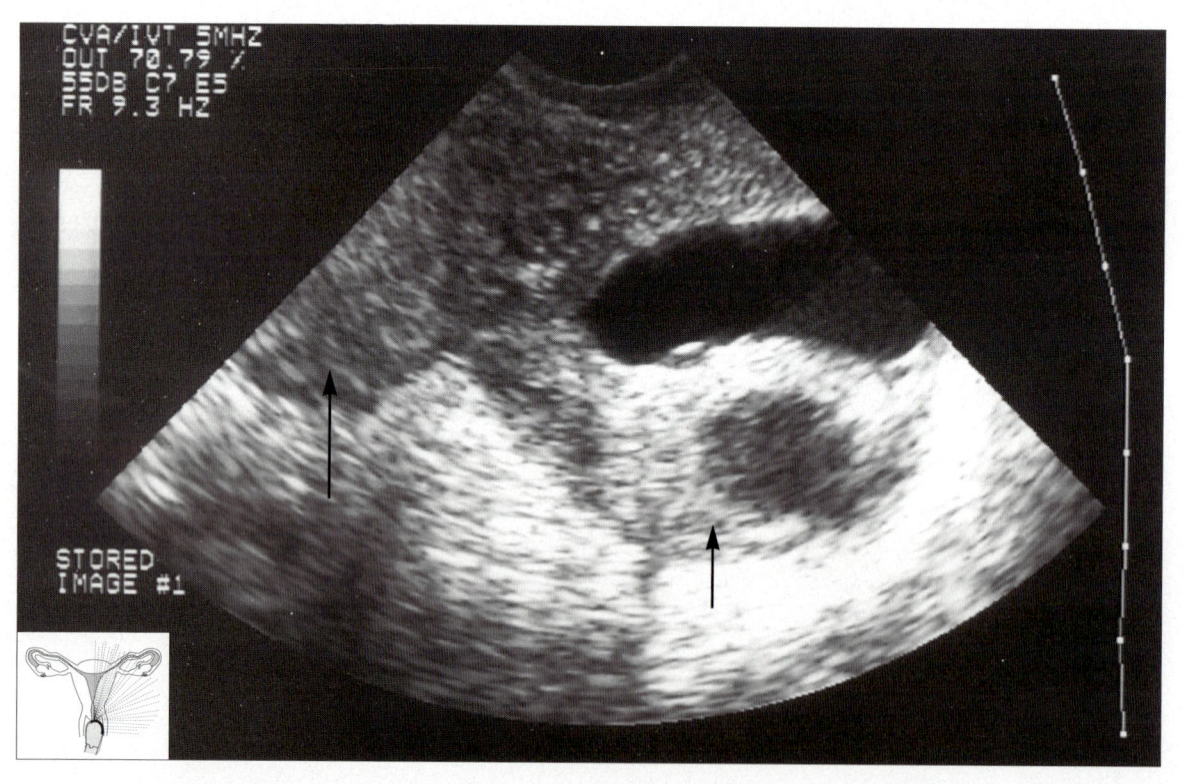

Figure 6~2. Sausage-shaped, anechoic distended fallopian tube lying above the ovary (small arrow) and lateral to the uterus (large arrow).

Fallopian Tube

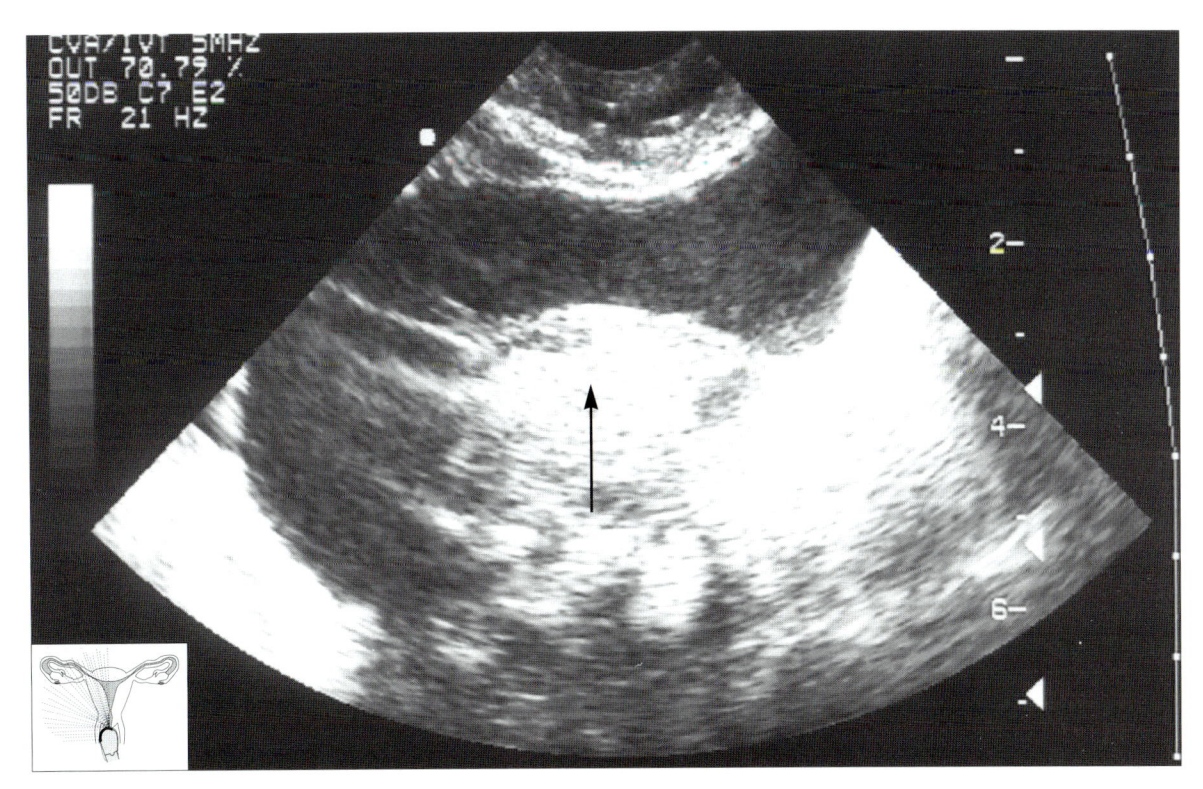

Figure 6-3. Grossly distended fallopian tube, wrapped around the ovary (arrow), forming a tubo-ovarian mass in a patient with pelvic inflammatory disease.

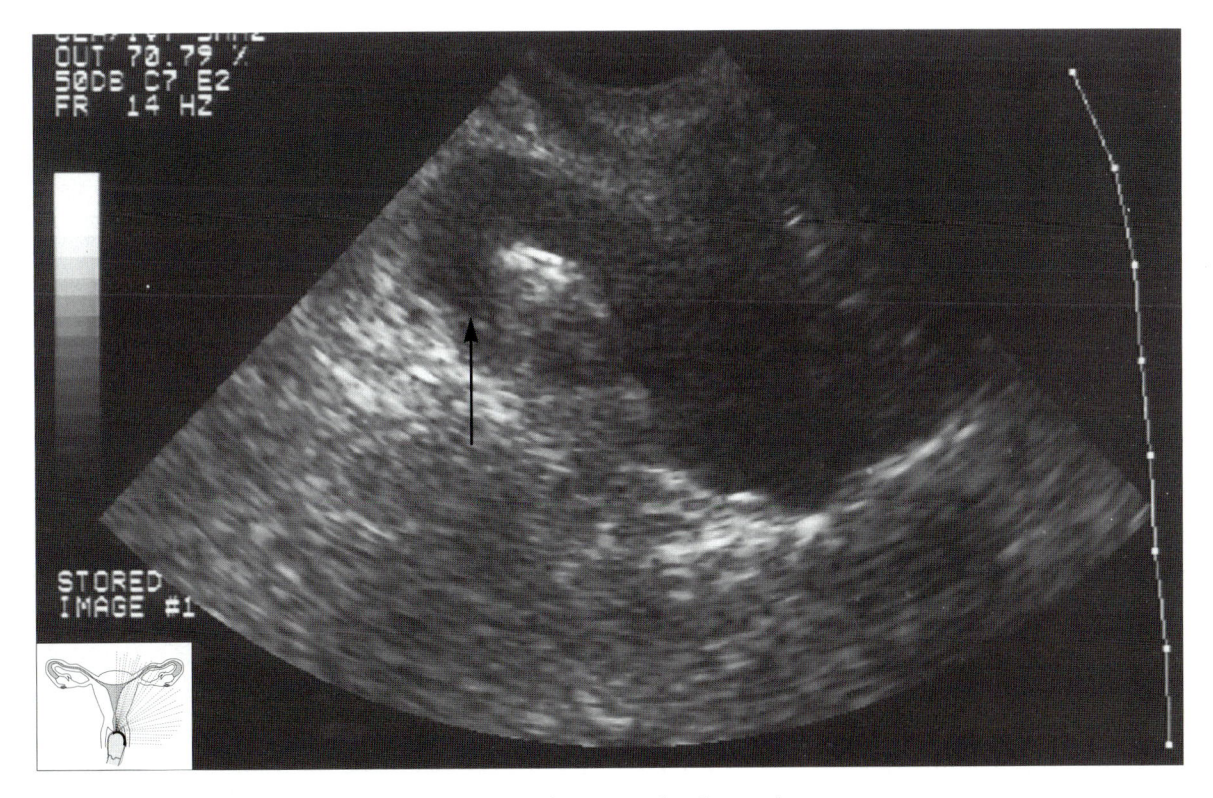

Figure 6-4. Hydrosalpinx (arrow) in a patient undergoing infertility work-up.

An Atlas of Transvaginal Sonography

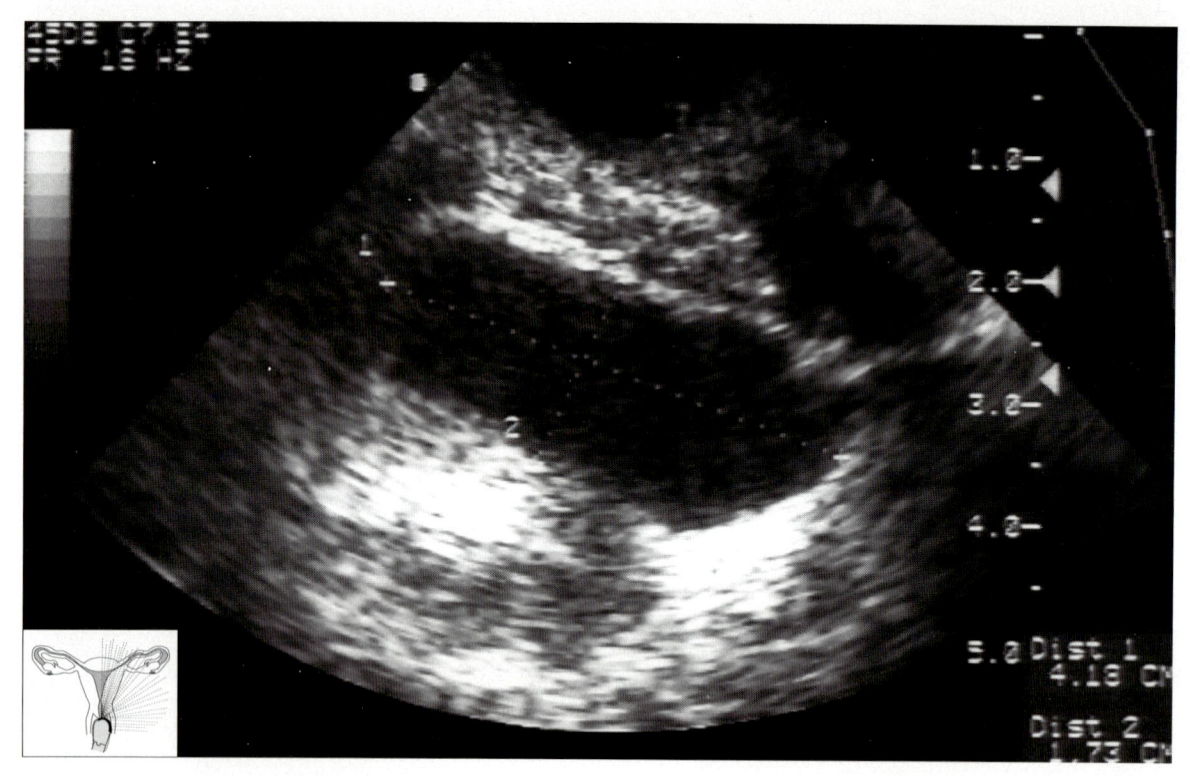

Figure 6-5. Sausage-shaped hydrosalpinx overlying the ovary.

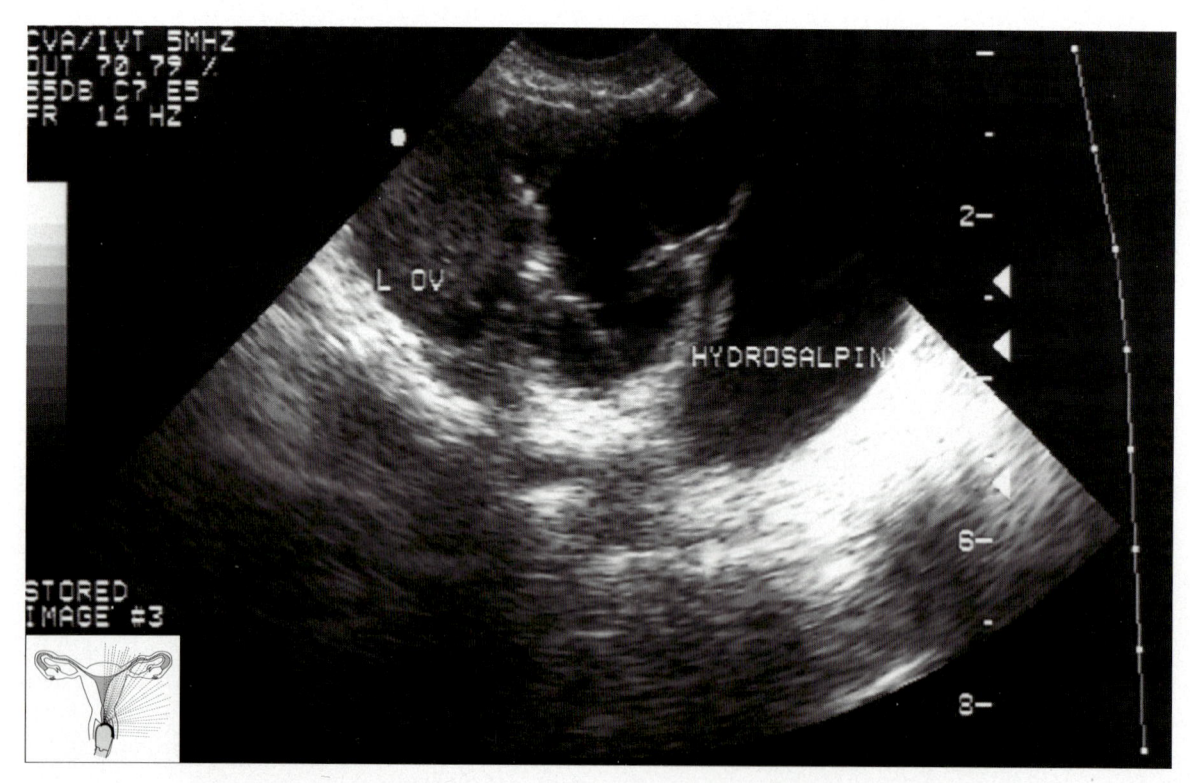

Figure 6-6. Complex hydrosalpinx adjacent to the ovary, demonstrating delicate mucosal pattern.

7   *Ovary*

The normal ovary is a 3.5 x 2.5 x 1.0 cm nodular organ weighing 4-7 gm. It is attached to the broad ligament on either side of the uterus. Each ovary is suspended from the posterolateral cornua of the uterus by the utero-ovarian ligament, and from the pelvic side wall by the infundibulopelvic ligament, which contains the ovarian artery, vein, and lymphatics.

Scan Findings

Although their size, shape, and morphology can change dramatically throughout each cycle, they sonographically appear as almond-shaped isochoic structures on the lateral pelvic side wall, just medial to the internal or external iliac vein. In premenopausal women the presence of small, clear follicular cysts easily distinguishes the ovary from surrounding structures.

Ovarian volume is calculated by applying the formula for a prolate ellipse, where volume = $(\pi/6) \times D_1 \times D_2 \times D_3$ and D_1, D_2 and D_3 represent the maximum anteroposterior, transverse and longitudinal diameters. Many factors influence ovarian size or volume. These include age, parity, obesity, menstrual status, and use of hormone replacement therapy.

Premenopausal ovarian volume is influenced by the menstrual cycle. Preovulatory volumes vary from 5.1 cm^3 to 6.2 cm^3, while the postovulatory ovarian volume averages about 3.2 ± 1.7 cm^3. Ovarian volume in postmenopausal women tends to be about half that of premenopausal women and should be no larger than 3.0 cm^3. After menopause there is a sharp decrease in ovarian volume. An early menopause is associated with smaller ovaries throughout the remainder of life. In premenopausal women, intraovarian blood flow is altered throughout the cycle. In the early proliferative part of the cycle, ovarian artery and intraovarian blood flow is characterized by a high resistance, vasoconstricted, low-flow bed. Blood flow is increased to the ovary containing the dominant follicle and corpus luteum. There is increased diastolic flow and lowered PI indicating a low-resistance vascular bed.

An Atlas of Transvaginal Sonography

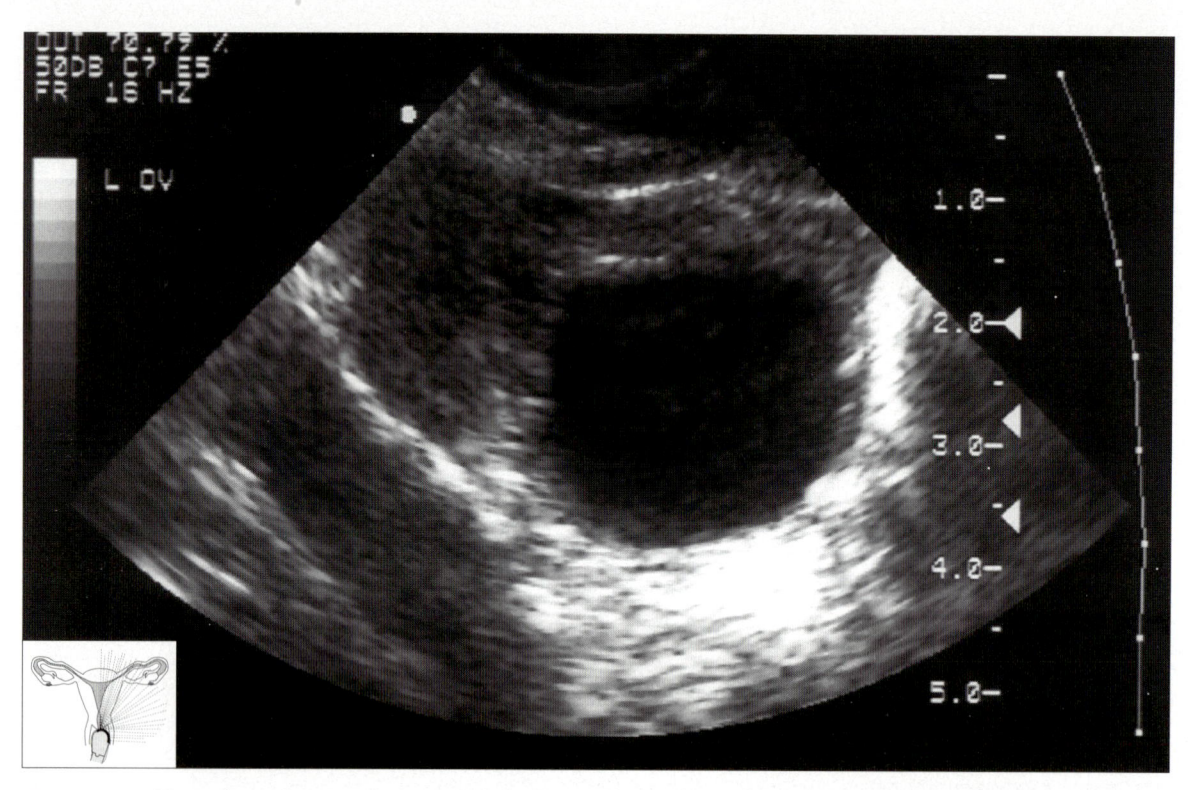

Figure 7-1. *Normal ovary containing corpus luteal cyst. The ovarian stroma has normal morphology.*

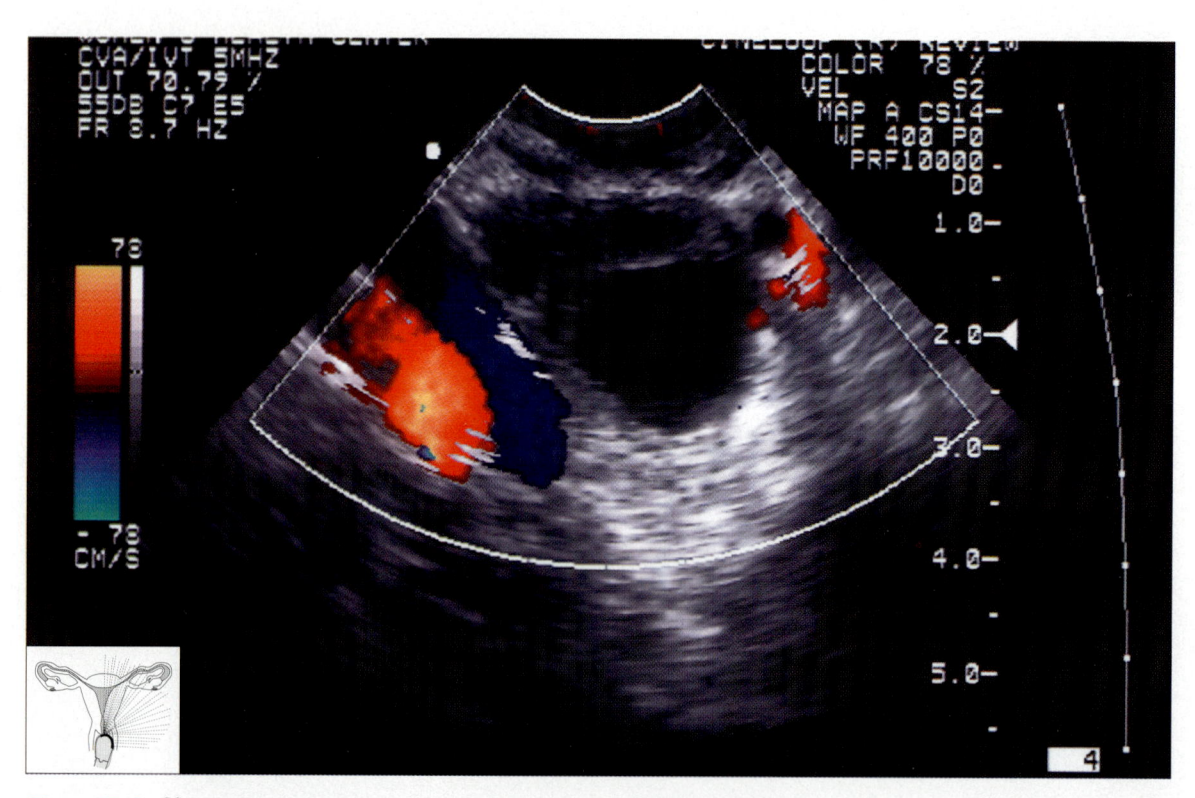

Figure 7-2. *Characteristic position of the ovary overlying the iliac vessels.*

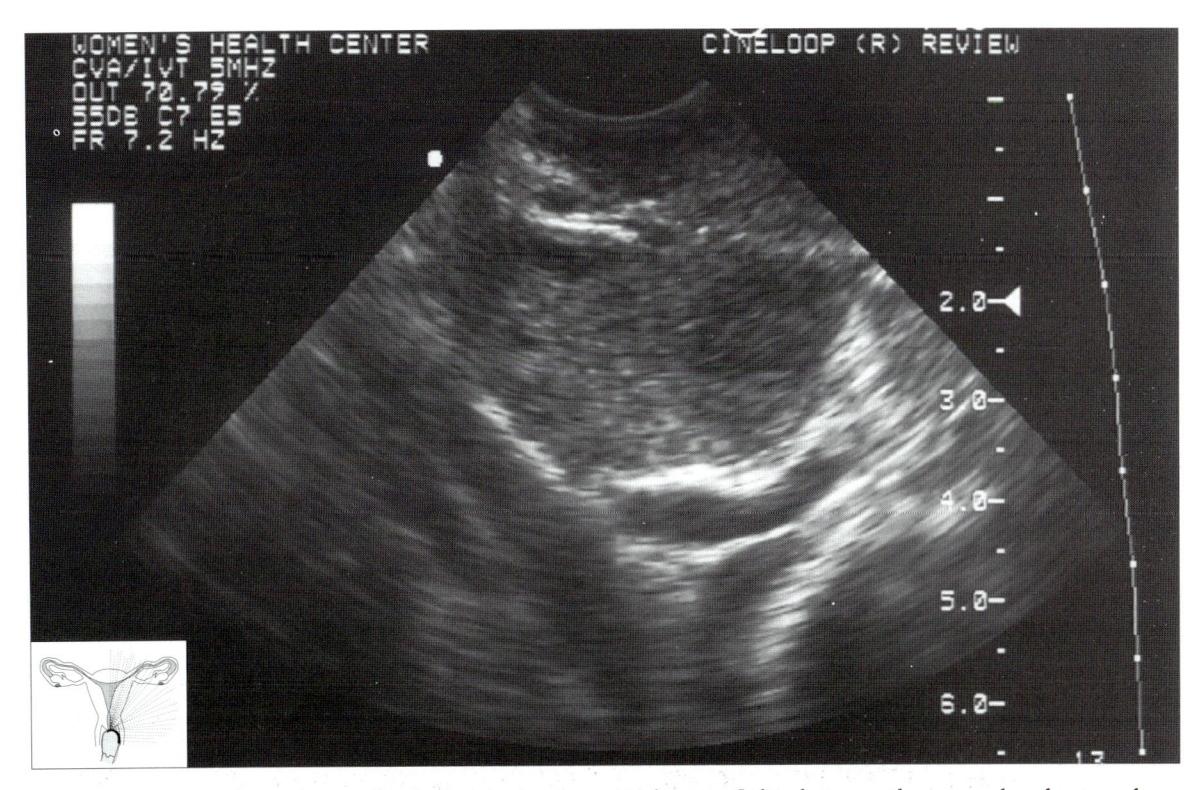

Figure 7-3. Normal ovary containing a hemorrhagic corpus luteum. It lies between the internal and external iliac vessels.

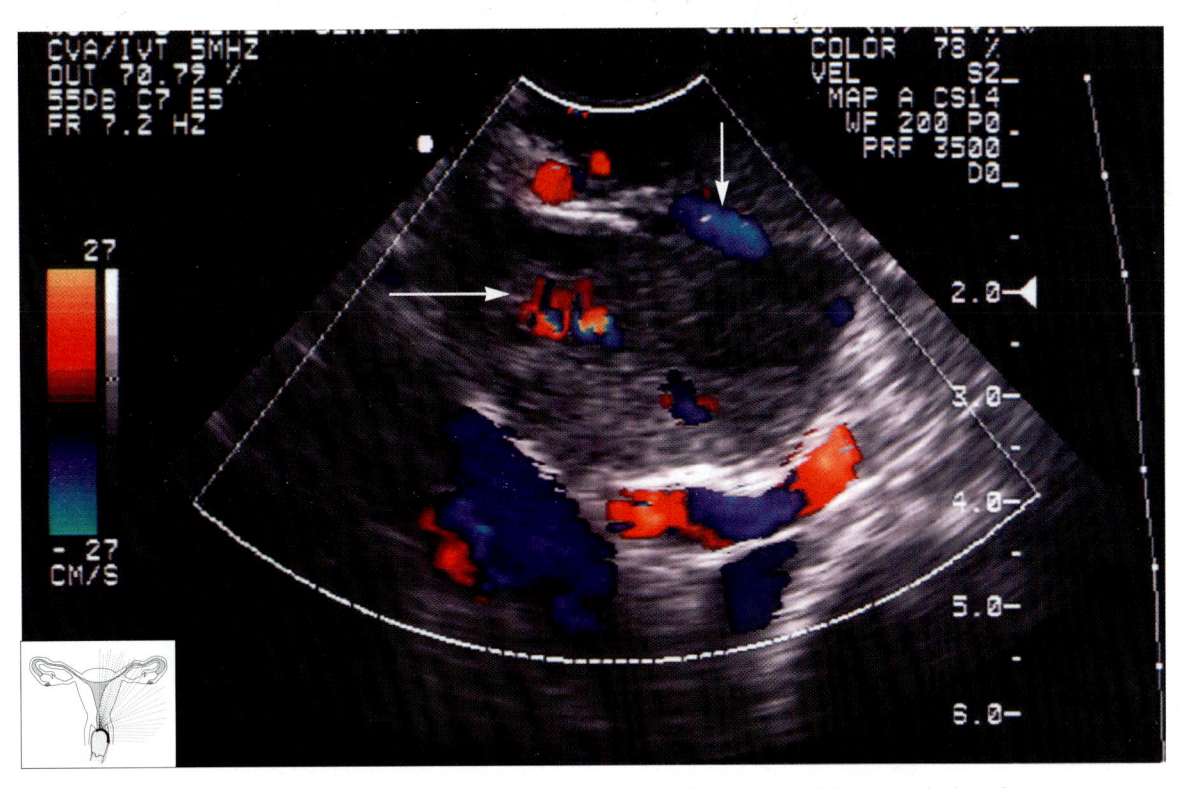

Figure 7-4. Color flow Doppler demonstrating not only the internal and external iliac vessels, but also intraovarian flow (large arrow) and segments of the uterine vessels (small arrow) within the broad ligament.

An Atlas of Transvaginal Sonography

Benign Ovarian Pathology

Benign lesions that may be imaged include functional cysts, polycystic ovaries, endometriomas, cystadenomas, mature cystic teratomas (dermoid cysts), paraovarian cysts, theca-lutein cysts, ovarian torsion, and a variety of solid ovarian tumors.

Functional Ovarian Cysts

Follicular and corpus luteum cysts consist of a fluid-filled sac, lined by a single layer of cells. They are formed as a result of ovulation. Follicular maturation can result in a follicular cyst prior to ovulation or a corpus luteum after ovulation. The latter may persist even in the absence of pregnancy; it occurs almost exclusively in menstruating women. Most are asymptomatic, and resolve spontaneously within one to three menstrual cycles. They should not reach sizes greater than 3 cm diameter. They are lined by an inner layer of granulosa cells and an outer layer of thecal cells.

Scan Findings

Sonographically follicular cysts are small clearly demarcated cysts without internal septa. After ovulation, an increase in internal echoes and layering of blood produces its characteristic sonographic appearance. Thin internal "pseudo-septa" can also be seen, which mimic a variety of ovarian tumors, including endometriomas and some epithelial tumors. Hemorrhagic corpora lutea will regress on follow-up scanning whereas ovarian tumors and endometriomas will not.

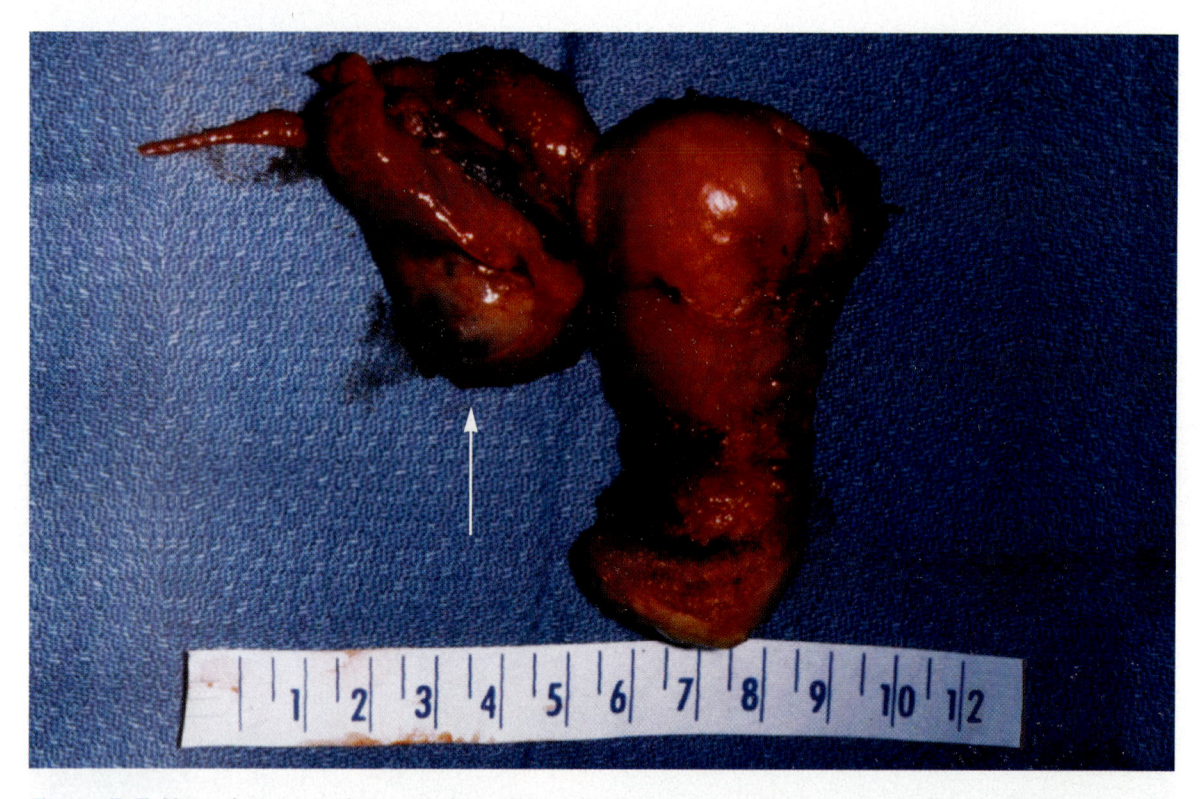

Figure 7-5. Normal uterus and ovary with small, simple, functional ovarian cyst on the lower pole (arrow).

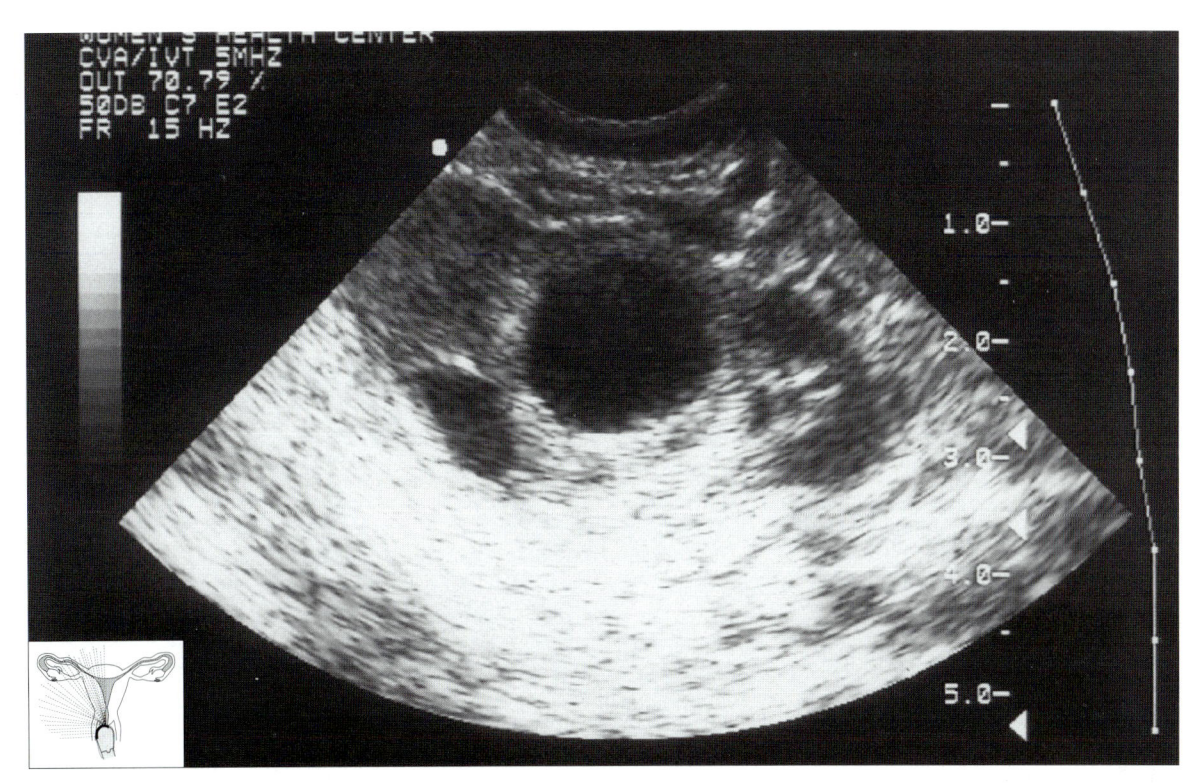

Figure 7-6. Clear "punched-out" follicular cyst.

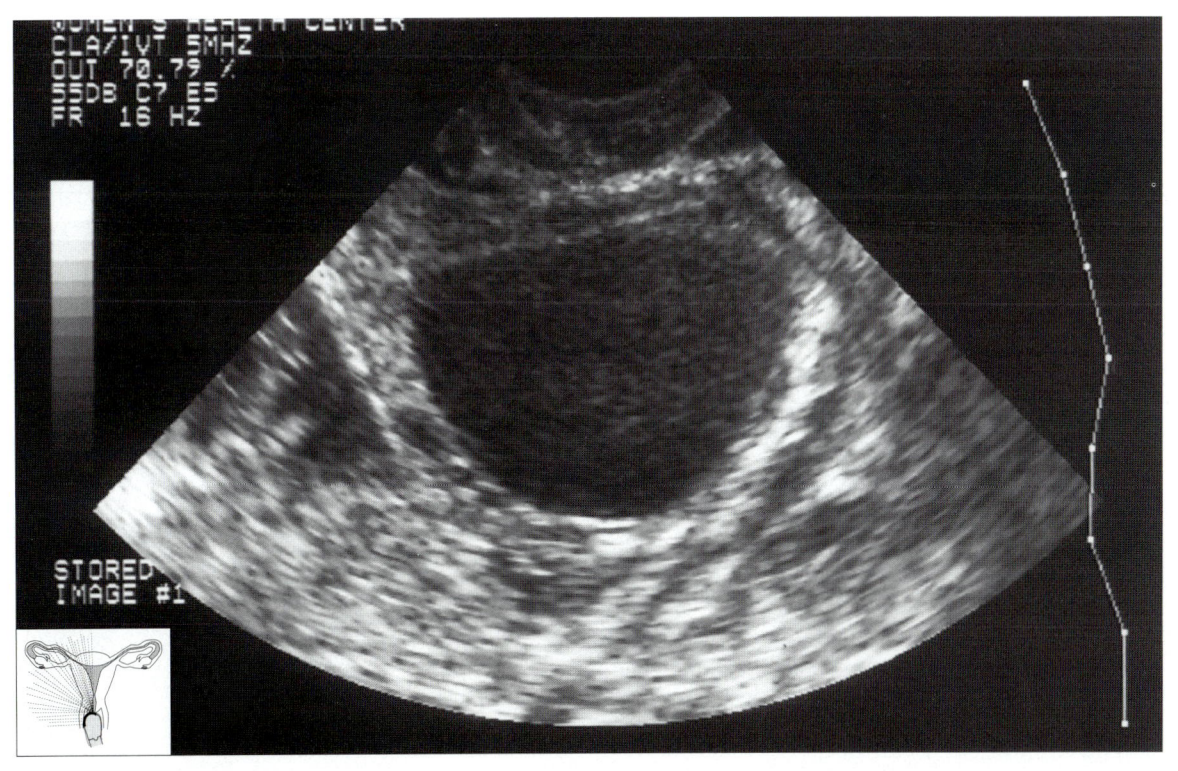

Figure 7-7. Hemorrhagic corpus luteum. Echoes within the cyst fluid correspond to blood-stained fluid. The surrounding ovarian cortex is normal.

An Atlas of Transvaginal Sonography

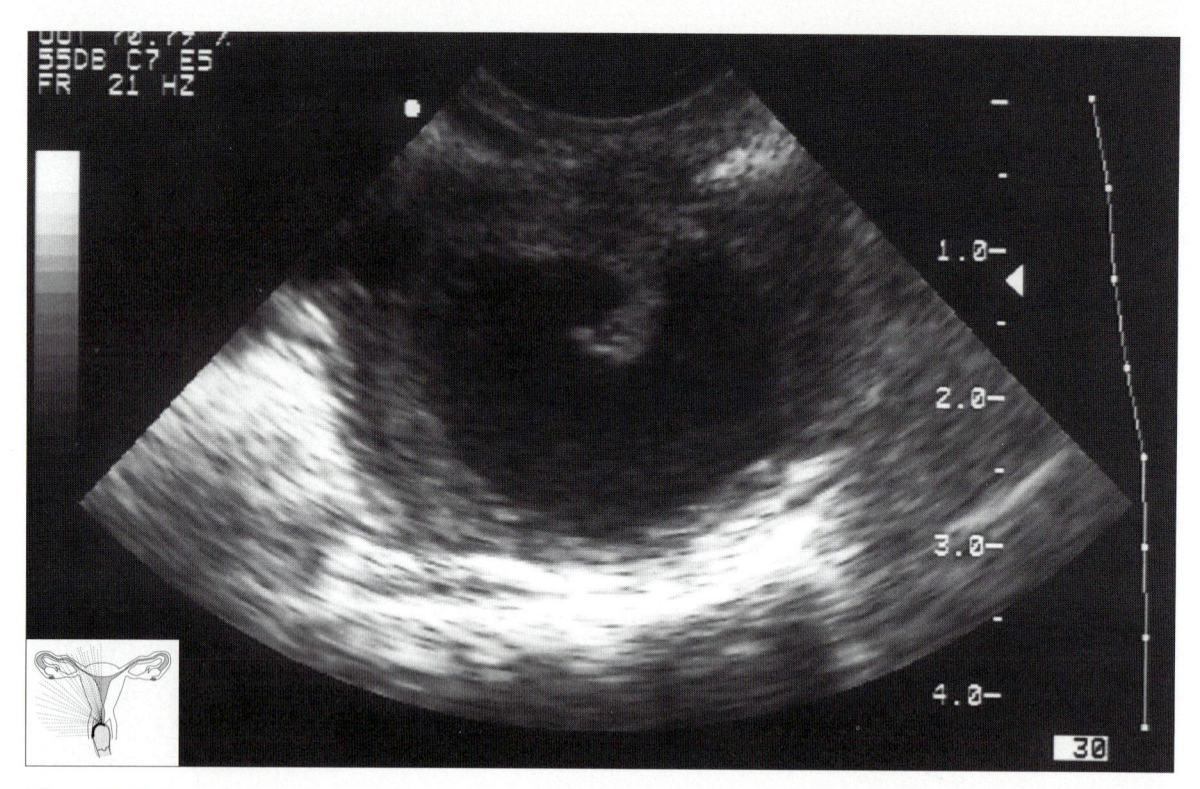

Figure 7~8. *Cystic ovarian mass with an apparent internal papillation. This is a hemorrhagic corpus luteum and the "papillation" represents the initiation of clot formation.*

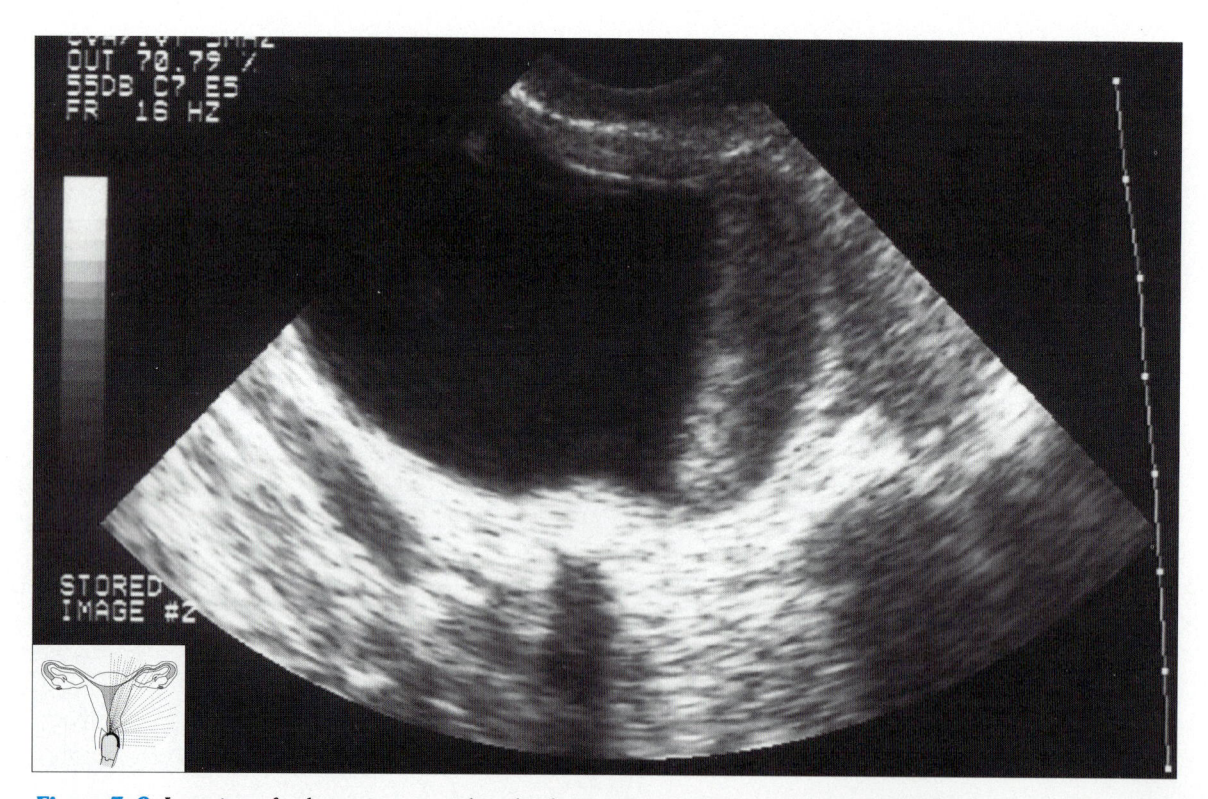

Figure 7~9. *Layering of echogenic material in this large ovarian cyst is consistent with blood.*

Ovary

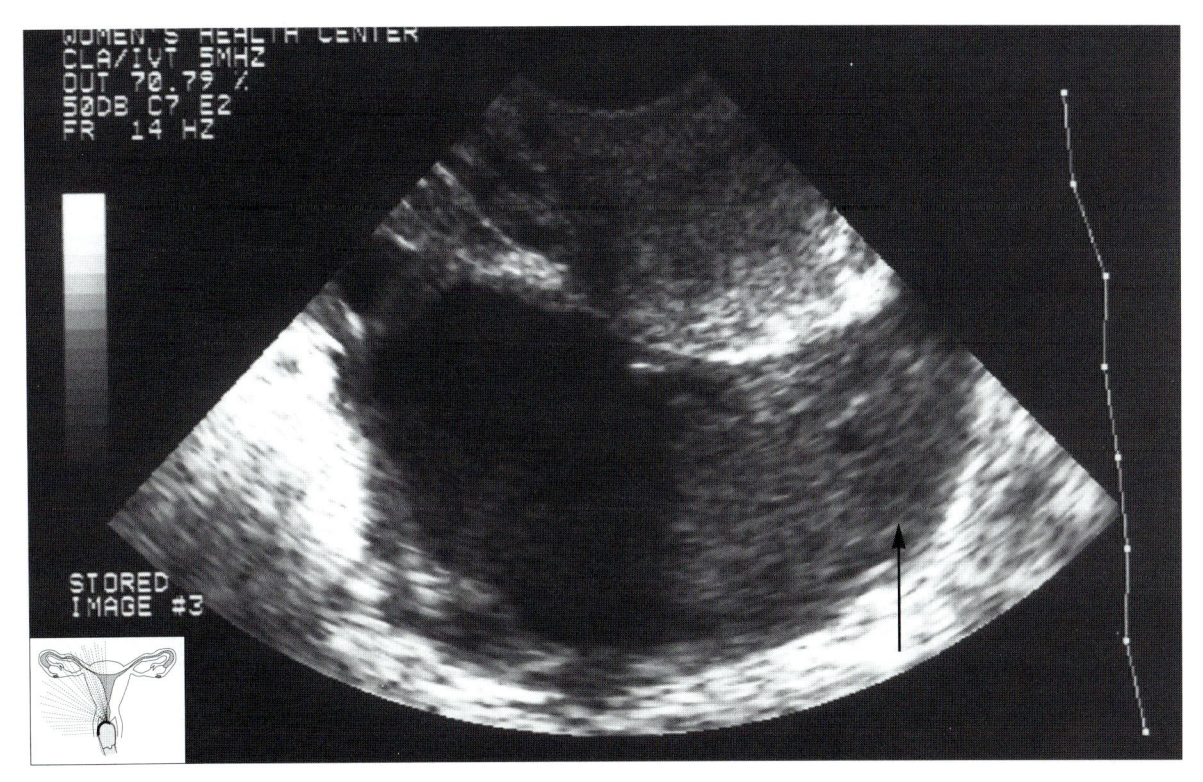

Figure 7-10. Increasing clot formation (arrow) in corpus luteal cyst.

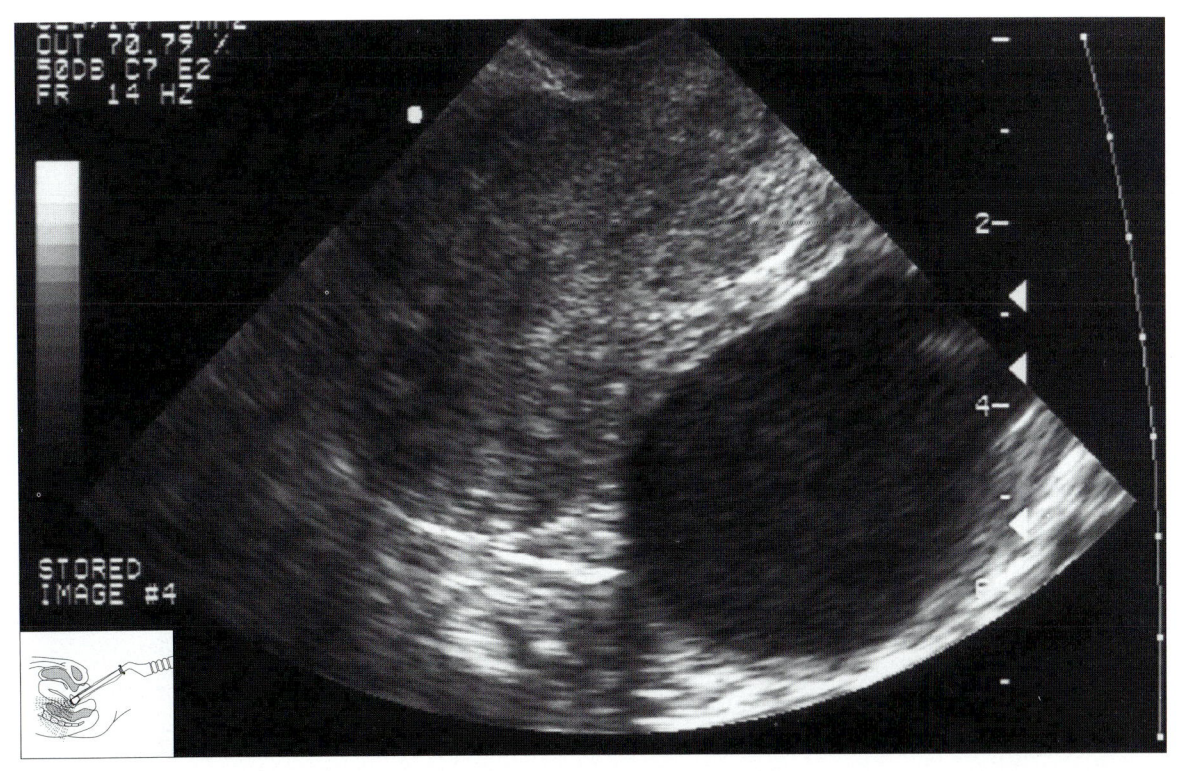

Figure 7-11. Hemorrhagic corpus luteum behind an anteverted uterus. The sonographic appearance is also consistent with an endometrioma, but resolution of the sonographic findings confirmed its true nature.

73

An Atlas of Transvaginal Sonography

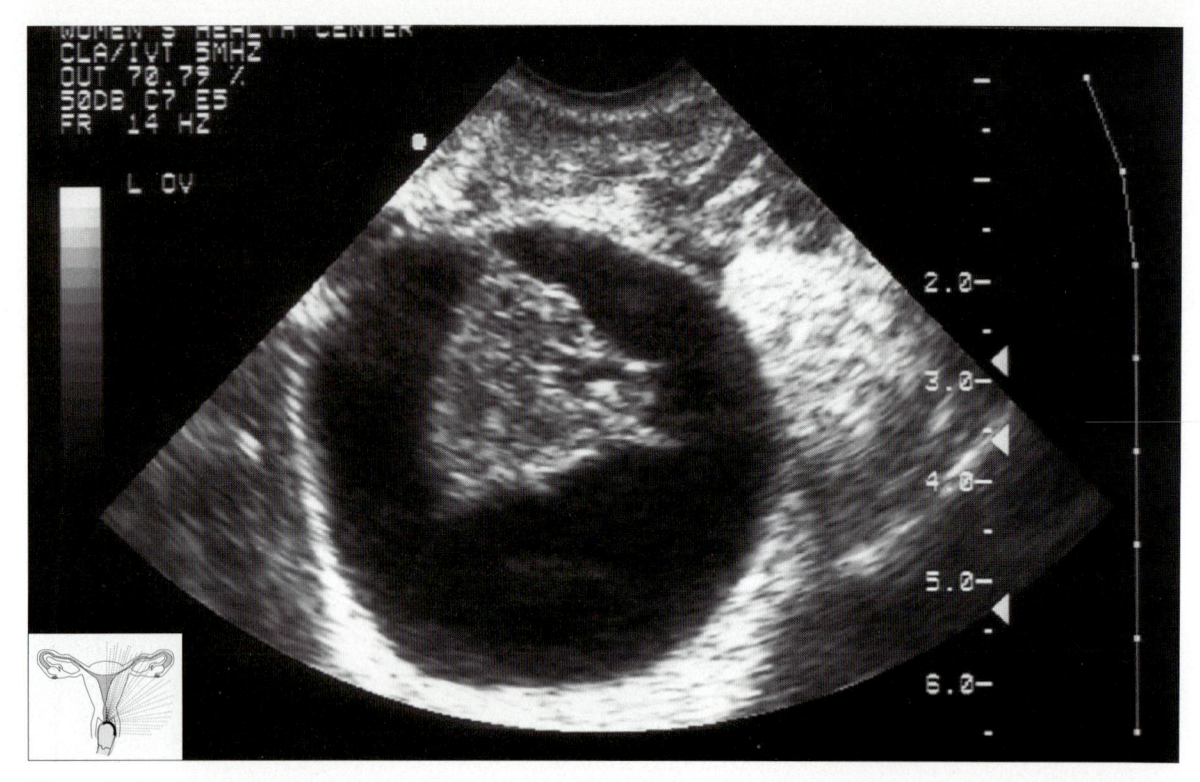

Figure 7-12. Clot formation within an otherwise simple cyst. This phenomenon is seen commonly in corpus luteum cysts. The appearance needs to be distinguished from complex malignant tumors.

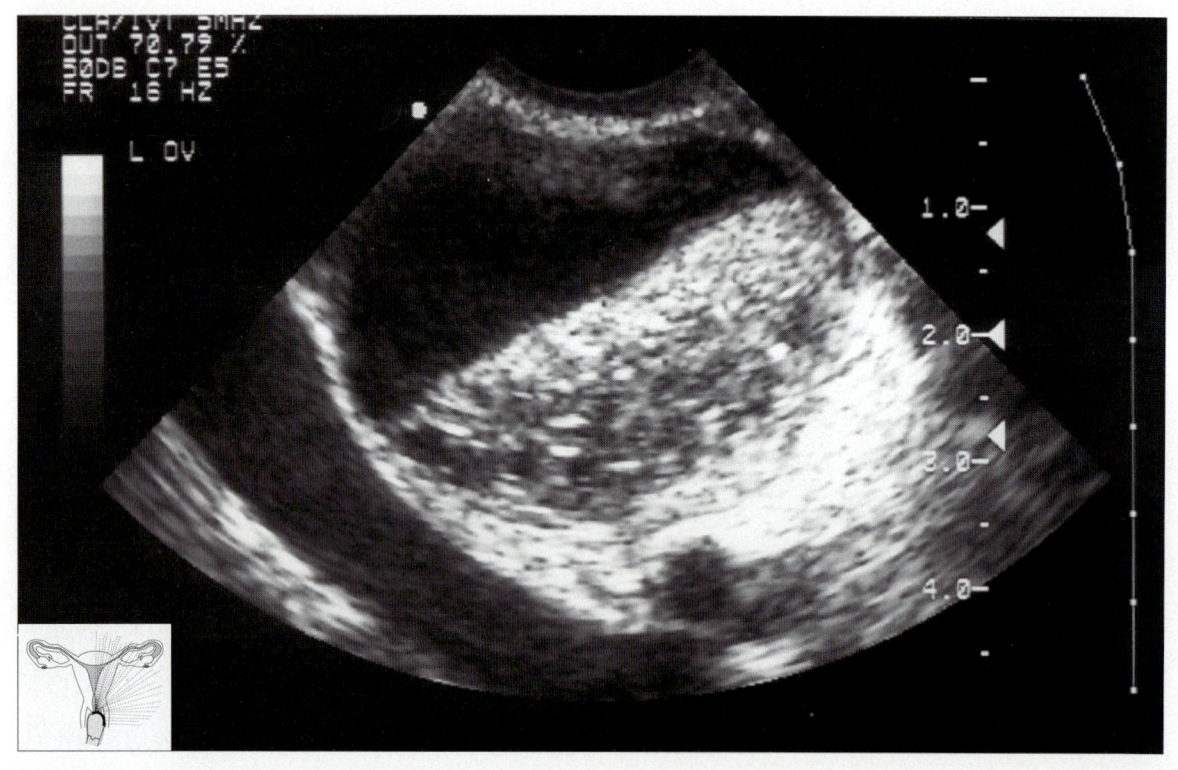

Figure 7-13. Layering effect of blood in a large cystic ovary. Color flow Doppler failed to demonstrate flow within the "solid" portion of this mass.

Ovary

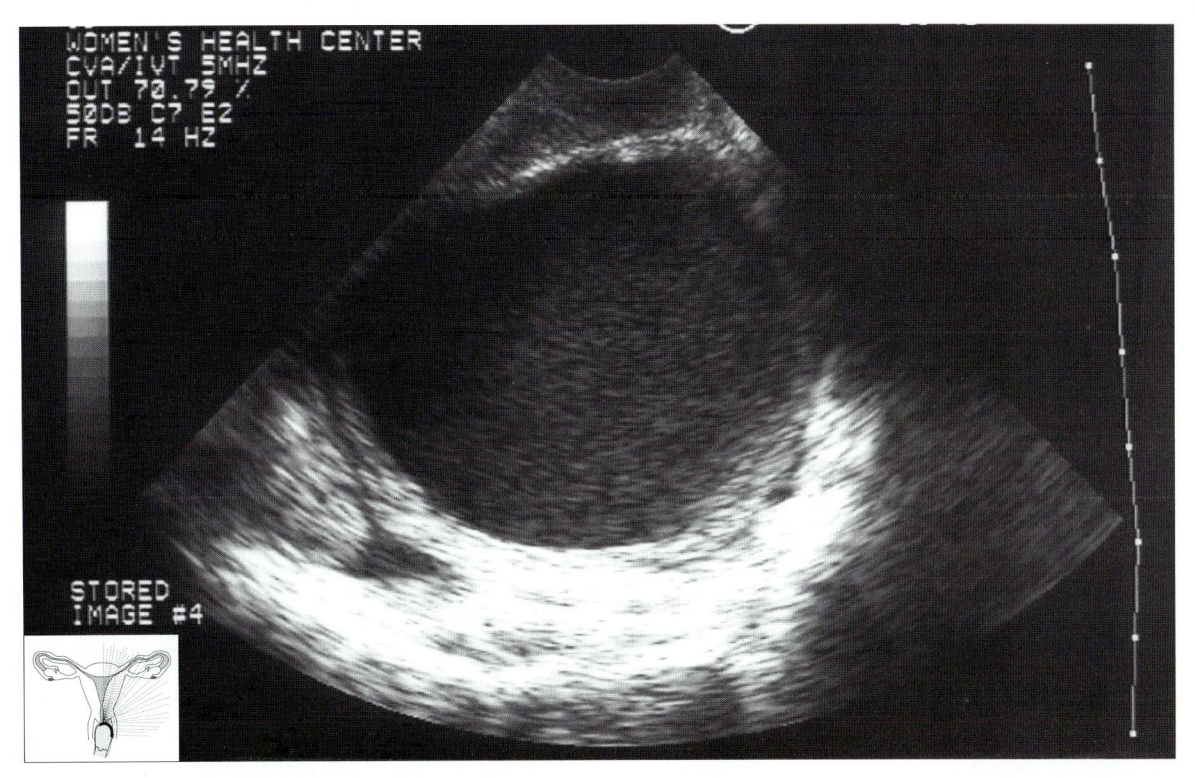

Figure 7-14. A large but otherwise uncomplicated hemorrhagic corpus luteum. Fine, echogenic cystic contents are bounded by normal ovarian stroma.

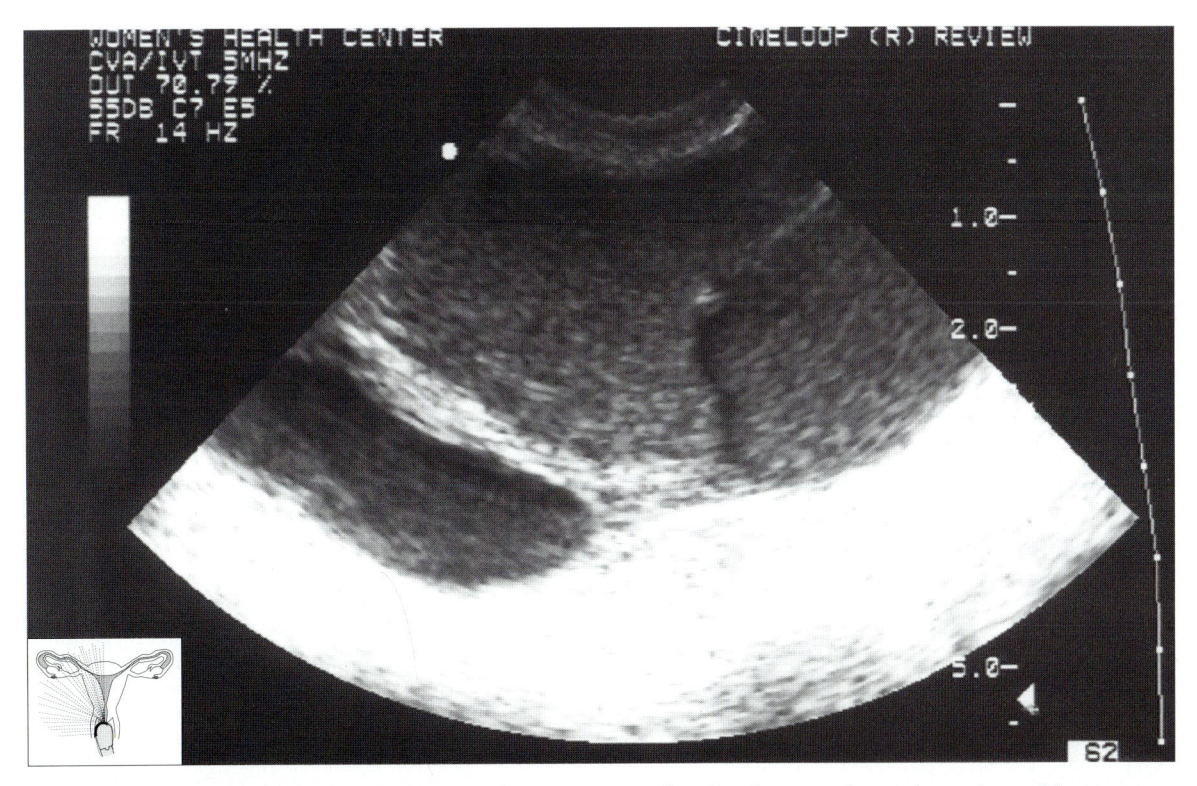

Figure 7-15. The multicystic mucinous cystadenoma was confused with a complex endometrioma. Mucinous material may also appear sonographically as fine homogenous echoes.

An Atlas of Transvaginal Sonography

Polycystic Ovary Syndrome

Polycystic Ovary Syndrome (PCOS) is a clinical syndrome consisting of hirsutism, obesity, and amenorrhea in association with enlarged polycystic ovaries. Most patients present with infertility, hirsutism, amenorrhea, and obesity. The diagnosis is confirmed by hormonal assays. There is a 2:1 reversal of the LH/FSH ratio. Androgens are also increased with an elevation in free testosterone and adrenal-derived DHEAS.

Scan Findings

The ovaries are enlarged to about twice normal size with a smooth white surface and thickened capsule. Sonographically multiple small, subcortical cysts are easily demonstrated on TVS.

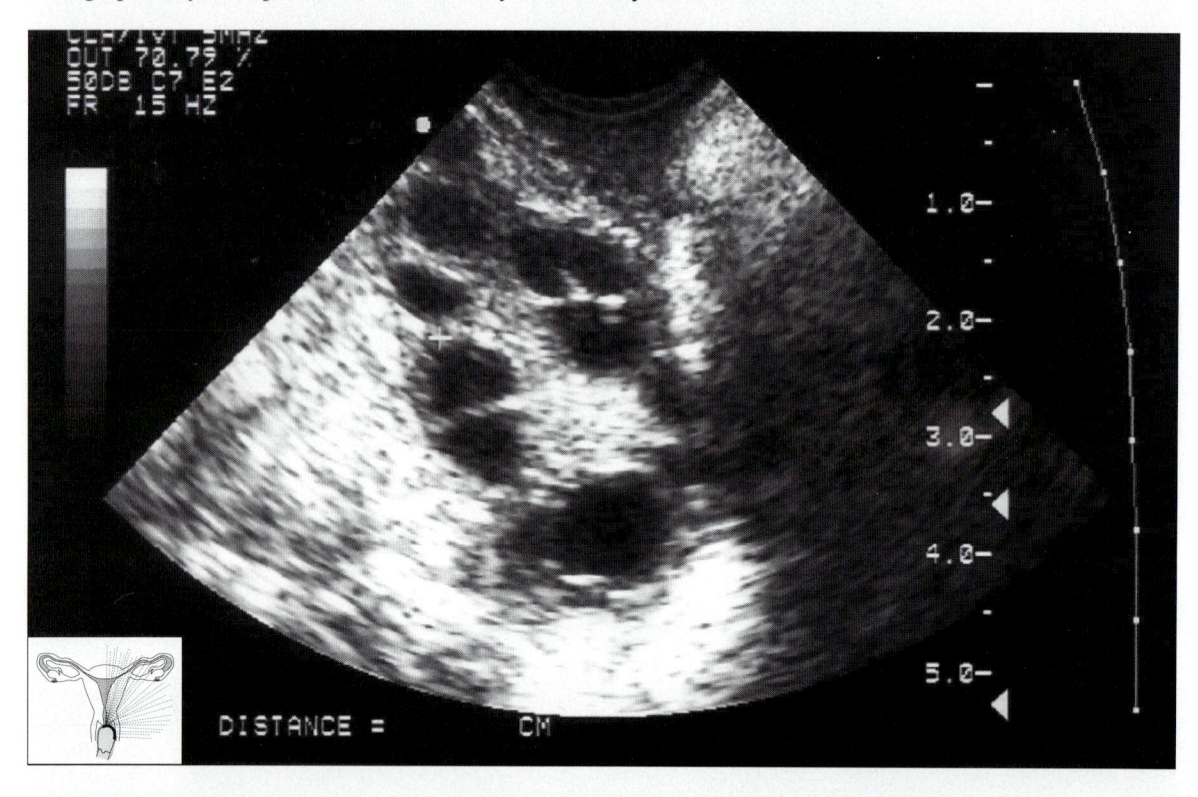

Figure 7-16. Multiple subcortical cysts are characteristic of the polycystic ovary syndrome.

Ovary

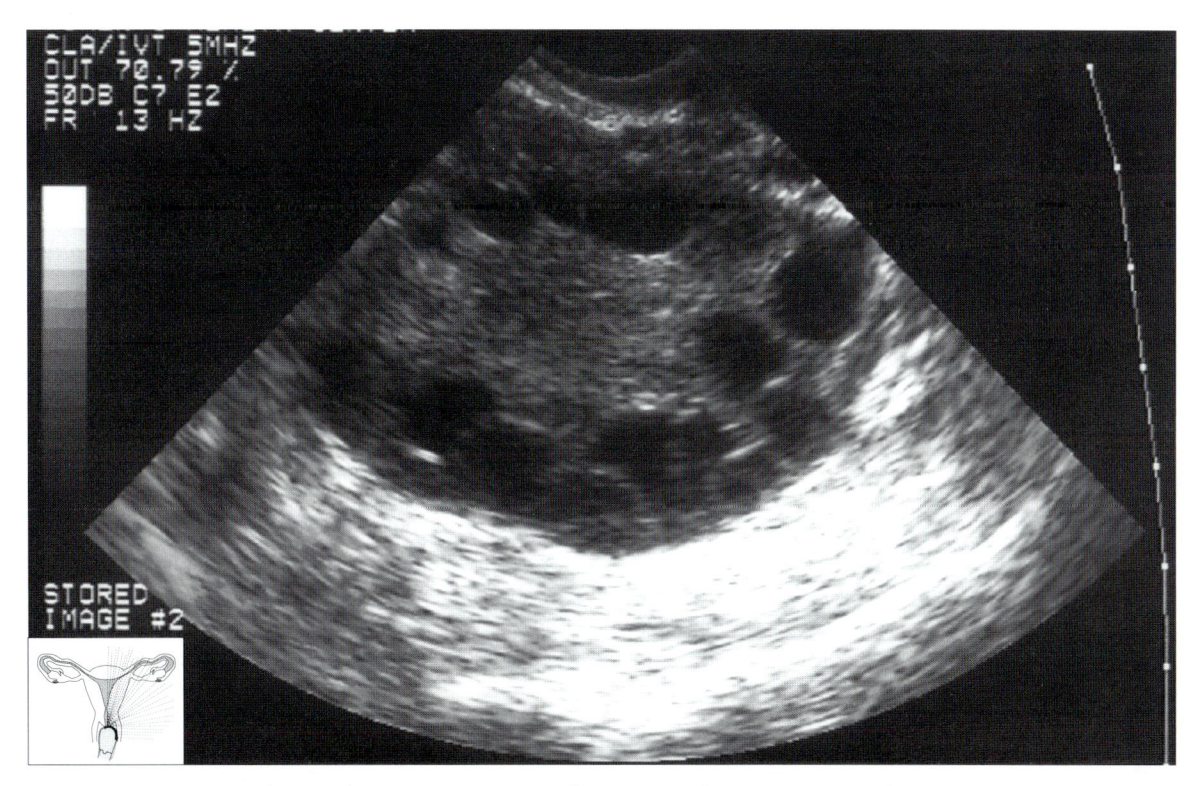

Figure 7-17. *Large subcortical ovarian cysts, typically seen in polycystic ovary syndrome.*

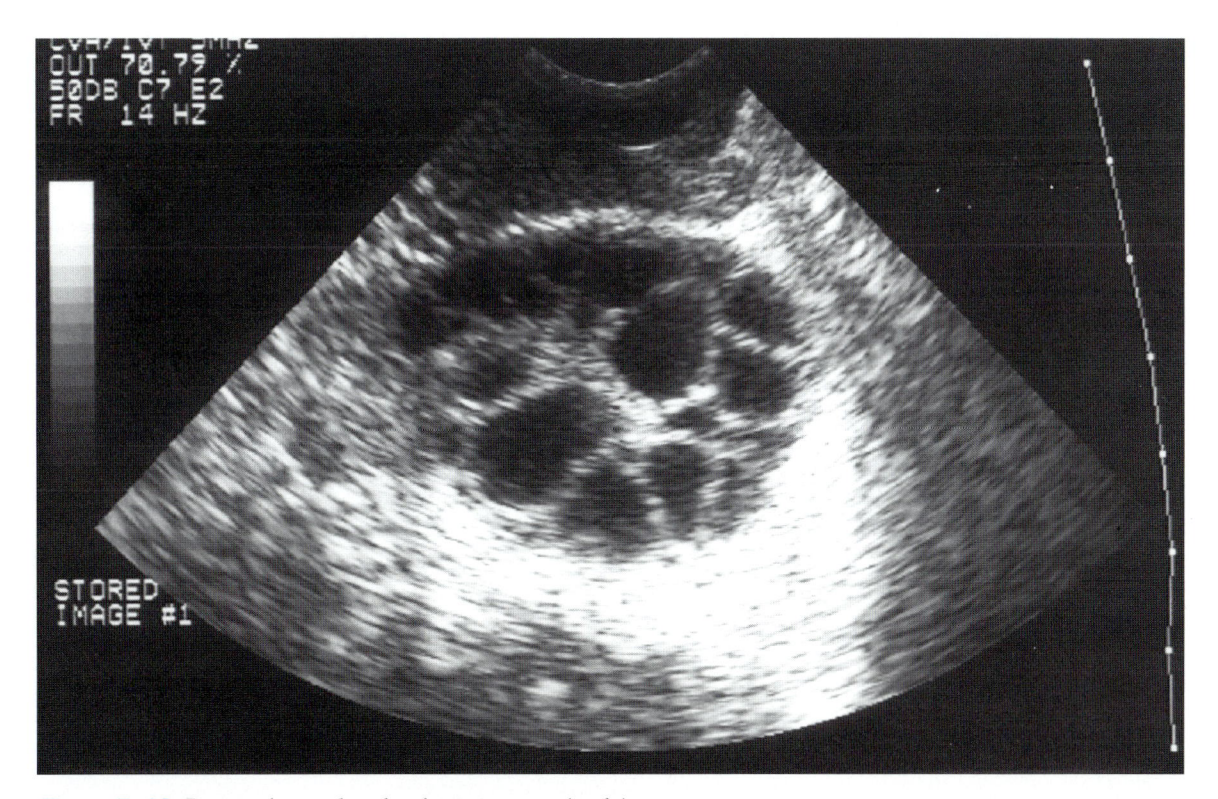

Figure 7-18. *Pergonal-stimulated polycystic ovary (early).*

An Atlas of Transvaginal Sonography

Endometriomas

Endometriosis is a common condition that primarily affects reproductive age women. It consists of functional endometrial glands and stroma in an extrauterine location, most commonly the ovary, although any peritoneal surface can be involved. The etiology is unknown but is likely due to either retrograde menstruation or celomic metaplasia.

Cyclic hemorrhage into foci of ovarian endometriosis can result in the formation of a thin-walled "chocolate cyst" or endometrioma, which usually is densely adherent to surrounding structures and is easily ruptured during attempted surgical removal. Most patients complain of pelvic pain, particularly dysmenorrhea and dyspareunia, and infertility. Less common symptoms include irregular menses, sacral backache, and painful defecation. Laparoscopy with biopsy of endometrial implants is needed to confirm the diagnosis.

Scan Findings

Endometriosis cannot be visualized on sonography until cyst formation occurs. The sonographic appearance is variable. Smooth adnexal cysts filled with echogenic fluid are commonly seen. They can be indistinguishable from a hemorrhagic corpus luteum with low-level echoes being returned from clotted blood. Rupture of an endometrioma may rarely produce acute abdominal pain, fever, and leukocytosis. Endometrioma may be confused not only with corpora lutea, but also a variety of epithelial and solid ovarian tumors. "Pseudo-septa" can mimic cystadenomas or cystadenocarcinomas. Solid components can be confused with solid components of cystadenocarcinomas or solid ovarian tumors. Color flow is absent within the "solid" and "pseudo-septa." Ovarian artery flow, if measured, can paradoxically reveal a low pulsatility index (PI) and resistance index (RI) depending on the phase of the menstrual cycle.

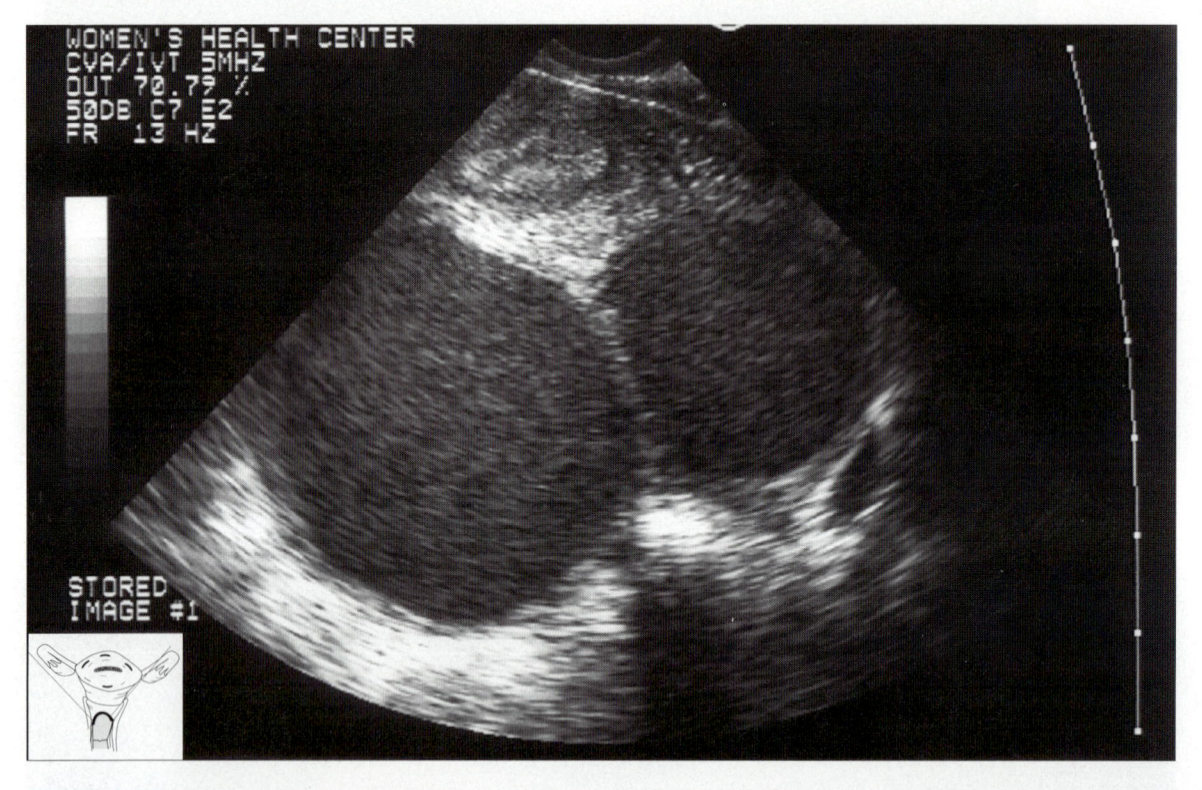

Figure 7-19. Transverse scan through uterus and large cul-de-sac mass. This polycystic mass, with echoic fluid is consistent with endometriomas. The ovarian cortex is otherwise normal.

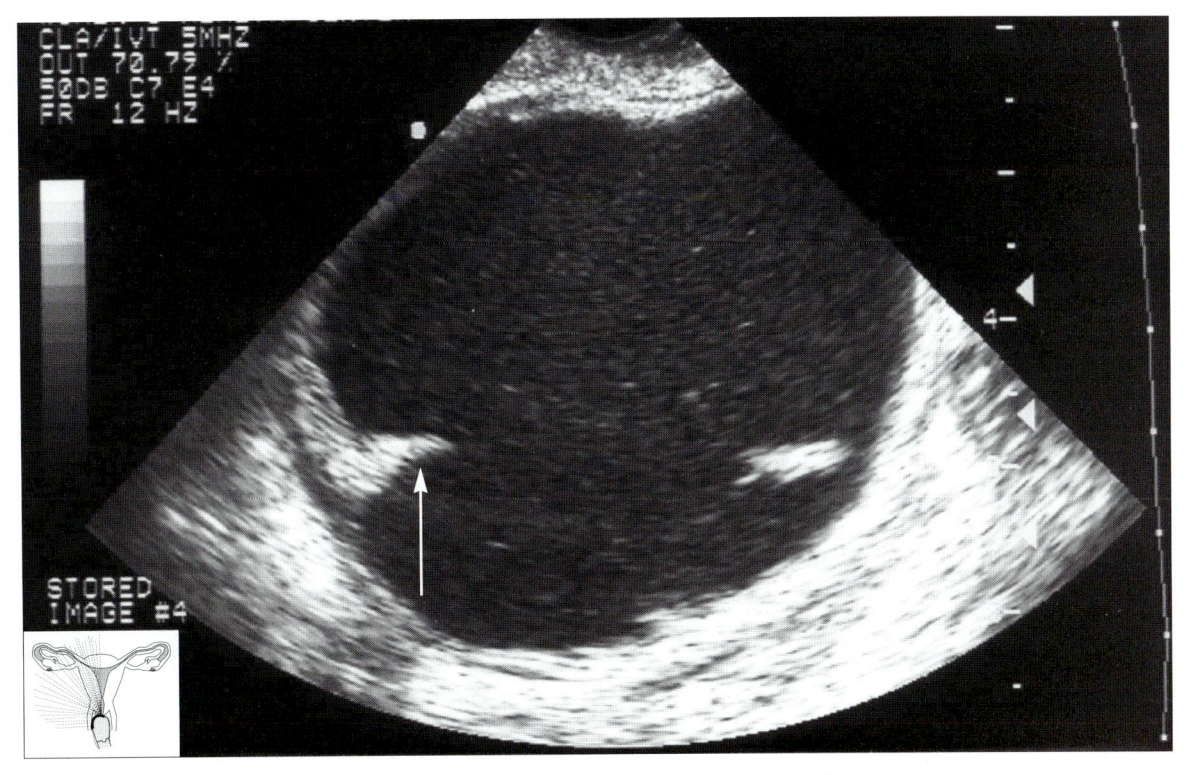

Figure 7-20. Large echogenic cystic ovary with development of pseudo septa (arrow).

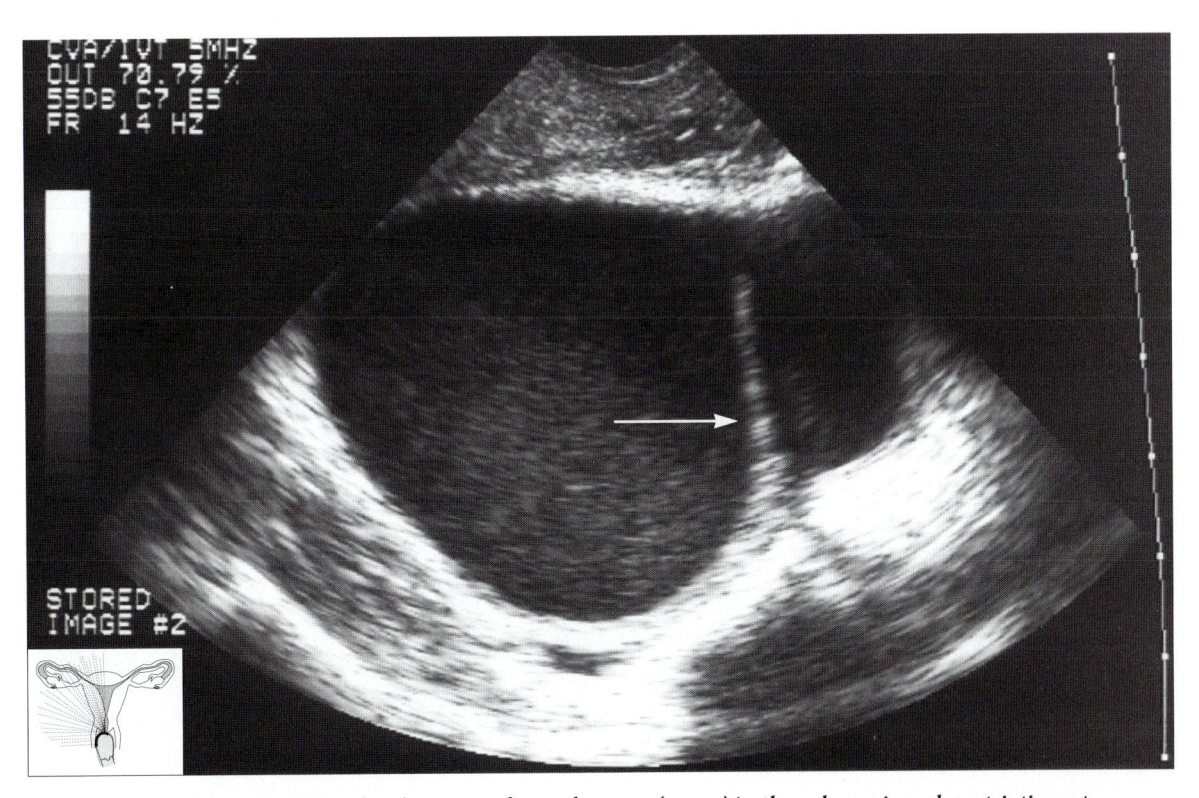

Figure 7-21. Almost complete development of pseudo septa (arrow) in the echogenic endometriotic cyst.

An Atlas of Transvaginal Sonography

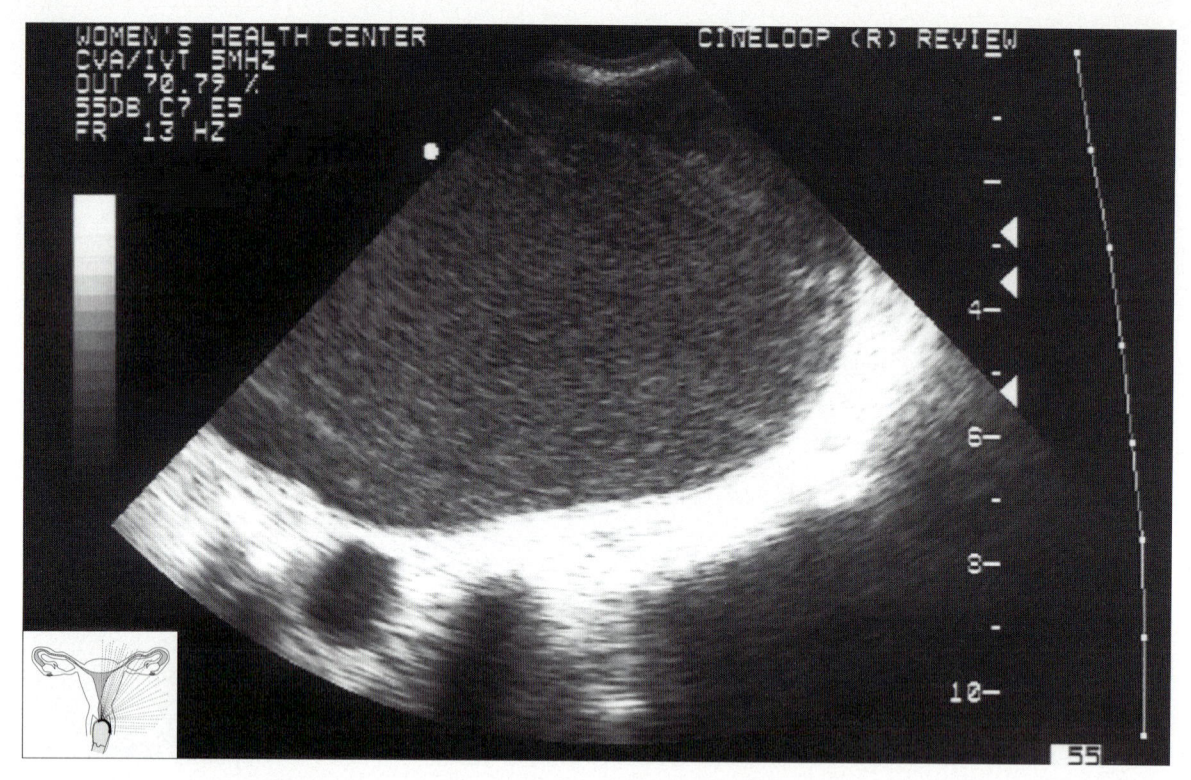

Figure 7-22. *Large endometrioma containing echogenic fluid.*

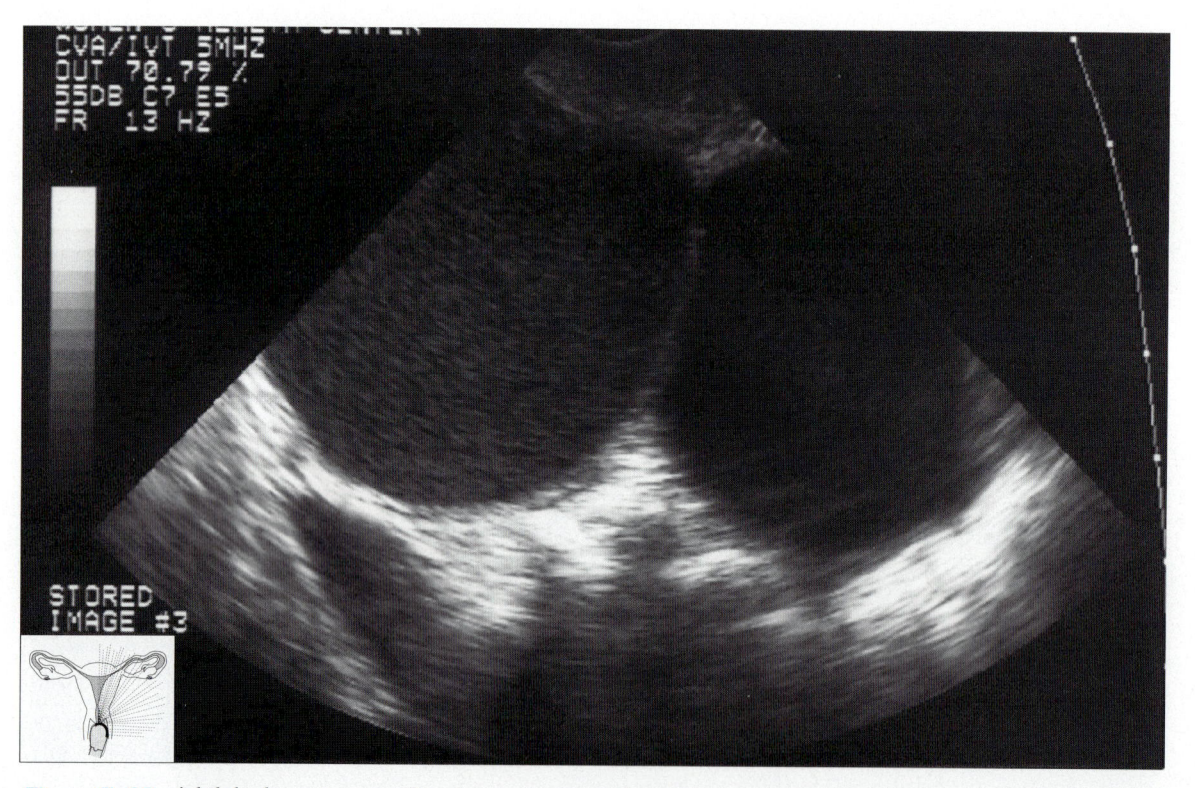

Figure 7-23. *A bilobed ovarian cyst. The left cyst is an endometrioma containing echogenic cystic fluid while the right cyst is anechoic.*

Ovary

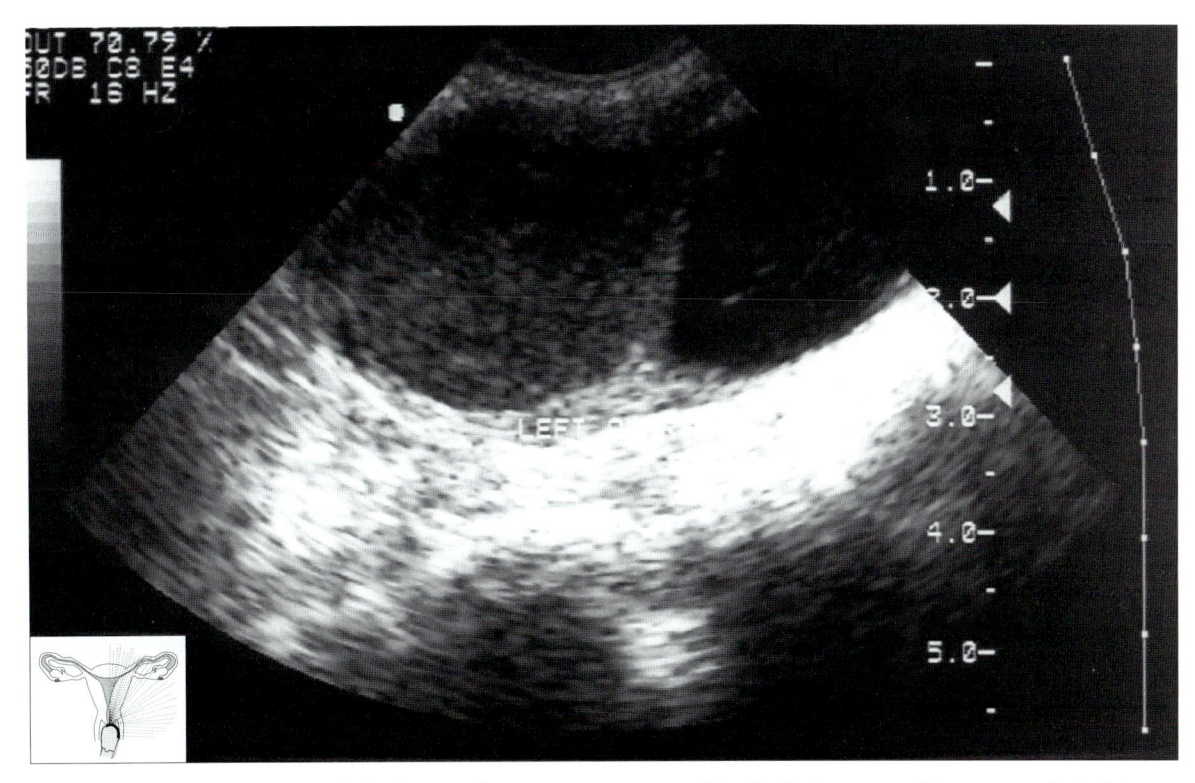

Figure 7~24. Cystic ovary with thick septa between two sonographically distinct cysts. The cyst on the left has dense homogenous echoes, and represents a "chocolate cyst" while the cyst on the right has multiple fine echoes that resolved on subsequent scanning.

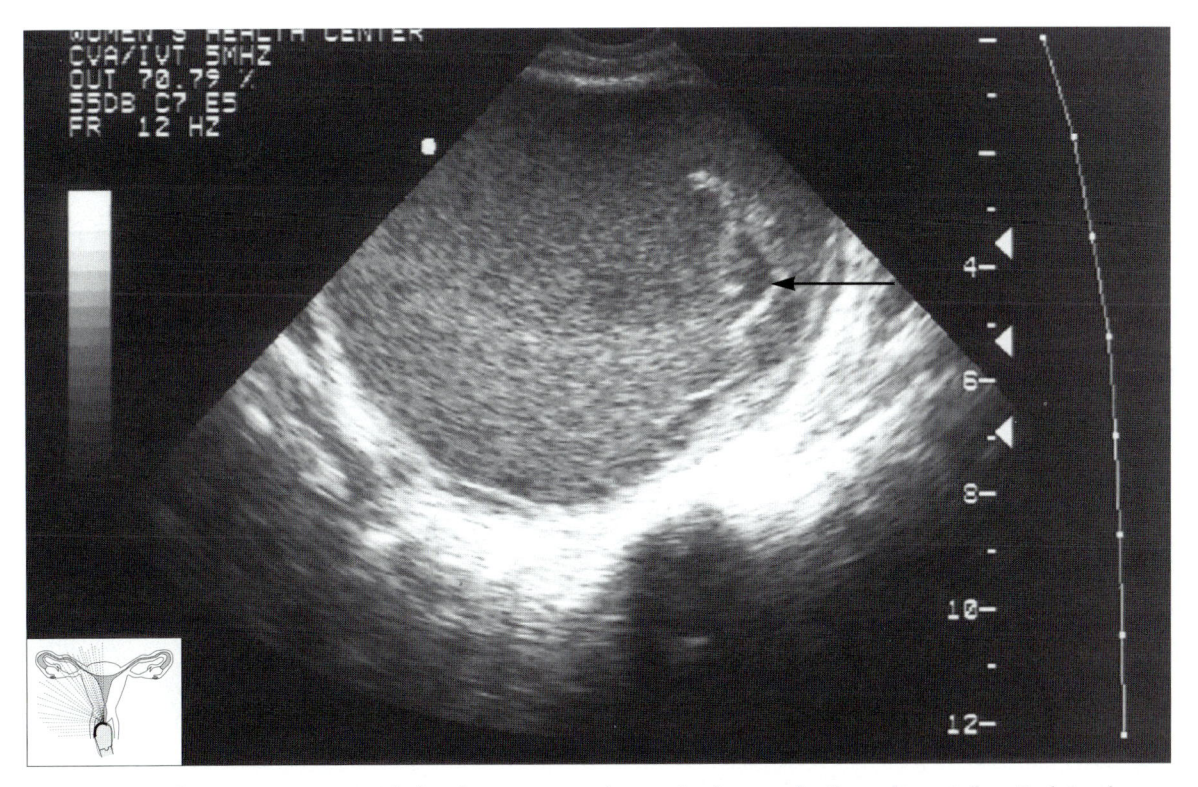

Figure 7~25. Large cystic ovary with fine homogeneous internal echoes and a "pseudo-septa" on its lateral margin (arrow).

An Atlas of Transvaginal Sonography

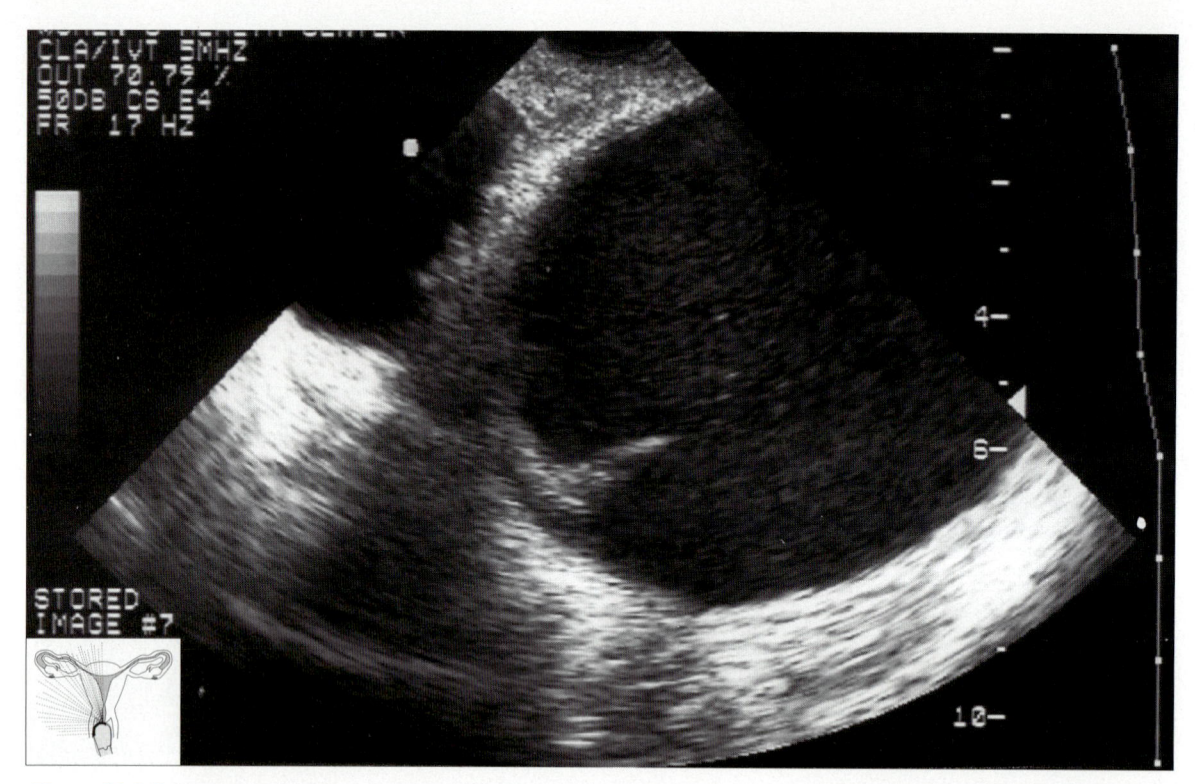

Figure 7-26. *Benign endometriotic cysts with very thick intraovarian septa, with small papillations and development of pseudo-septa.*

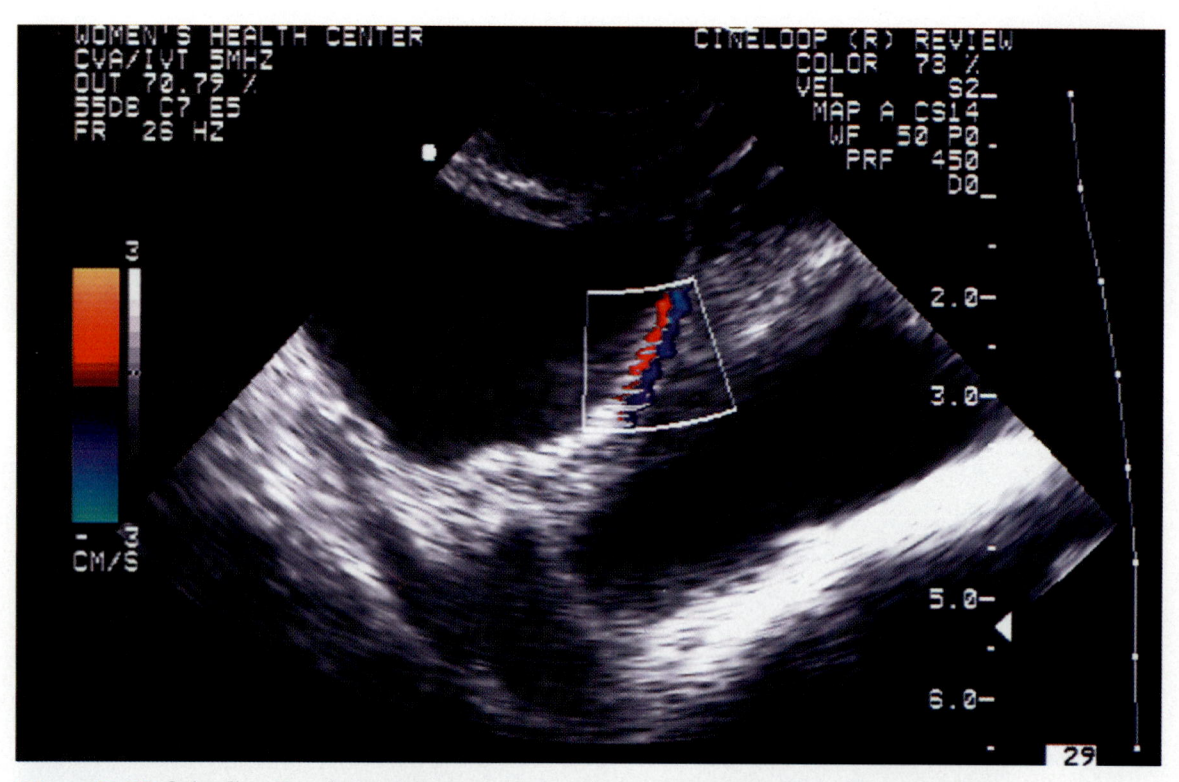

Figure 7-27. *Color flow Doppler reveals normal linear flow in this septa.*

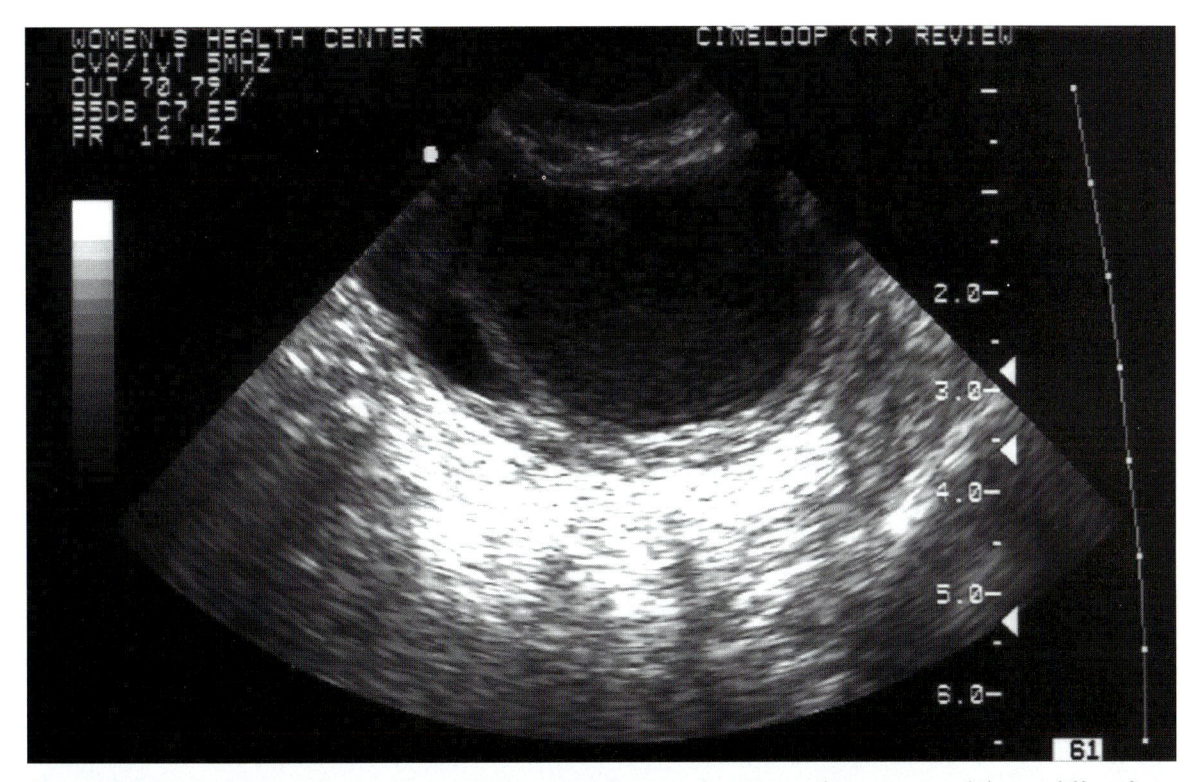

Figure 7-28. *Although similar to a hemorrhagic corpus luteum, this is an endometrioma exhibiting diffuse fine internal echoes consistent with blood.*

Ovarian Cystadenomas

Ovarian cystadenomas (serous, mucinous, clear cell, and endometrioid) are the most common benign ovarian neoplasms, accounting for up to 25% of all ovarian tumors. Despite their benign nature, they can attain a large size and are bilateral in 15-25% of cases. They are simple ovarian cysts lined by a single layer of cells of either serous, mucinous, clear cell, or endometrioid cell types. The fluid within the cysts is either proteinaceous or mucinous. Thin-walled regular septa can form.

Scan Findings

Unilocular or multilocular ovarian cysts of variable size may be seen. There should be no solid component within the tumor. The thin-walled, regular septa can usually be demonstrated by ultrasound. Color flow may be demonstrated within these septa, but is typically not increased.

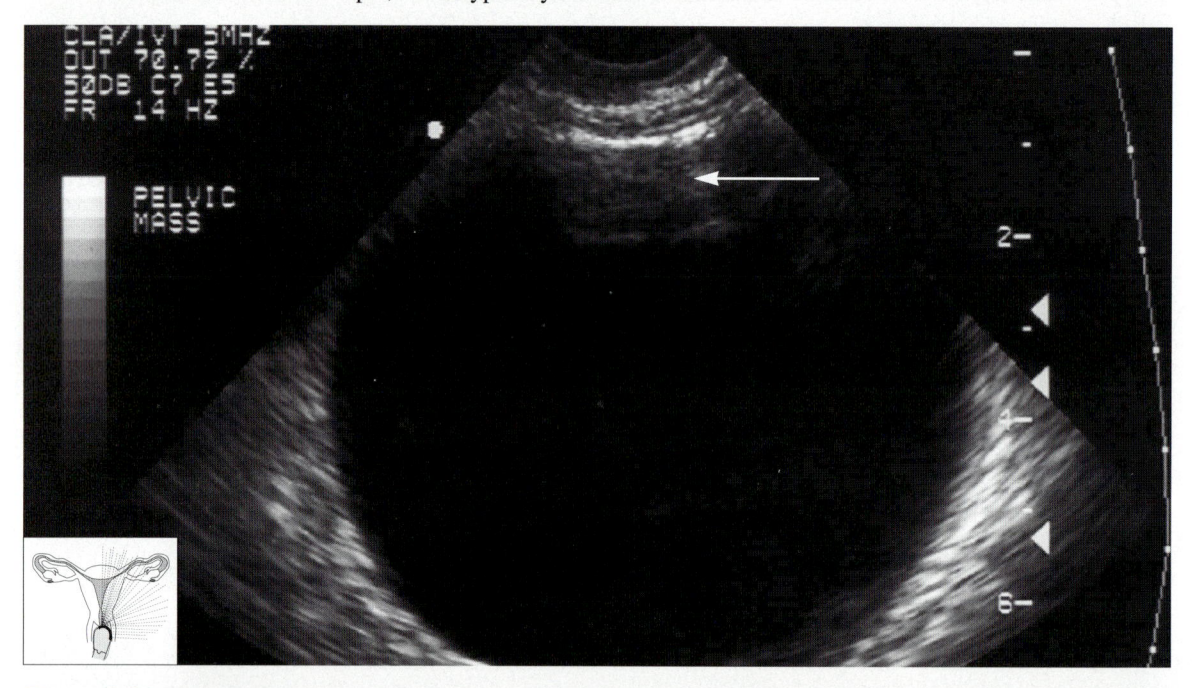

Figure 7-29. Large simple anechoic benign cyst. Near field or reverberation artifact (arrow) is seen in the proximal portion of the cyst.

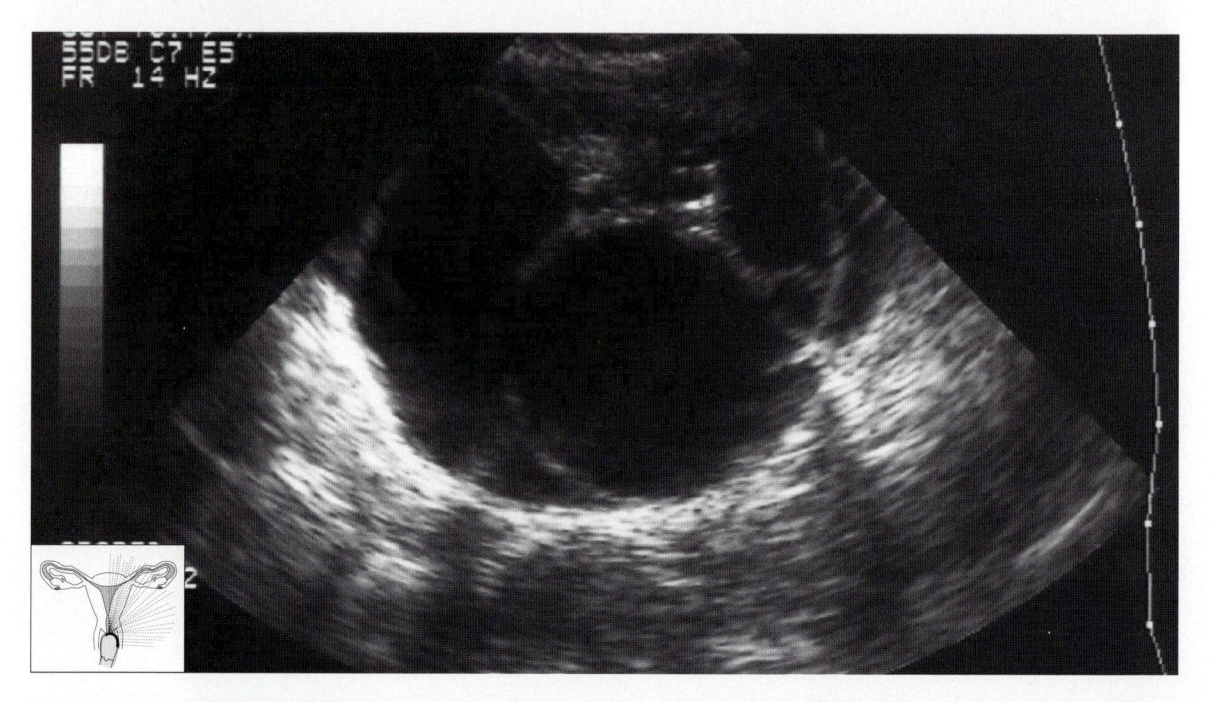

Figure 7-30. Multicystic mucinous cystadenoma. Cyst walls are thin, the solid portion has normal morphology, and the cysts are anechoic.

Ovary

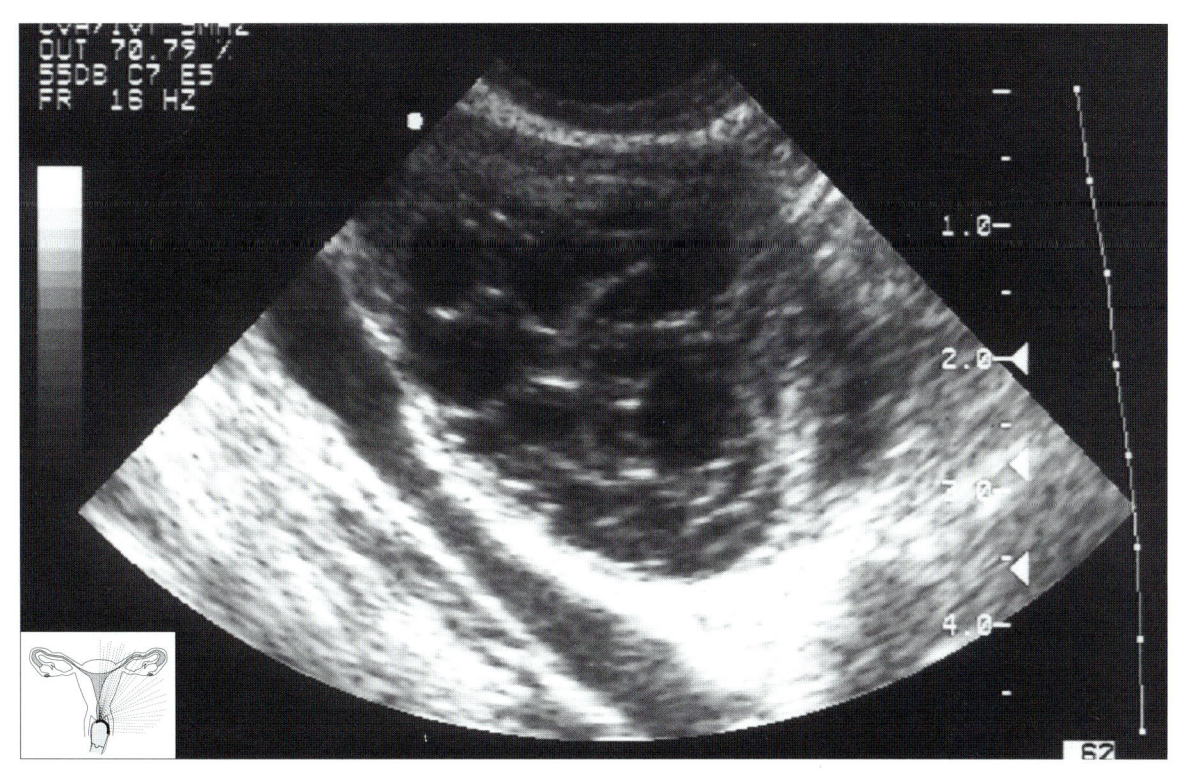

Figure 7-31. Small multicystic mucinous cystadenoma overlying iliac vein.

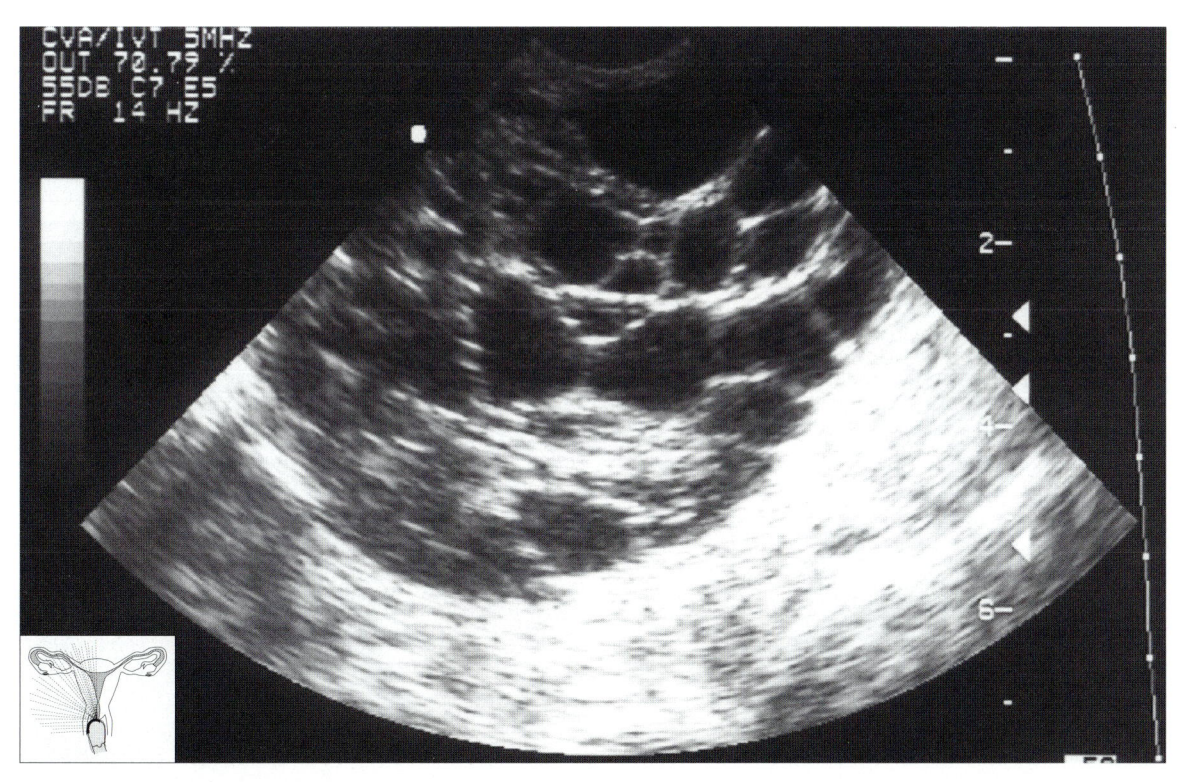

Figure 7-32. Honey-combed multicystic serous cystadenoma.

An Atlas of Transvaginal Sonography

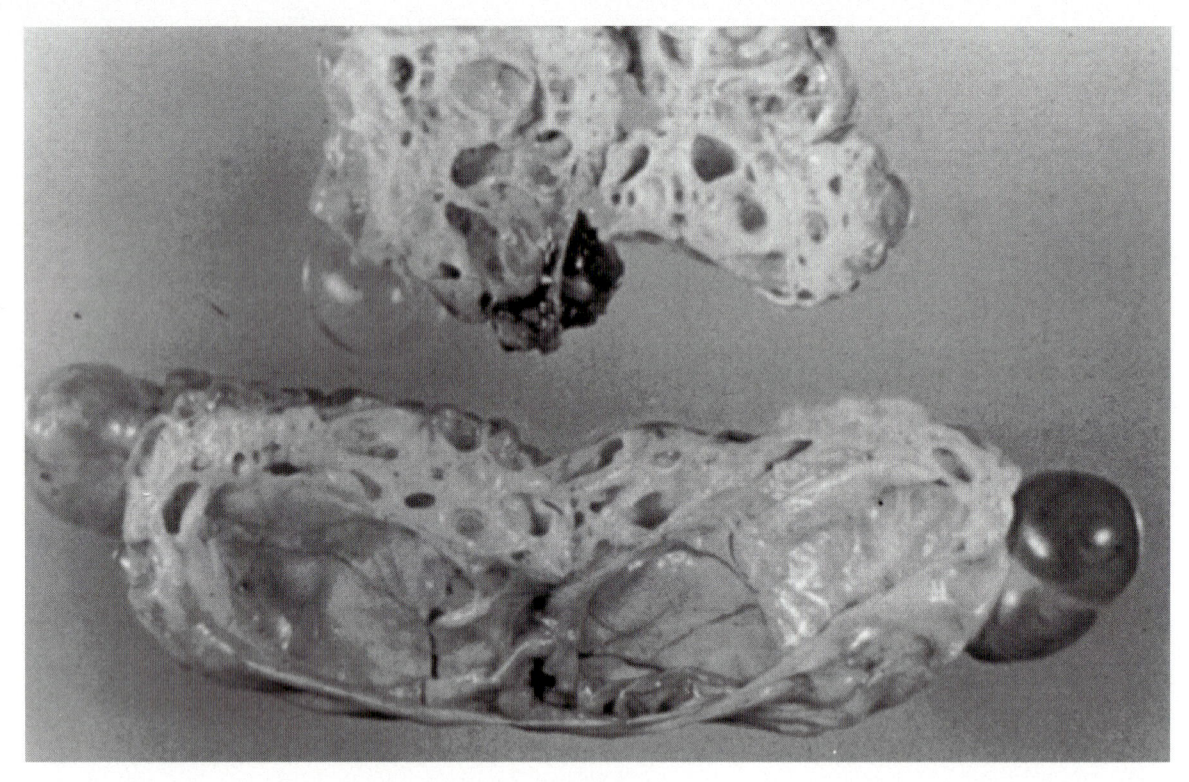

Figure 7-33. Honey-combed multicystic serous cystadenoma.

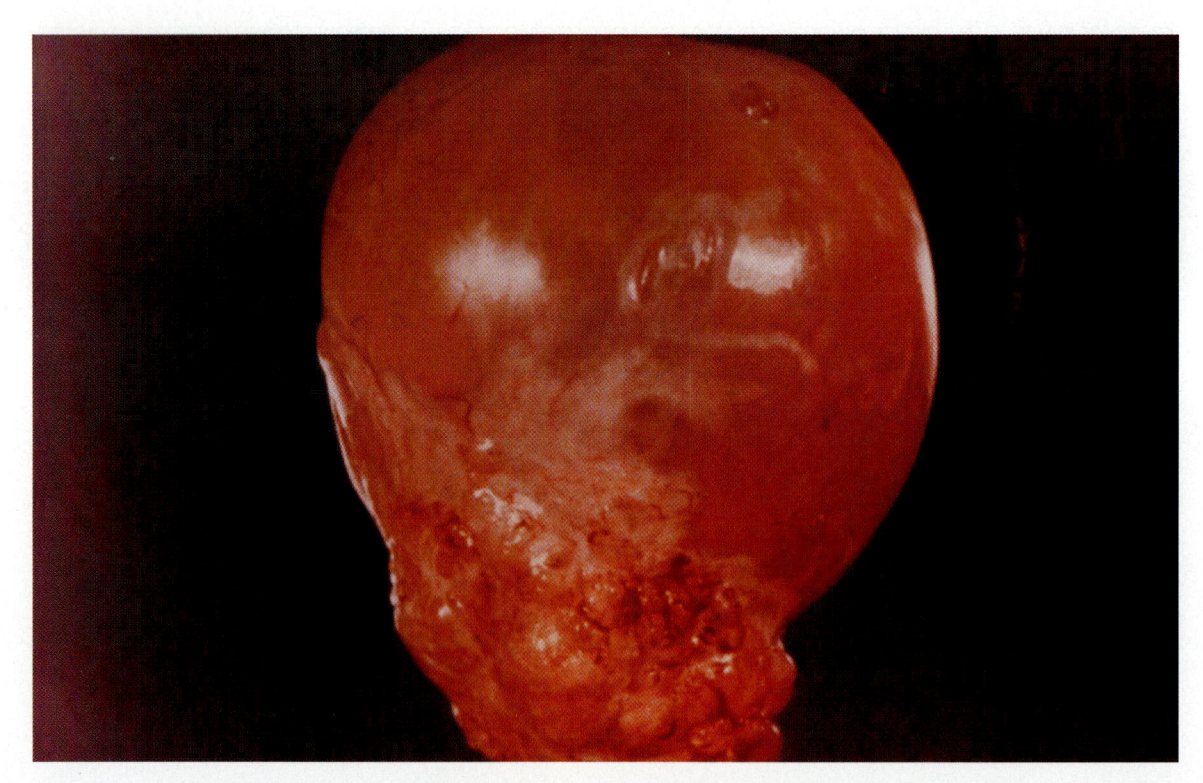

Figure 7-34. Simple cystic serous cystadenoma.

Ovary

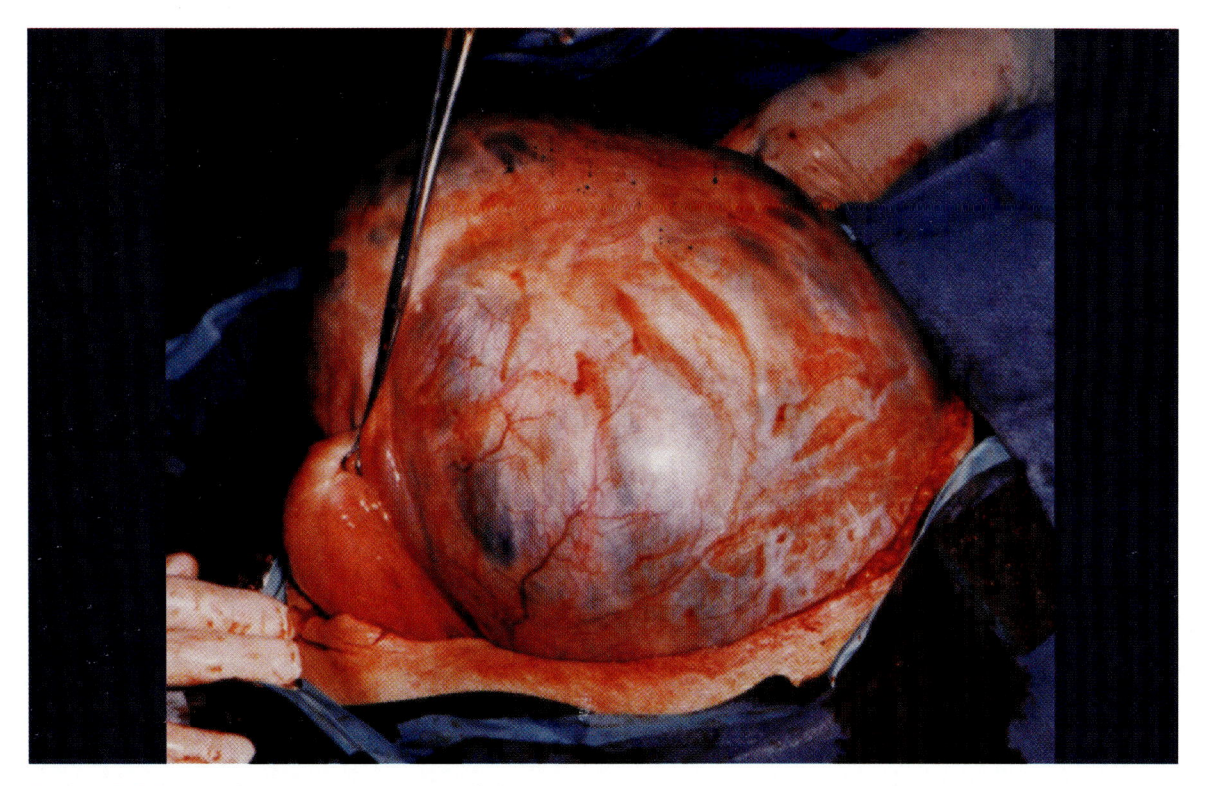

Figure 7-35. *Huge benign mucinous cystadenoma.*

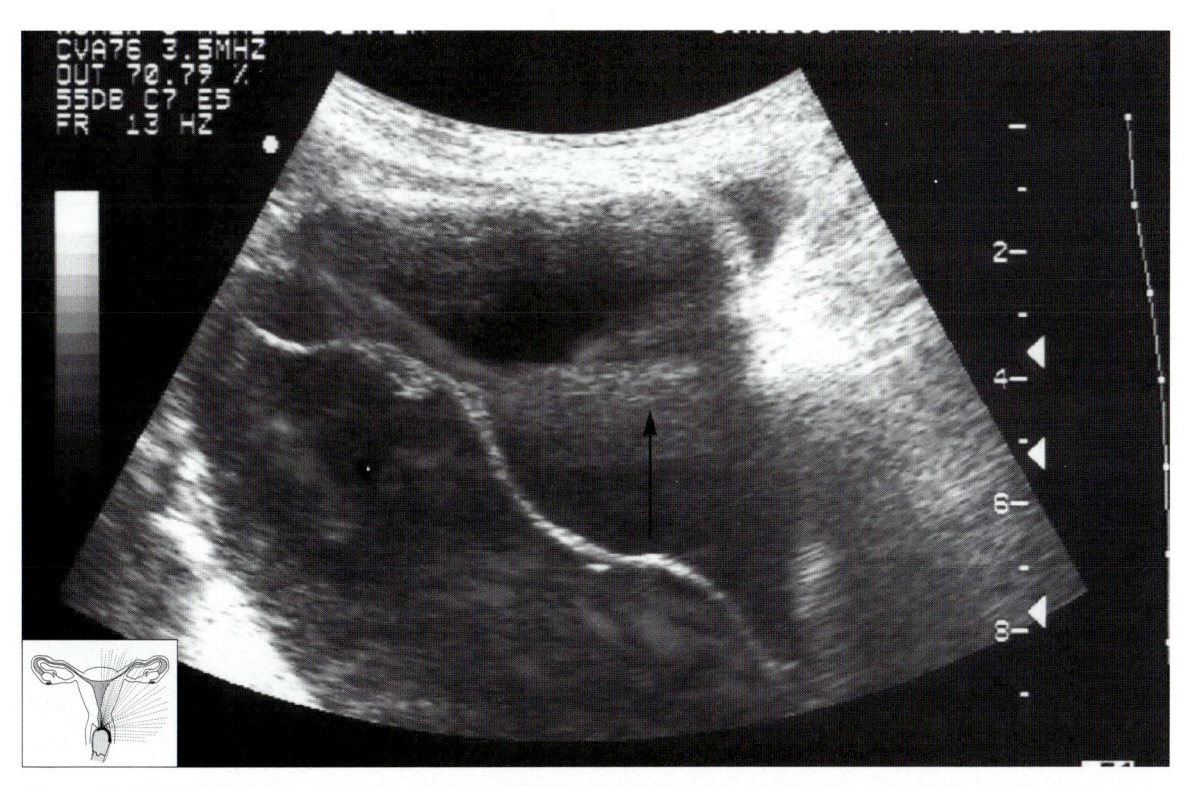

Figure 7-36. *Large cystic ovary with thin mobile septa. Reverberation artifact (arrow) mistakenly gives the impression of echoic cyst fluid.*

An Atlas of Transvaginal Sonography

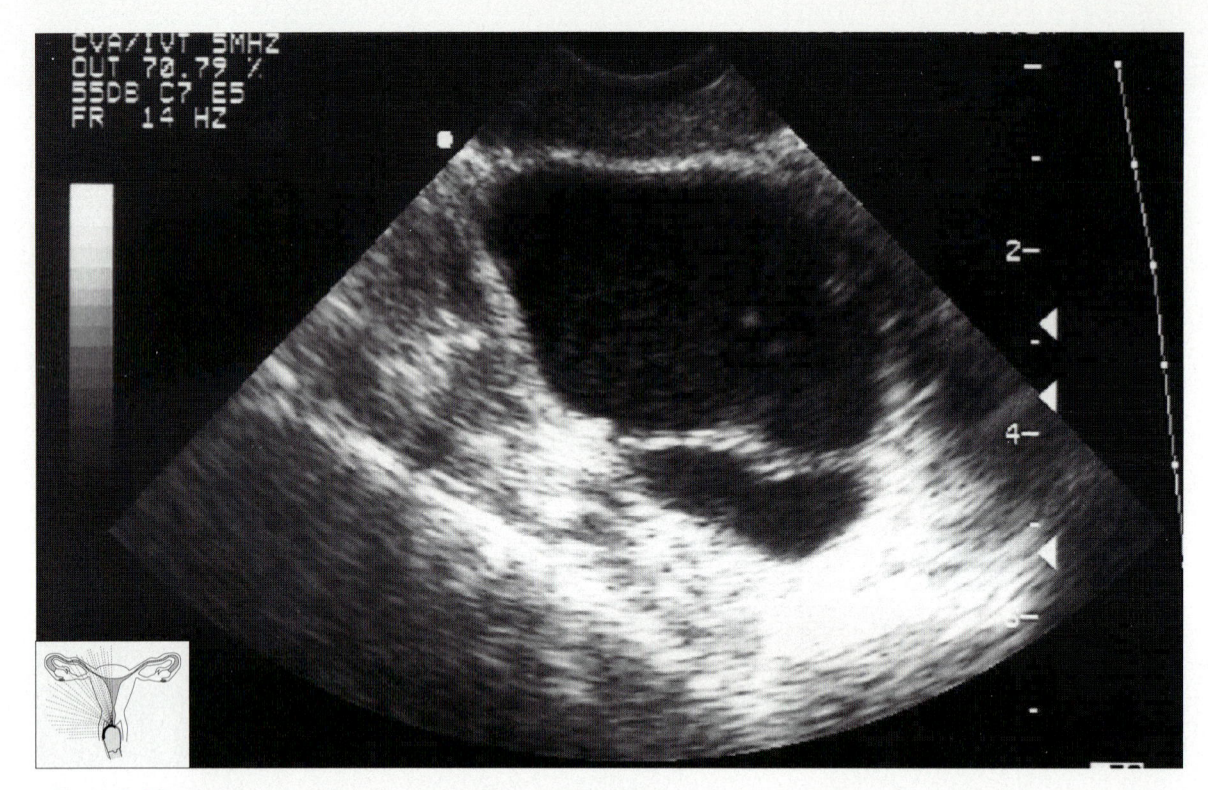

Figure 7-37. Thin septa in an otherwise simple ovarian cyst.

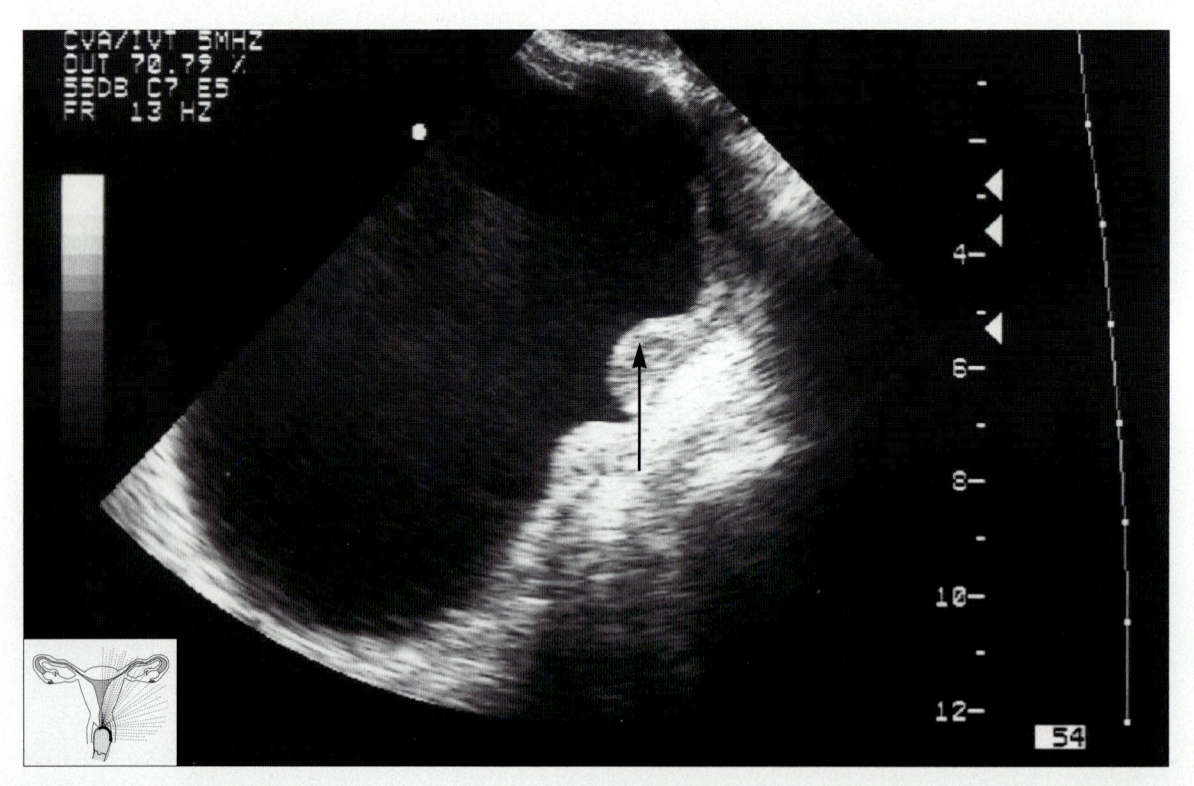

Figure 7-38. Large "simple" serous cystadenoma with a degree of thickening of the internal capsule (arrow). Color flow Doppler was negative.

Ovary

Mature Cystic Teratomas (Dermoid Cysts)

Mature cystic teratomas (dermoid cysts) are the most common type of teratoma and most common of all germ cell tumors. They are also one of the most common of all ovarian neoplasms, representing up to 10% in some series. Although it is commonly diagnosed during the reproductive years, it can be found during infancy, in postmenopausal women, and during pregnancy.

These cysts are composed of mature tissue derived from all the three germ cell layers, but predominantly ectoderm, and are completely benign. Any one of these mature cell layers can undergo malignant change, but it is rare. Malignant changes occur in < 2% of all cases and usually in postmenopausal women. Mature cystic teratomas are bilateral in 15% of cases. Grossly, they have a smooth, glistening surface and a soft consistency with solid areas on palpation. When sectioned, sebaceous material, hair, and teeth may be recognized. Within the cyst wall a dominant mass or nodule, Rokitansky's protuberance could be noted, usually in that part of the dermoid that contains cartilage or teeth.

Most dermoid cysts are asymptomatic. Complications include torsion and rupture with chemical peritonitis. Unusual complications include infection, usually with salmonellae or coliform bacteria, autoimmune hemolytic anemia, which resolves following surgical resection, and malignant transformation.

Scan Findings

These tumors have a characteristic sonographic pattern of sharply defined fluid levels (lipid), dense echoes (hair and teeth), and cystic areas. As dermoids typically contain fatty material, distal acoustical shadowing is often seen. Large fatty dermoids may blend into the background of bowel gas and a clear sonographic image may be difficult to obtain. Except in the rare metabolically active dermoids, color flow is either normal or absent.

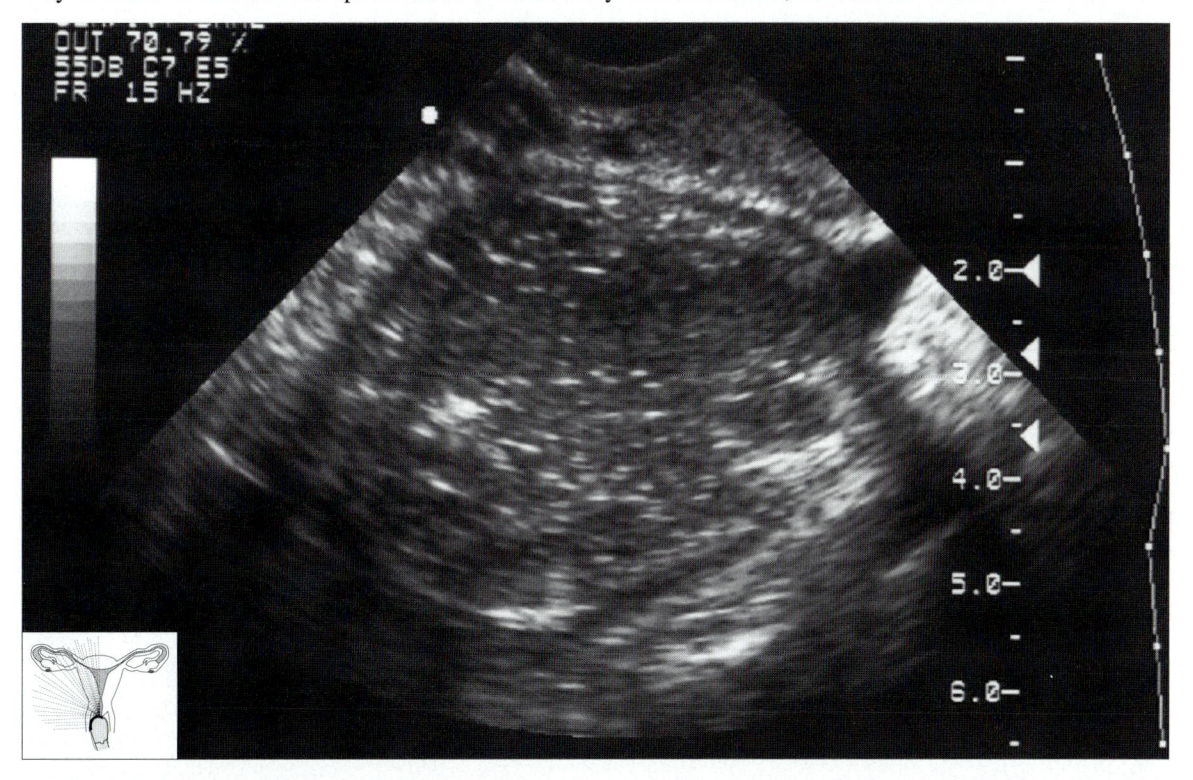

Figure 7-39. Mixed echogenic ovarian dermoid cyst.

An Atlas of Transvaginal Sonography

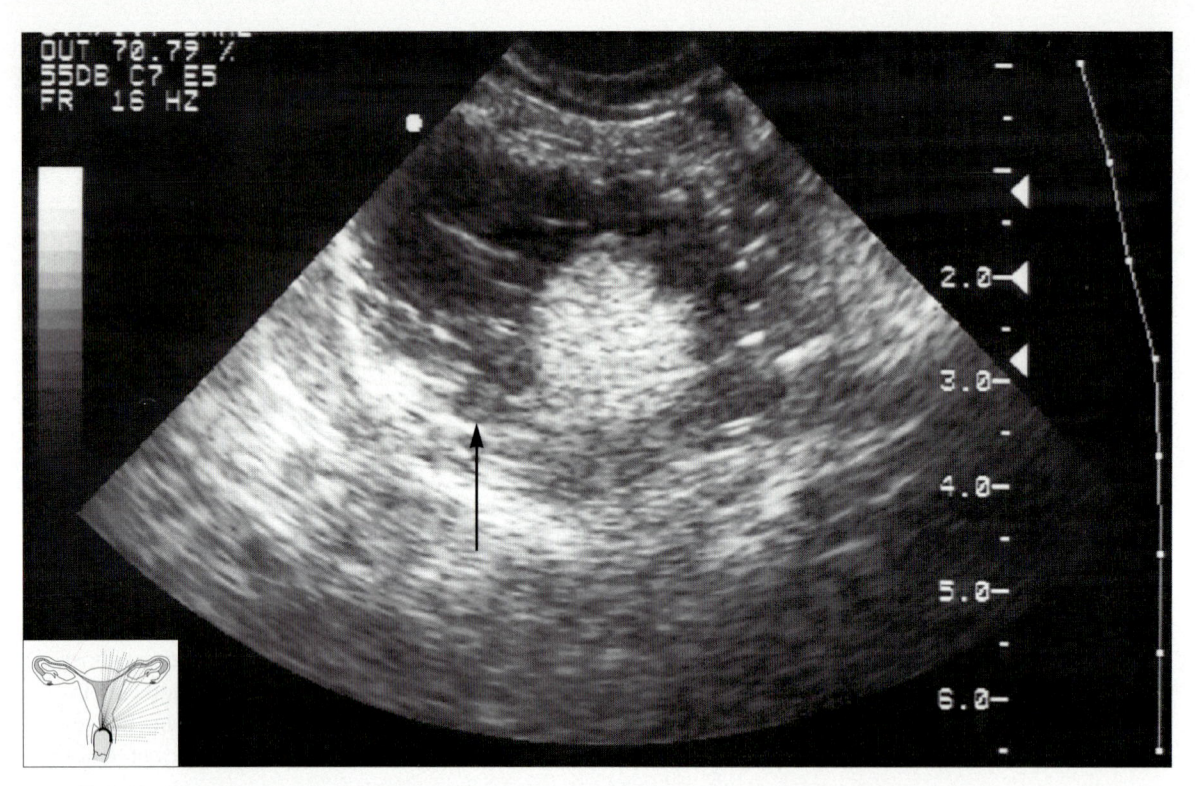

Figure 7-40. Ovarian dermoid cyst demonstrating central echoic area, corresponding to sebaceous material. "Dirty echoes" from within the dermoid (arrow) result in an obscuring of the posterior wall.

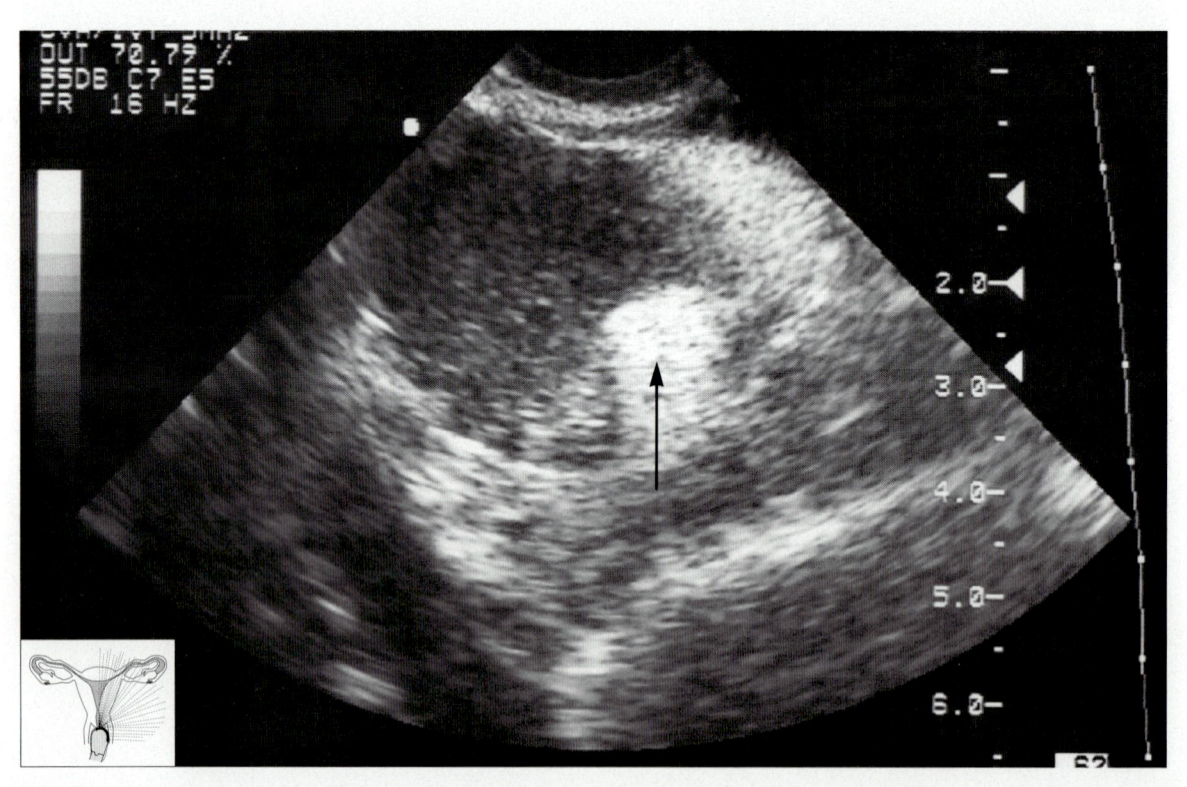

Figure 7-41. Rokitansky's protuberance (arrow), seen as an echogenic region on the lower margin of this dermoid cyst.

Ovary

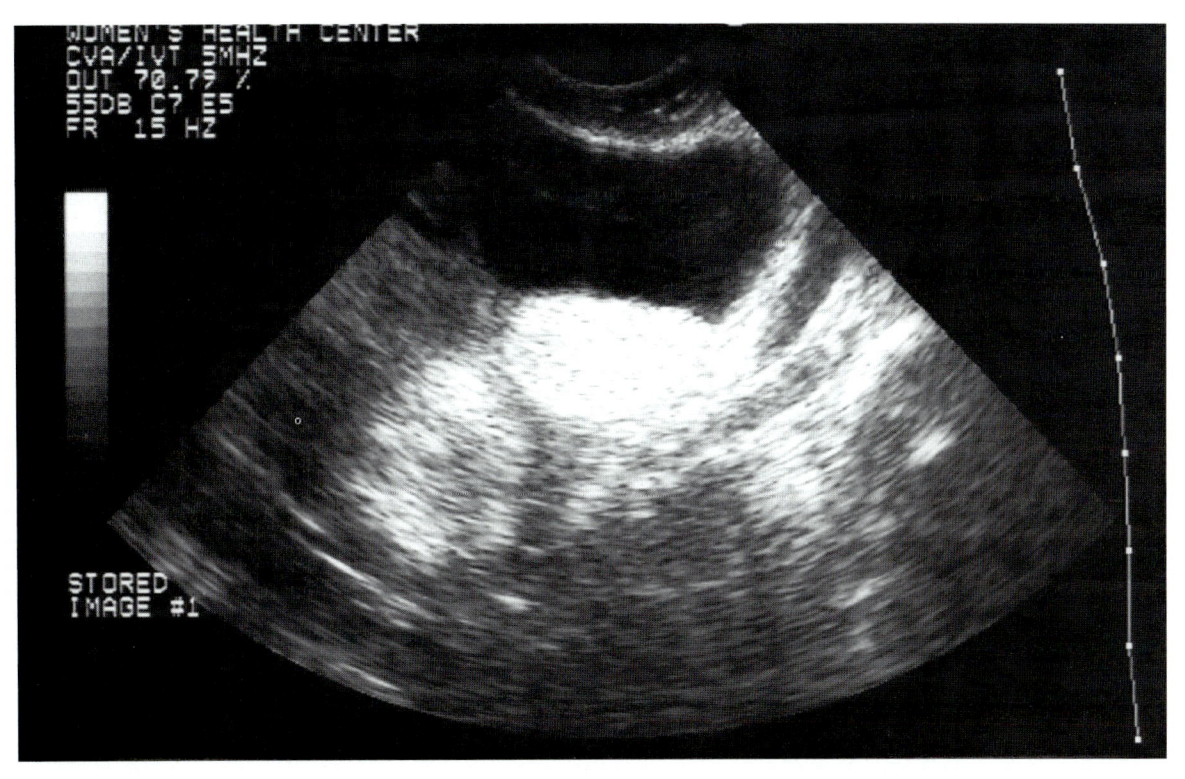

Figure 7-43. A combination of fatty and sebaceous material results in the mixed echogenic appearance of this dermoid cyst.

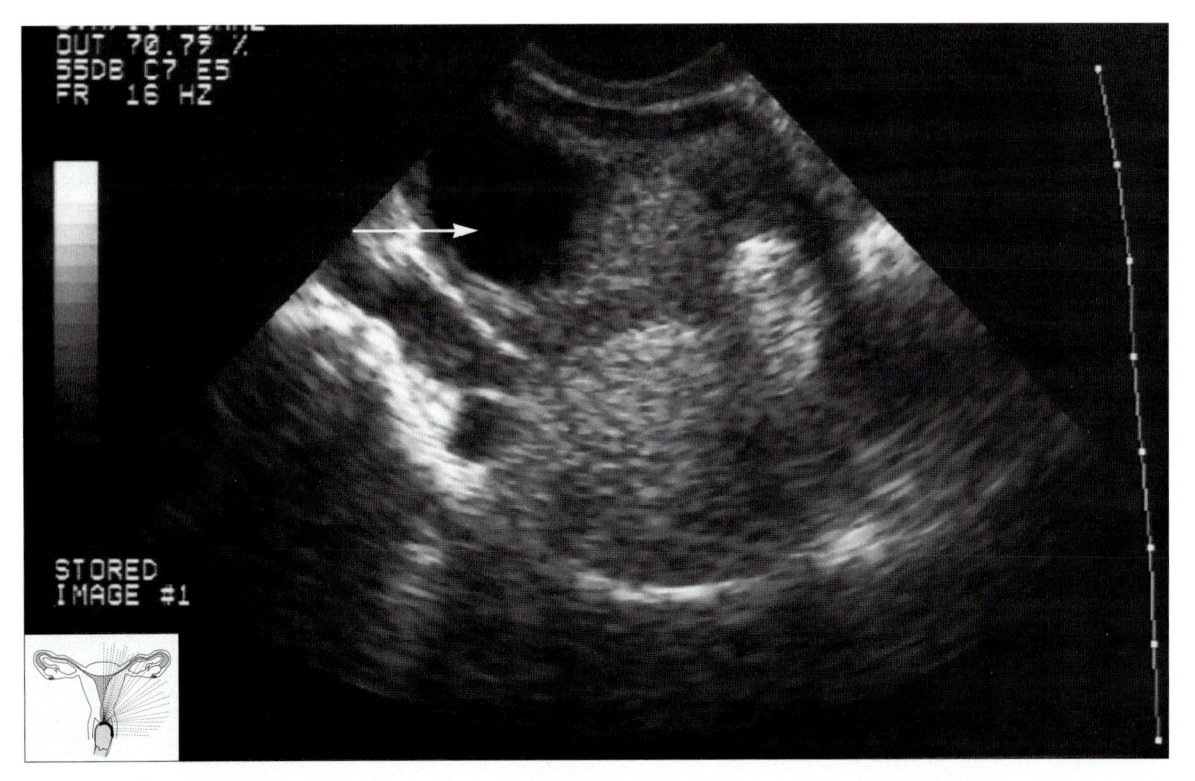

Figure 7-43. Corpus luteal cyst (arrow) arising from functioning normal ovarian tissue around this dermoid cyst.

An Atlas of Transvaginal Sonography

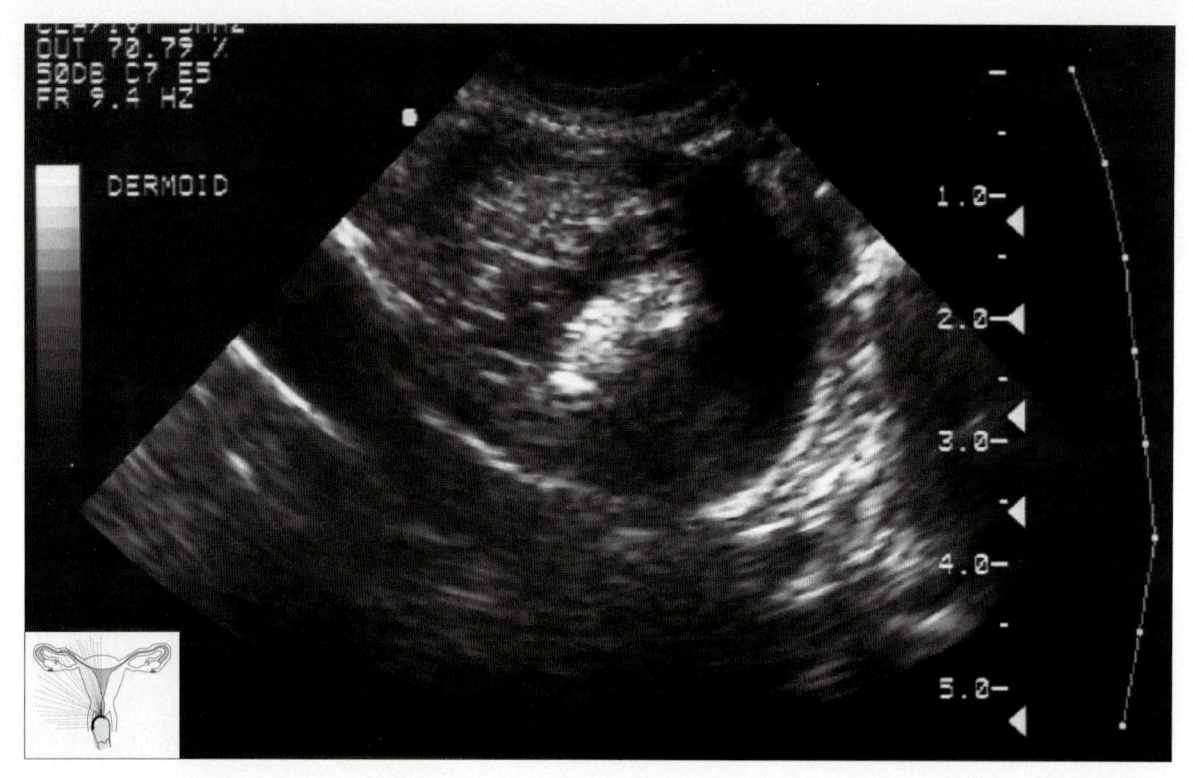

Figure 7-44. Mixed echogenic dermoid cyst overlying iliac vein.

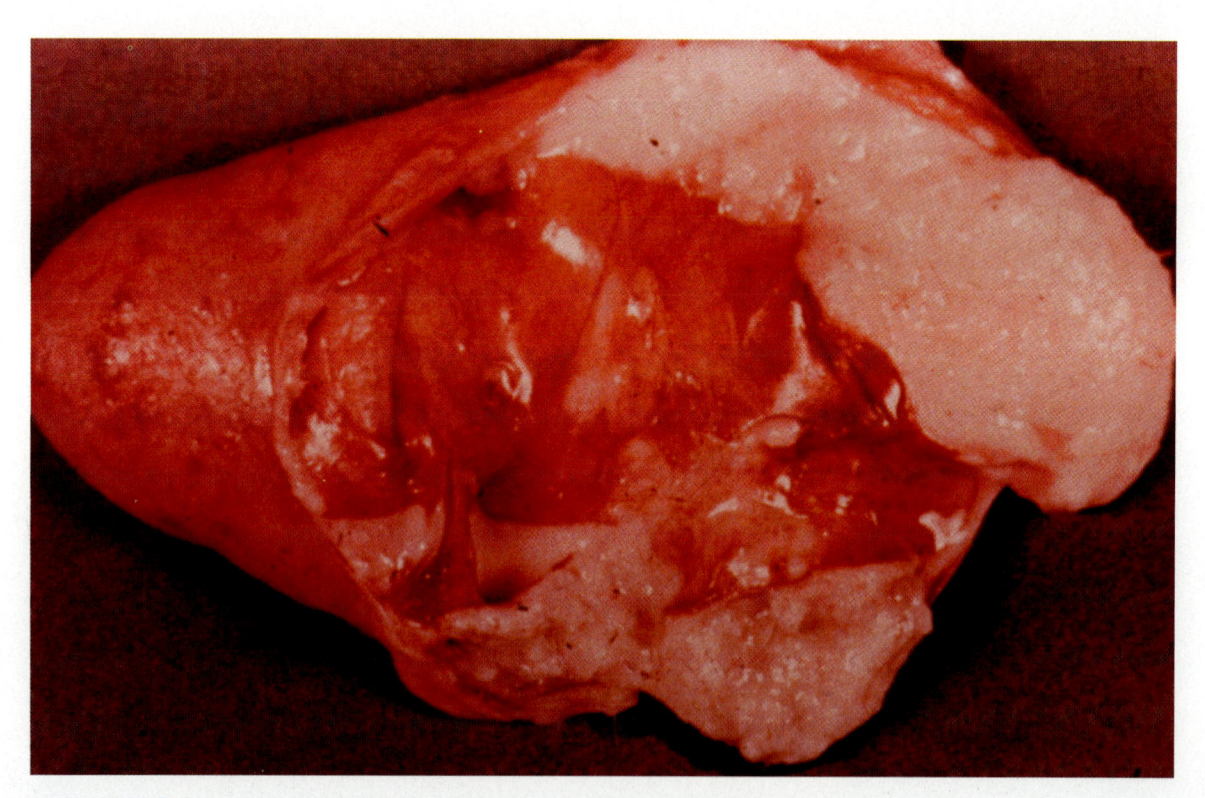

Figure 7-45. Ovarian dermoid, demonstrating thick sebaceous material.

Ovary

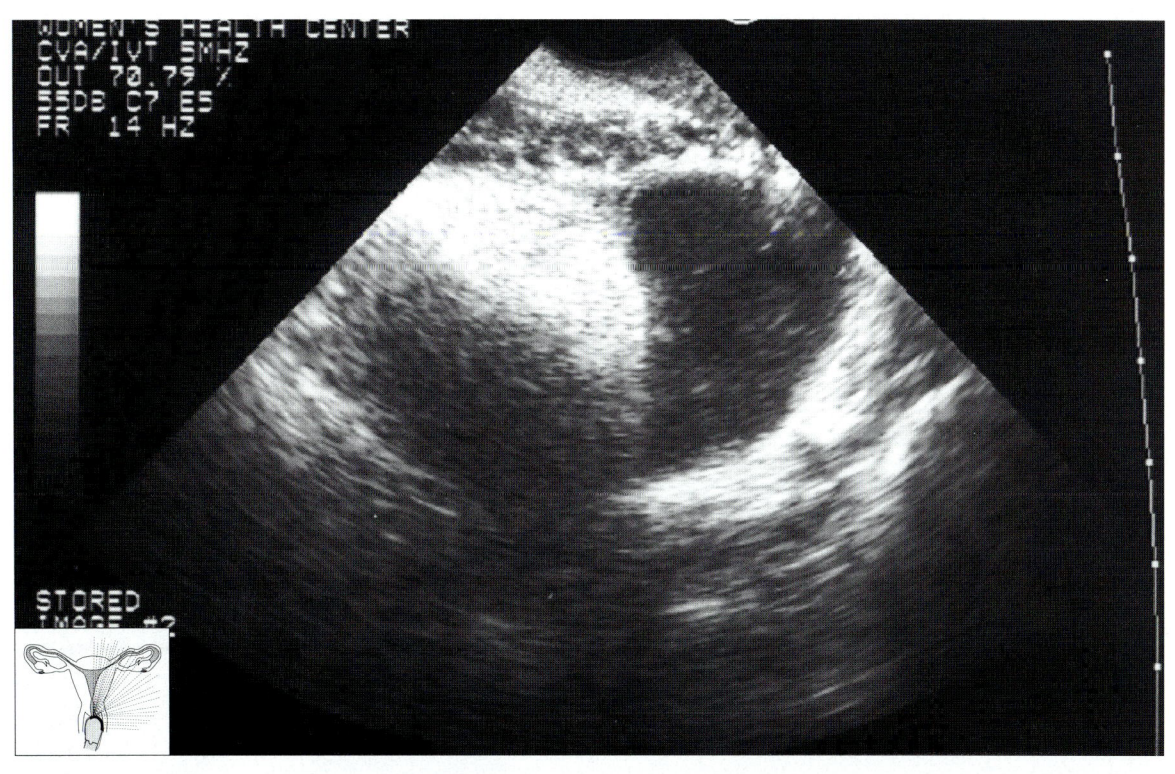

Figure 7-46. *Echogenic fatty material layered out in this ovarian dermoid cyst.*

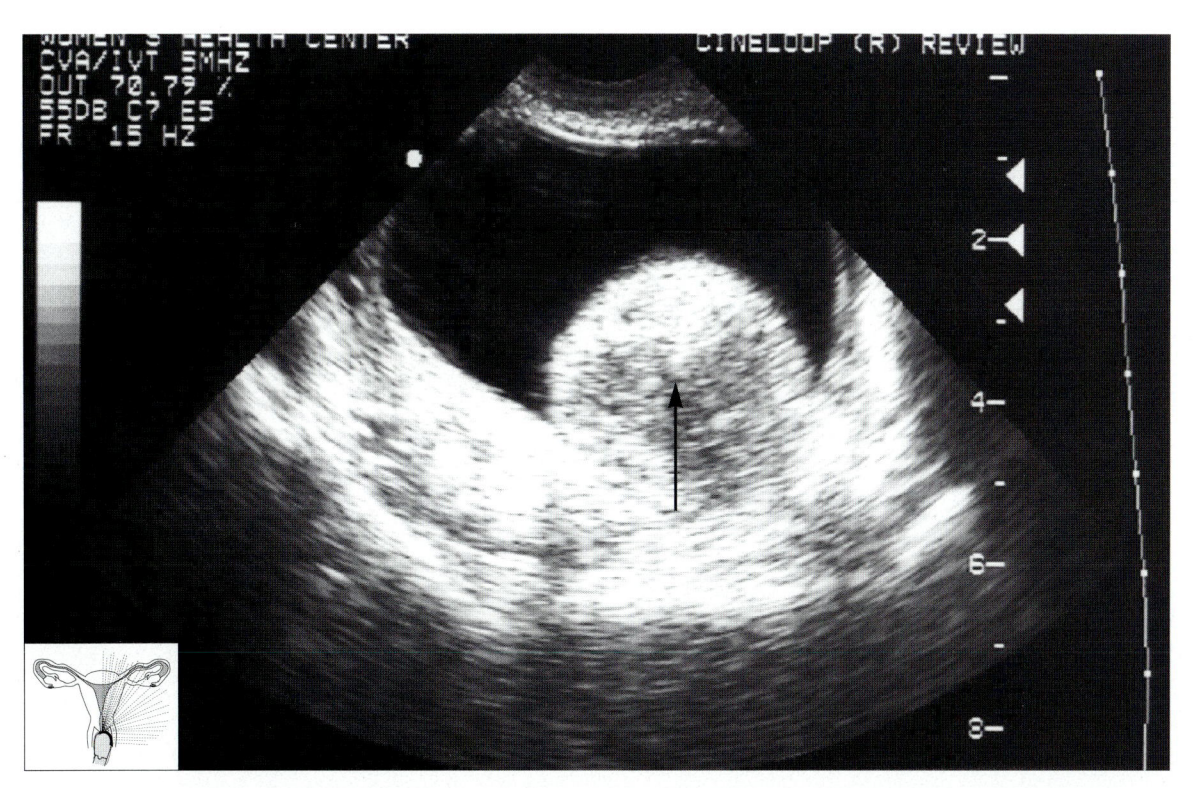

Figure 7-47. *Complex ovarian tumor containing a mucinous cystadenoma, and echogenic solid component (arrow), confirmed to be a dermoid.*

Paraovarian Cysts

Paraovarian cysts are simple cystic structures that arise in the broad ligament and are derived from either paramesonephric (Mullerian) or mesonephric (Wolffian) duct remnants. A smaller percentage arise as simple peritoneal inclusion cysts. Most are asymptomatic and are usually diagnosed on routine pelvic examination. Only rarely do they become complicated.

Scan Findings

Ultrasound reveals a simple anechoic cyst that can be confused with a functional ovarian cyst. Paraovarian cysts can be demonstrated to move independently of the adjacent ovary by gently balloting the cyst with the vaginal transducer.

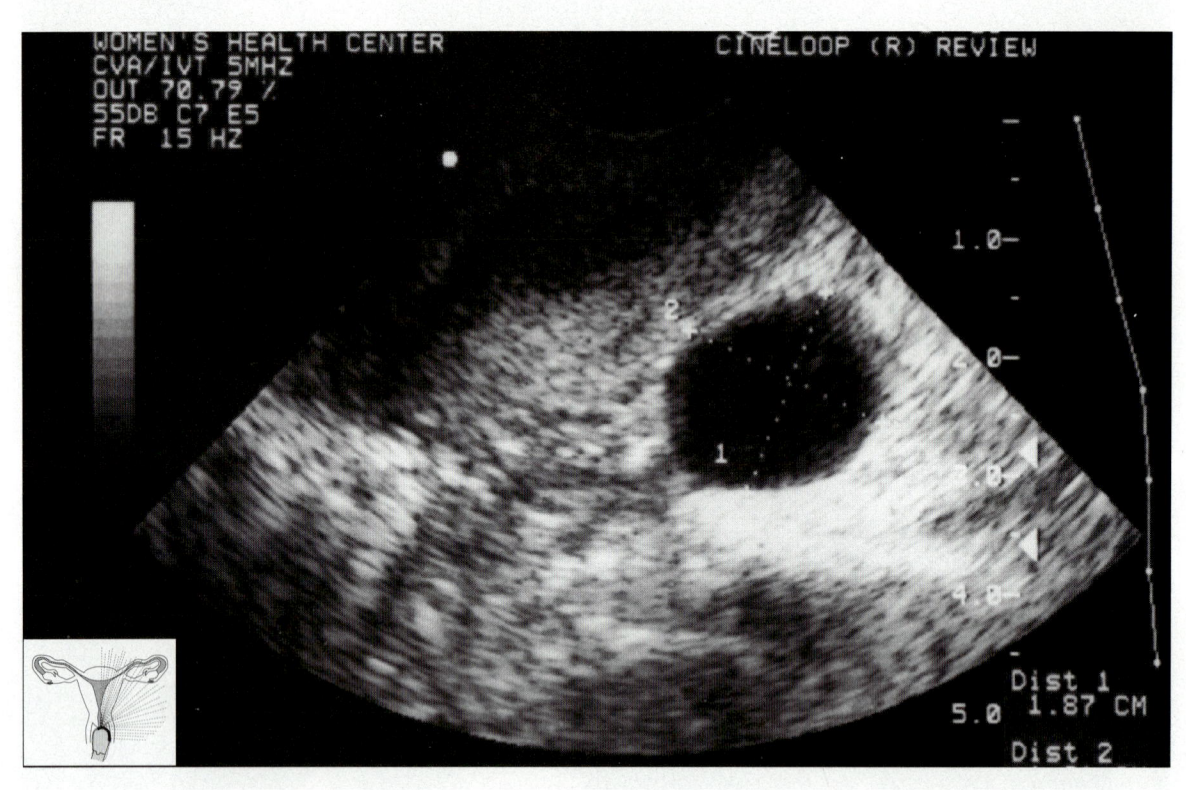

Figure 7-48. Small cystic structure on pelvic side wall is consistent with an ovarian cyst or para ovarian cyst.

Ovary

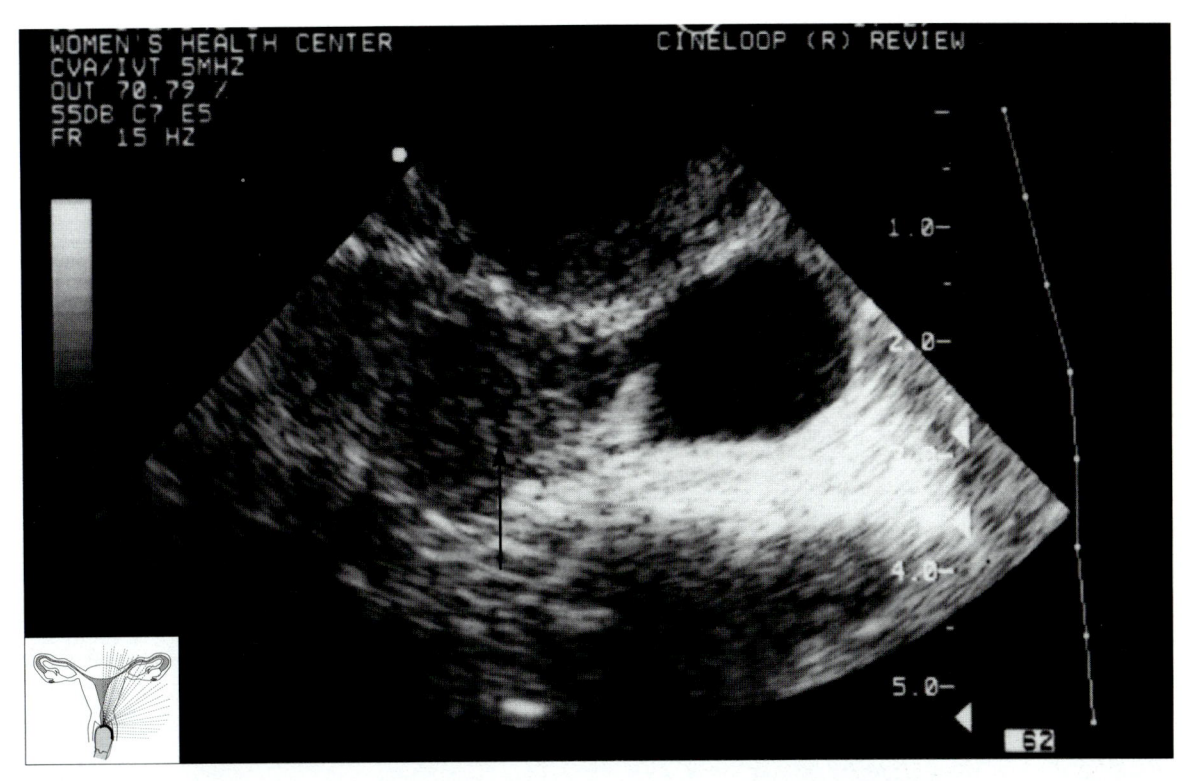

Figure 7-49. *The para ovarian cyst is clearly separate from the ovary (arrow) on the left.*

An Atlas of Transvaginal Sonography

Theca-Lutein Cysts

Theca-lutein cysts are non-neoplastic sonolucent ovarian enlargements consisting of multiple grossly enlarged follicular cysts that contain luteinized theca cells. They are probably the result of excessive stimulation by high levels of hCG from (1) molar pregnancies, (2) Pergonal for ovarian stimulation, (3) multiple pregnancy, severe hypertensive disease of pregnancy (HDP) or Rh isoimmunization. Severe cases can be associated with ascites, pleural effusions and cardiovascular collapse.

Scan Findings

Sonography reveals large, tender, multicystic ovaries with ascites. Color flow tends to be prominent and can paradoxically reveal increased diastolic flow and abnormally low PI and RI. They have a similar appearance to hyperstimulated ovaries.

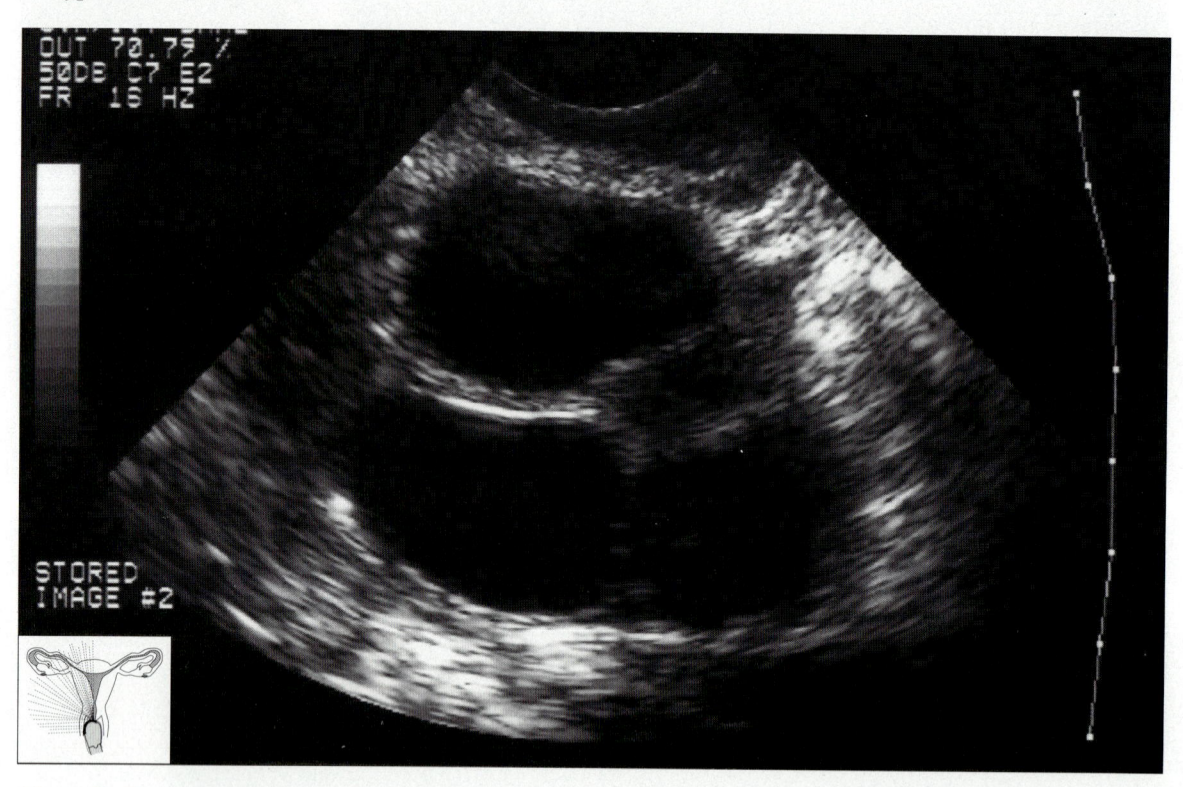

Figure 7-50. A large polycystic theca luteal cyst. It is similar in appearance to a hyperstimulated ovary.

Ovary

Ovarian Torsion

A mobile ovary may rotate on its vascular pedicle resulting in ischemic necrosis and ultimate infarction. Ovarian torsion can be confused with tender, swollen, simple ovarian cysts or hemorrhagic cysts.

Scan Findings

Sonographically the ovary is enlarged, tender to "palpation" by the vaginal transducer and charatcristically will be devoid of blood flow on color flow Doppler. Unfortunately, these criteria are not pathognomonic, as the ovary has a dual blood supply, from the adnexal branch of the uterine artery and the ovarian artery. Torsion affecting only one of these arterial supplies can result in the presence of arterial flow on color flow Doppler.

Solid Ovarian Tumors

Solid ovarian tumors should be considered malignant until proved otherwise, regardless of patient age. Tumors that are cystic and solid also have a much greater chance of being malignant than cystic tumors and should be considered sufficient indication for exploratory laparotomy. There are several solid or partly solid ovarian neoplasms that are not malignant and are common. They include the ovarian fibromas, germ cell tumors, and the metastatic ovarian cancers.

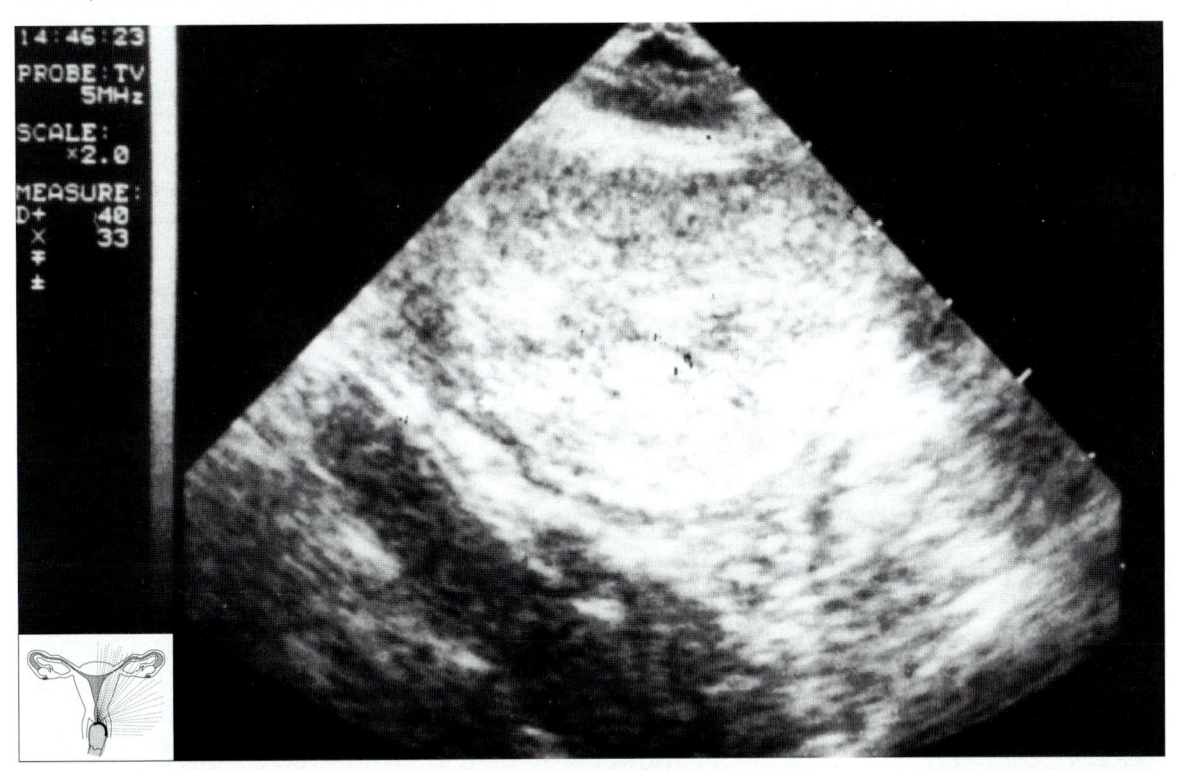

Figure 7-51. Solid echogenic ovarian tumor overlying iliac vein.

An Atlas of Transvaginal Sonography

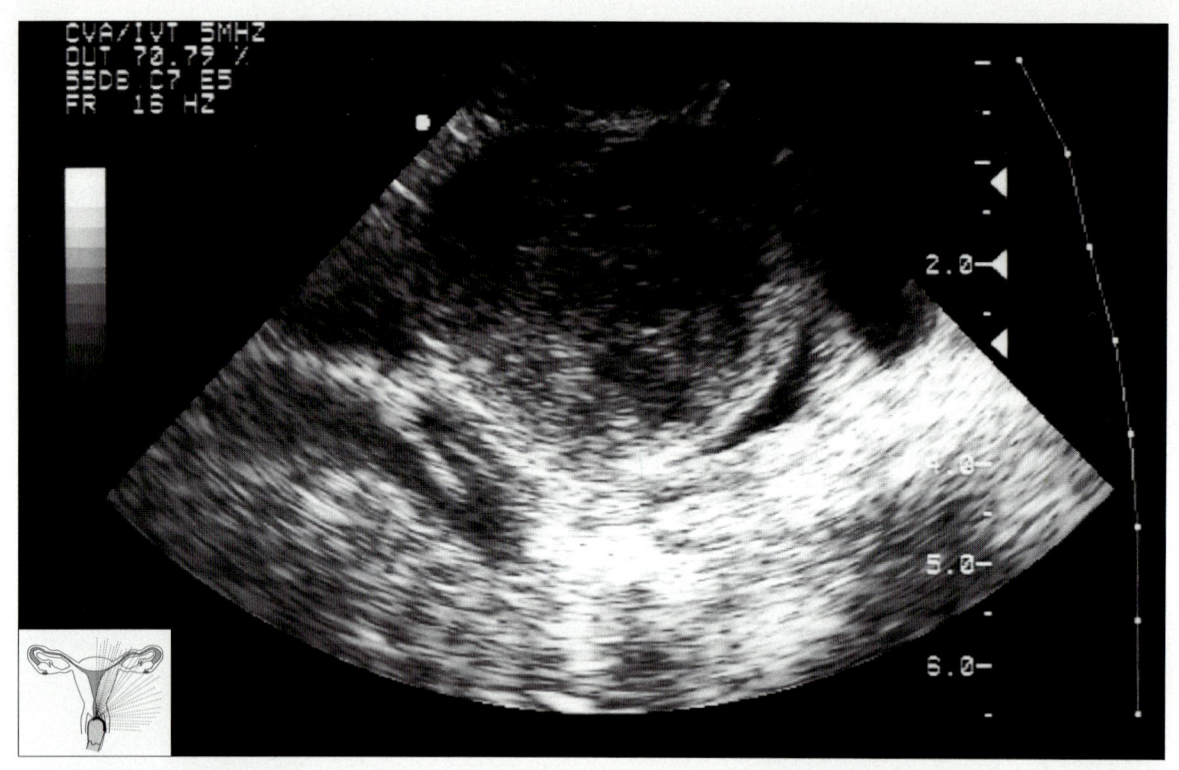

Figure 7-52. Solid ovarian dysgerminoma, demonstrating mixed echogenicity.

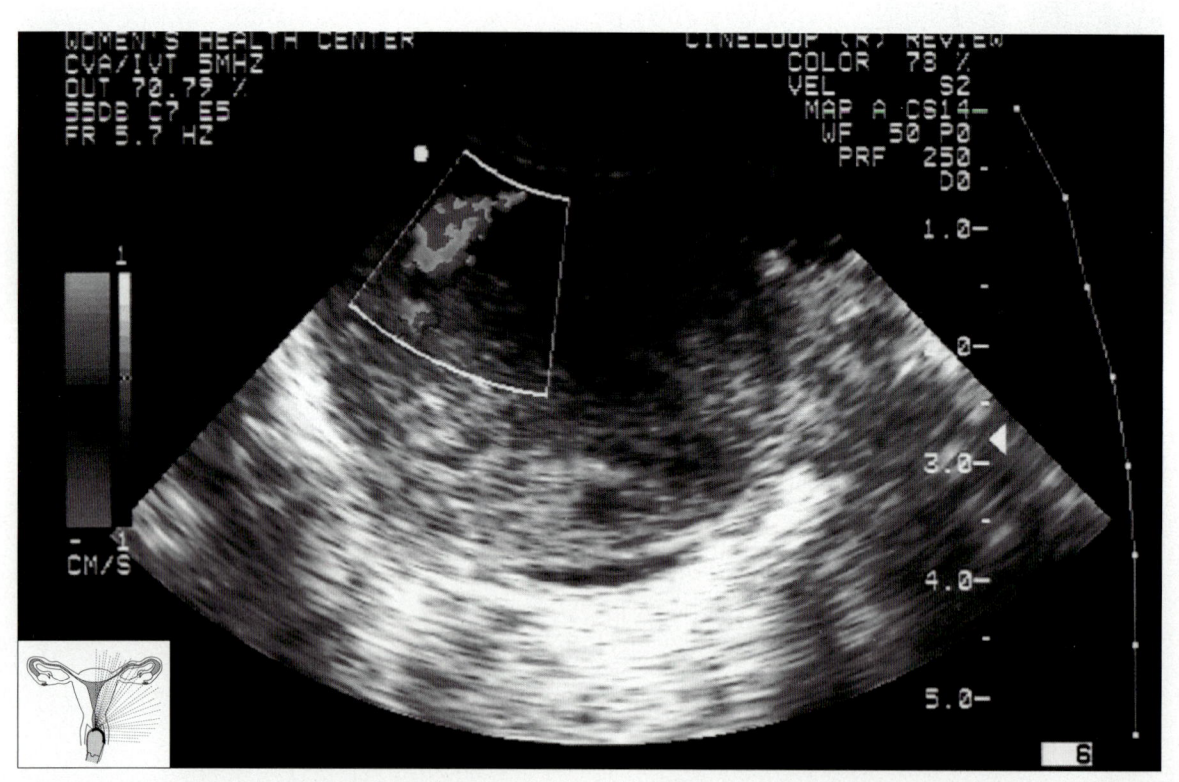

Figure 7-53. Color flow Doppler reveals essentially peripheral flow.

Fibroma

Ovarian fibromas are the most common solid benign ovarian tumor, accounting for 20% of all solid ovarian tumors. Most ovarian fibromas are detected on routine clinical examination. They rarely are larger than 6-8 cm, and only 10% are bilateral. These tumors are not hormonally active. Calcification may be noted on KUB. Five percent of ovarian fibromas are associated with Meigs' syndrome, characterized by the presence of ascites and right-sided hydrothorax, which resolves following resection of the fibroma.

Scan Findings

Ultrasound demonstrates a smooth, solid ovarian tumor, although a cystic area may be noted if fibromas attain great size and portions of the tumor undergo necrosis and liquefaction. Ascites may be seen in cases of Meigs' syndrome.

Germ Cell Tumors

Germ cell tumors comprise a group of tumors derived from primitive germ cells. These tumors typically affect young women and girls. The younger the woman, the greater likelihood the tumor is malignant.

Scan Findings

Germ cell tumors are usually solid or complex ovarian tumors that may be bilateral if dysgerminoma is the tumor type. The internal morphology is variable, depending on histologic type. Color flow Doppler reveals increased color flow and analysis of the spectral wave form confirms spectral broadening and low polsatelety and resistance indices.

Metastatic Ovarian Tumors

The ovary is commonly the site of metastic spread from malignancies originating in the colon, stomach or breast. These metastases are often referred to as Krukenberg's tumors, but this is, in fact, a histologic diagnosis.

Scan Findings

Characteristically, the ovaries are enlarged and irregular. The ovaries have a solid internal morphology, but rarely they have a cystic component. The disease process tends to affect both ovaries and the presence of ascites is common. Color flow Doppler confirms increased flow, while analysis of the spectral waveform confirms spectral broadening and resultant pulsatility and resistance indices.

An Atlas of Transvaginal Sonography

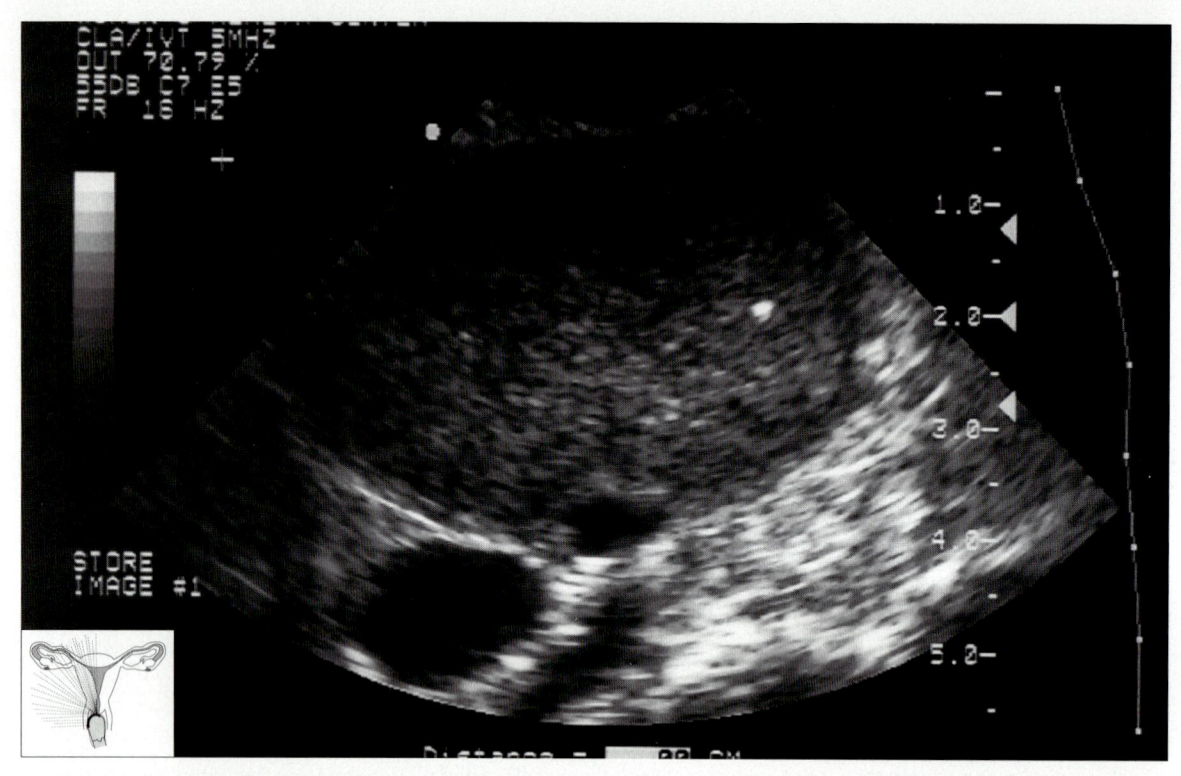

Figure 7-54. *Ovarian fibroma. Sonographically, it has a similar appearance to uterine fibroids.*

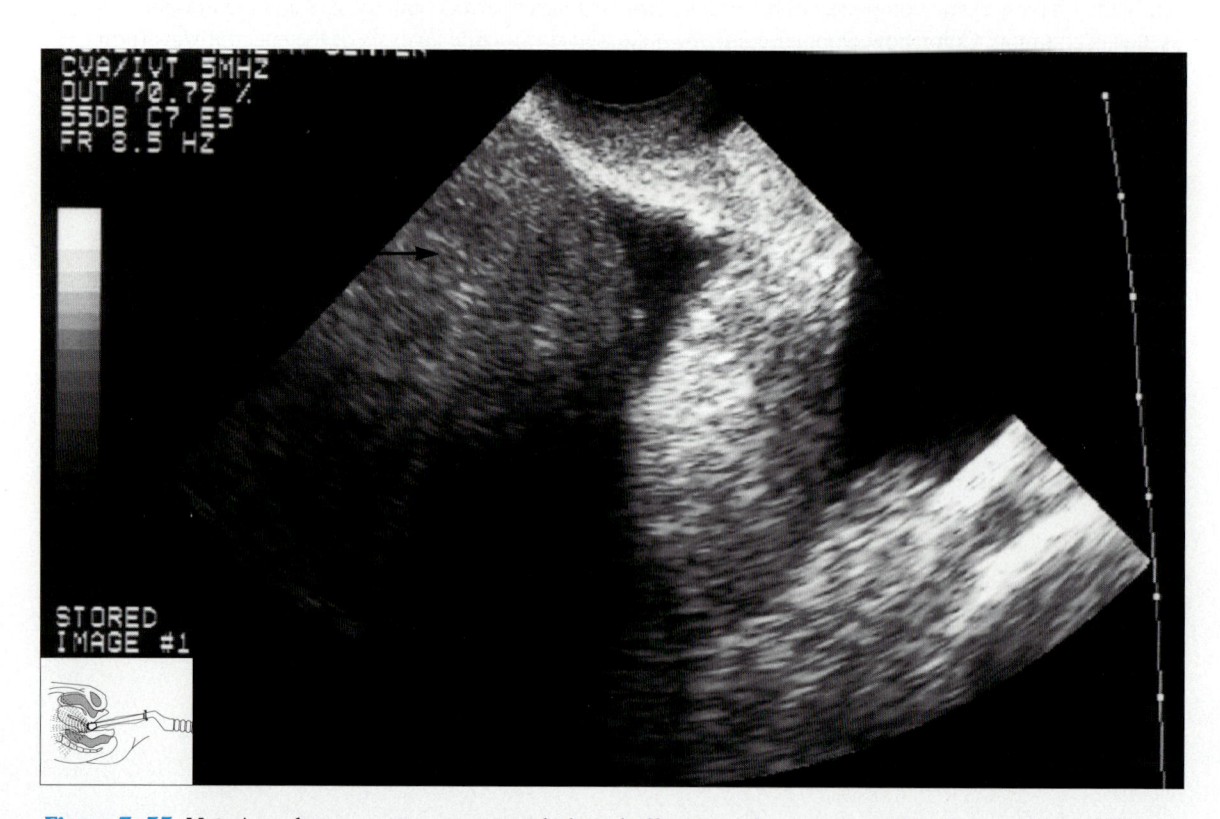

Figure 7-55. *Meigs' syndrome, ascites, associated pleural effusion with an ovarian fibrothecoma (arrow). The uterus is retroverted and appears to be suspended within the ascitic fluid.*

8   Normal Early Pregnancy

Due to the higher frequency transducers and their proximity to the pelvic organs, transvaginal sonography is able to identify embryonic developmental milestones approximately one week earlier than transabdominal sonography.

Fetal Development

The first sonographic appearance suggestive of intrauterine pregnancy is thickening of the choriodecidua, which occurs at about four weeks. Around five weeks the chorionic sac is visible as a small hypoechoic area, surrounded by the echogenic choriodecidua. This corresponds to a ß-hCG titer of 500 mIU/ml (2nd Int Stand). At five-six weeks the yolk sac/embryo complex can be seen within the gestational sac. Fetal heart motion can be detected by TVS in embryos that are over 5 mm or five-six weeks gestation. Initially slow in early pregnancy (70-90 beats per minute), the fetal heart rate increases during the first trimester to 120 beats per minute by 8-10 weeks gestation. Between six-eight weeks, fetal movement can be depicted, consisting of flexion and extension of the body and extremities. At around seven weeks the rhombencephalon appears as a hypoechoic area within the posterior aspect of the fetal head, corresponding to the developing fourth ventricle. The normal physiologic herniation of the small intestines occurs at eight-nine weeks and should have spontaneously regressed by the end of the first trimester.

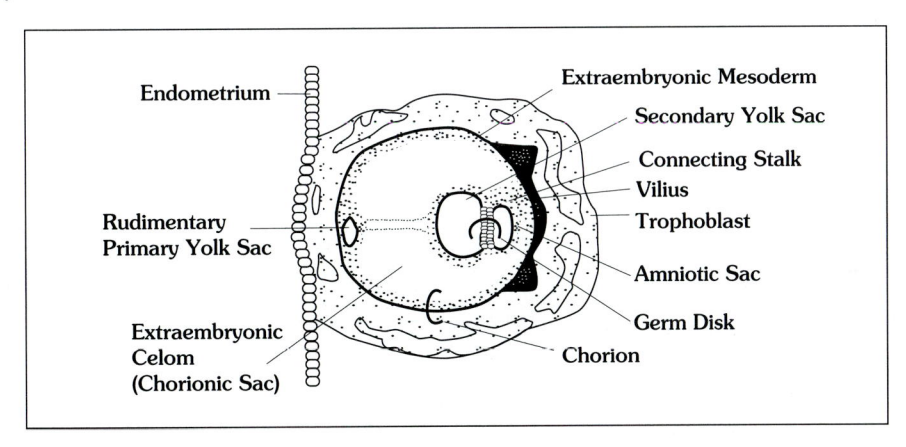

Figure 8-1. Blastocyst at approximately 14 days post-menstruation with remnants of the primary yolk sac and the newly formed secondary yolk sac.

An Atlas of Transvaginal Sonography

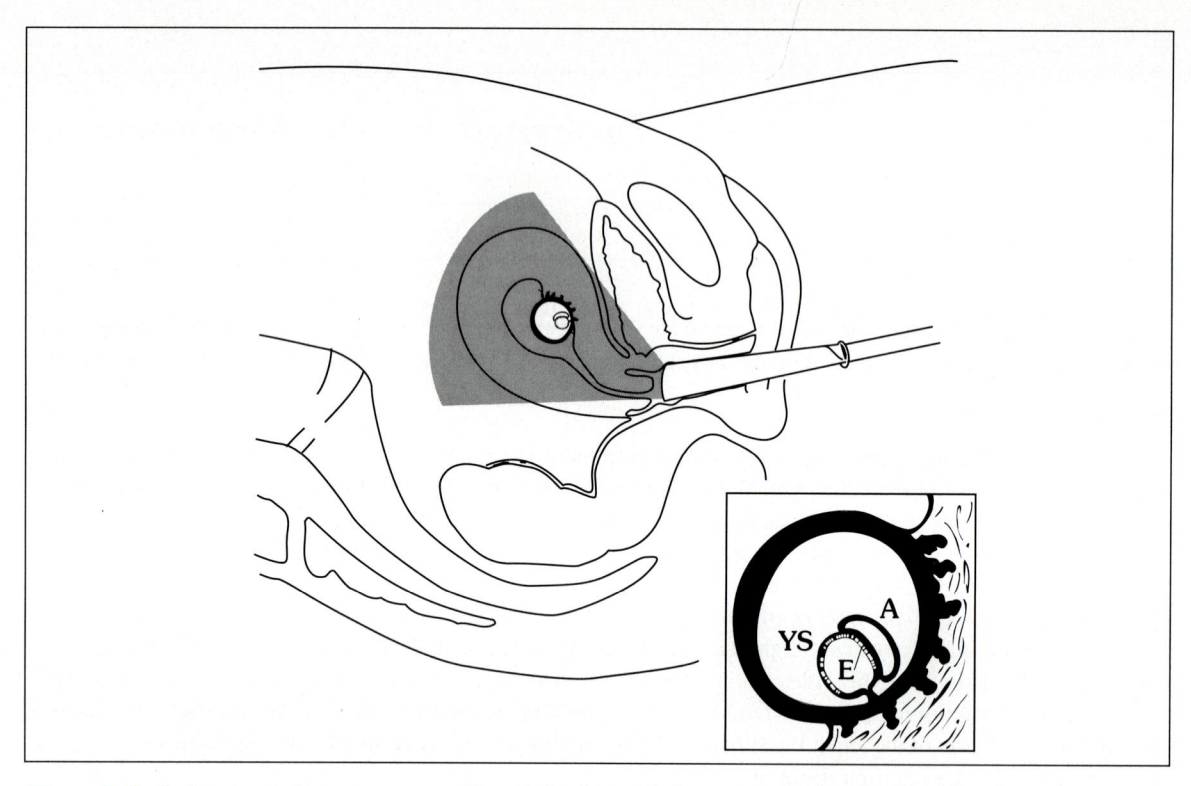

Figure 8-2. Early intrauterine pregnancy and its relationship with the transvaginal probe. Note that the embryonic disk (E) lies between the developing amnion (A) and yolk sac (YS).

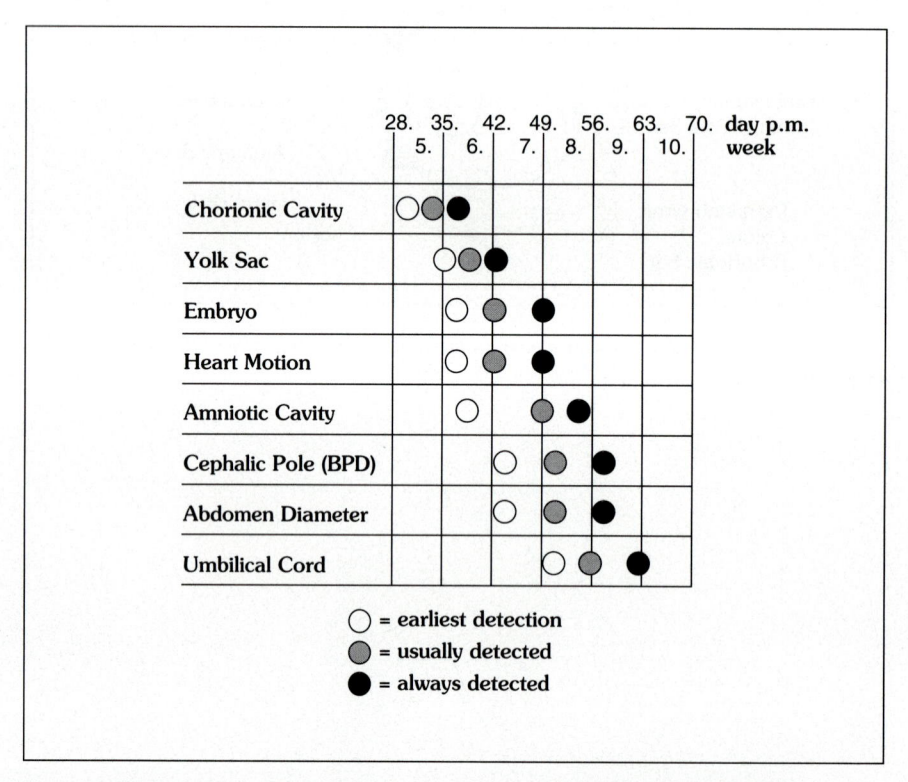

Figure 8-3. Detectability of various parameters in early pregnancy by transvaginal sonography.

Normal Early Pregnancy

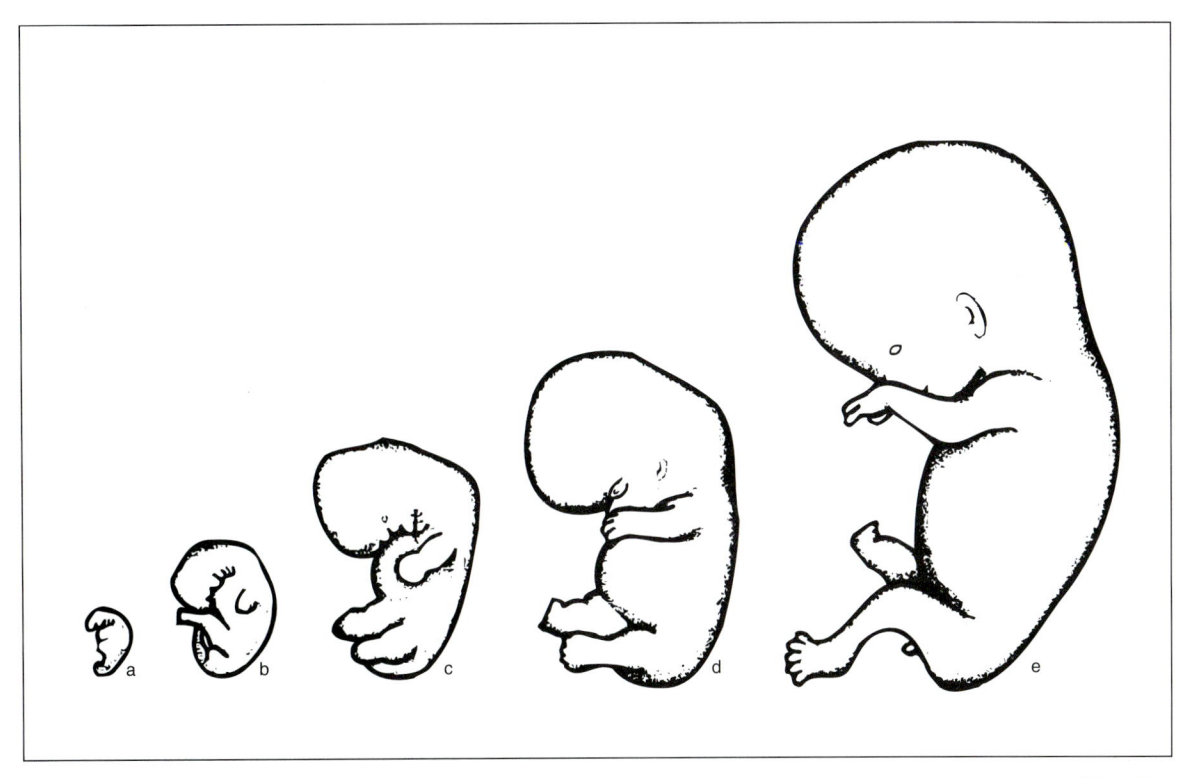

Figure 8-4. Schematic drawings of an embryo: a) on post-menstrual day 42, CRL= 3mm; b) on post-menstrual day 49, CRL= 7mm; c) on post-menstrual day 56, CRL= 13mm; d) on post-menstrual day 63, CRL= 18mm; e) on post-menstrual day 70, CRL = 30mm.

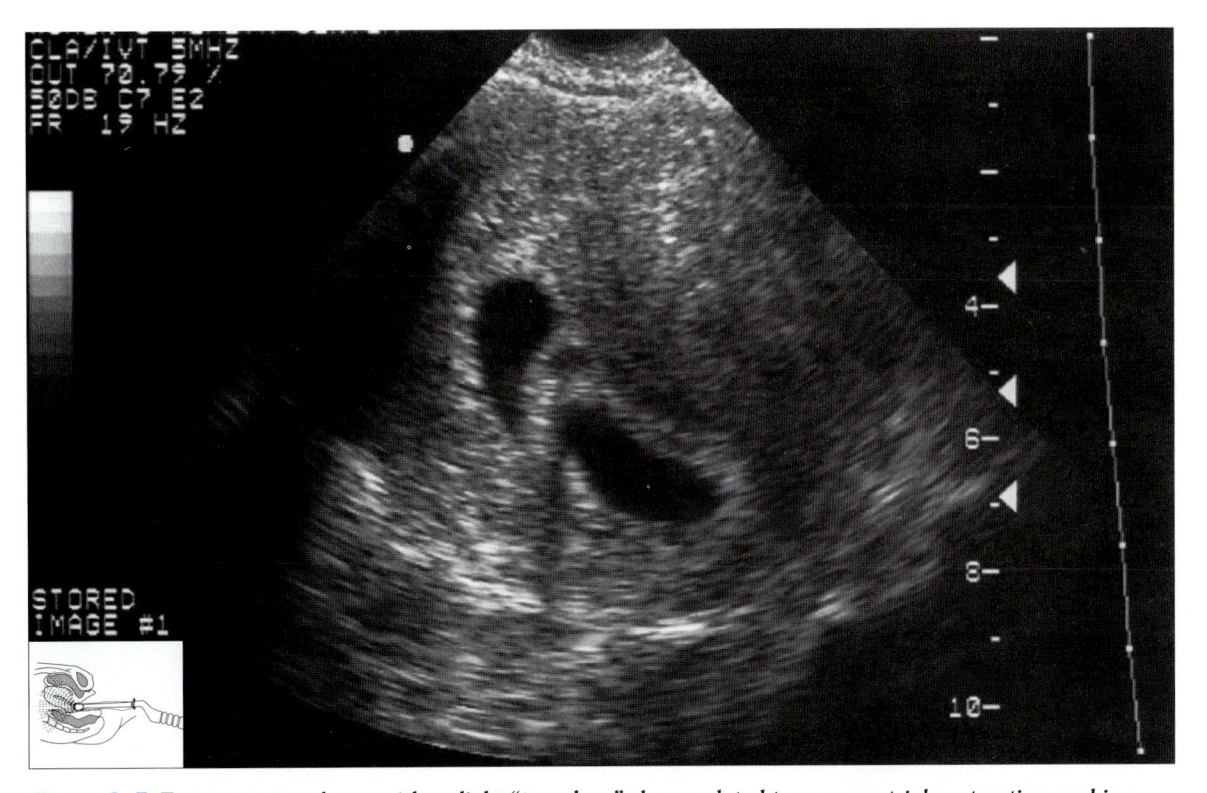

Figure 8-5. Twin gestational sacs with a slight "tear-drop" shape related to a myometrial contraction pushing down on the sac.

An Atlas of Transvaginal Sonography

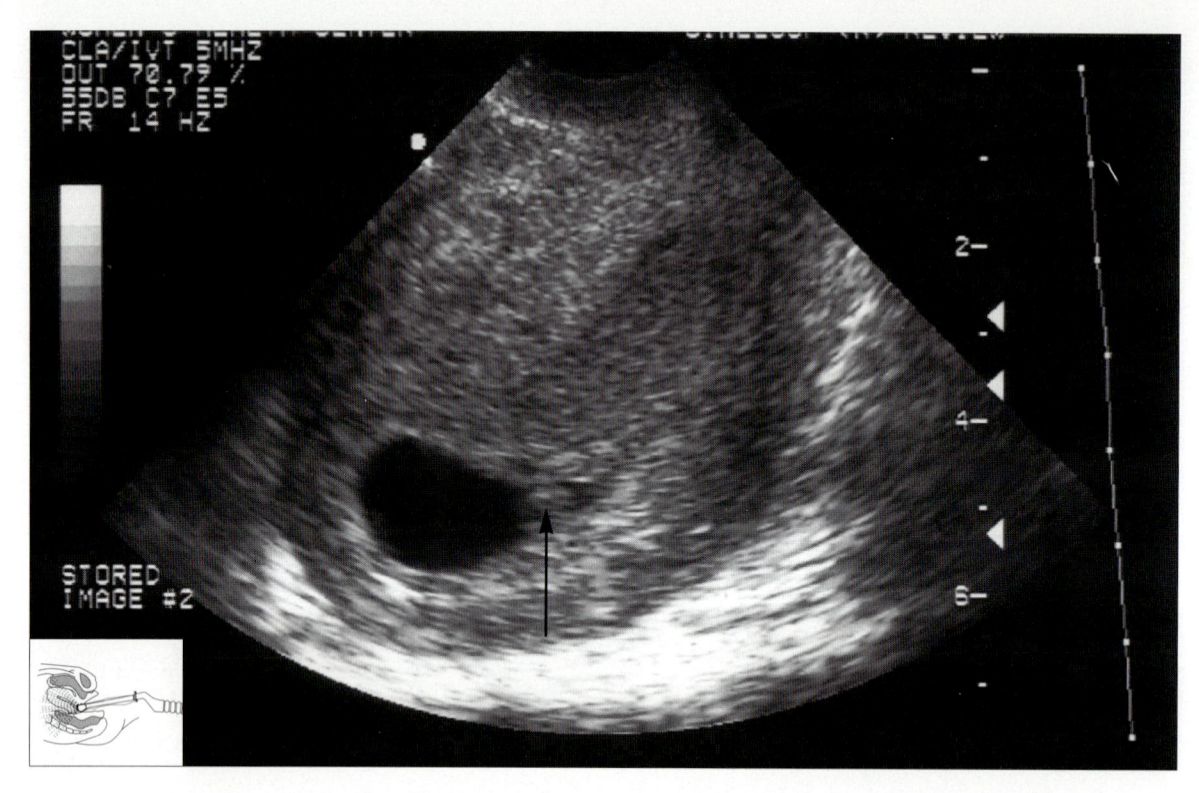

Figure 8-6. *Fetus-yolk sac complex (arrow) just visible in the inferior portion of this "teardrop"-shaped gestational sac.*

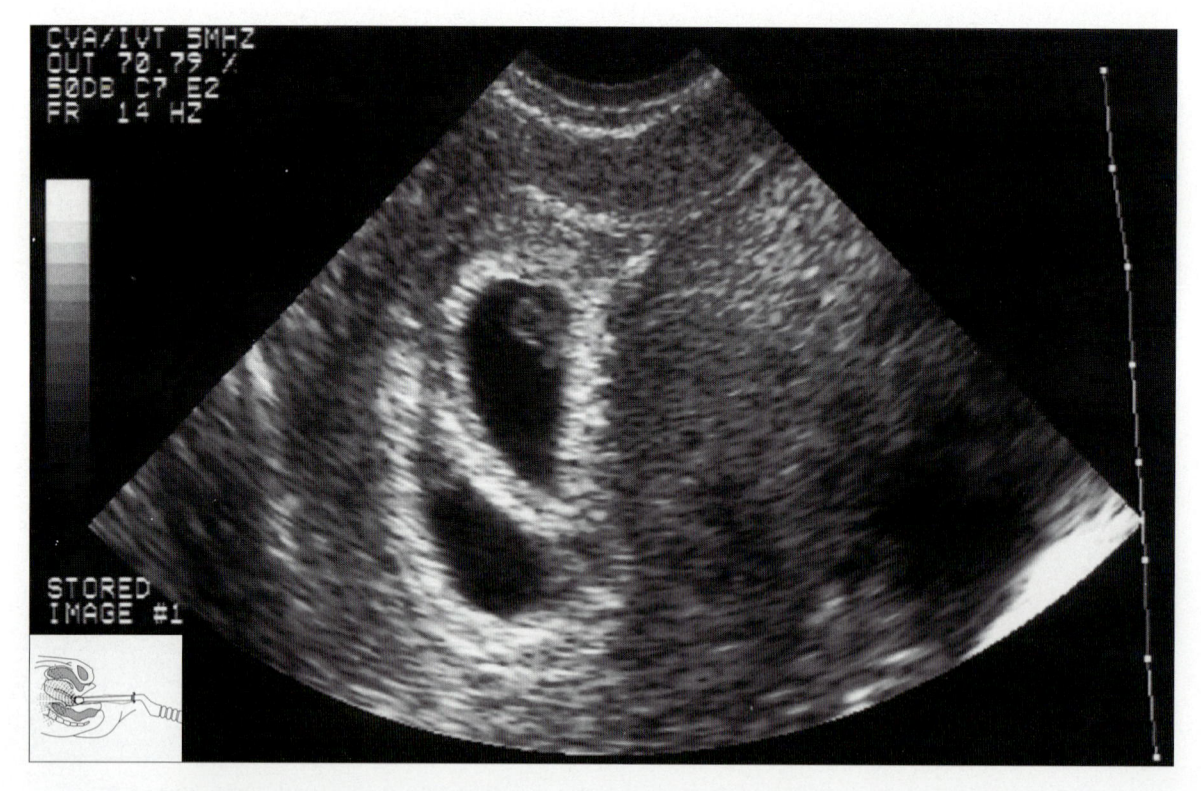

Figure 8-7. *Twin gestational sacs demonstrating the embryo-yolk sac complex, echogenic choriodecidual reaction, and a closed cervix.*

Normal Early Pregnancy

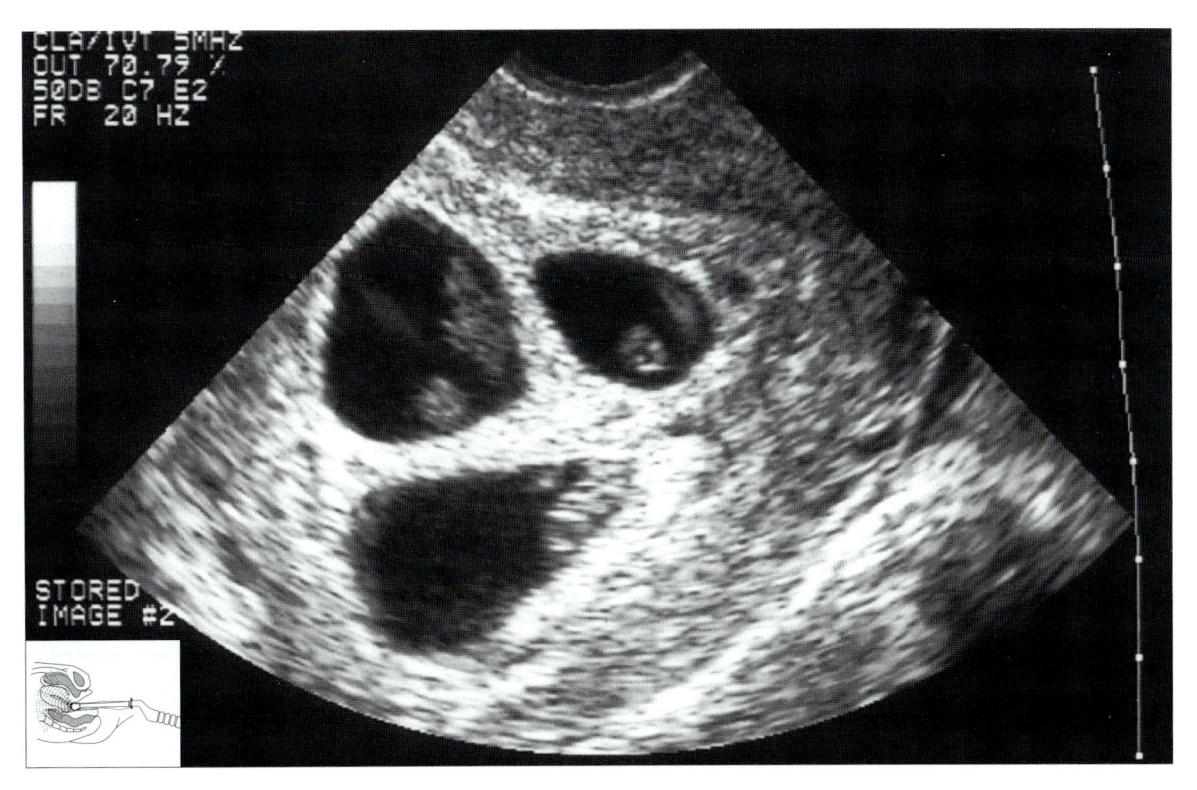

Figure 8-8. Early triplet pregnancy demonstrating clear distinction between the fetus and yolk sac. When less well-defined, the yolk sac can be incorrectly measured as part of the fetus.

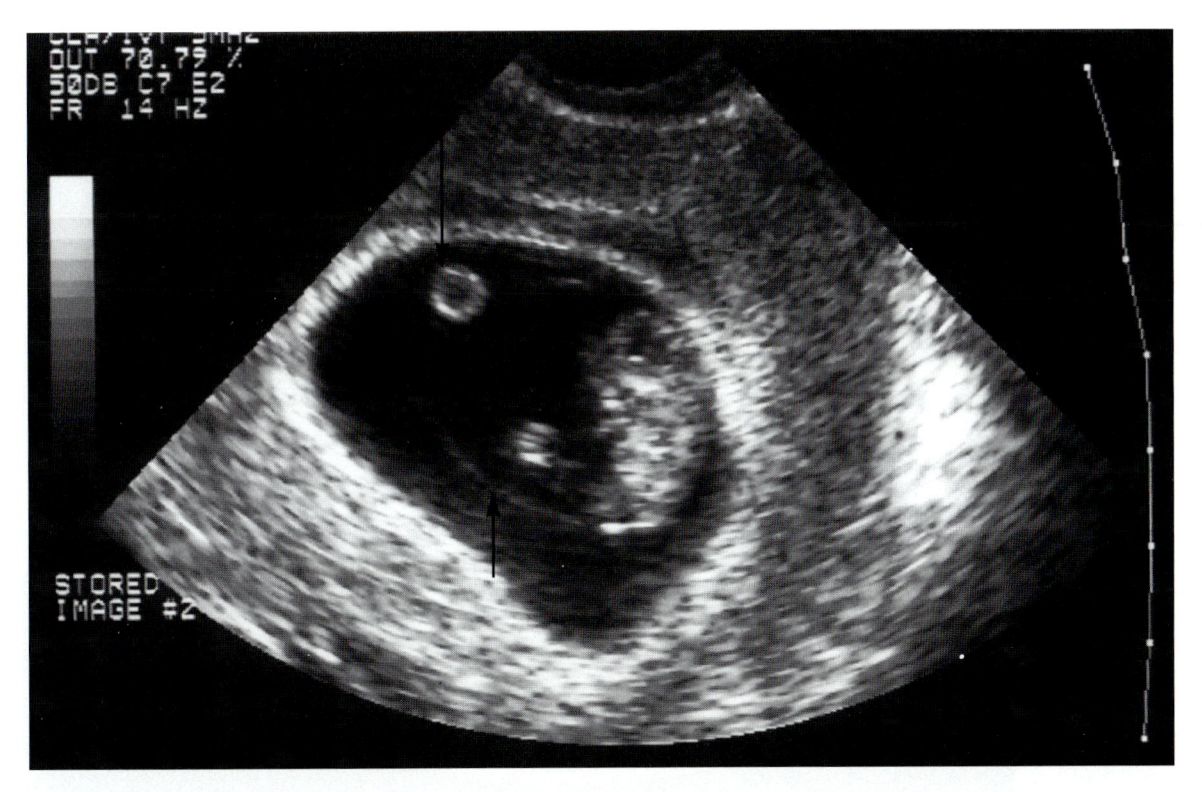

Figure 8-9. Singleton early pregnancy with a thin amniotic membrane (small arrow) visible surrounding fetus. The echogenic yolk sac is seen (large arrow). Outside the amniotic cavity is the extraembryonic celom or chorionic cavity.

An Atlas of Transvaginal Sonography

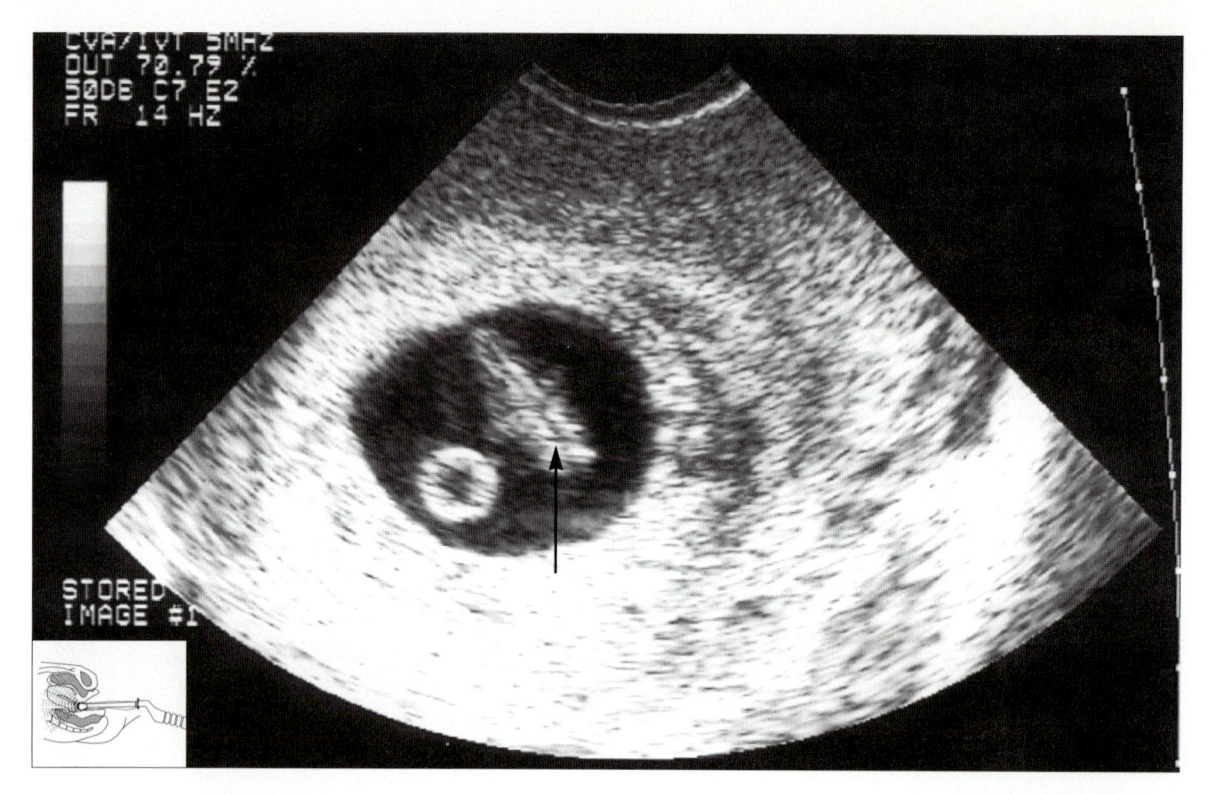

Figure 8-10. At 7.5 weeks the fetus and intensely echogenic yolk sac are clearly seen. The parallel echogenic lines (arrow) in the fetus represent the developing neural tube.

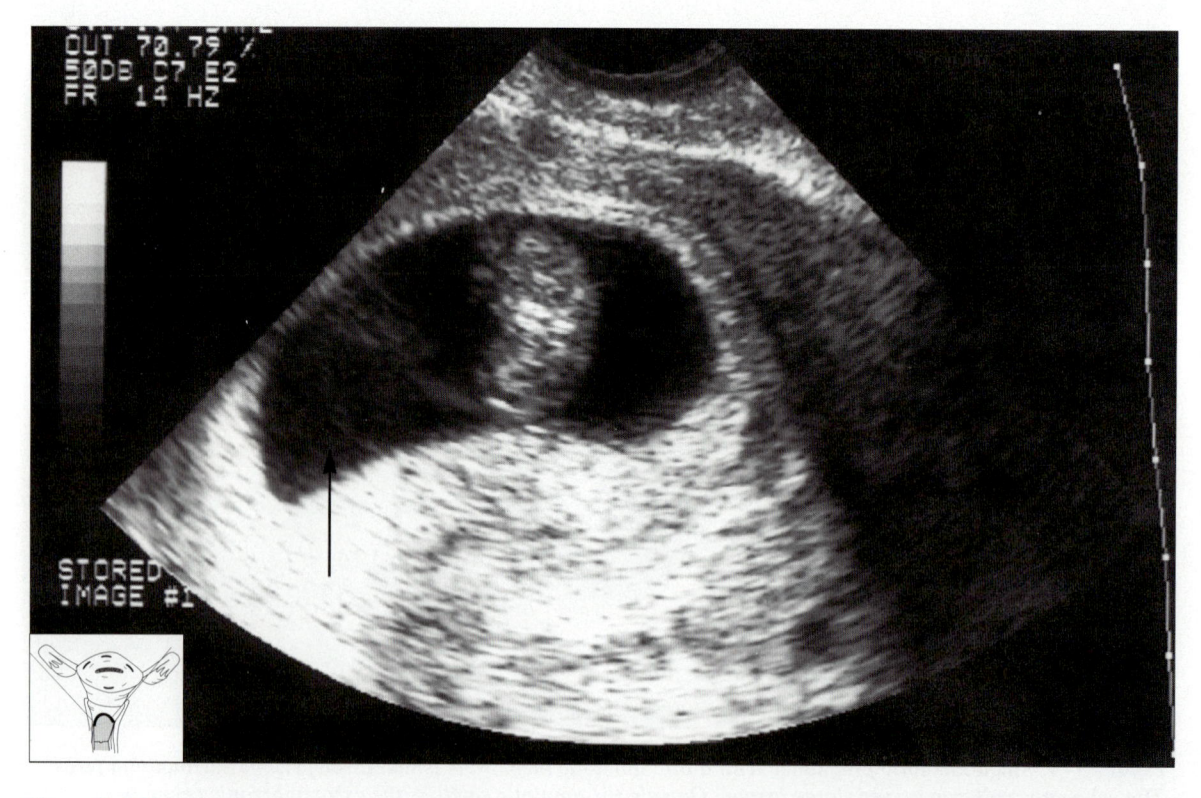

Figure 8-11. Fetus with an anechoic gestational sac, surrounded by a slightly more echogenic chorionic cavity (arrow).

Normal Early Pregnancy

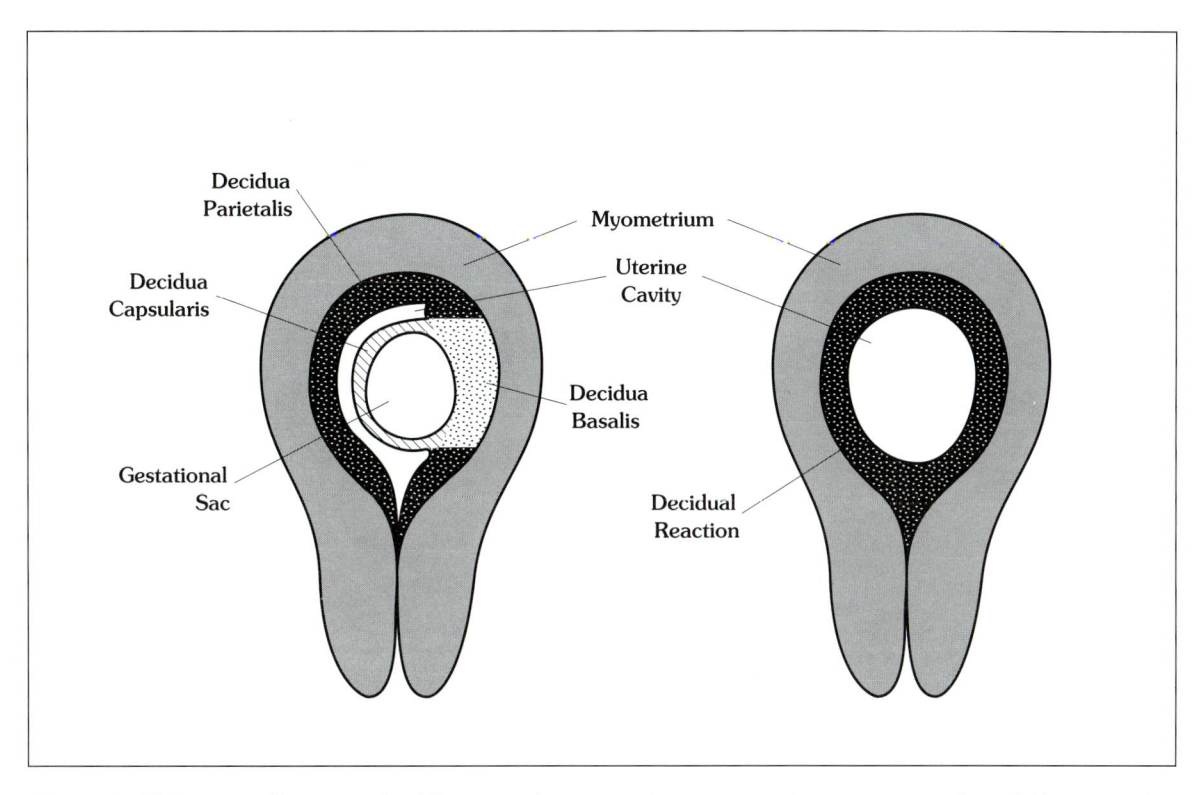

Figure 8-12. Diagram illustrating the difference in location and appearance of a true gestational sac (left) compared with a pseudo gestational sac (right).

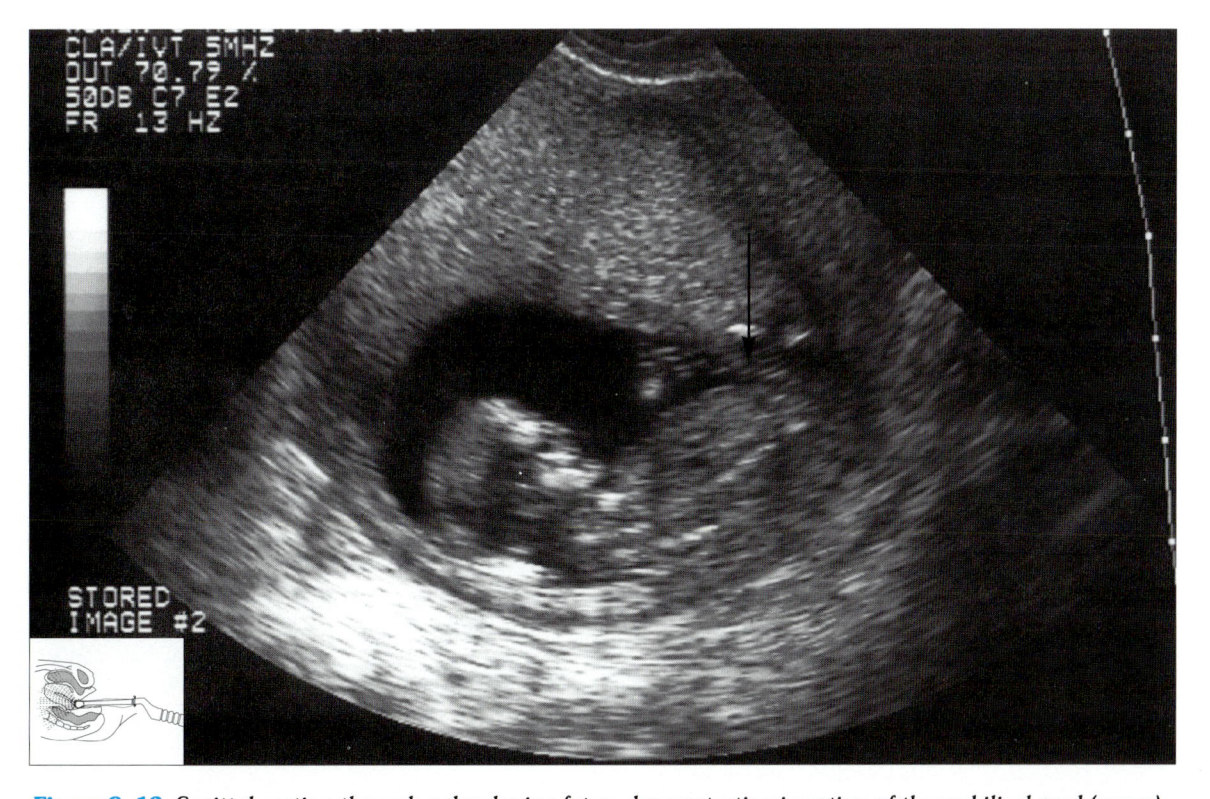

Figure 8-13. Sagittal section through a developing fetus, demonstrating insertion of the umbilical cord (arrow).

107

An Atlas of Transvaginal Sonography

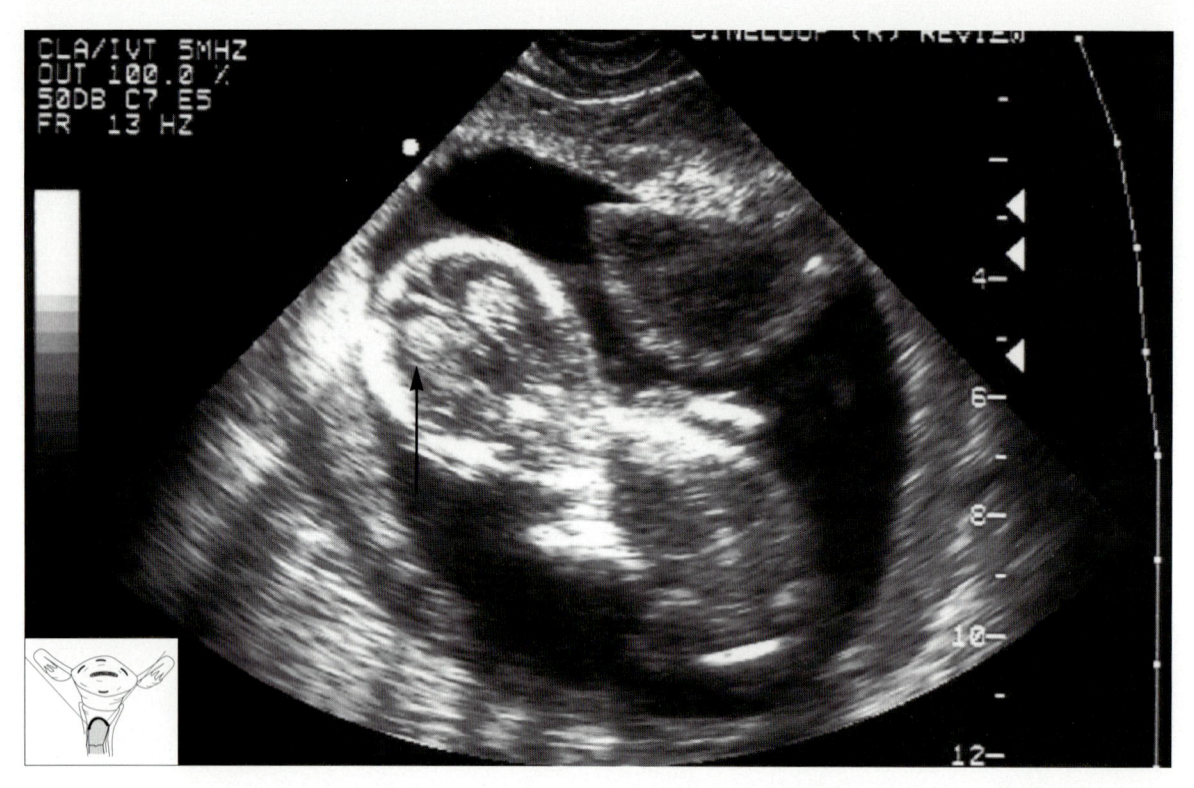

Figure 8-14. Echogenic choroid plexus (arrow) seen within the lateral ventricles.

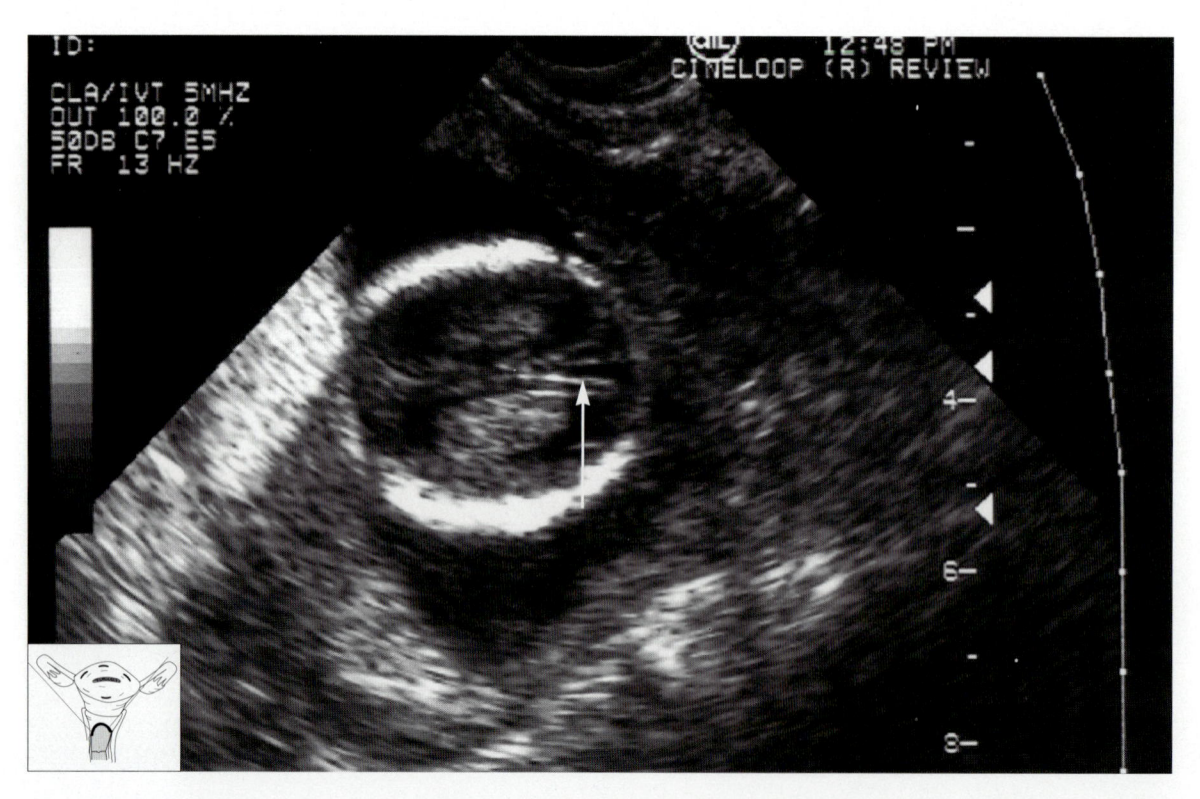

Figure 8-15. Echogenic choroid plexus seen within the lateral ventricles, and separated by the thin falx (arrow).

108

Normal Early Pregnancy

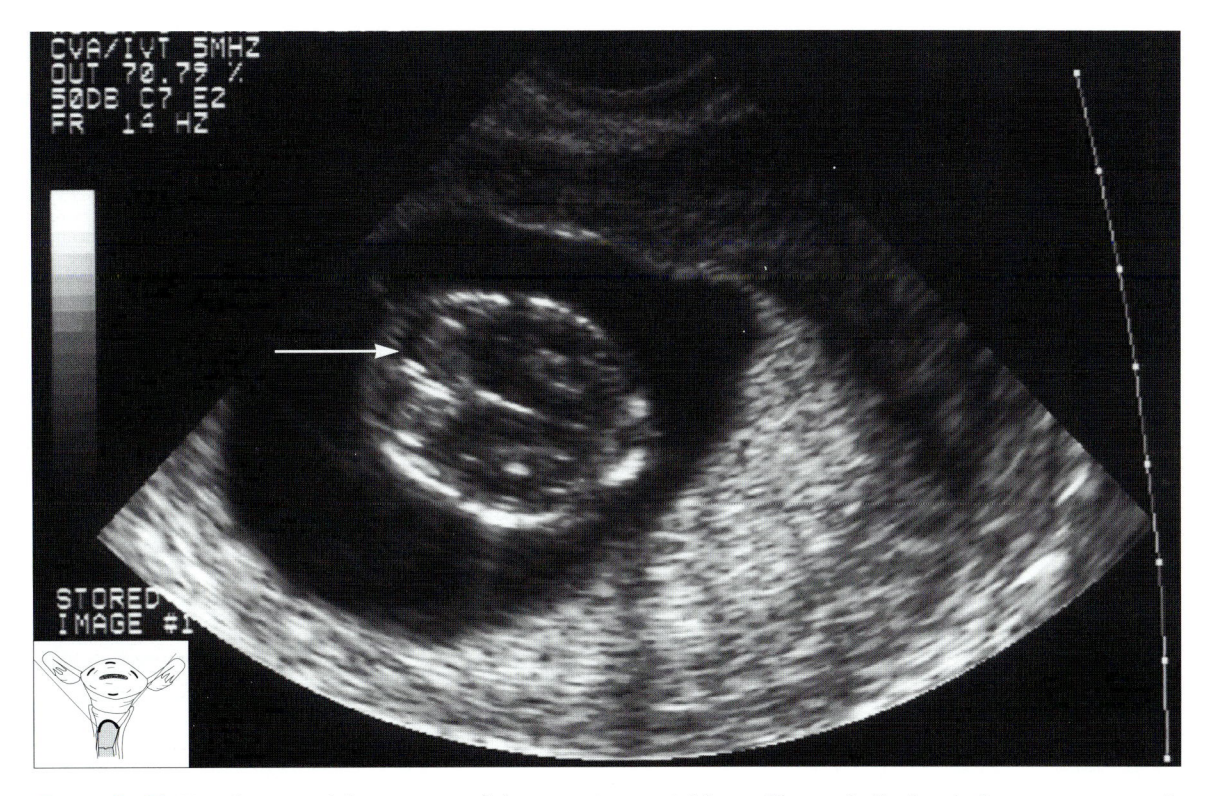

Figure 8~16. Visualization of the contents of the posterior cranial fossa. The cerebellar hemispheres are separated by the falx cerebelli and lie adjacent to the occipital sinus (arrow).

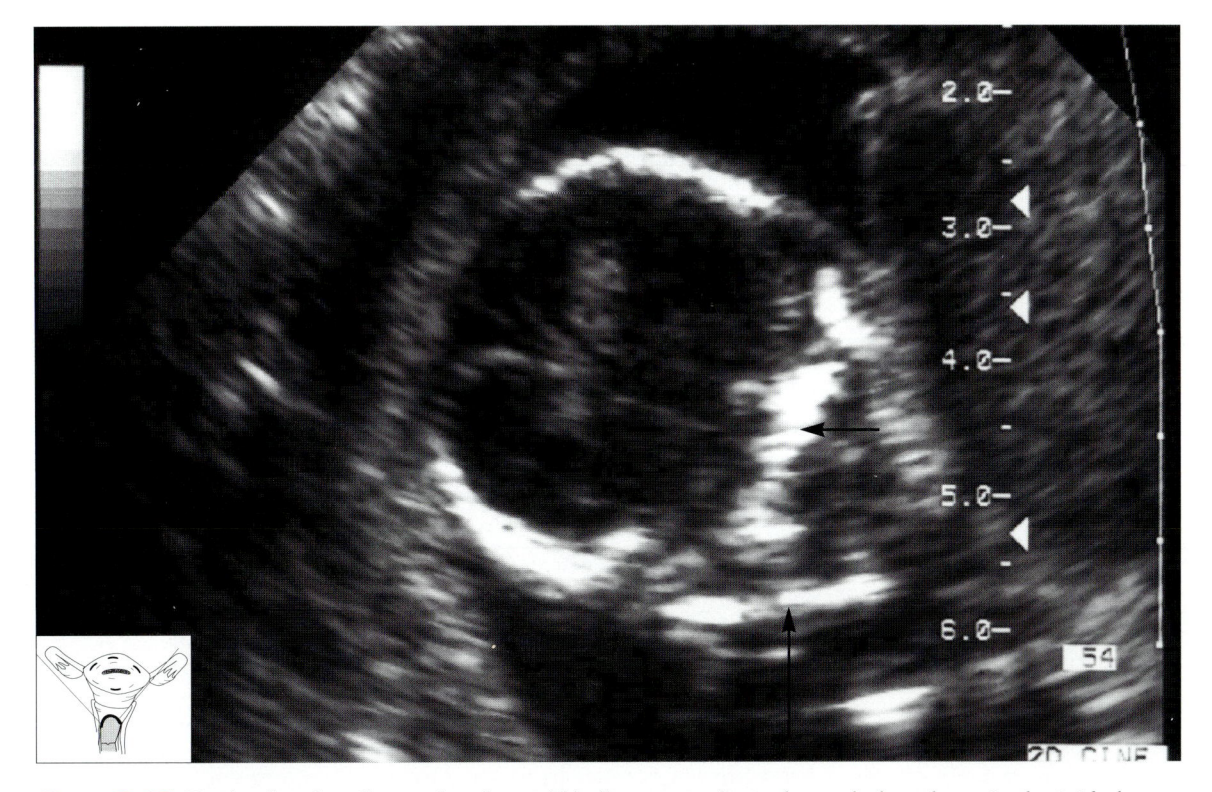

Figure 8~17. Hard palate (small arrow) and mandible (large arrow) seen beneath the echogenic chorioid plexus in the lateral ventricles.

An Atlas of Transvaginal Sonography

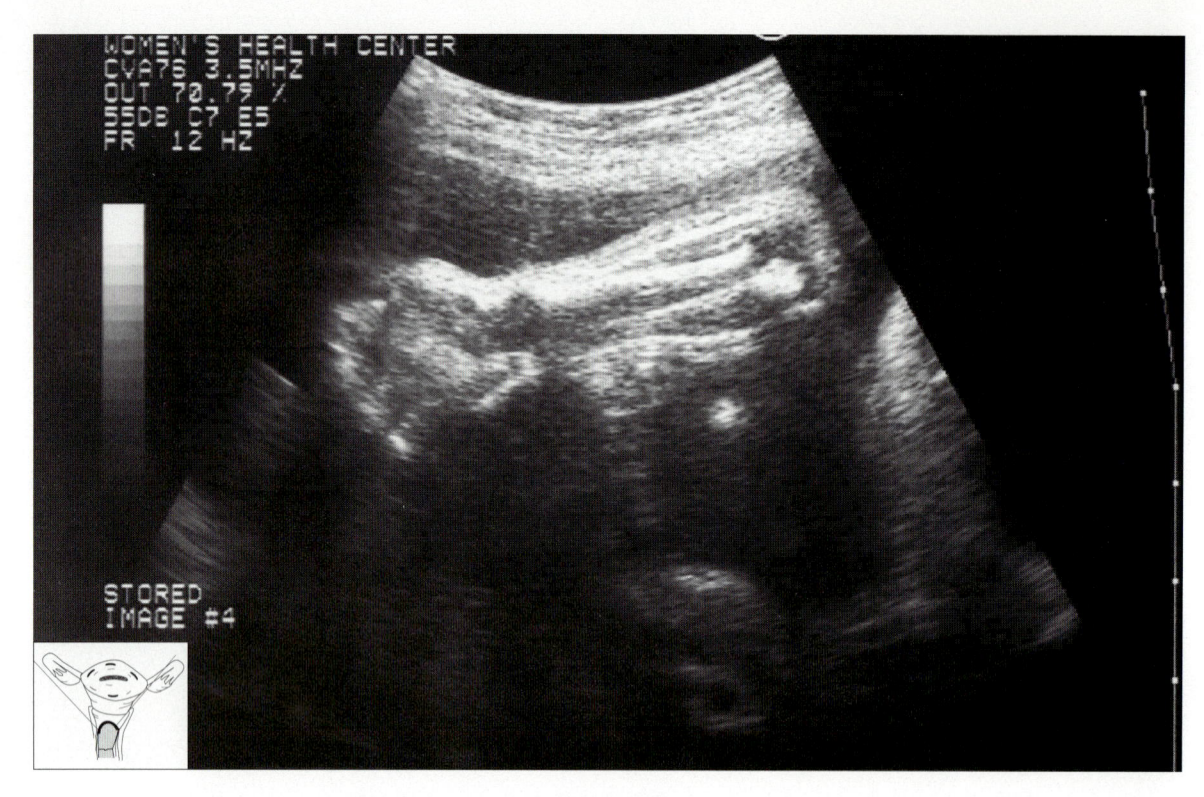

Figure 8-18. *Sonogram of fetal forearm and outstretched hand.*

9   *Abnormal Early Pregnancy*

The most common abnormalities occurring in the first trimester of pregnancy include abortions and ectopic pregnancies. Transvaginal sonography plays an indispensable role in diagnostic and management decisions.

Abortion

Abortion is the termination of pregnancy by any means prior to 20 weeks of gestation. It is classified as (i) threatened, (ii) inevitable, (iii) incomplete, (iv) complete, (v) missed, (vi) septic and (vii) habitual. Although the usual quoted incidence is 10-20%, many are unreported.

Scan Findings

A threatened abortion is recognized sonographically as an area of retro chorionic hemorrhage that is relatively hypoechoic. Embryonic death frequently precedes bleeding into the decidua basalis, separation of the placenta, and delivery of the products of conception. Echogenic tissue retained within the uterine lumen after a spontaneous abortion is characteristic of retained choriodecidua, and confirms the diagnosis of incomplete abortion. In such cases, often the internal cervical os can be visualized as being dilated. Complete abortions obviously lack any echogenic tissue within the uterine lumen.

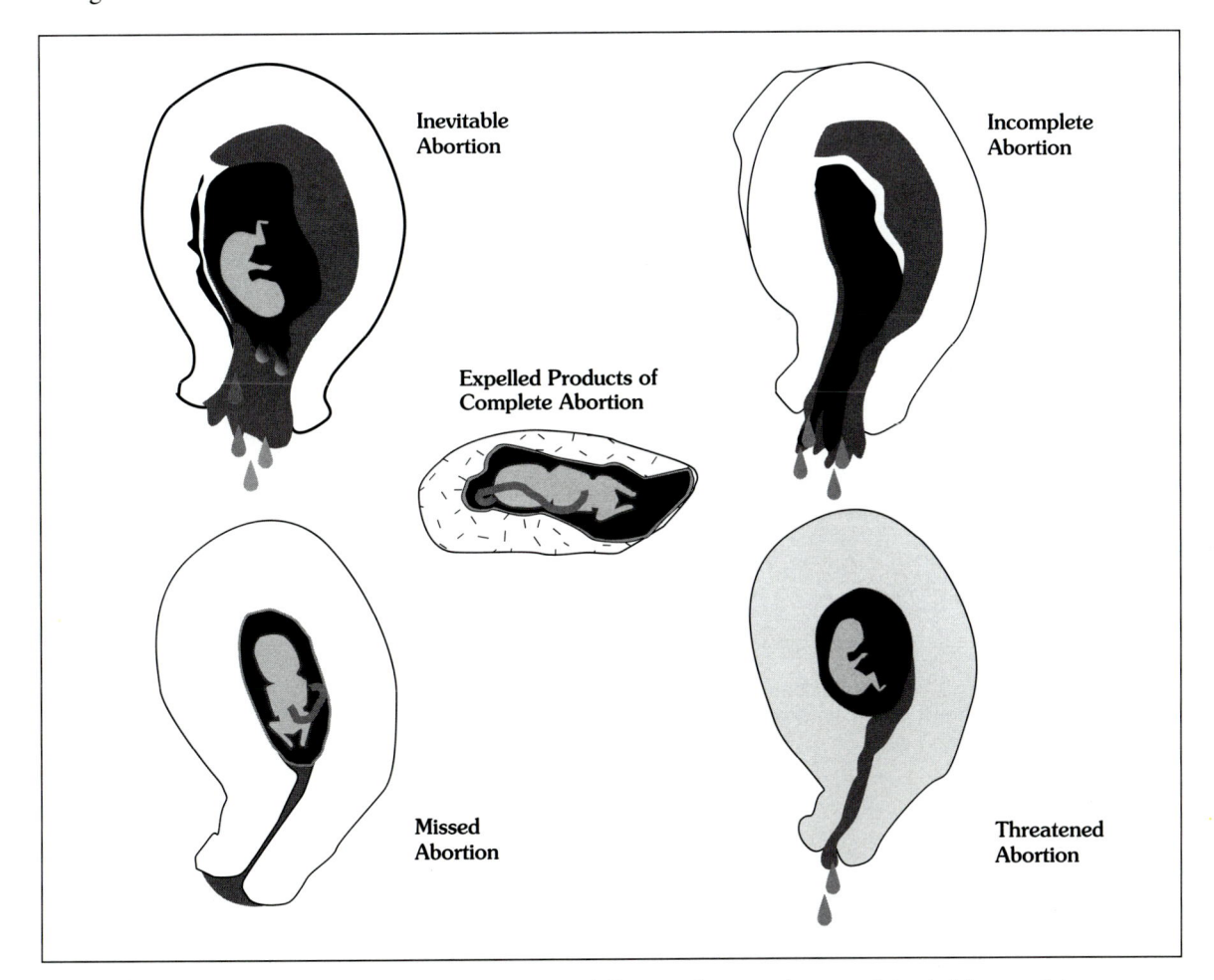

Figure 9-1. Diagrammatic illustrations demonstrating differences between threatened, inevitable, complete, incomplete and missed abortions.

An Atlas of Transvaginal Sonography

Ectopic Pregnancy

Ectopic pregnancy is a pregnancy occurring outside the uterine cavity. It is classified according to site, with most occurring in the fallopian tube. Implantation occurs most commonly in the ampullary and isthmic regions of the tube. The reported incidence has currently increased to 1:90 pregnancies.

The ectopic pregnancy undergoes hemorrhage, then detachment from the tube, followed by absorption or extrusion out of the tubal ostium, or rupture through the tubal wall. The hormonal production results in uterine enlargement and decidual reaction in the endometrium.

Scan Findings

Sonography confirms an empty uterus and the absence of an intrauterine gestational sac. This finding, though, does not exclude a very early, normal intrauterine pregnancy. The endometrial stripe/decidual reaction is characterized by a fine midline echoic echo. Fluid within the uterus can distort this echo, producing a saclike structure, resembling a gestational sac. This appearance has been termed a "pseudogestational sac." Although sonography is unable to differentiate this intrauterine fluid from PID, decidual reaction or early intrauterine pregnancy, with the appropriate history, a high index of suspicion may be reached. The presence of an adnexal mass is not necessary for the diagnosis, nor is it confirmatory. If an adnexal mass is present and contains fetal echoes with fetal movement, the diagnosis is confirmed. A "tubal ring" may be present, consisting of an echogenic rim and a hypoechoic center. The fallopian tube may be visualized as a distended, fusiform structure, containing echogenic fluid (blood), and if rupture has occurred, fluid may be seen in the cul-de-sac.

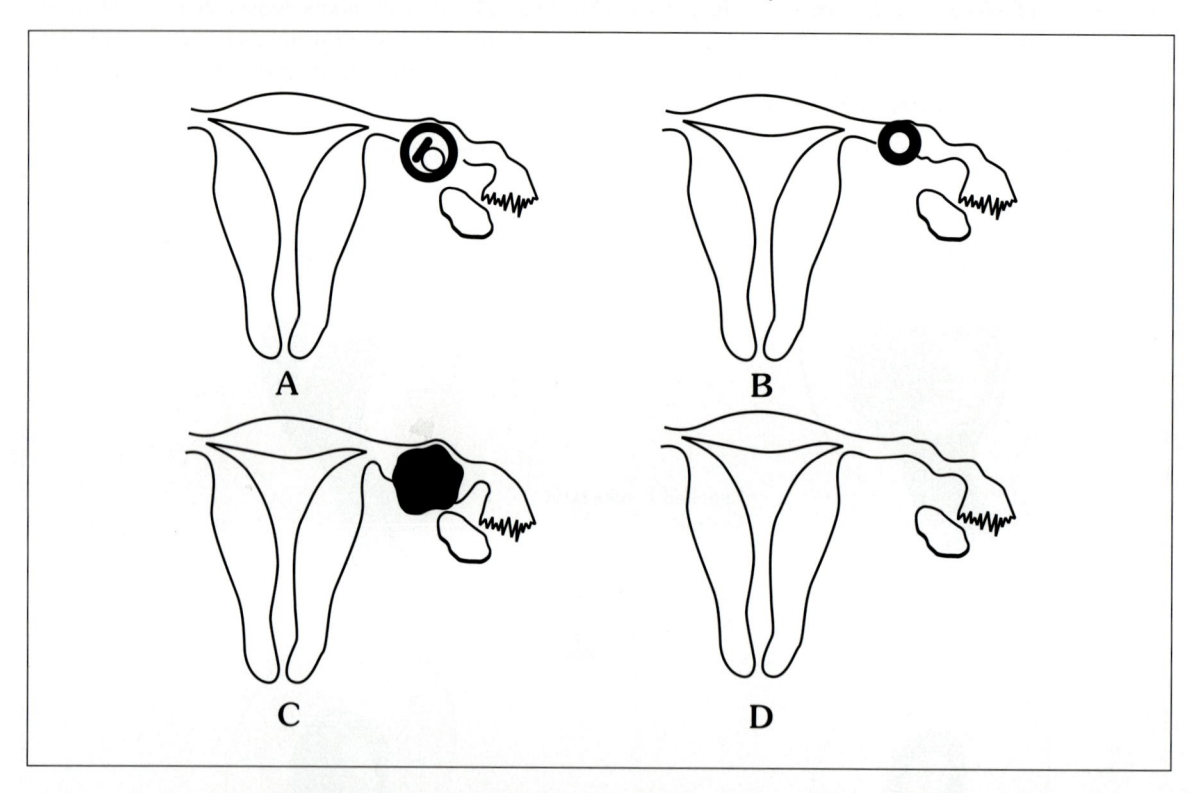

Figure 9-2. Drawings illustrating the adnexal findings that may be seen by transvaginal sonography in a patient with an ectopic pregnancy. A) living extrauterine embryo, B) extrauterine sac with or without a yolk sac or non-living embryo, C) adnexal mass, and D) no specific adnexal findings.

Abnormal Early Pregnancy

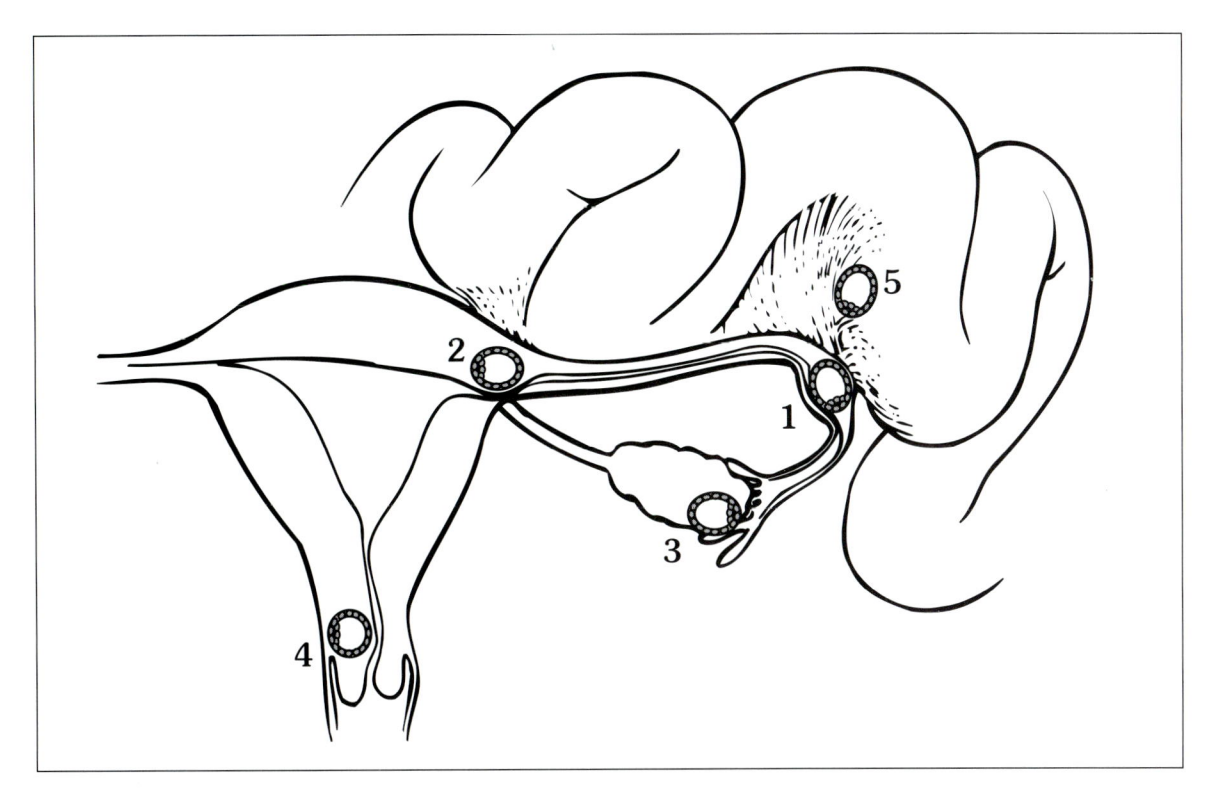

Figure 9-3. Sites of ectopic pregnancy. 1) tubal, 2) isthmic, 3) ovarian, 4) cervical and 5) peritoneal.

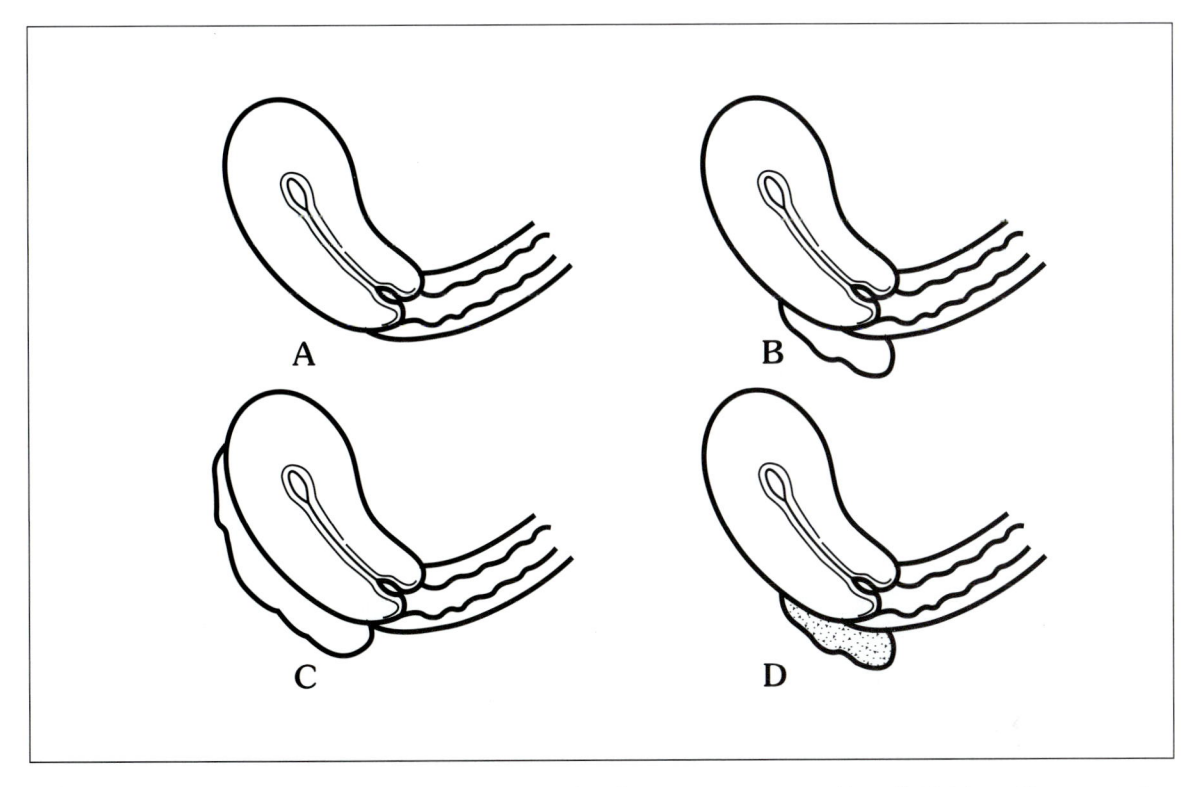

Figure 9-4. Drawing of cul-de-sac findings associated with ectopic pregnancy. A) no fluid, B) small amount of fluid, C) moderate to large amount of fluid and D) echogenic fluid.

113

An Atlas of Transvaginal Sonography

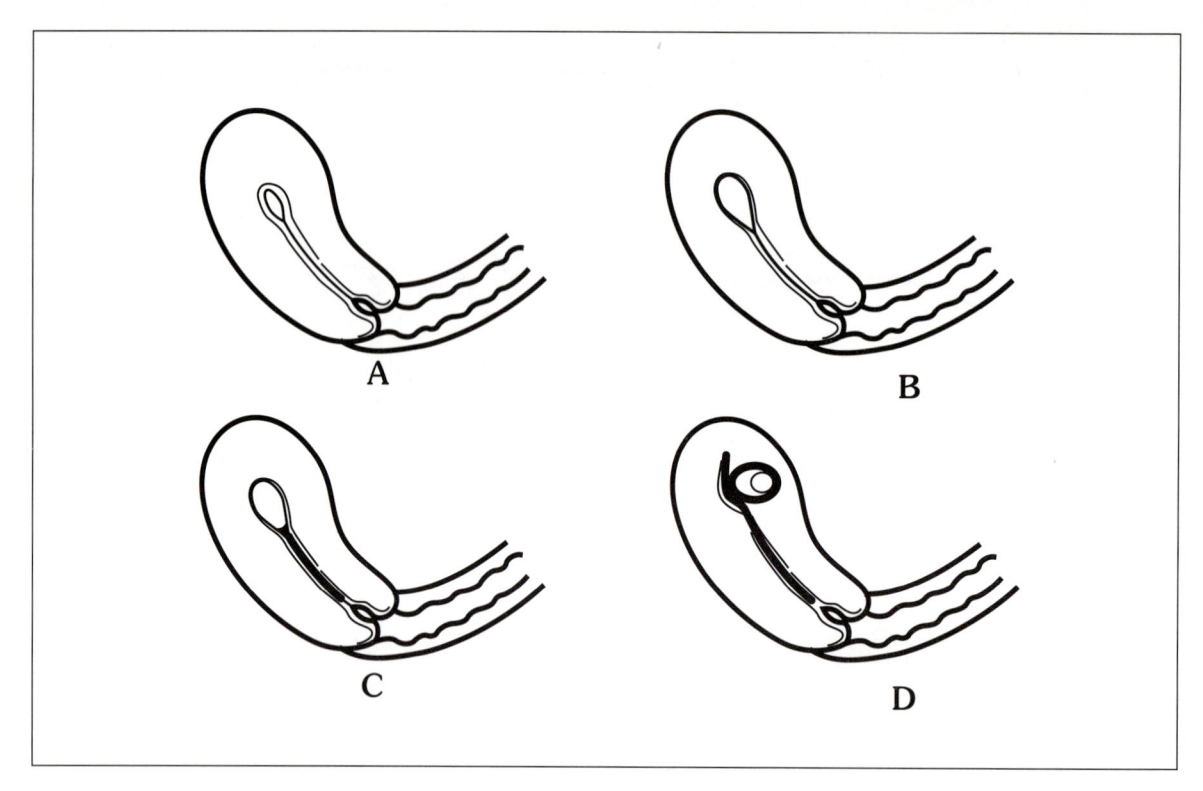

Figure 9-5. Intrauterine sonographic findings that may be associated with ectopic pregnancy. A) empty uterus, B) decidual reaction, C) pseudogestational sac, D) concurrent intrauterine pregnancy.

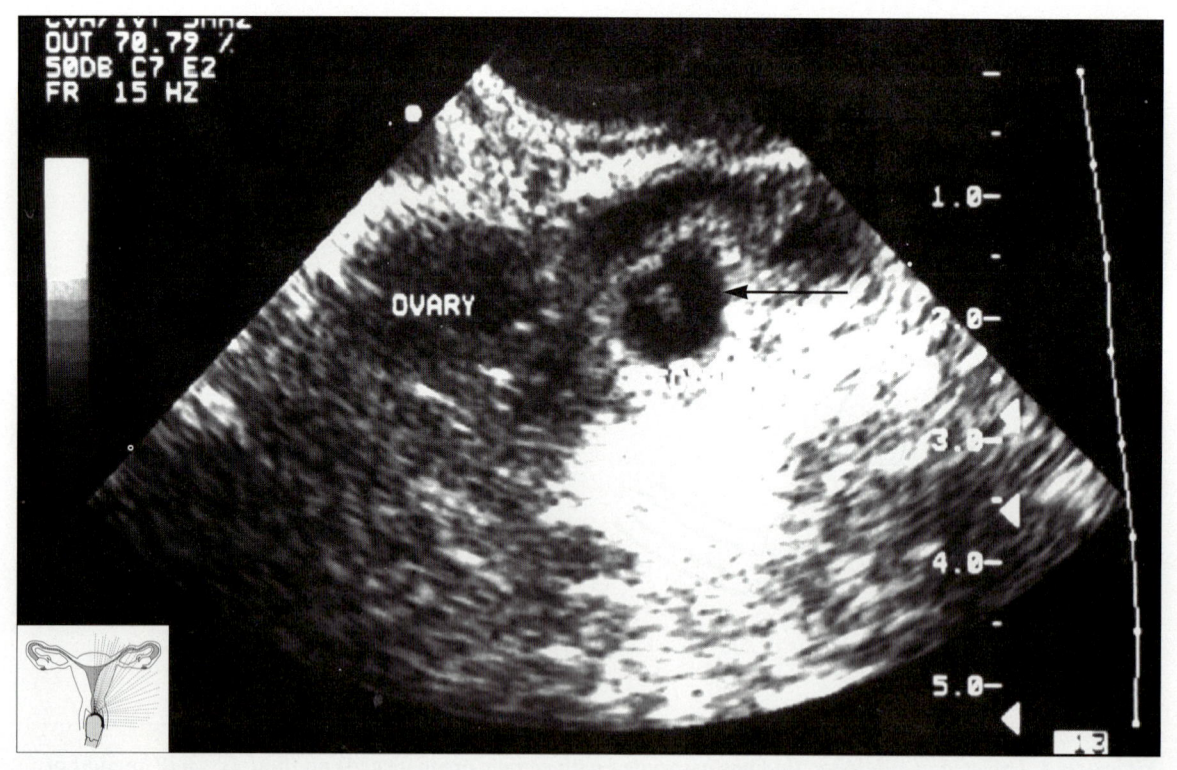

Figure 9-6. Transverse scan of the left adnexa demonstrating an extrauterine gestational sac and fetal pole (arrow) adjacent to the ovary.

Abnormal Early Pregnancy

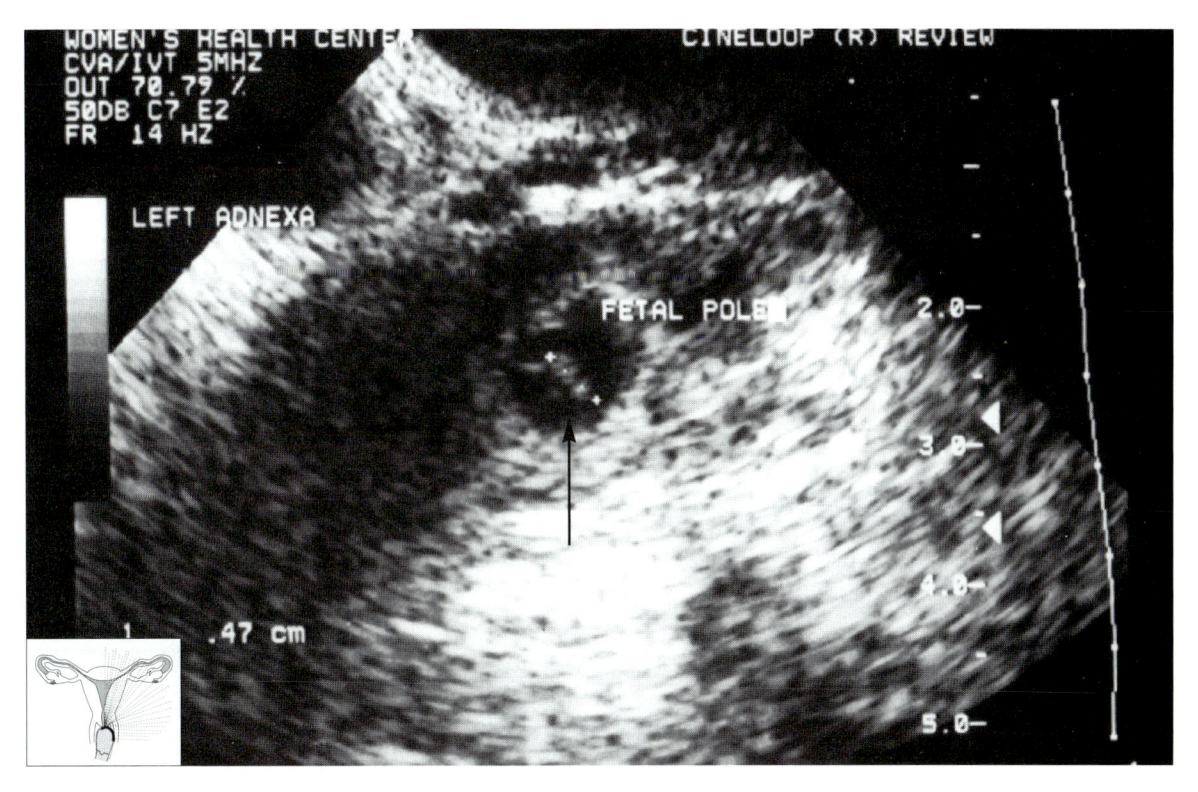

Figure 9-7. Ectopic pregnancy confirmed by demonstrating a fetal pole (arrow) with cardiac activity within the extrauterine gestational sac.

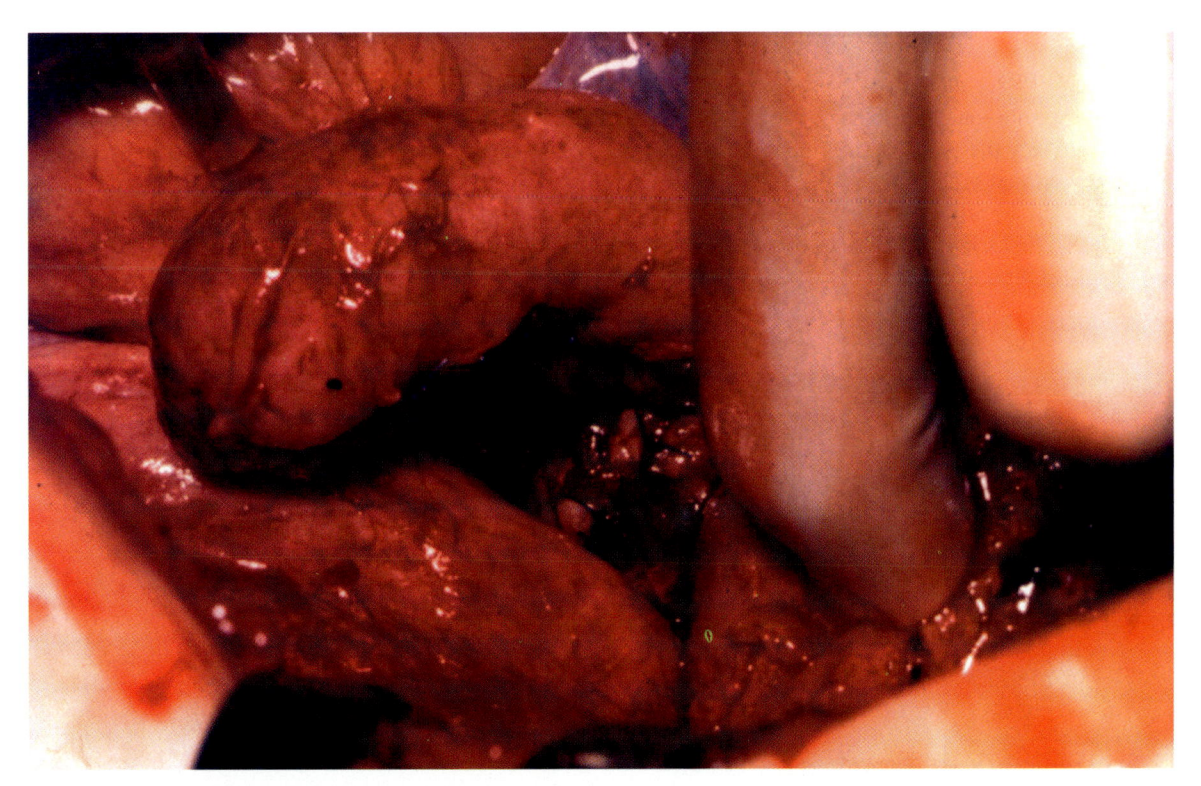

Figure 9-8. "Clubbed" fimbrial end of fallopian tube, distended with an ectopic pregnancy. The broad ligament has been transsected prior to definitive treatment.

An Atlas of Transvaginal Sonography

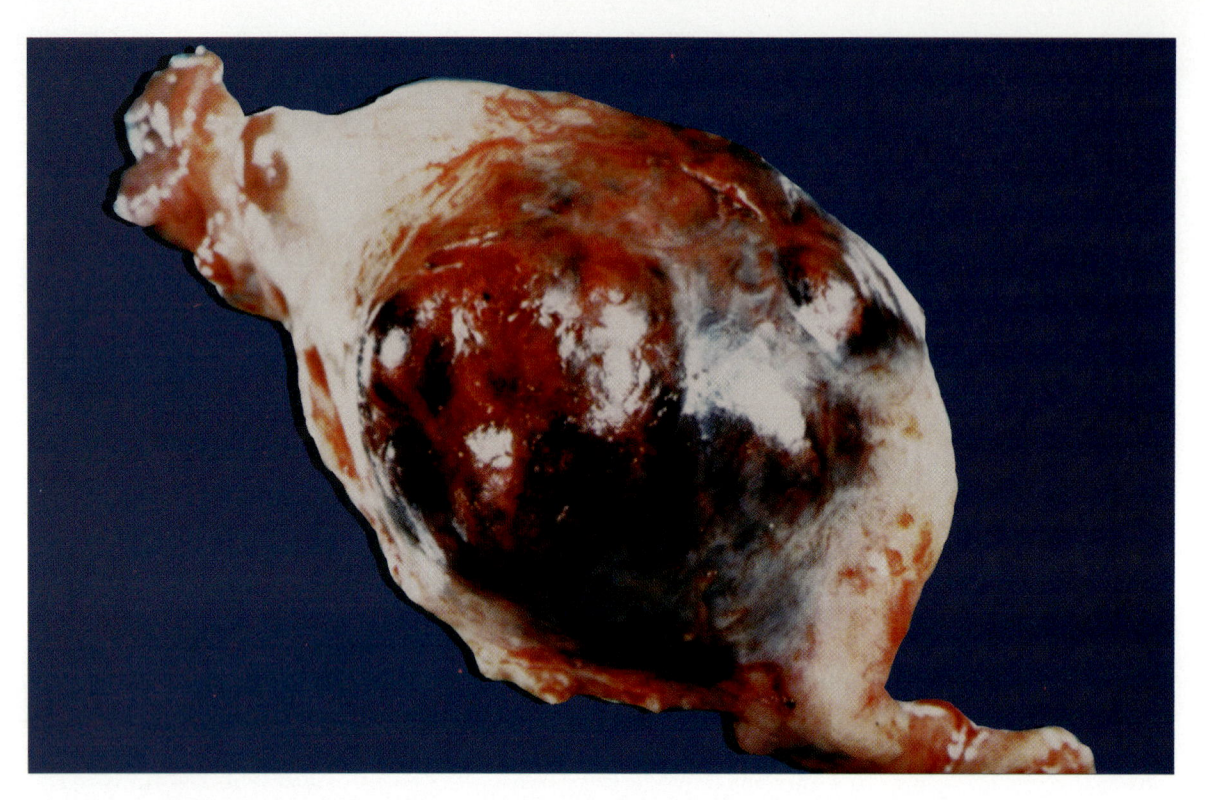

Figure 9-9. High-power view of an unruptured tubal ectopic pregnancy.

Fetal Death

The diagnosis of fetal death is often difficult to make on clinical grounds. Subtle changes in uterine growth may be appreciated by the obstetrician, but usually the diagnosis needs to be confirmed by sonography.

Scan Findings

Fetal, or embryonic, death has a variety of sonographic appearances, depending upon gestational age. In early pregnancy the yolk sac and embryo may not be present sonographically and thus all that is seen is an empty gestational sac. This by itself is not confirmatory evidence of fetal/embryonic death, but on serial scanning there be will lack of enlargement of the sac, and failure of development of the fetal pole. In the early to mid first trimester, absence of a fetal heart rate, coupled with a crumpled gestational and yolk sac is diagnostic of fetal demise.

Abnormal Early Pregnancy

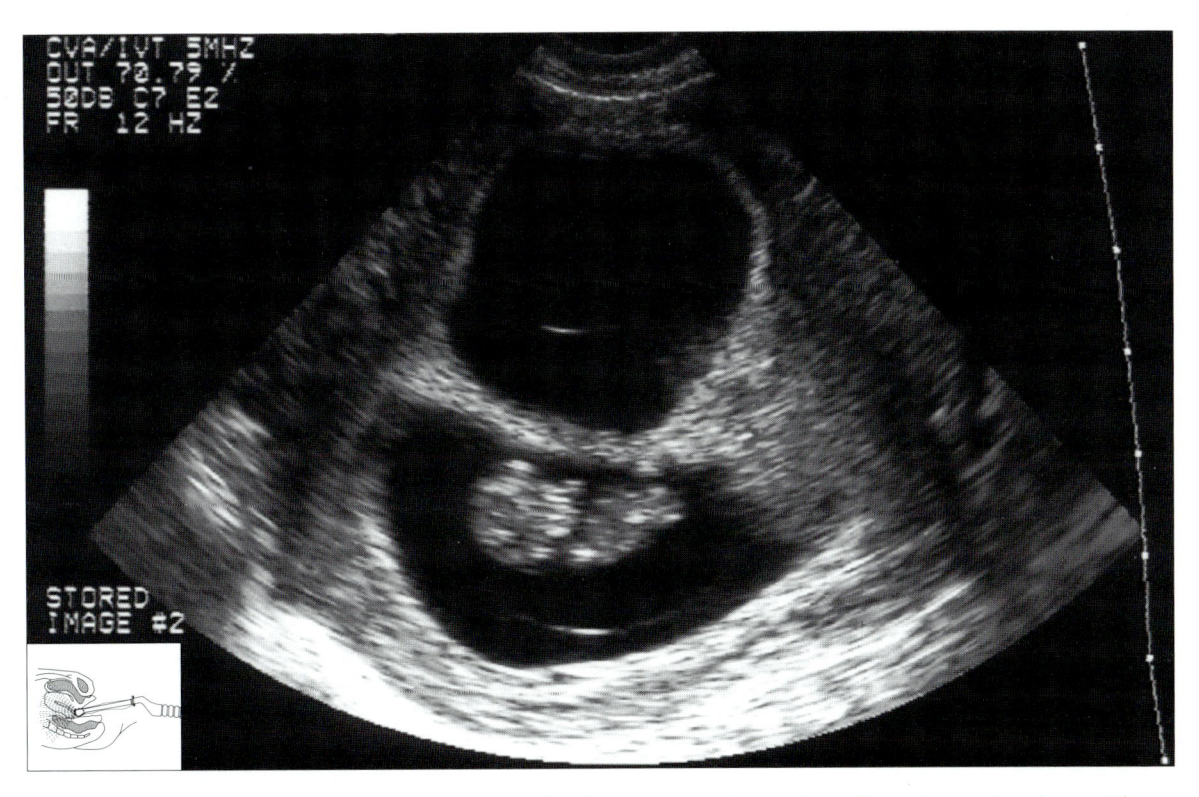

Figure 9-10. Twin pregnancy demonstrating a viable fetus and amnion and an adjacent gestational sac with a nonviable, blighted ovum. The thick wall separating the gestational sacs suggests a dichorionic gestation.

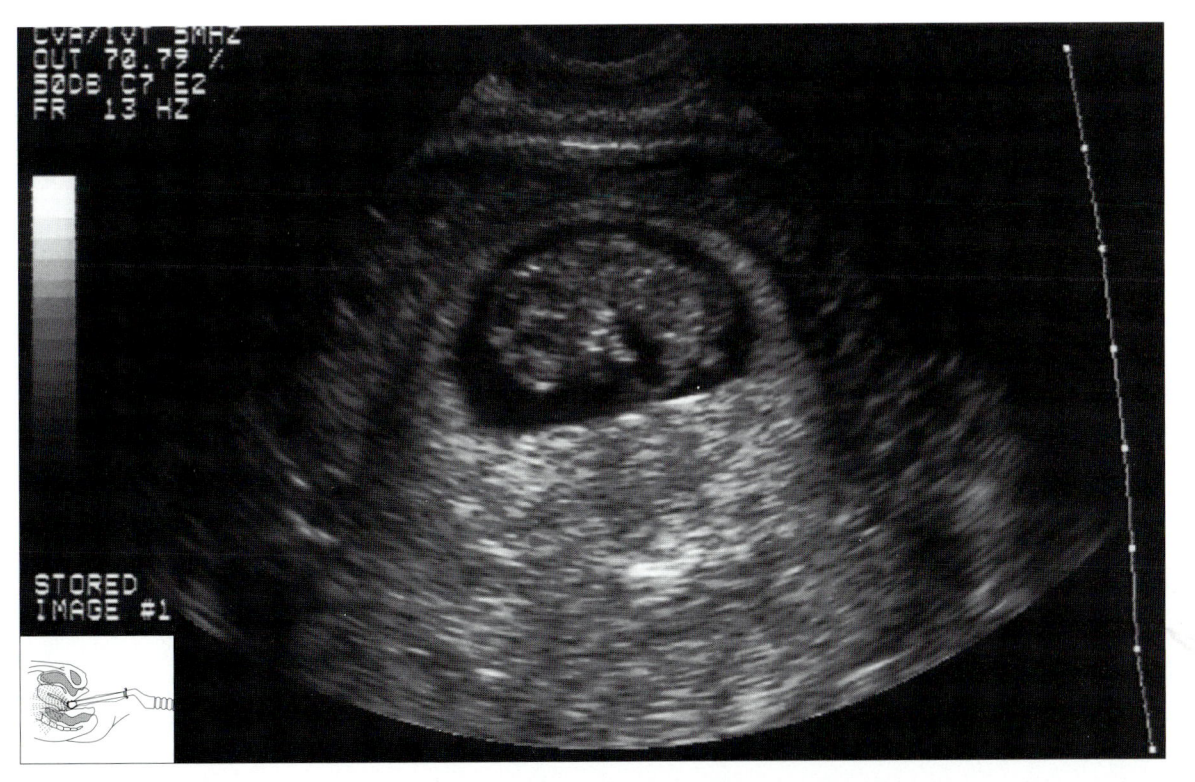

Figure 9-11. Fetal demise, with a reduction of amniotic fluid and on Doppler sonography, absent fetal heart tones.

10 Gestational Trophoblastic Disease

Gestational trophoblastic disease (GTD) encompasses four clinicopathologic forms of growth disturbance of the human trophoblast: (1) hydatidiform mole, (2) invasive mole, (3) choriocarcinoma, and (4) placental site trophoblastic tumor.

Hydatidiform Mole

Hydatidiform mole occurs in approximately 1 per 1,500 pregnancies. Repeat moles have a 0.5-2.6% recurrence rate and these patients also have a greater risk for developing invasive moles and choriocarcinomas. Complete or classical moles are characterized by vesicular swelling of placental villi, trophoblastic hyperplasia and the absence of an intact fetus. They usually have a 46XX karyotype, paternally derived. Partial moles are characterized by slowly progressive hydatidiform change in the presence of functioning villous capillaries that affects only some of the villi. It is associated with an identifiable abnormal fetus, fetal membranes or red blood cells. Trophoblastic immaturity is constant and there is only focal hyperplasia. They usually have a triploid karyotype.

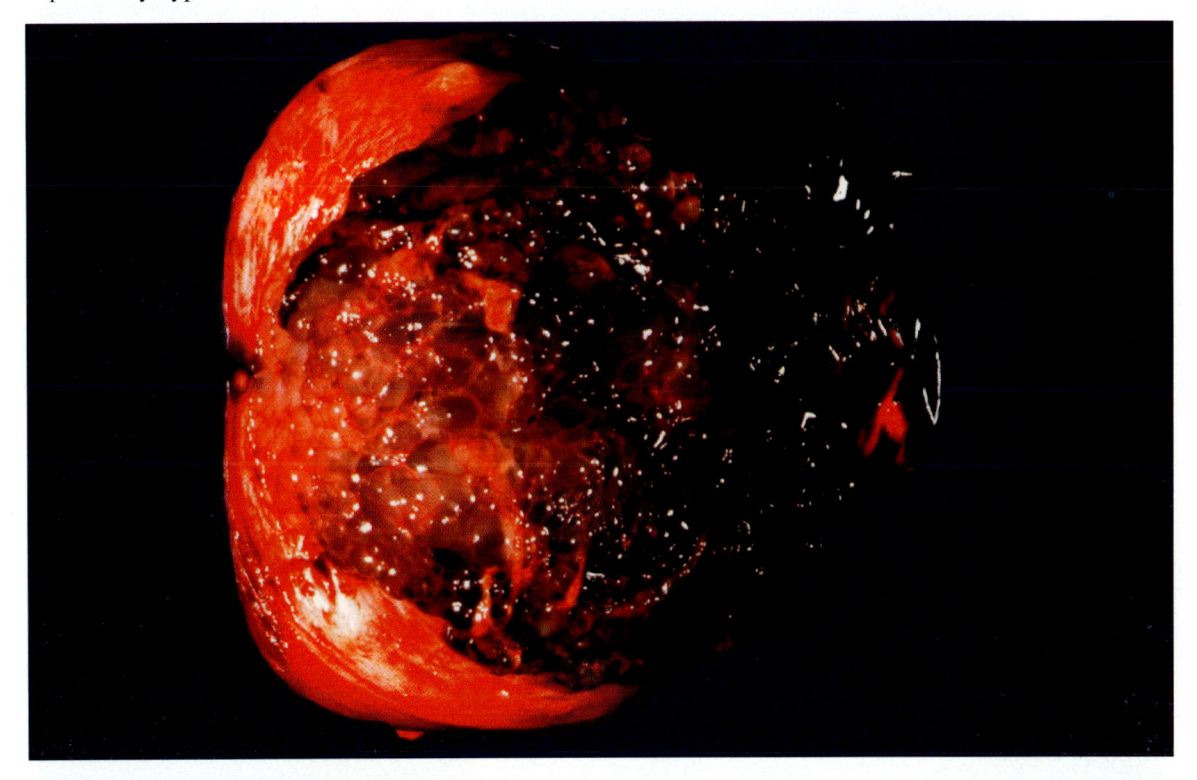

Figure 10-1. Hysterectomy specimen of a complete hydatidiform mole. The myometrium is distended by grape-like cystic vesicles and hemorrhage.

An Atlas of Transvaginal Sonography

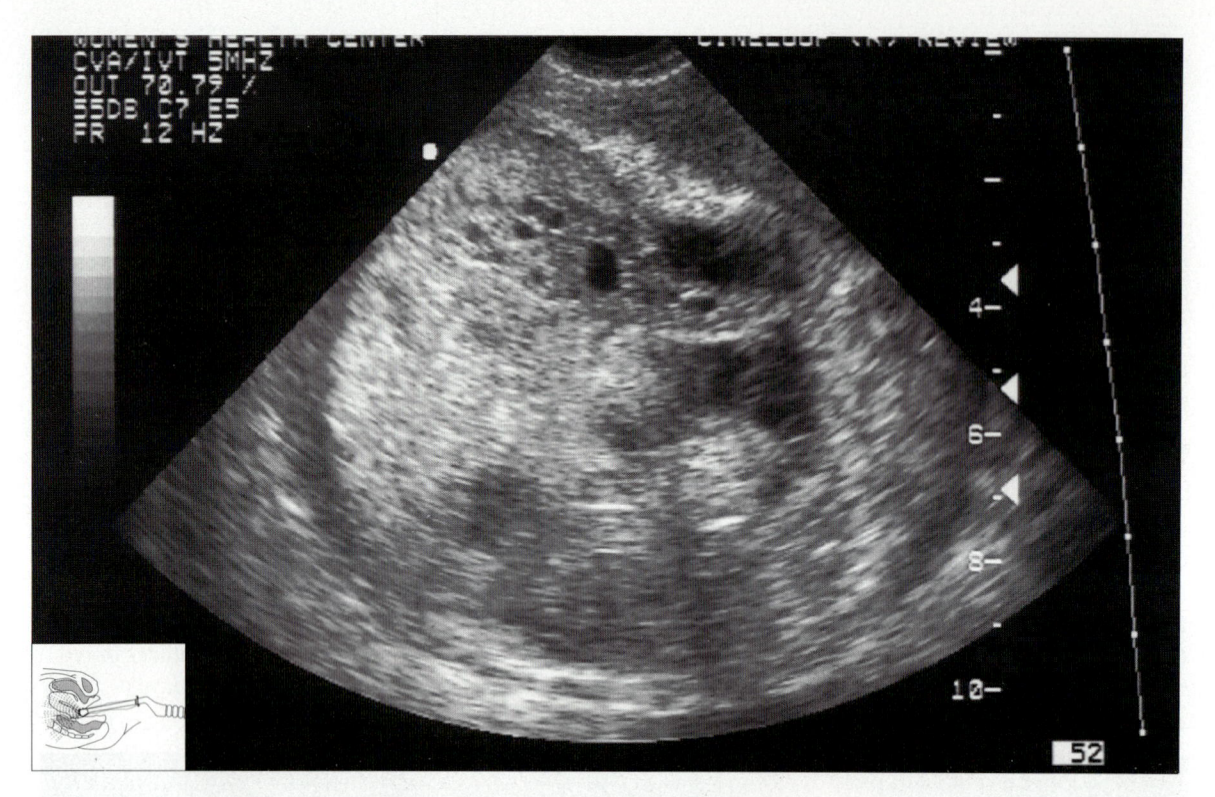

Figure 10-2. Distended uterine cavity by complete or "classical" hydatidiform mole.

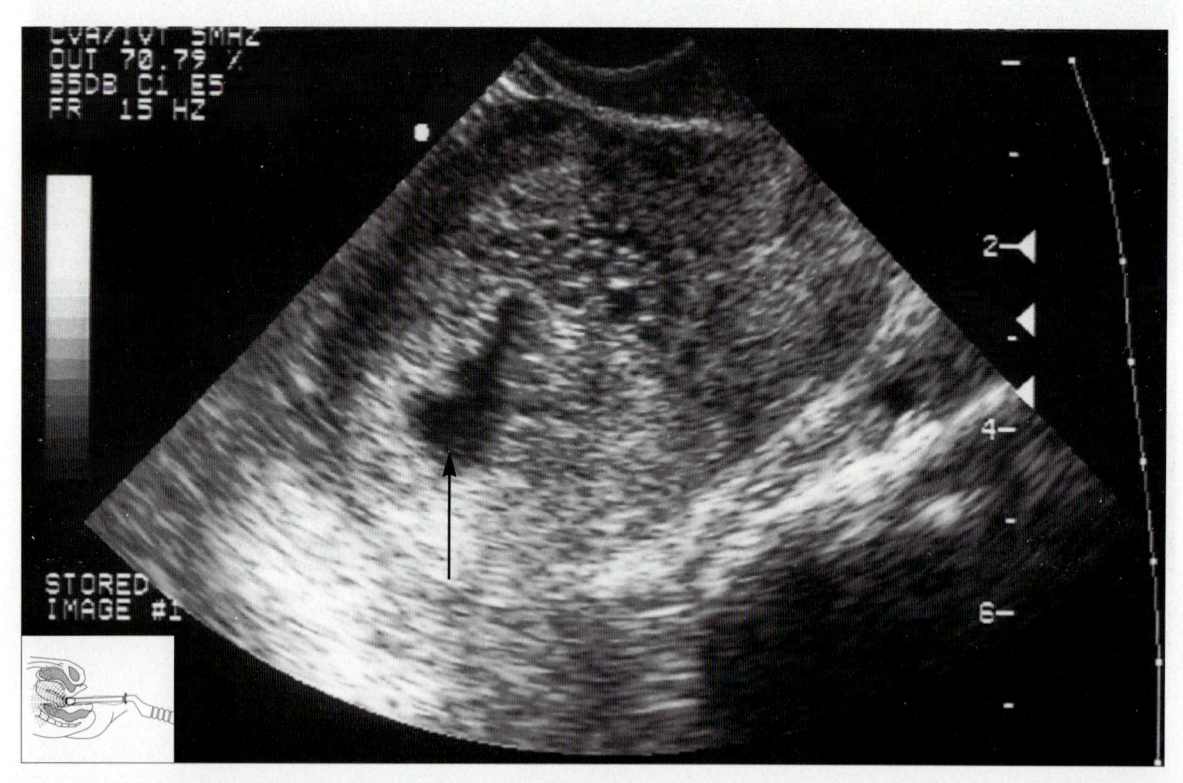

Figure 10-3. Echogenic choriodecidua, with sonolucent cystic areas and a rarely seen central chorionic sac (arrow).

120

Gestational Trophoblastic Disease

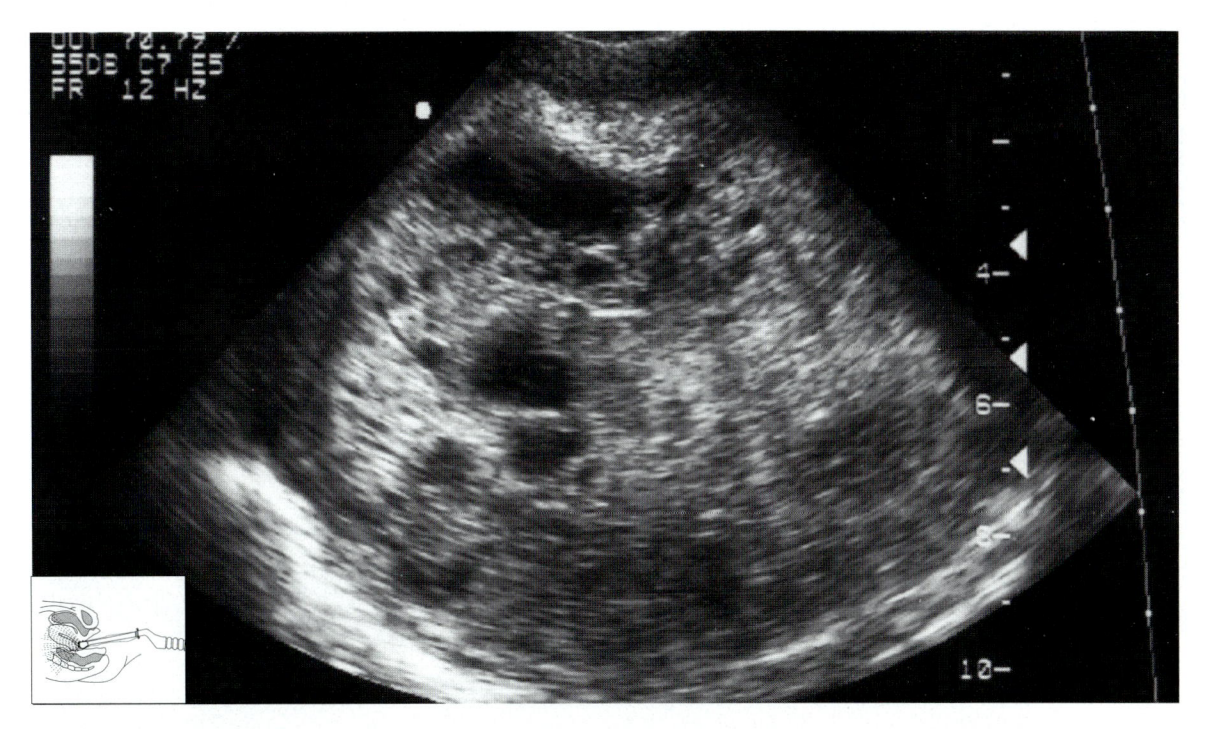

Figure 10-4. The entire uterine cavity is filled with an echogenic solid mass interspersed with cystic areas, corresponding to the hydatidiform vesicles or areas of hemorrhage.

Invasive Mole

Invasive moles occur in 1 per 15,000 pregnancies. Approximately 10-17% of hydatidiform moles result in invasive moles. A benign hydatidiform mole invades the myometrium by direct extension or by venous channels. It can metastasize to distant sites in 15% of cases, most commonly the lungs and vagina. The tumor is characterized by swollen villi and trophoblast hyperplasia and usually dysplasia located in sites outside the cavity of the uterus.

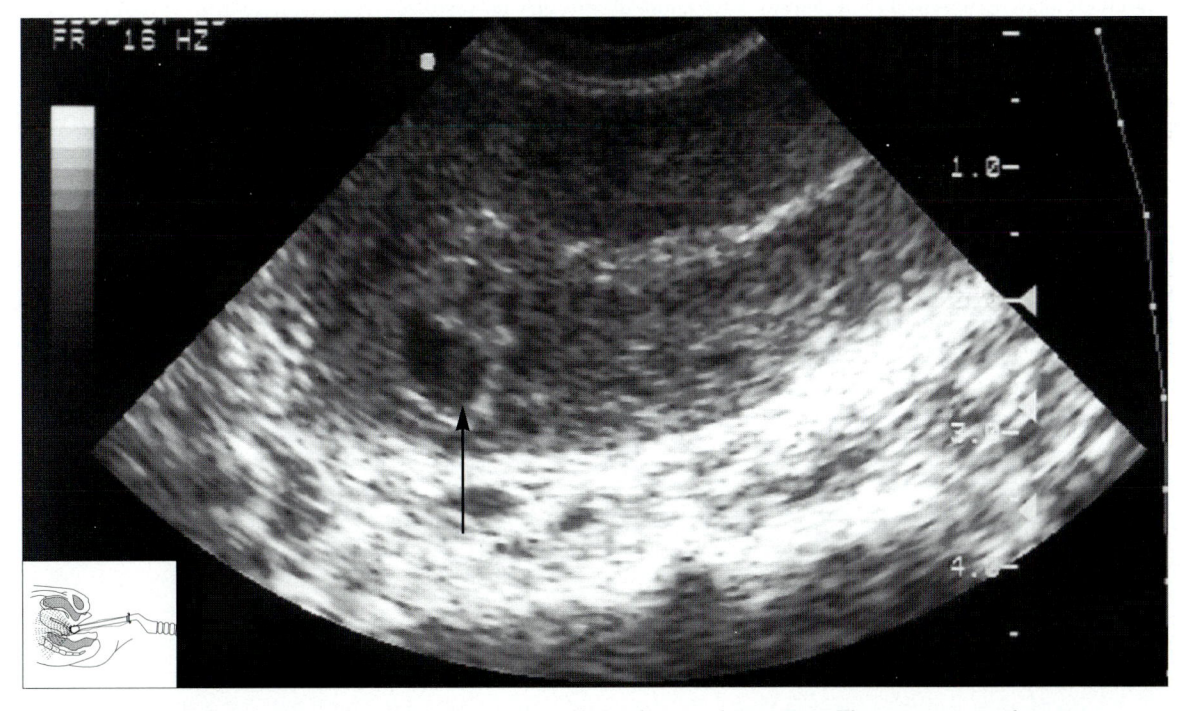

Figure 10-5. Sagittal section through uterus with a thin, echoic endometrium. The patient is undergoing evaluation for increasing B-hCG titers after mole evacuation. Deep within the fundal myometrium is an invasive gestational trophoblastic implant (arrow).

An Atlas of Transvaginal Sonography

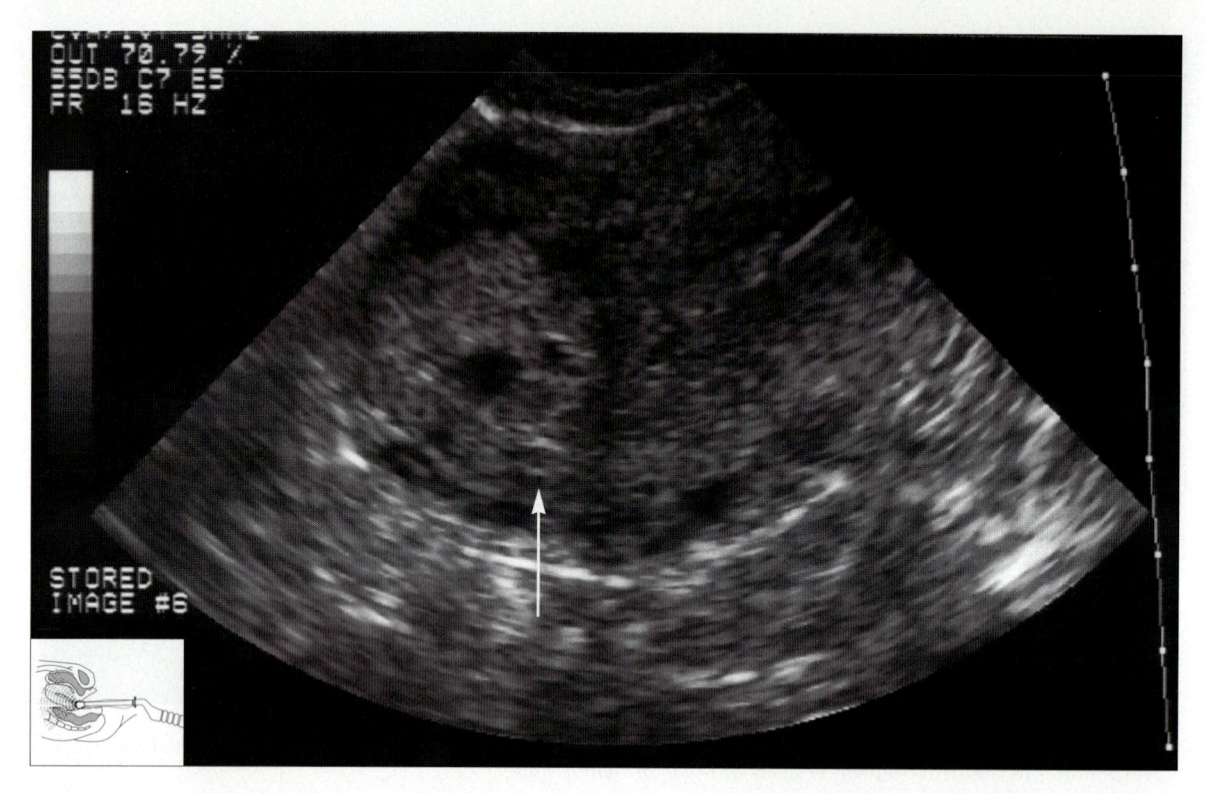

Figure 10-6. A large echogenic invasive mole (arrow) deep within the myometrium. Its morphologic sonographic features are similar to those of a complete mole, with small vesicles and areas of hemorrhage.

Choriocarcinoma

Choriocarcinomas are extremely rare, occurring in 1 per 40,000 pregnancies. Approximately 2-3% of hydatidiform moles progress to choriocarcinoma, which accounts for almost 50% of cases. These are highly malignant aggressive tumors that require chemotherapy for disease control.

Placental Site Trophoblastic Tumor

Placental site trophoblastic tumor is a rare and very malignant tumor derived from the intermediate cells of the placental bed. Unlike the other gestational trophoblastic diseases, B-hCG may not be a reliable tumor marker.

Scan Findings

The characteristic sonographic features of GTD include an enlarged uterus that is filled with complex echogenic vesicles. Hemorrhage into vesicles results in an increased echogenicity. Invasive moles show a discrete region deep within the myometrium with a hypoechoic center and an echoic rim, similar in appearance to the endometrium. Sometimes such clearly demarcated regions are not demonstrable. Color flow reveals increased flow deep within the myometrium and Doppler studies confirm low resistance to flow and resultant low PI. The lesions are able to be followed as measurable disease, regressing with therapy and in parallel with the declining titers of B-hCG.

Gestational Trophoblastic Disease

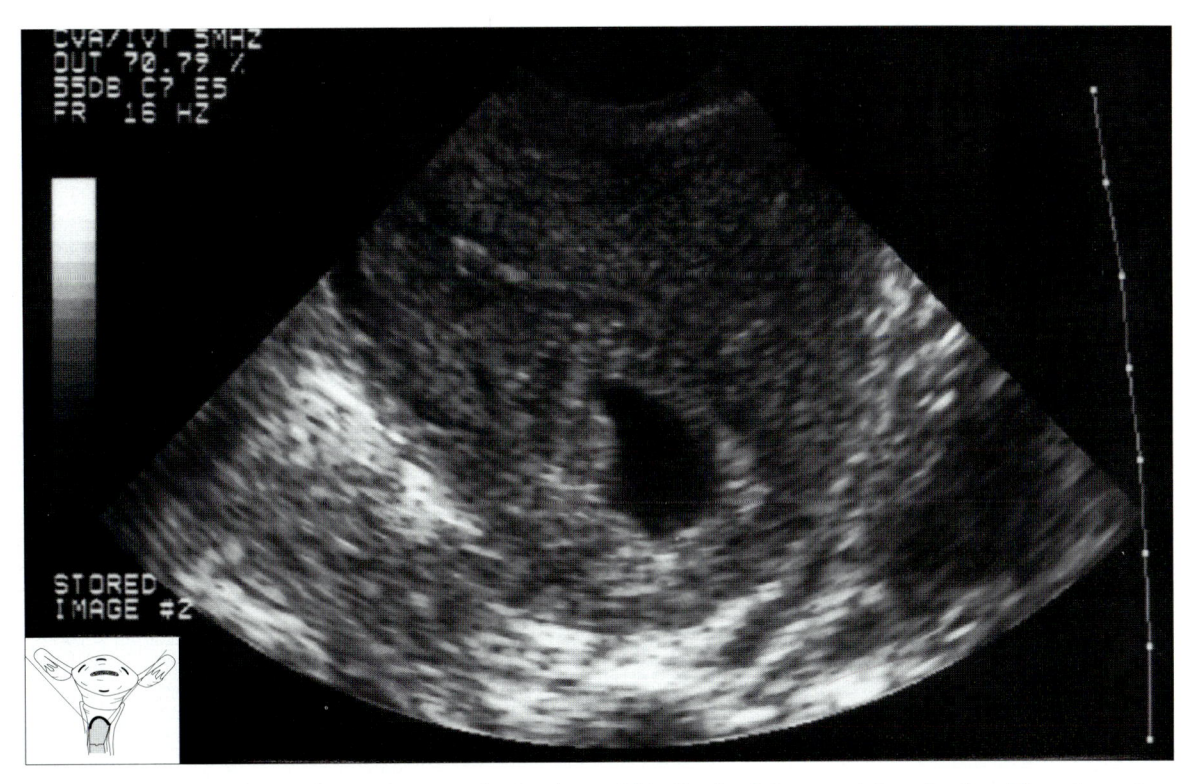

Figure 10-7. *A mainly anechoic invasive molar implant within the fundal myometrium, bordered by echogenic choriodecidua. The lesion is separate from the endometrial cavity.*

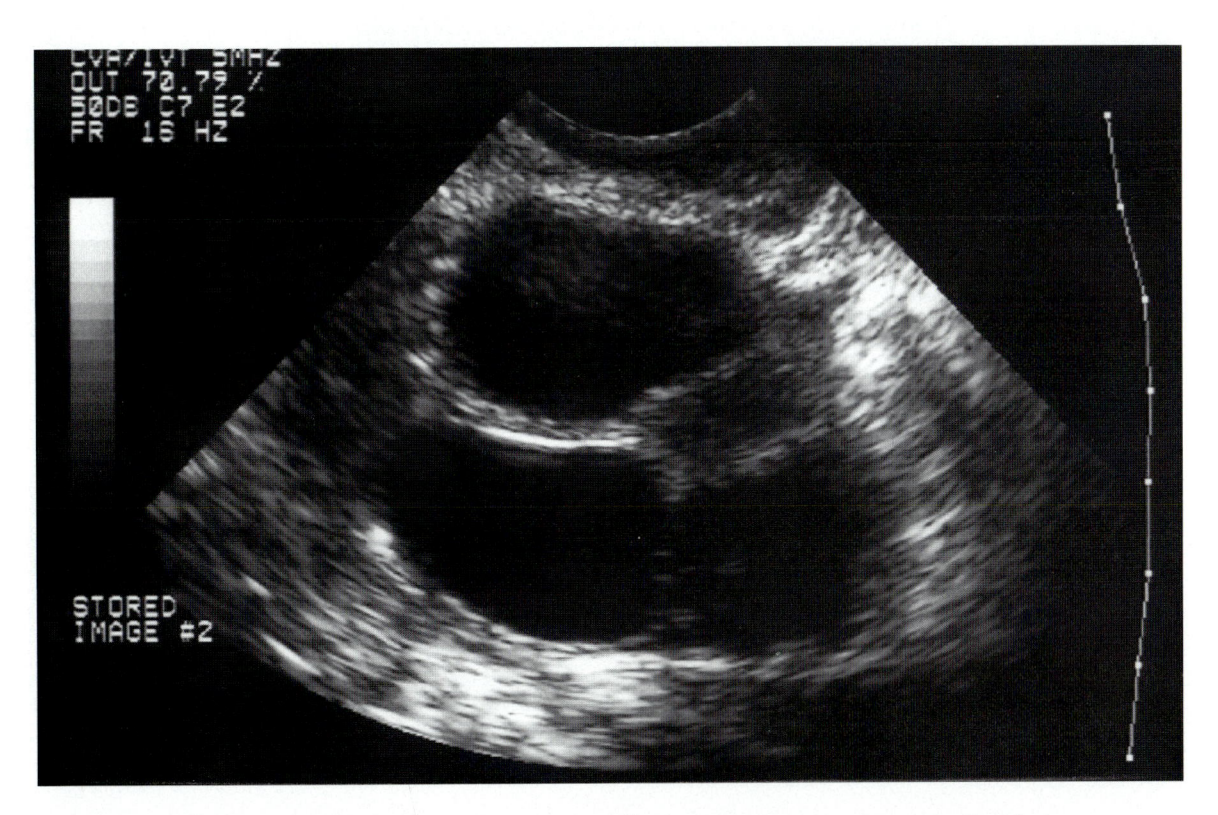

Figure 10-8. *A large polycystic theca luteal cyst. It is similar in appearance to a hyperstimulated ovary.*

An Atlas of Transvaginal Sonography

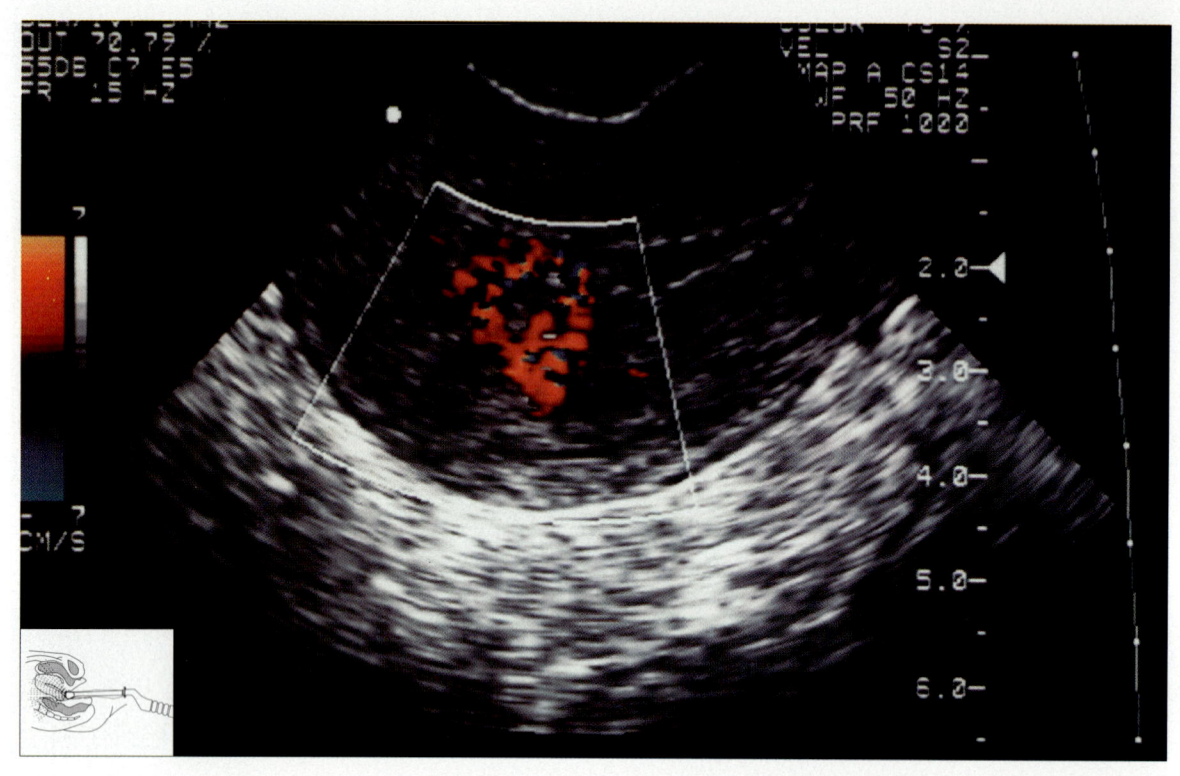

Figure 10-9. Color flow Doppler of a patient suspected of having persistent GTD. A small amount of residual trophoblast remains within the uterine cavity and demonstrates intense color flow. Early myometrial invasion is demonstrated.

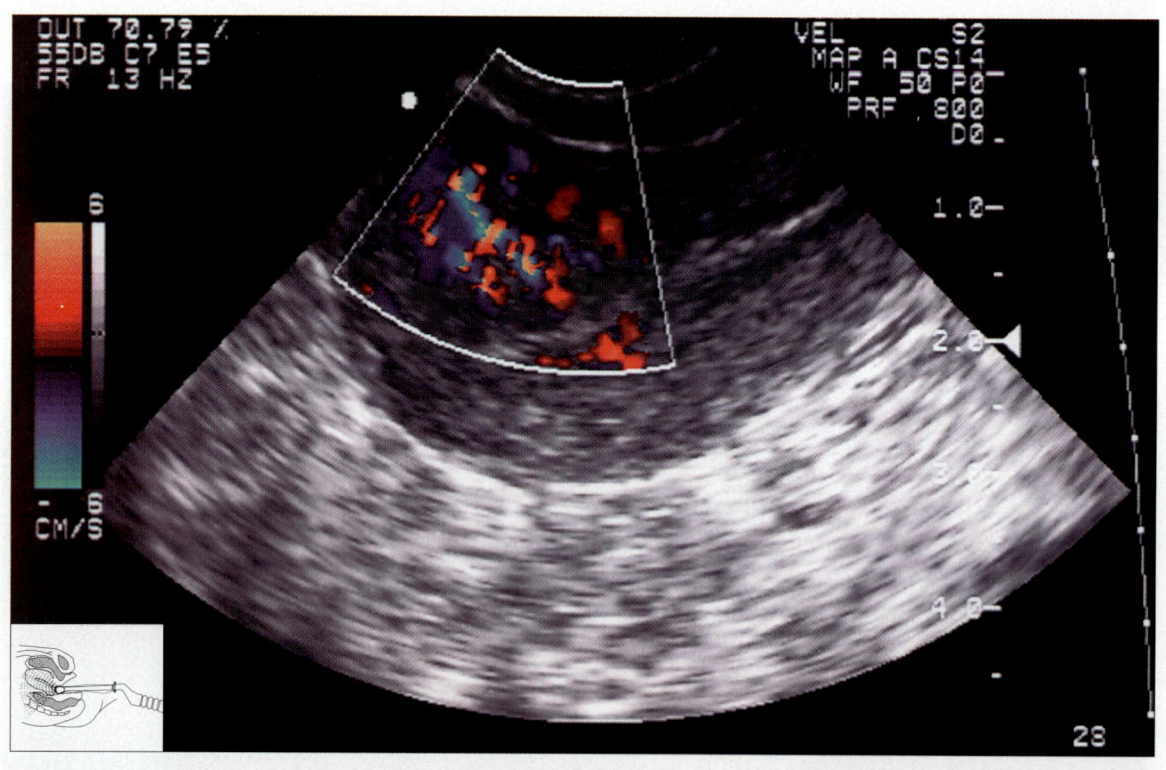

Figure 10-10. Increased color flow within the fundal myometrium of a patient with persistent GTD. The endometrium is thin and the uterine cavity empty.

Gestational Trophoblastic Disease

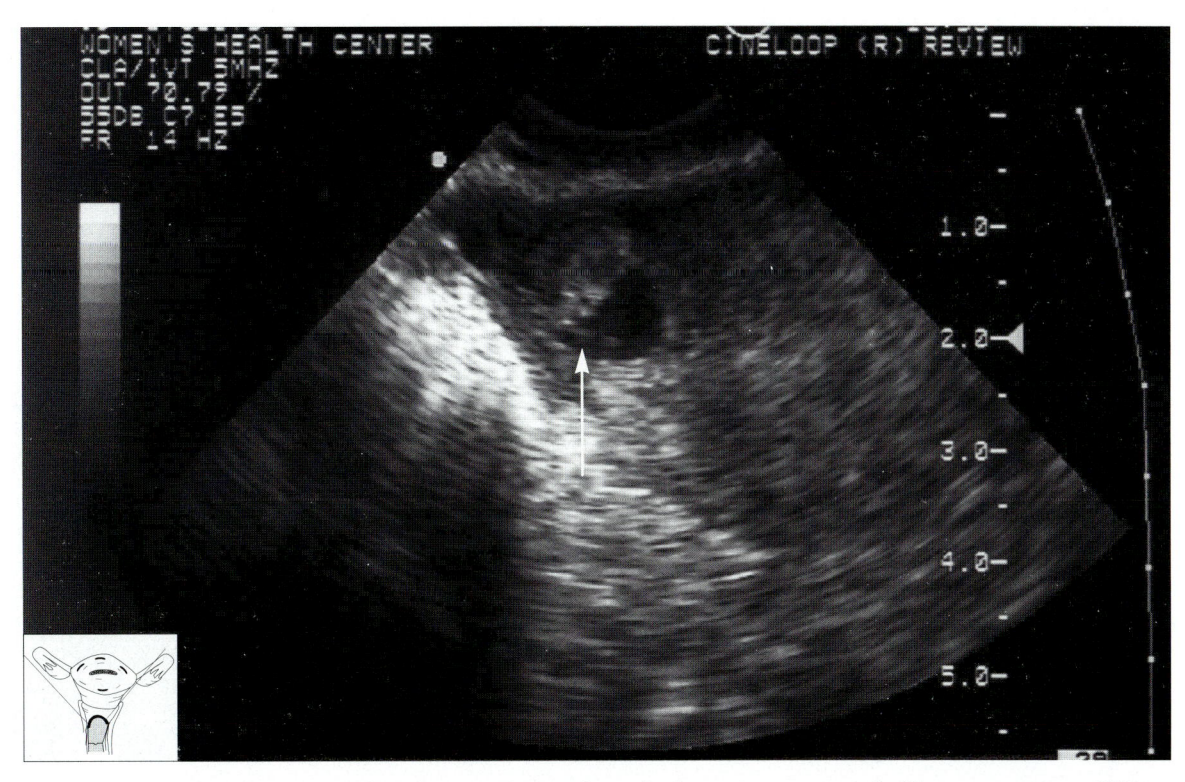

Figure 10-11. Complex mass within the myometrium (arrow) of a patient suspected of having persistent GTD.

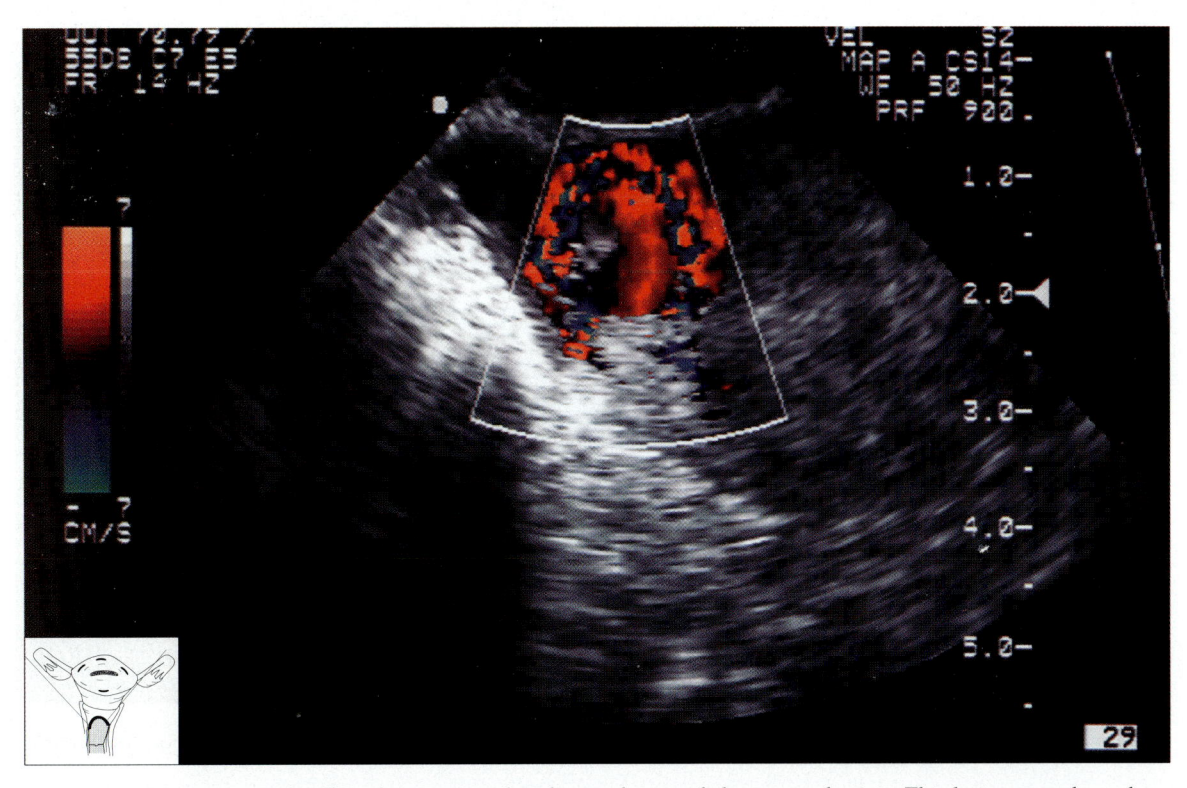

Figure 10-12. Intense color flow demonstrated within and around the tumor deposit. This lesion was the only demonstrable tumor in this patient, and served as a useful "marker" for a response to chemotherapy.

An Atlas of Transvaginal Sonography

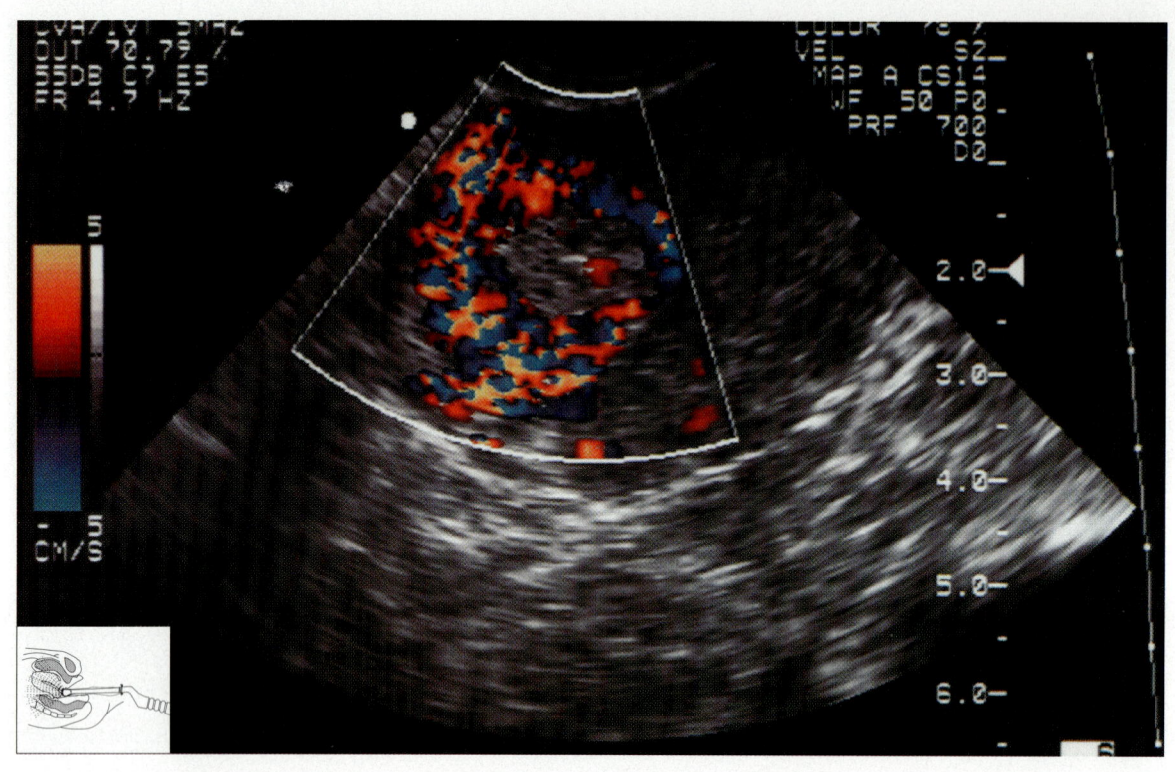

Figure 10-13. A large invasive mole implant demonstrating increased color flow.

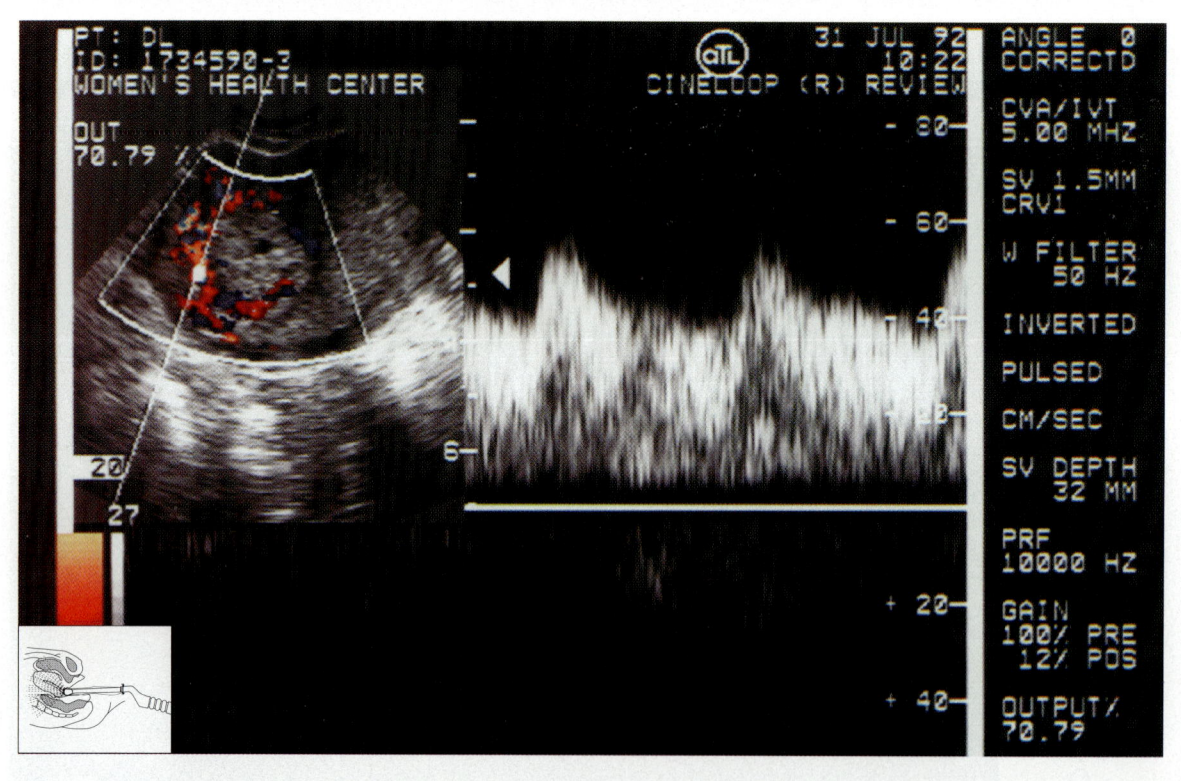

Figure 10-14. Spectral analysis confirms spectral broadening, increased diastolic flow and absence of diastolic notch.

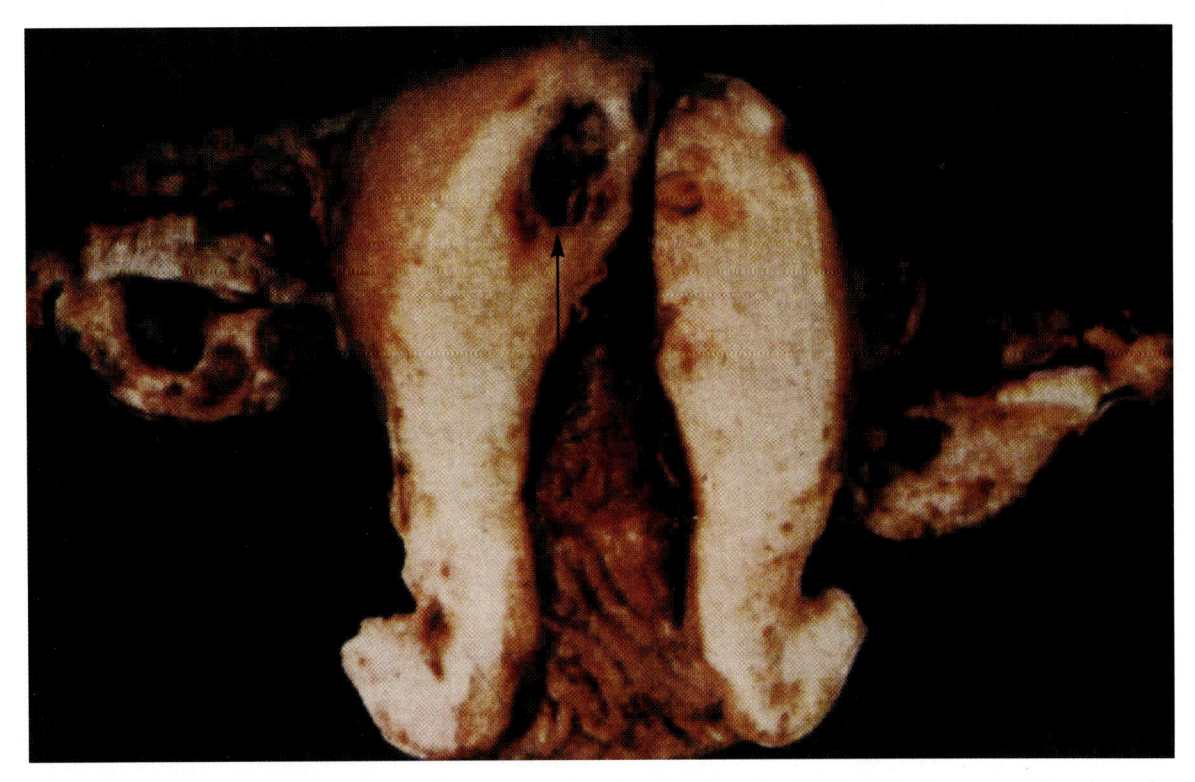

Figure 10-15. Hysterectomy specimen of a patient with an invasive deposit of GTD within the myometrium (arrow).

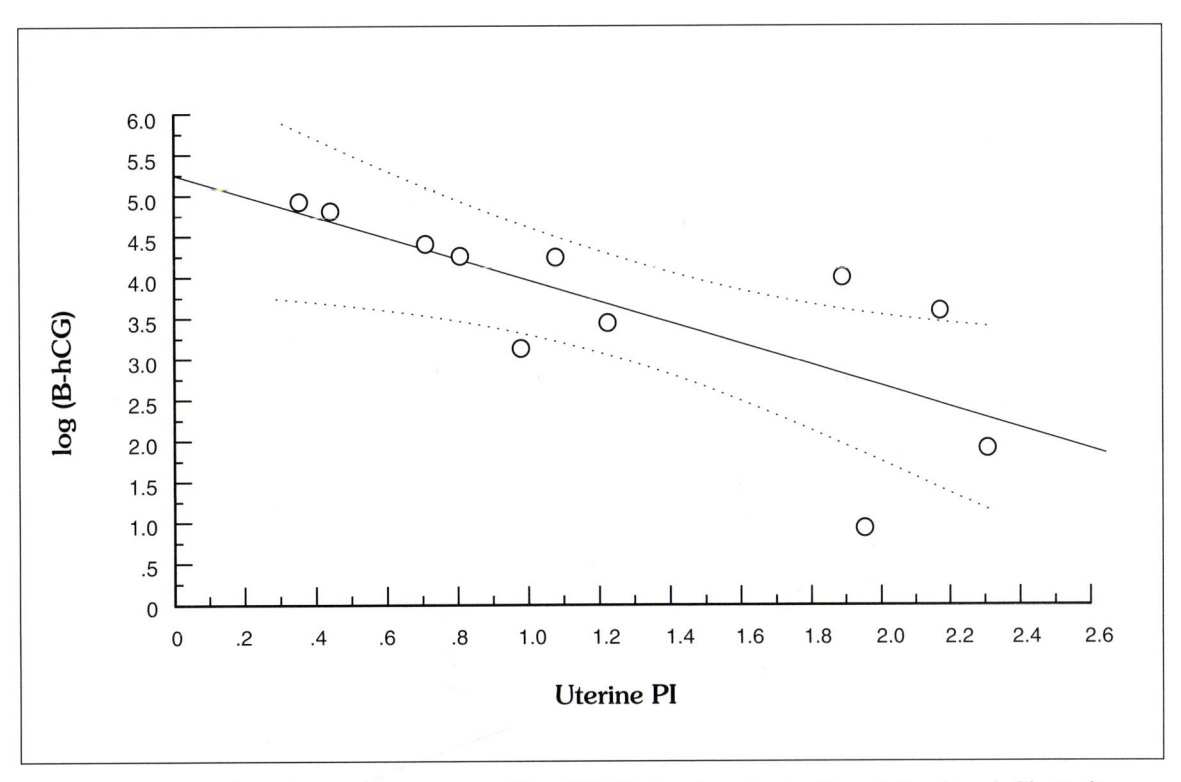

Figure 10-16. Correlation between uterine artery PI and B-hCG titers in patients with gestational trophoblastic disease.

An Atlas of Transvaginal Sonography

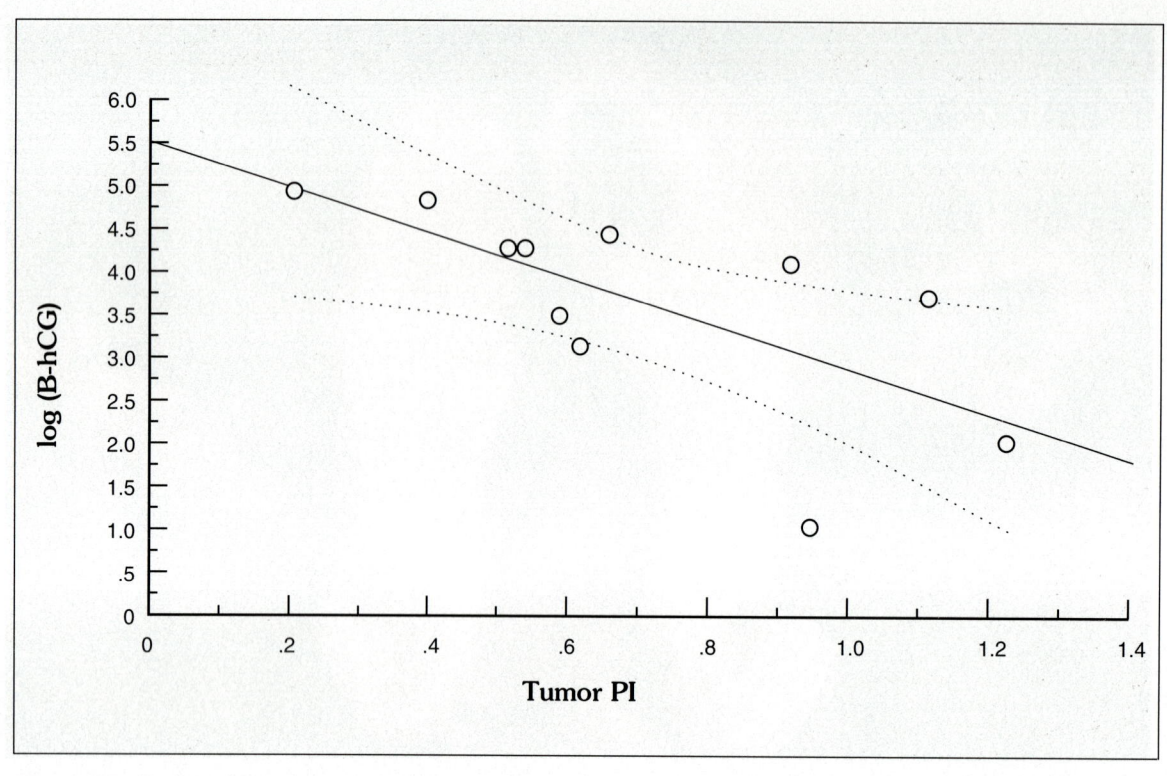

Figure 10-17. Correlation between intratumor PI assessment and B-hCG titers in patients with gestational trophoblastic disease.

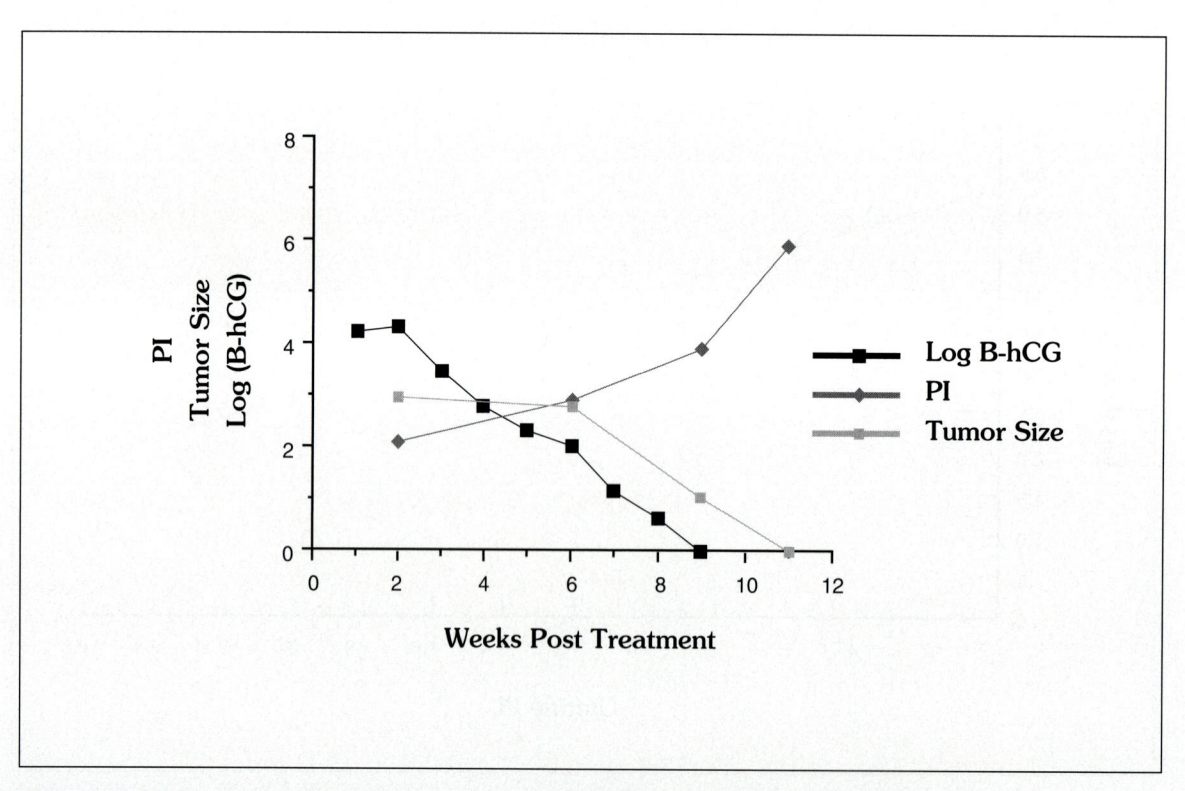

Figure 10-18. Graph depicting tumor size, PI and log B-hCG titers throughout therapy in a patient with an invasive mole.

11   Uterine Cancer

Endometrial Carcinoma

Endometrial adenocarcinoma is the most common of all gynecologic malignancies, but is one of the least common causes of death. In the United States, 34,000 cases are predicted yearly with 3,000 women annually dying of their disease. The low death rate is related to the fact that more than 80% of this type of cancer are clinically confined to the uterus at presentation. It is a disease of the middle and upper socio-economic groups with a median age of 60 years. One-quarter of all patients are premenopausal, with 5% under age 40 at the time of initial diagnosis.

Endometrial cancer is the result of unopposed estrogen stimulation on the endometrium, which induces endometrial proliferation, precancer, and finally endometrial cancer. Risk factors for the development of endometrial cancer include obesity, hormone replacement therapy (HRT), diabetes, nulliparity, early menarche, late menopause, polycystic ovary syndrome (PCOS), gall bladder disease, and the use of sequential oral contraceptives.

Scan Findings

Early invasive endometrial cancers are often indistinguishable from sonograms of patients with endometrial hyperplasia. The endometrial stripe is thickened and echoic with loss of the subendometrial halo. This hypoechoic halo is a layer of compact, vascular myometrium. Preservation of this halo usually indicates superficial invasion, while absence is frequently associated with deep myometrial invasion.

The presence of uterine fibroids can, unfortunately, render assessment of the entire uterine cavity impossible. Acoustical shadowing can leave large areas of the endometrium inaccessible to the vaginal transducer.

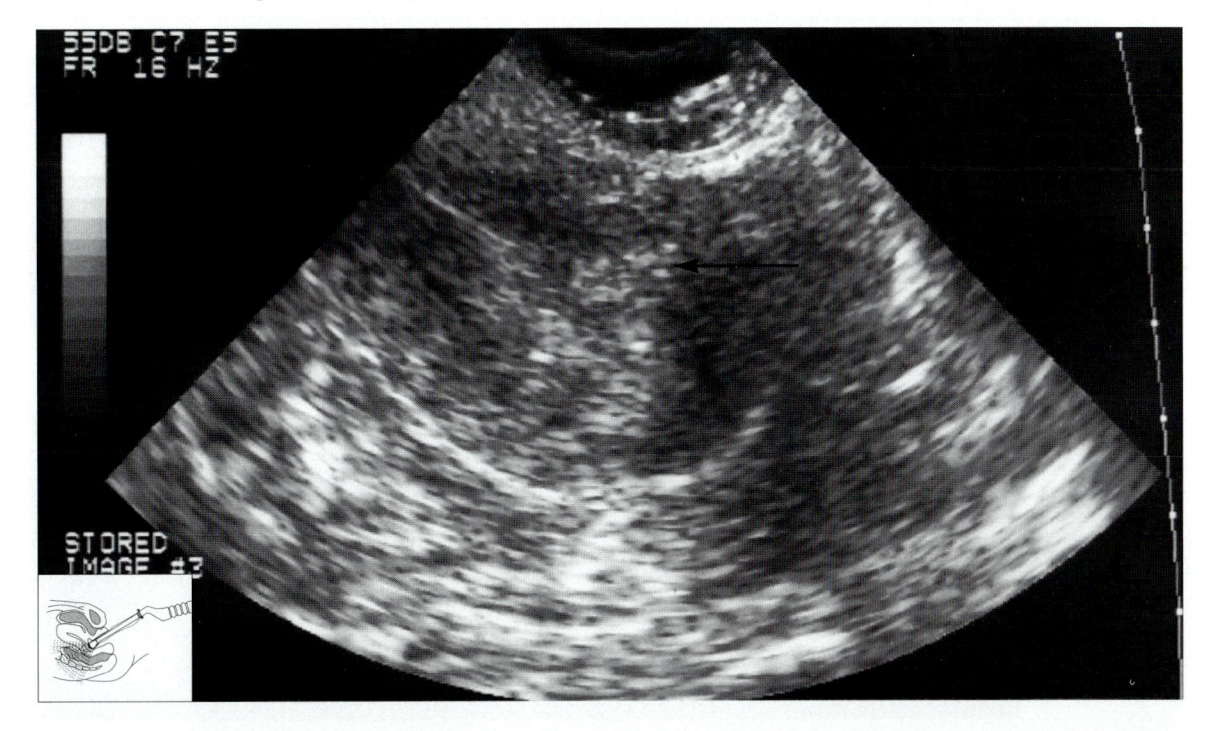

Figure 11-1. Retroverted uterus with invasive endometrial cancer. Echogenic endometrioid cancer invades into the adjacent myometrium, disrupting the subendometrial halo (arrow).

An Atlas of Transvaginal Sonography

Depth of myometrial invasion can also be directly measured. Fleischer used real-time sonography to measure depth of invasion. In 70% of cases, ultrasound accurately estimated the depth of invasion as compared to actual measurements on the gross specimen. Other findings indicative of endometrial cancer include an enlarged uterine cavity, and enlarged uterus with a mixed echogenic pattern, pyometra or a prominent or variably echogenic endometrium. In advanced cancers the endometrium may be irregular, with tongues of echoic tumor penetrating the myometrium. The endometrial/myometrial interface may be fuzzy. Color Doppler reveals an increased blood flow and lowered resistance. A uterine artery or intratumor PI of 2.0 gives a detection rate of 99% with a false positive rate of 2.6%.

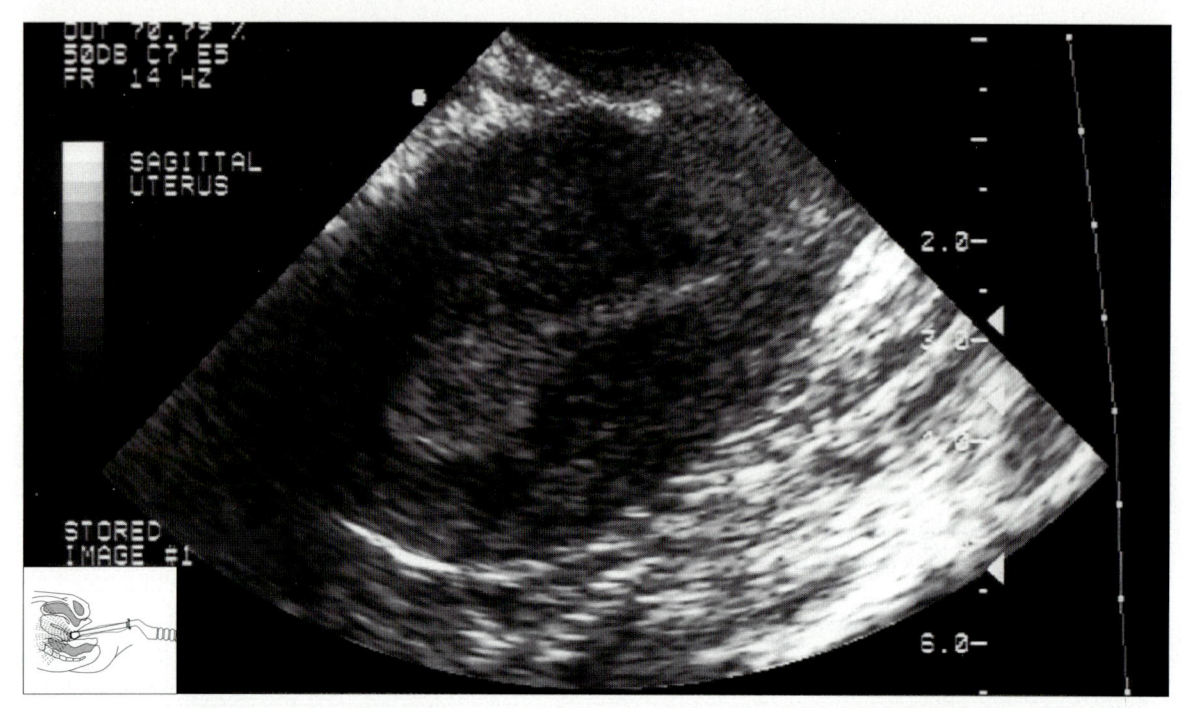

Figure 11-2. Superficially invasive uterine cancer. The endometrium is thickened and echoic.

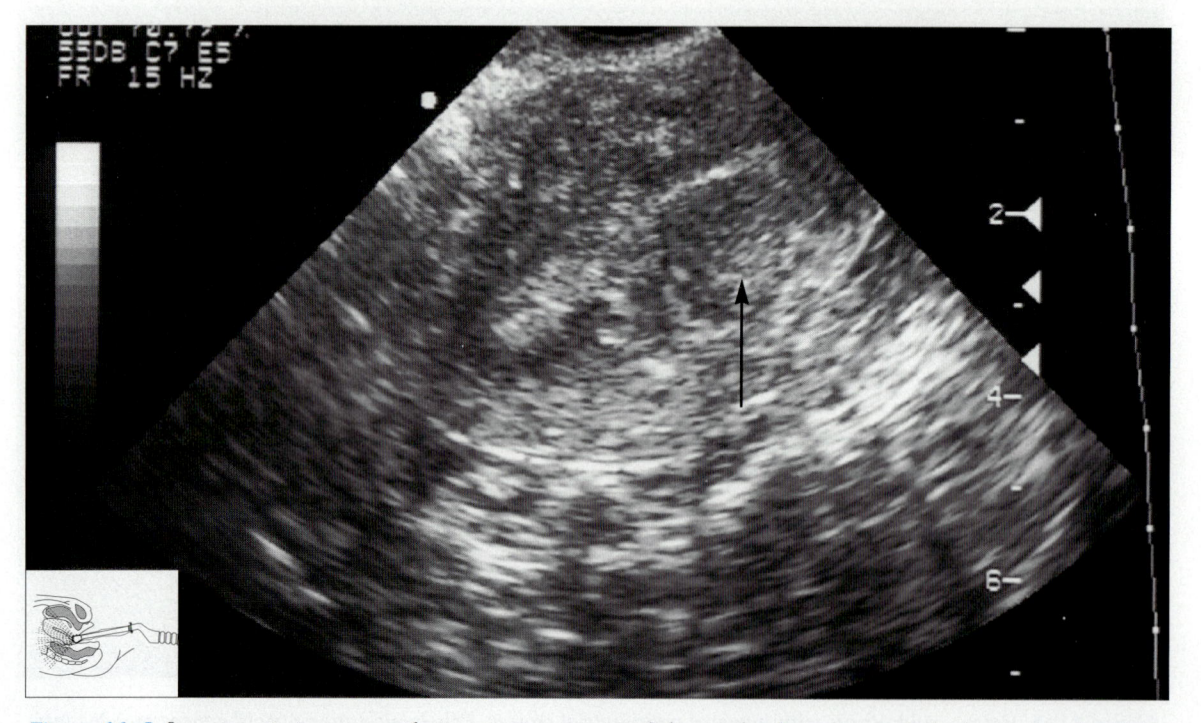

Figure 11-3. Invasive uterine cancer that was not appreciated due to the distortion and shadowing produced by the posterior wall fibroid (arrow).

Uterine Cancer

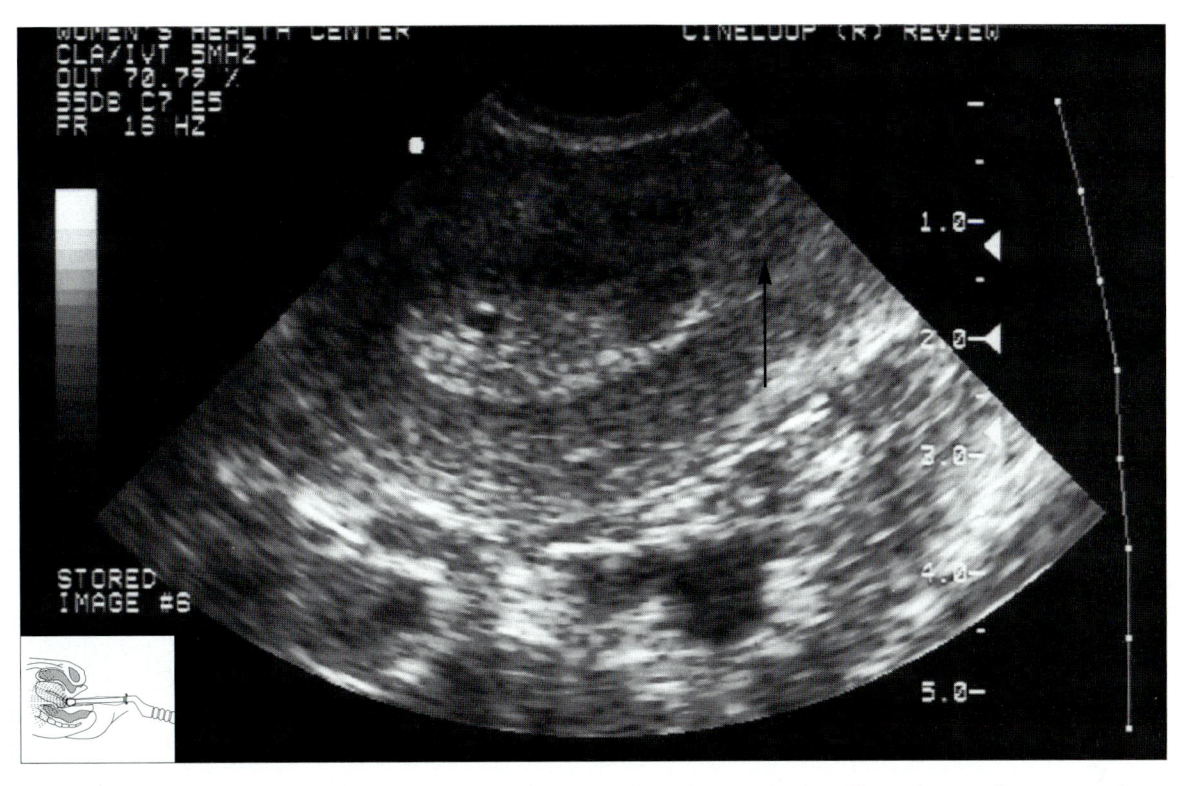

Figure 11-4. Coexisting superficially invasive uterine cancer and endometrial polyp. The endometrial cancer is echoic but is bounded by the subendometrial halo. An isoechoic polyp is prolapsing down into the endocervix (arrow).

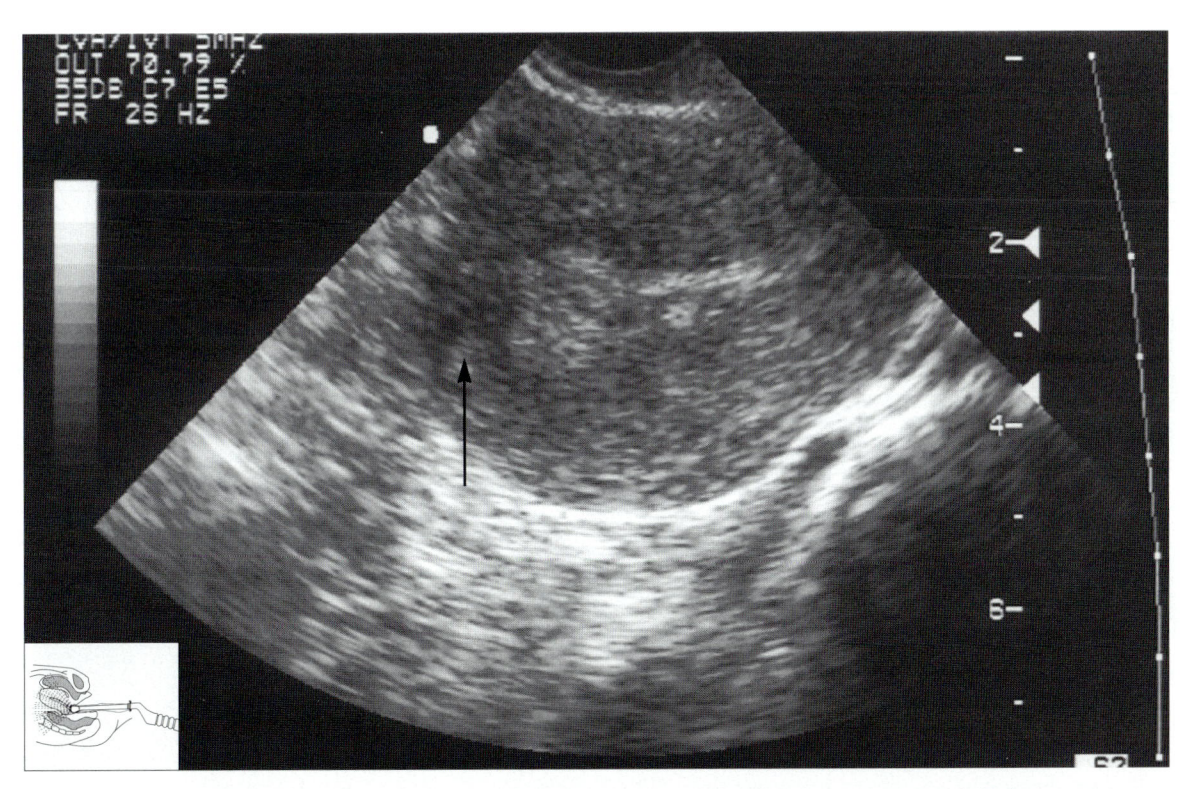

Figure 11-5. An echogenic endometrial cancer invading greater than 50% of the myometrial thickness, with a small deposit immediately adjacent to the fundal uterine serosa (arrow).

An Atlas of Transvaginal Sonography

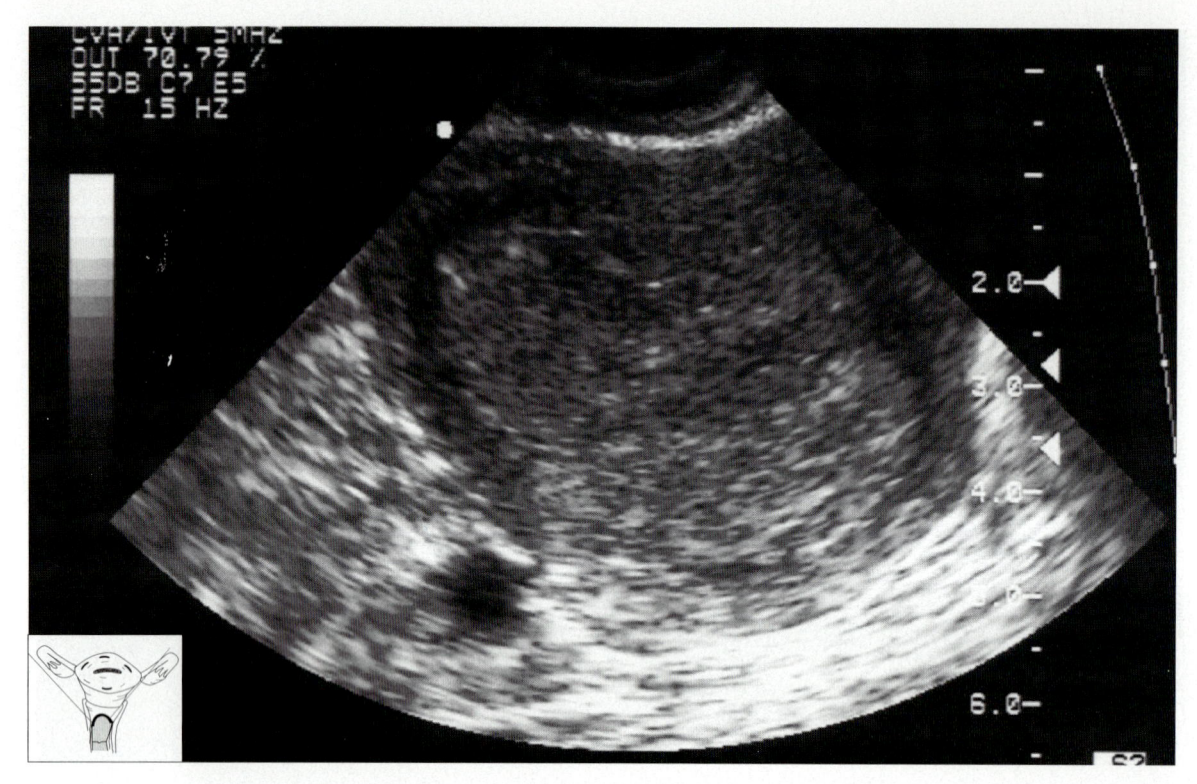

Figure 11-6. An isoechoic endometrial cancer distending the uterine cancer.

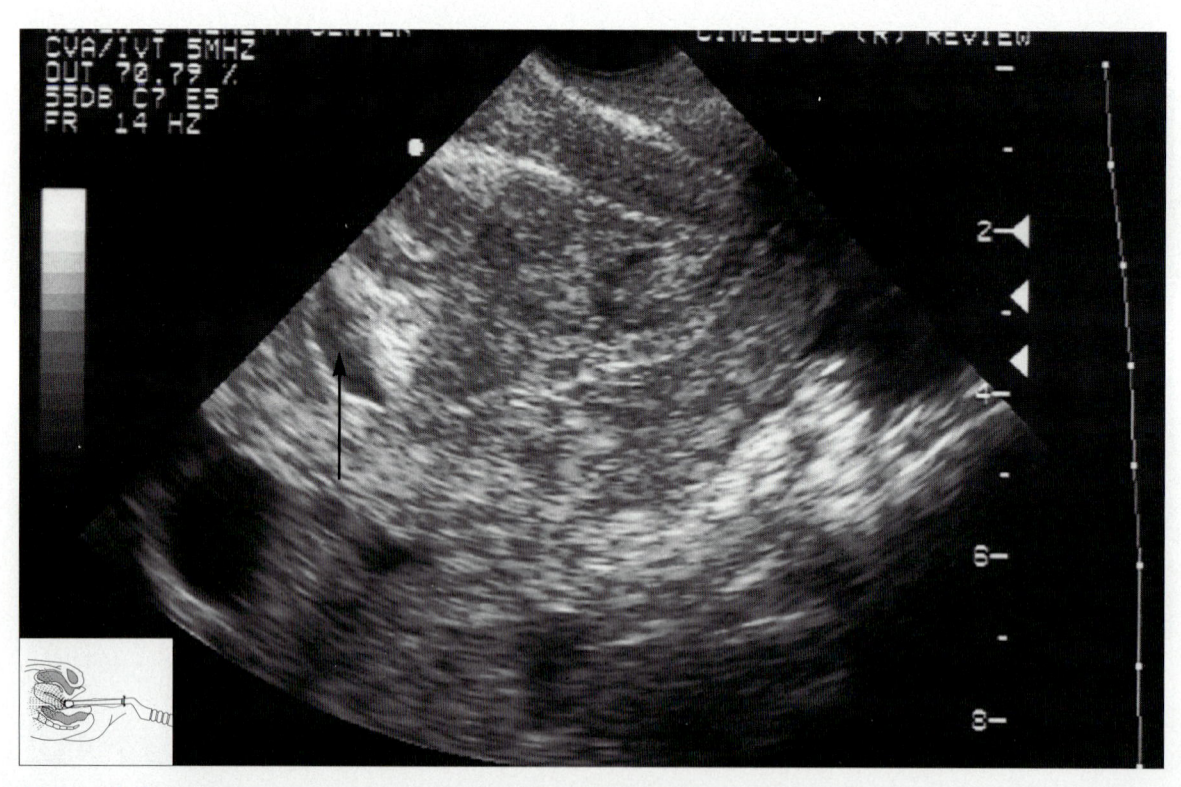

Figure 11-7. A uterine tumor arising from an endometrial polyp. The endometrium is thin and echoic while the tumor is of mixed echogenicity. A small area of hemorrhage (arrow) lies behind the tumor.

Uterine Cancer

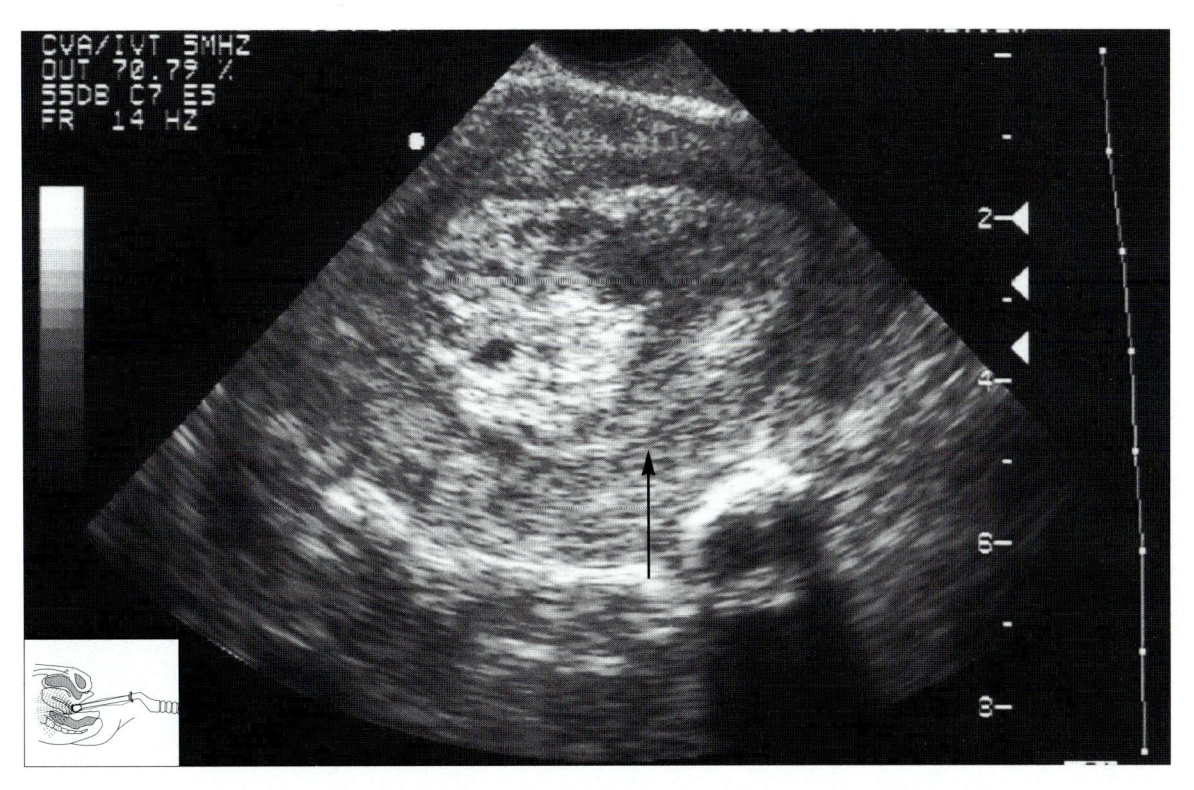

Figure 11-8. Fundal site of origin of endometrial cancer, showing loss of subendometrial halo (arrow). The remainder of the uterine cavity shows a clear layer of compact myometrium or "subendometrial halo."

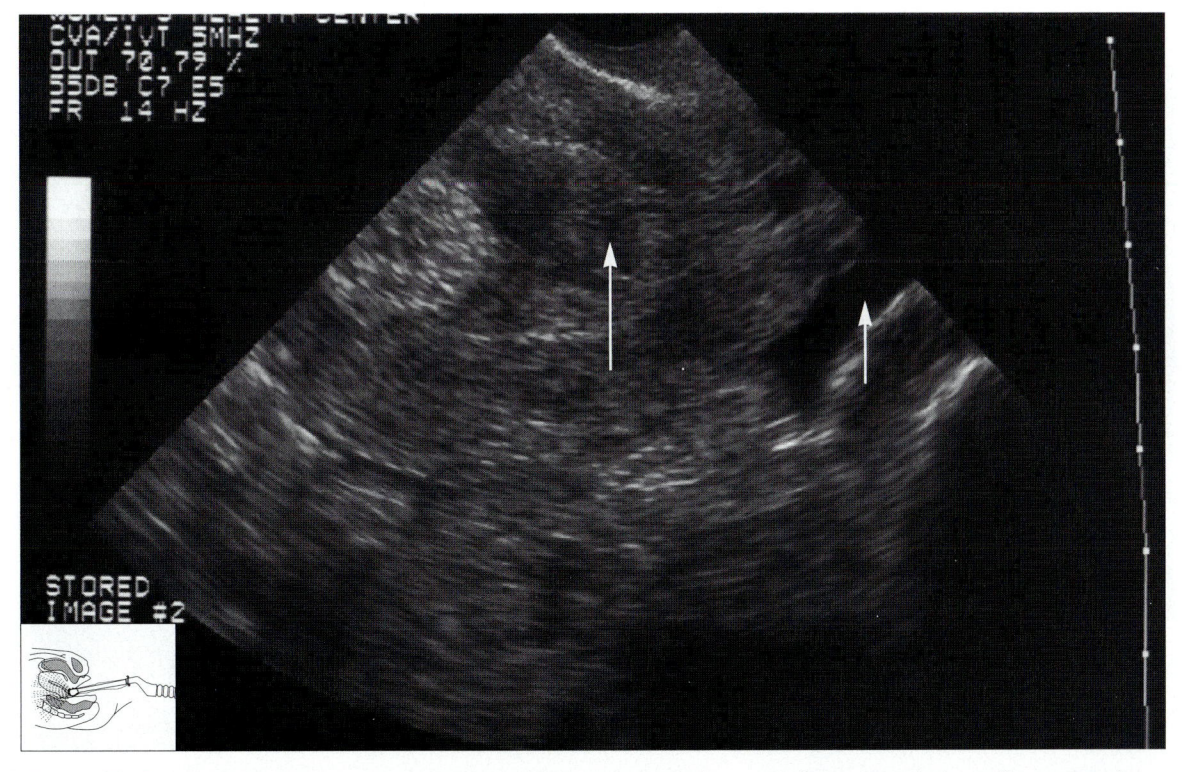

Figure 11-9. Mixed echogenic uterine cancer prolapsing through the cervix (large arrow). A small amount of fluid is present within the cul-de-sac (small arrow).

An Atlas of Transvaginal Sonography

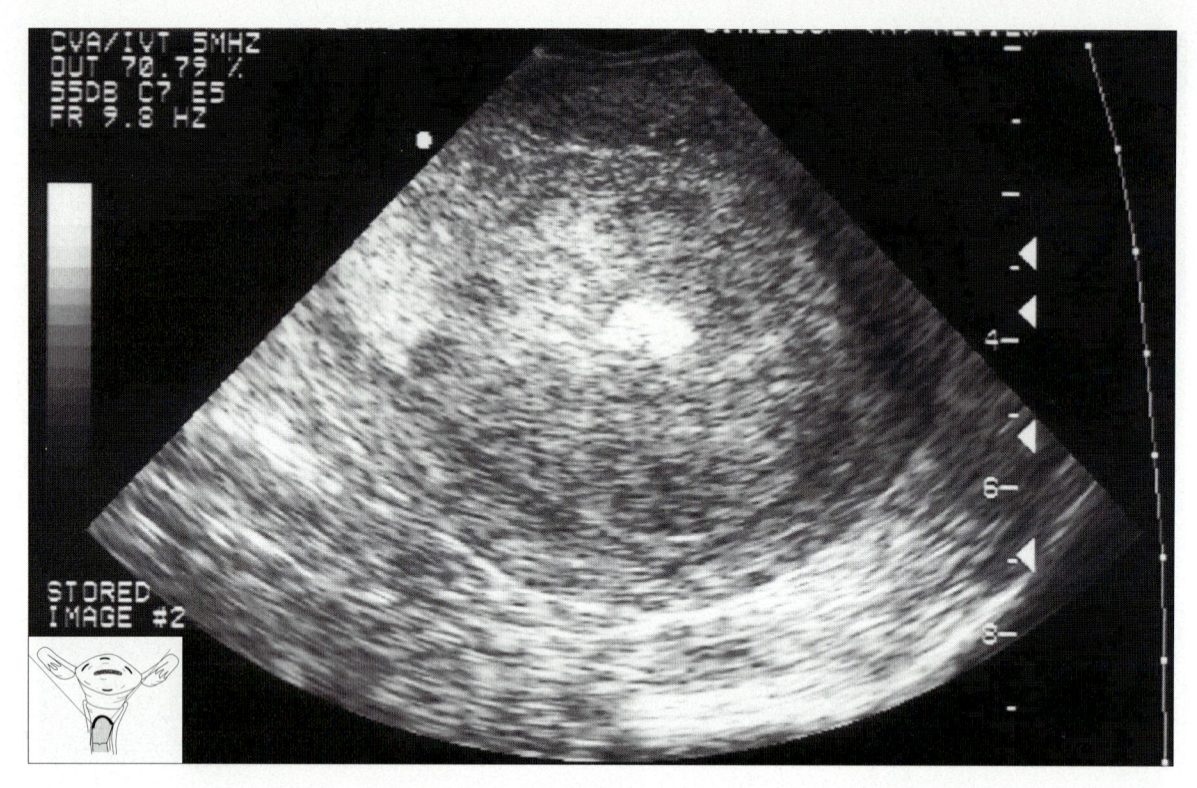

Figure 11-10. Large, essentially isoechoic, endometrial cancer distending the uterine corpus. Echoic areas represent areas of hemorrhage.

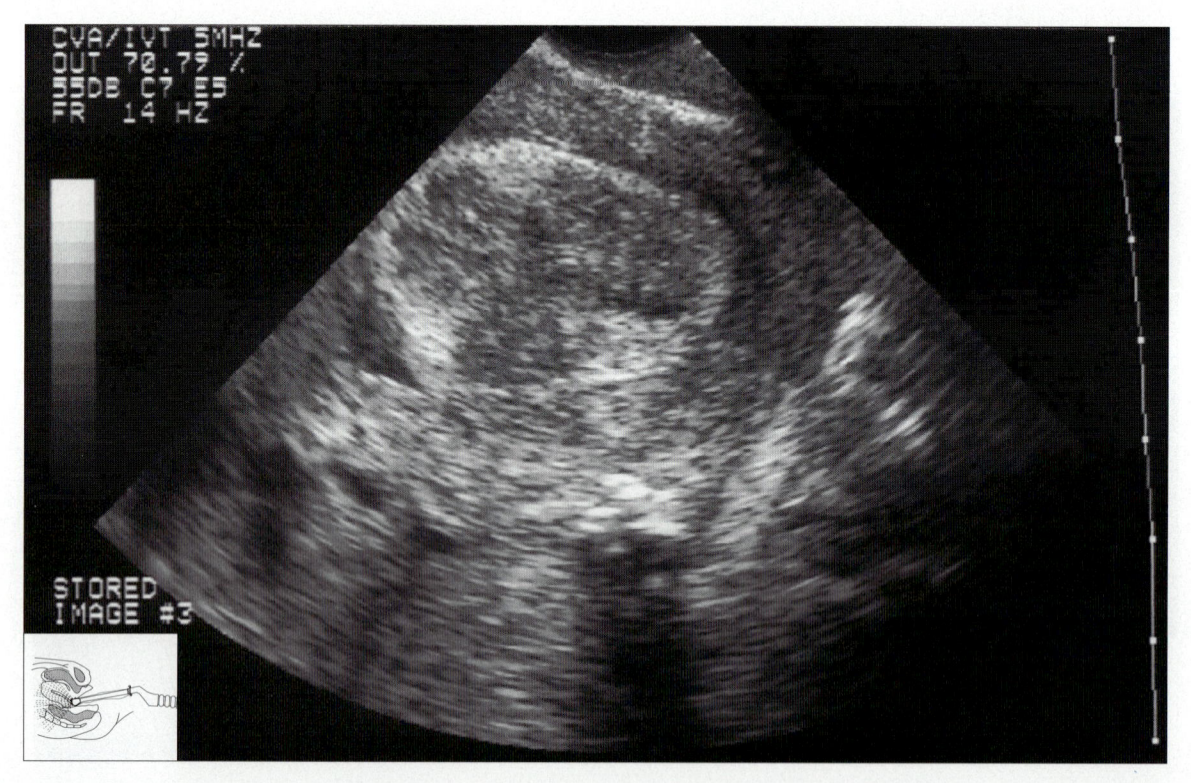

Figure 11-11. Coronal view through uterus and large, mixed, echogenic, uterine cancer.

Uterine Cancer

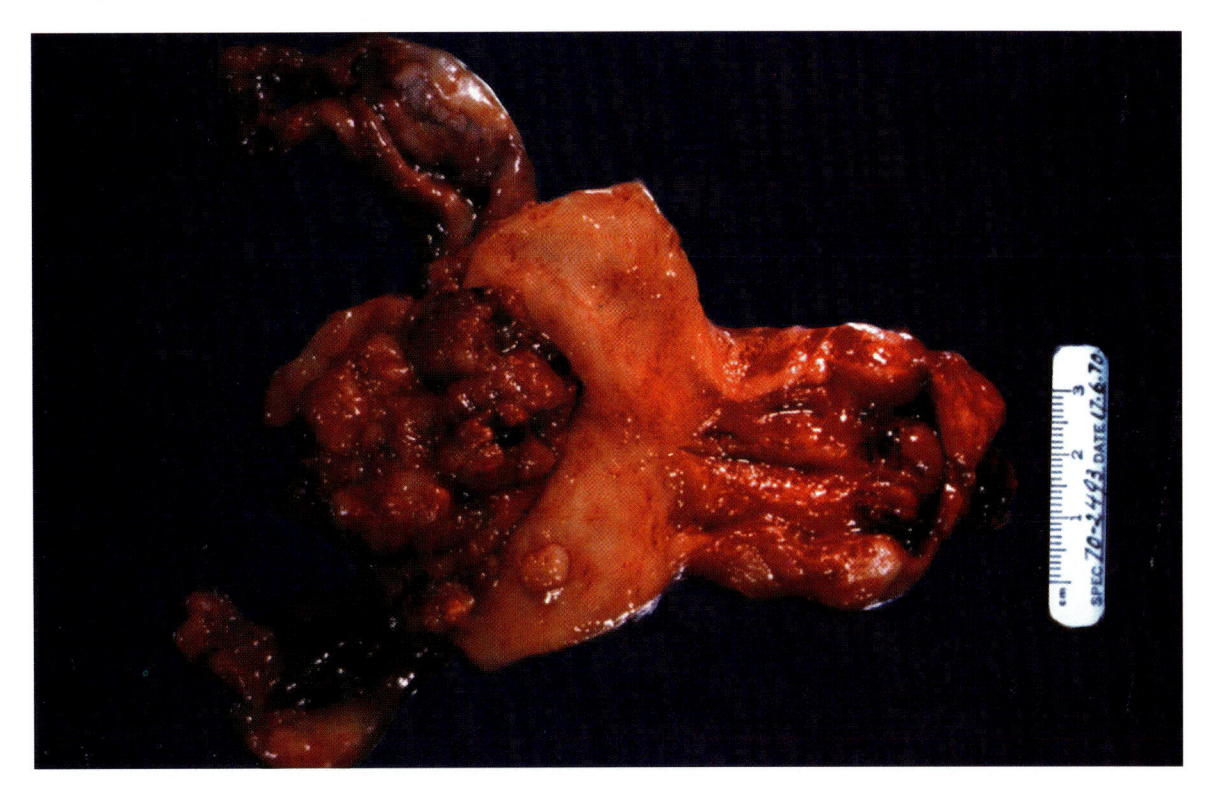

Figure 11-12. Exophytic polyoid uterine cancer.

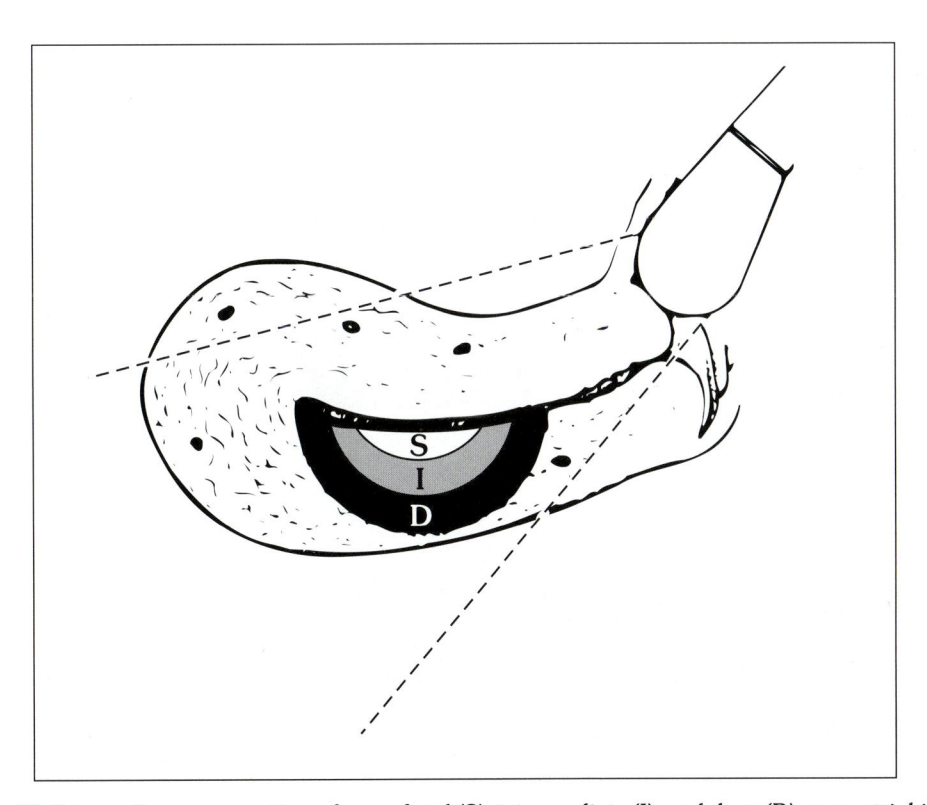

Figure 11-13. Schematic representation of superficial (S), intermediate (I), and deep (D) myometrial invasion as seen in the sagittal transvaginal plane.

An Atlas of Transvaginal Sonography

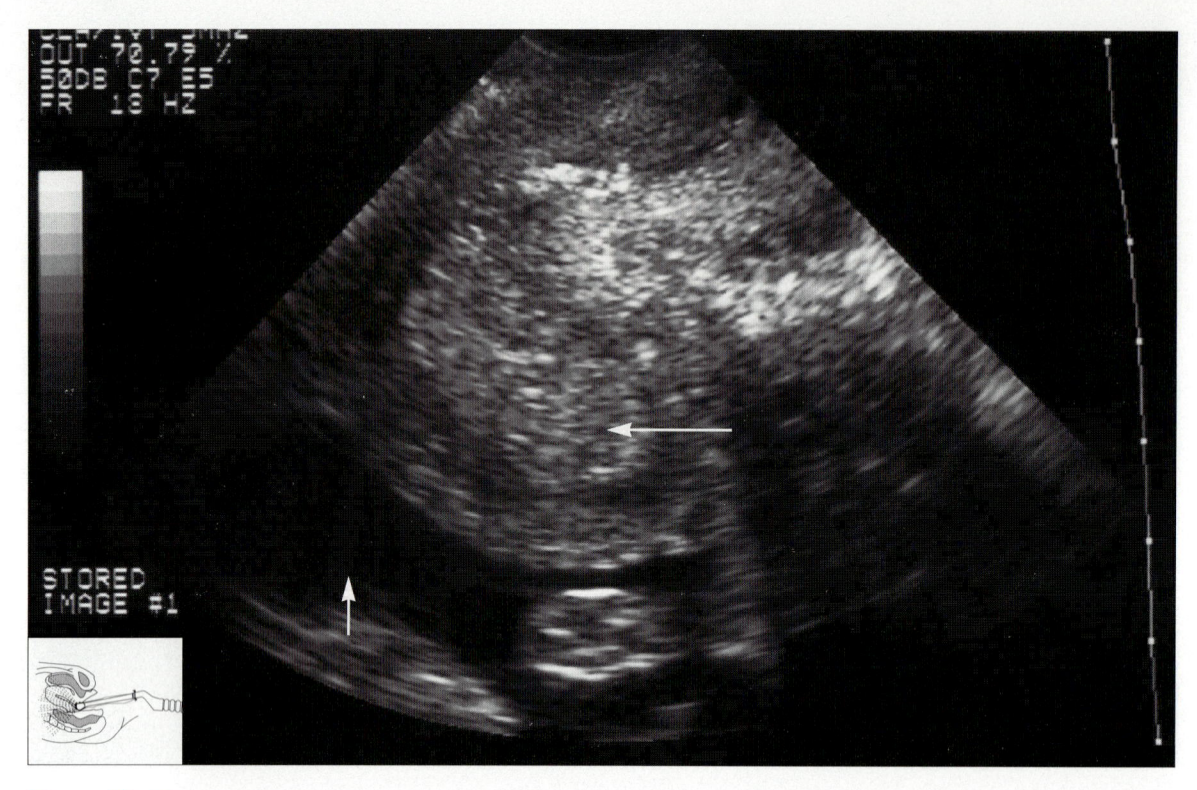

Figure 11-14. Advanced uterine cancer. Retroverted uterus with a voluminous endometrial cancer (large arrow) bathed in ascitic fluid (small arrow), positive for malignant cells.

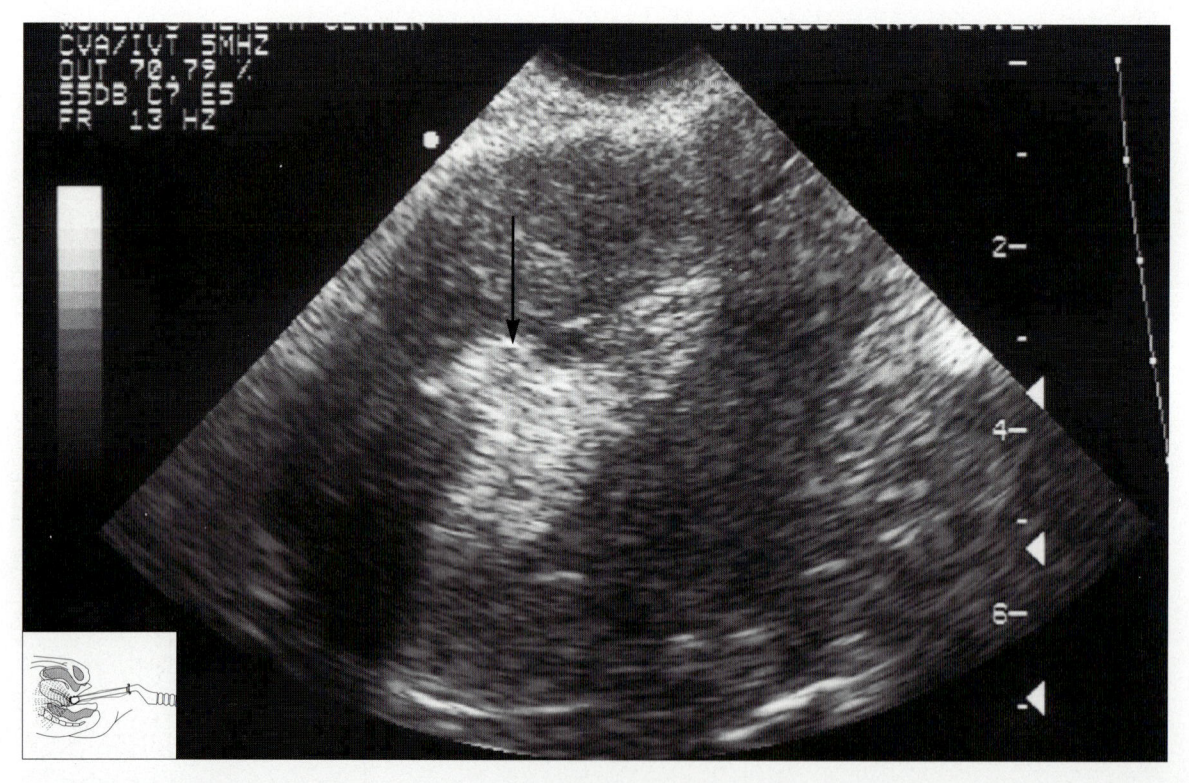

Figure 11-15. Echogenic endometrial cancer clearly demonstrating invasion to 50% (arrow) of the myometrial thickness.

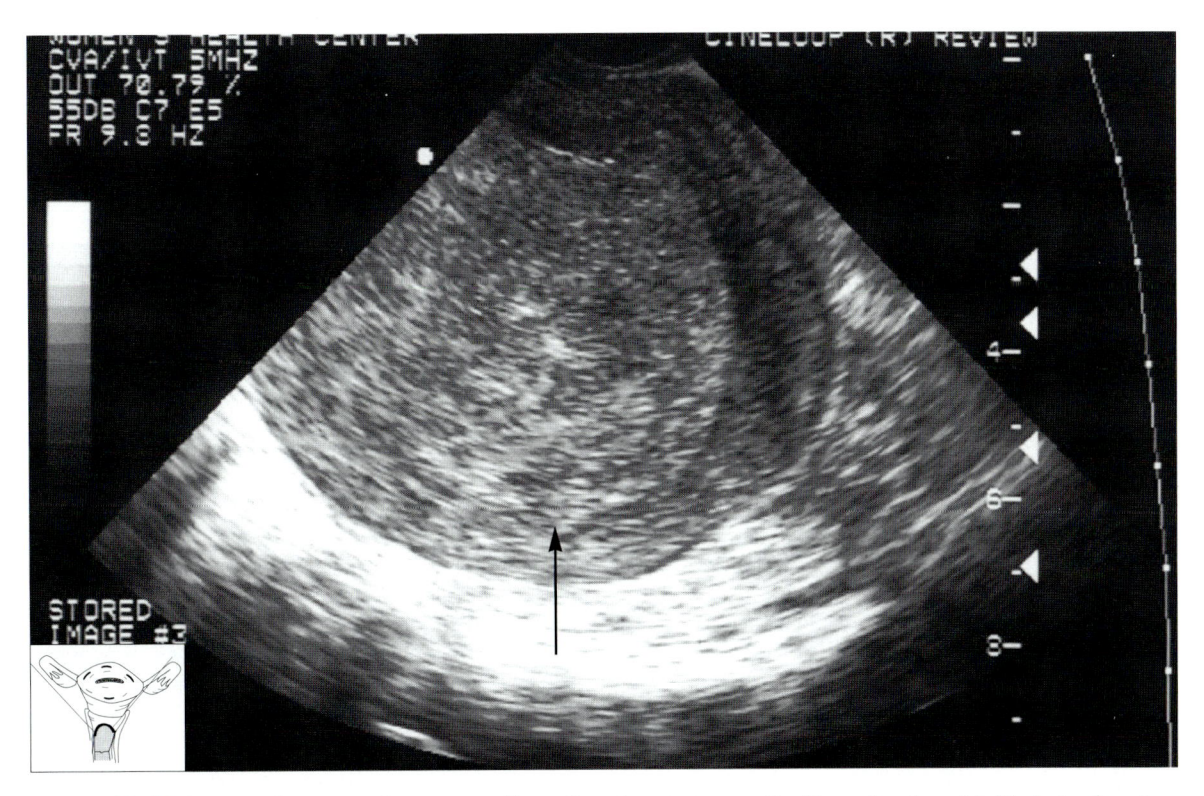

Figure 11-16. Large-volume isoechoic tumor distending the uterine cavity. The subendometrial halo is absent posteriorly (arrow).

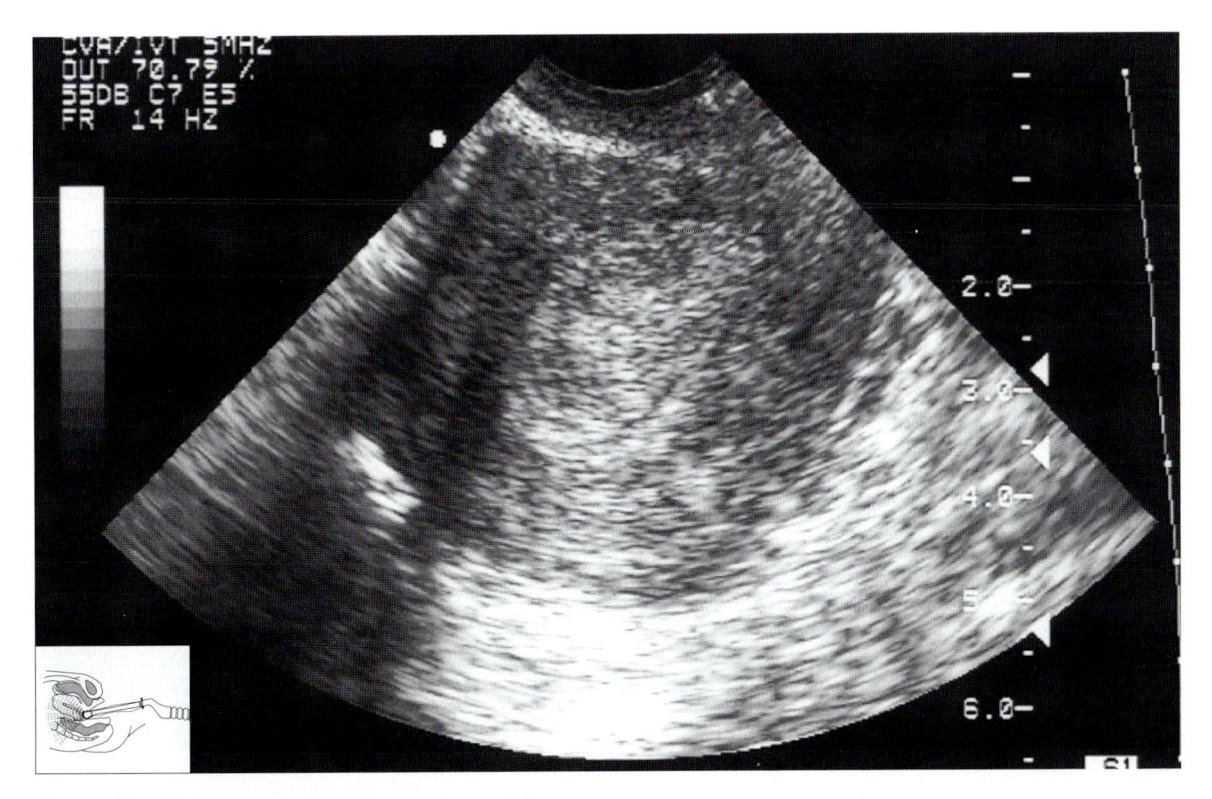

Figure 11-17. Early invasive echoic endometrial cancer.

An Atlas of Transvaginal Sonography

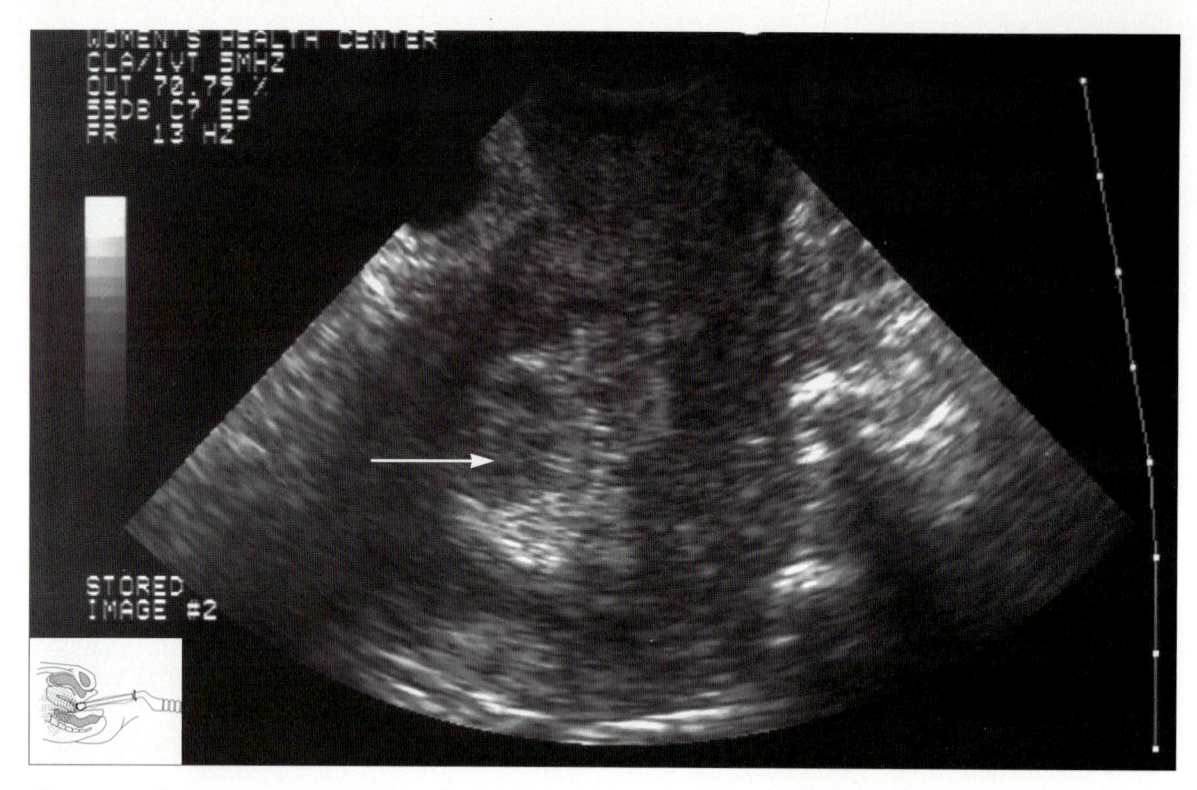

Figure 11-18. Deeply invasive echoic endometrial cancer, with a shaggy irregular endometrial outline. An associated isoechoic endometrial polyp (arrow) is seen from the anterior uterine wall.

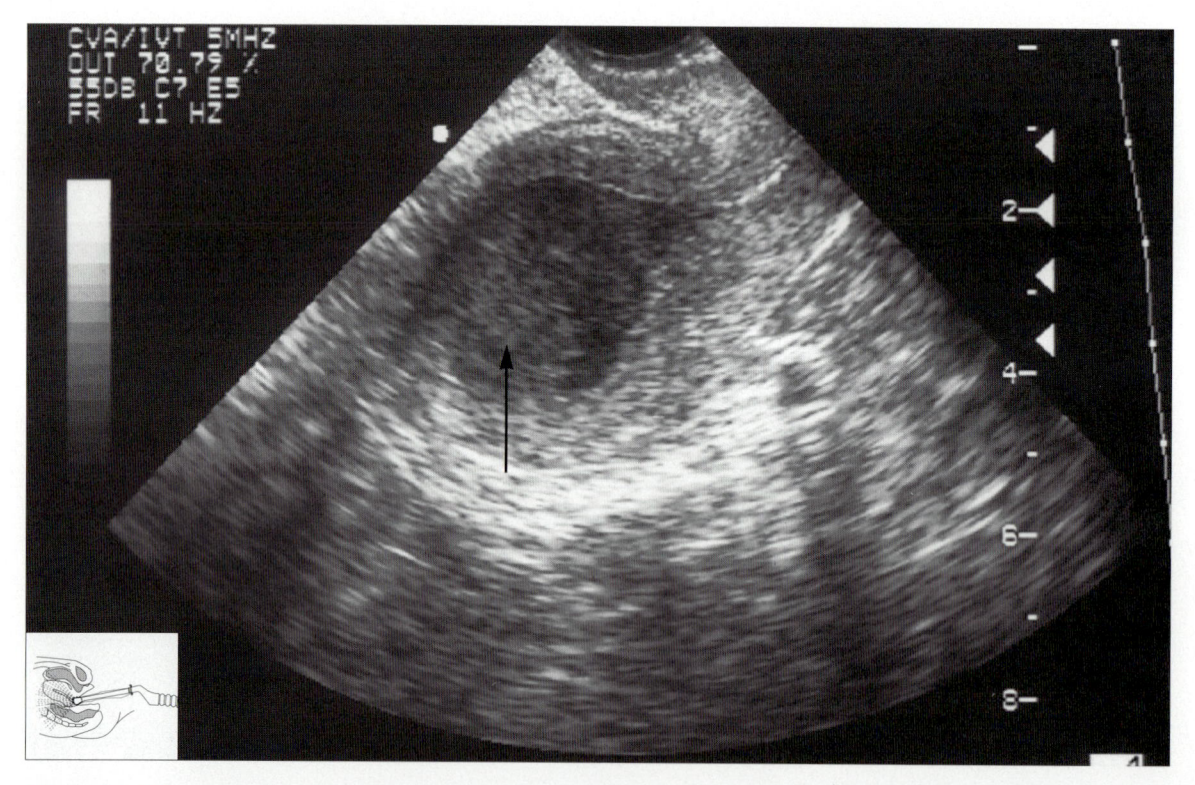

Figure 11-19. An atrophic postmenopausal uterus. Hematometra is present and distends the uterine cavity and outlines an isoechoic invasive uterine tumor (arrow).

Uterine Cancer

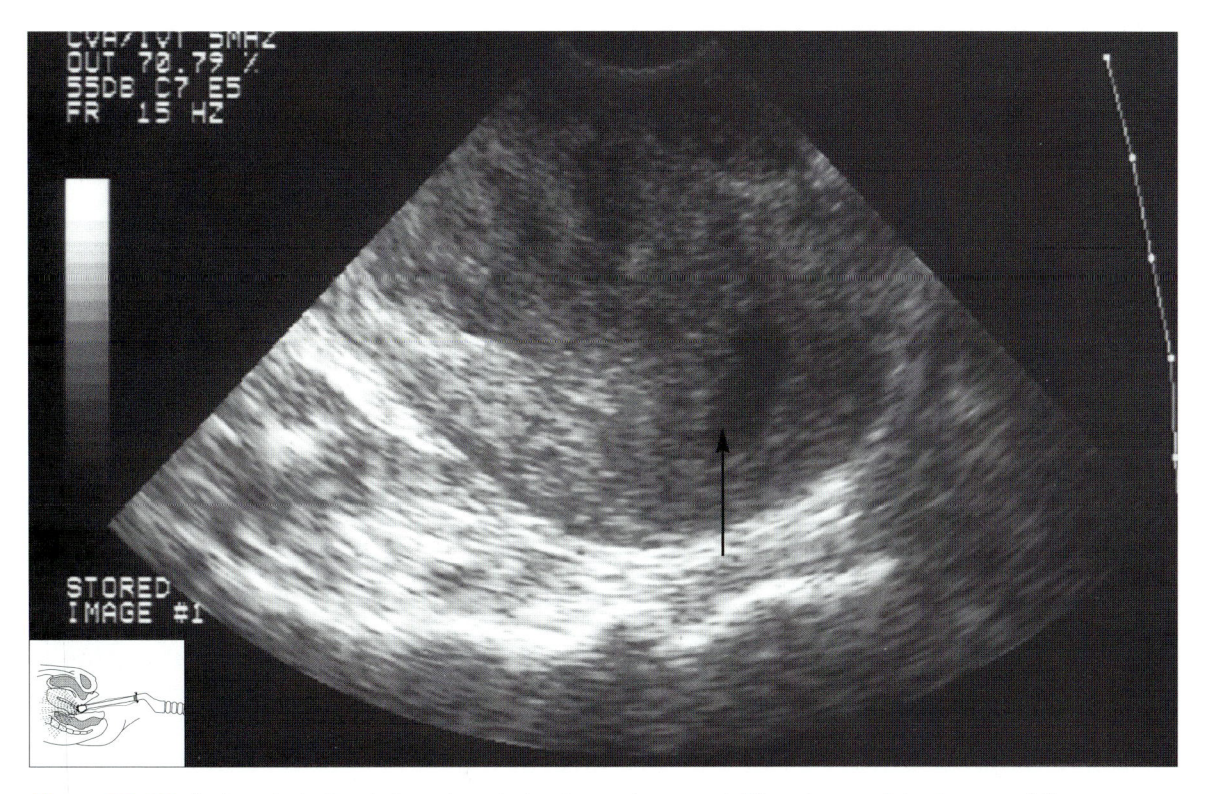

Figure 11-20. An isoechoic deeply invasive uterine tumor is present. There is complete absence of the subendometrial halo. Hypoechoic regions (arrow) of hemorrhage and tumor necrosis are visible.

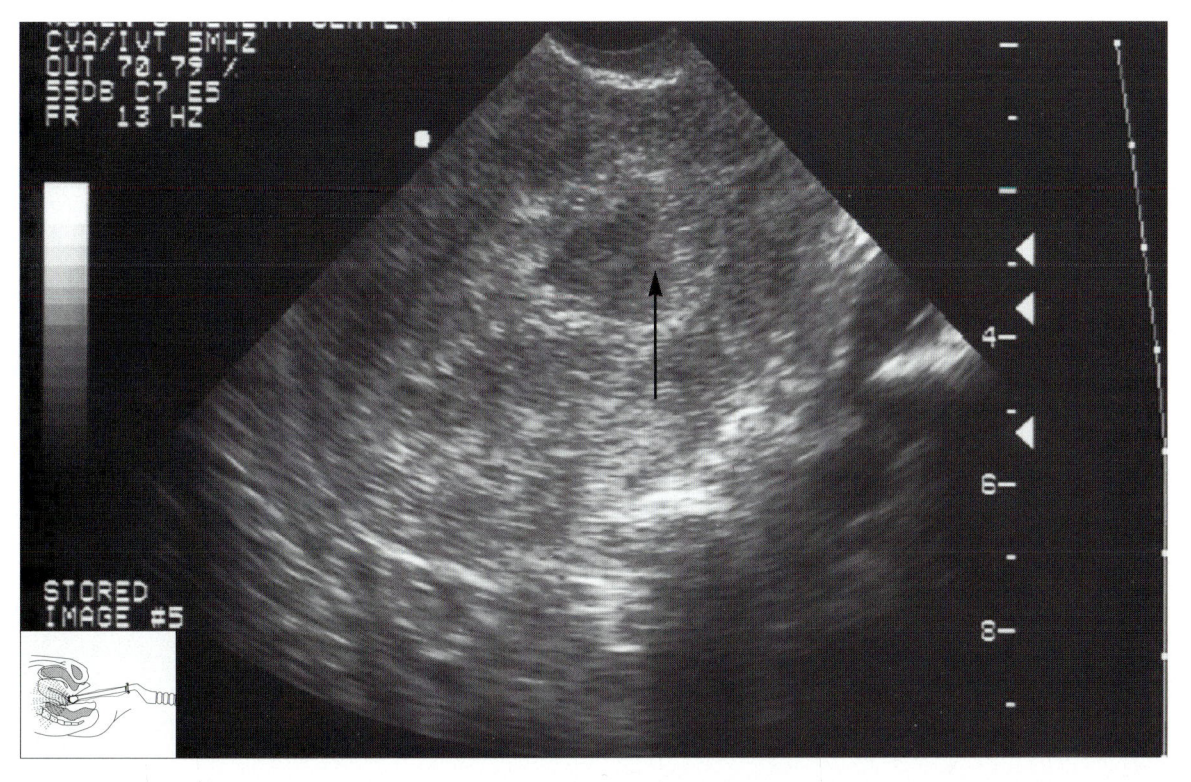

Figure 11-21. Invasive uterine tumor with large area of hemorrhagic necrosis (arrow) in the lower uterine segment.

An Atlas of Transvaginal Sonography

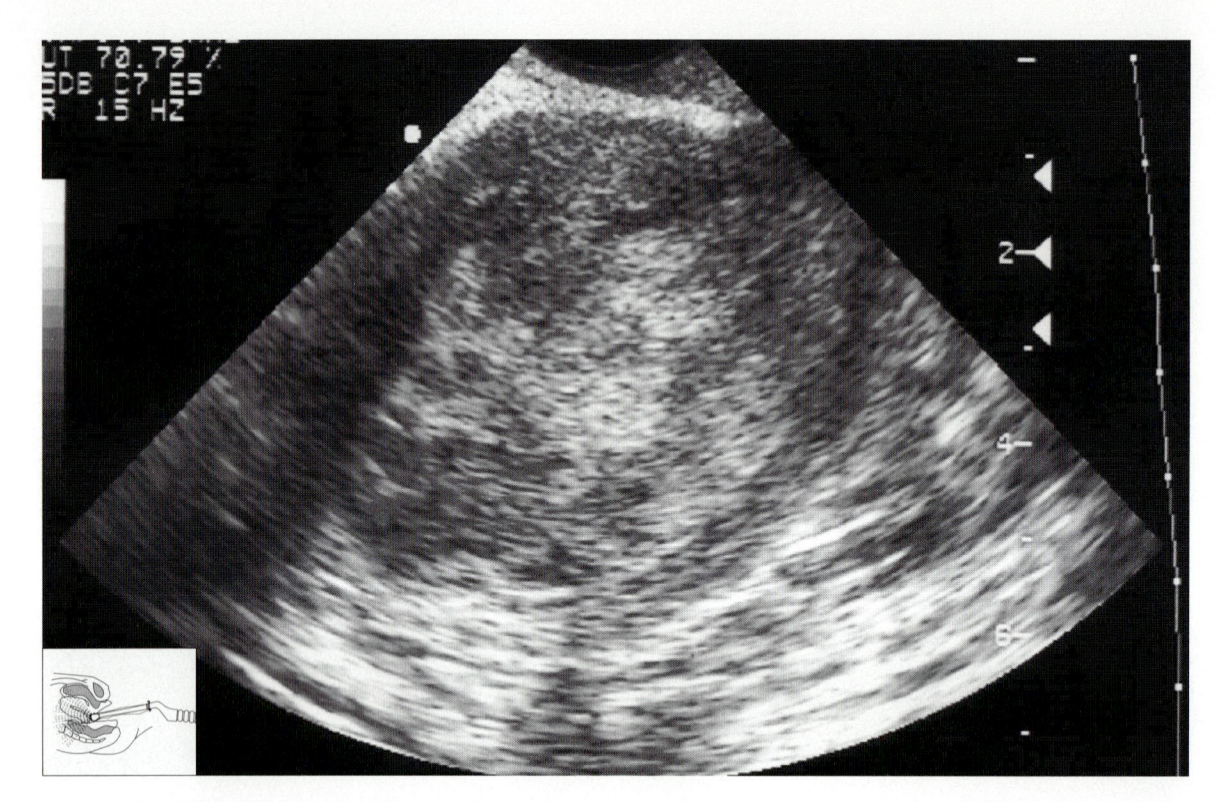

Figure 11-22. Deeply invasive endometrial cancer.

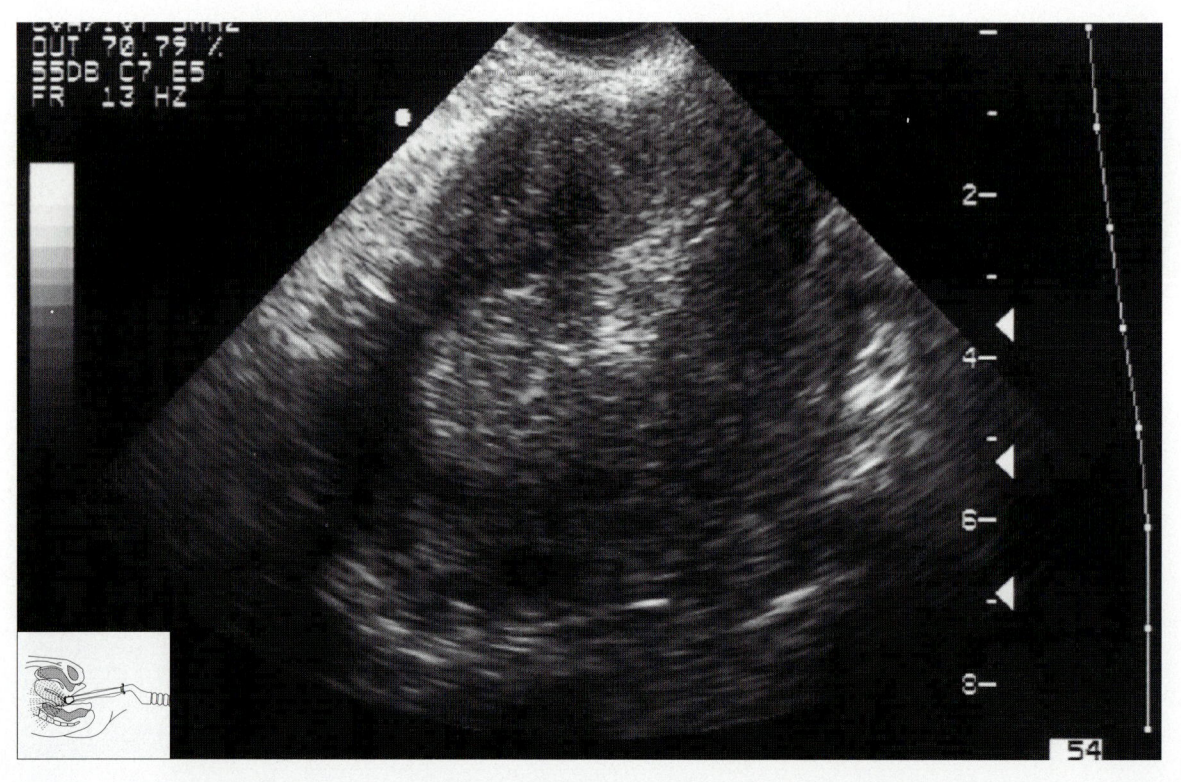

Figure 11-23. Superficially invasive, echogenic, endometrial cancer in a postmenopausal woman.

Uterine Cancer

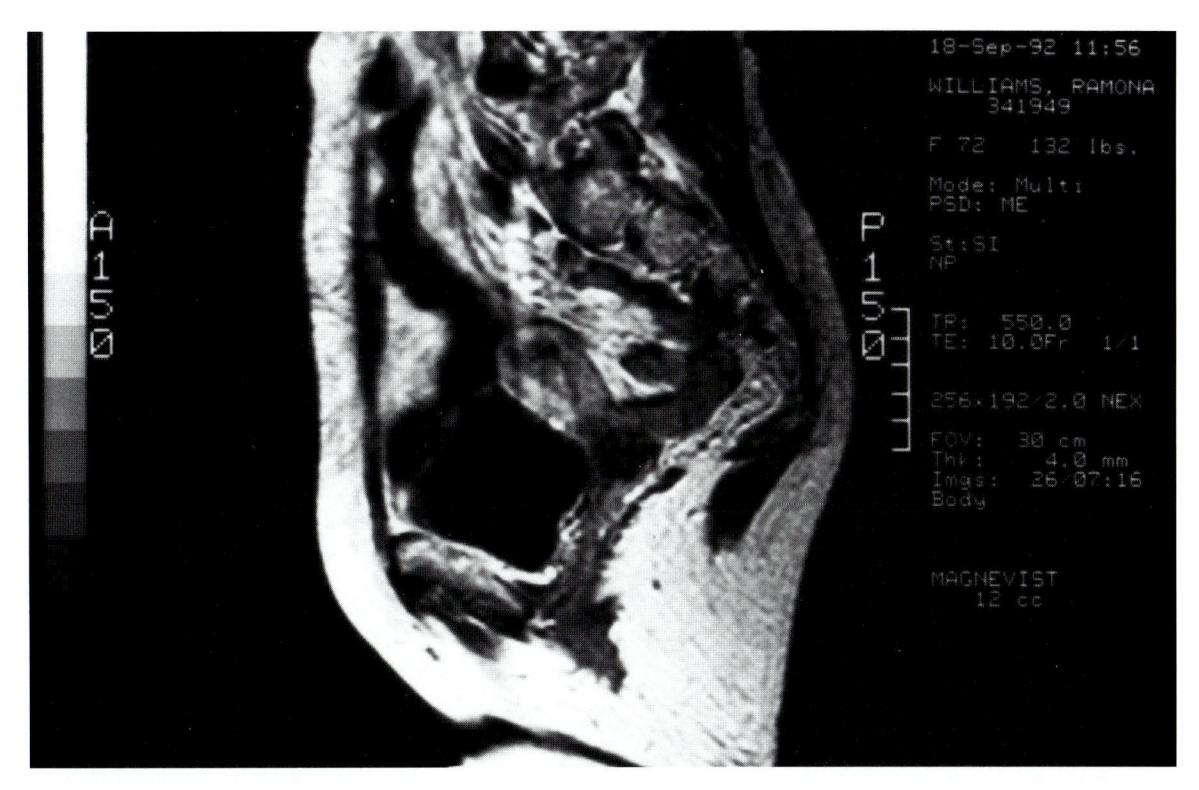

Figure 11-24. T_1 *weighted MRI image of patient with invasive uterine cancer. Uterine image resolution is clearly inferior to high resolution scans obtained from TVS.*

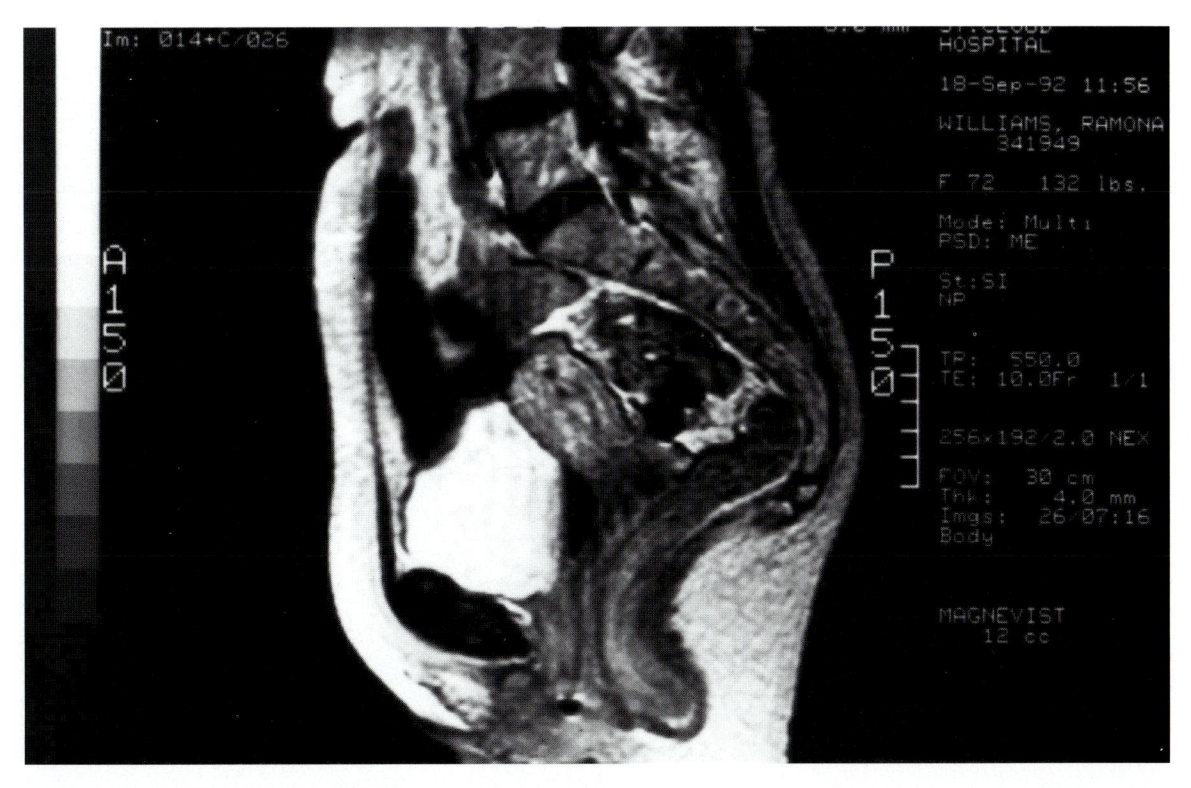

Figure 11-25. T_2 *weighted MRI image of patient with invasive uterine cancer. Uterine image resolution is clearly inferior to high resolution scans obtained from TVS.*

An Atlas of Transvaginal Sonography

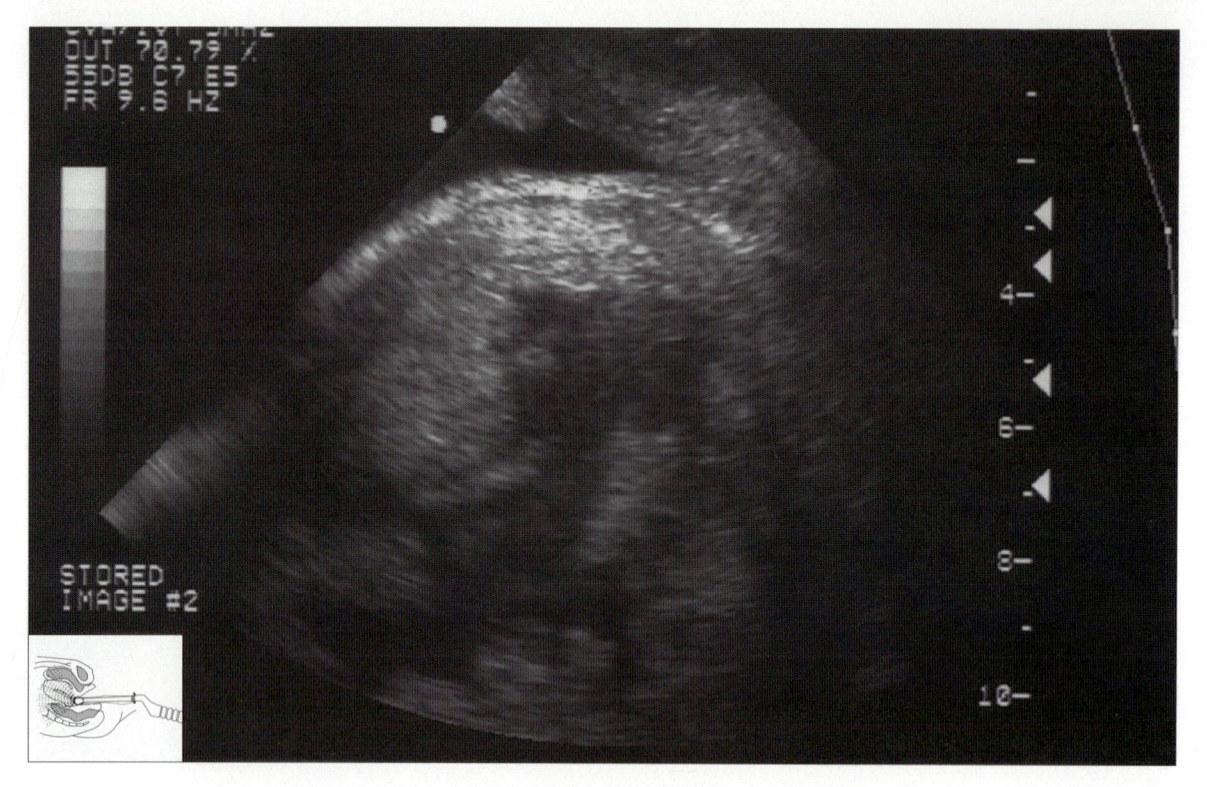

Figure 11-26. Large, complex, uterine cancer, pushing the bladder wall anteriorly.

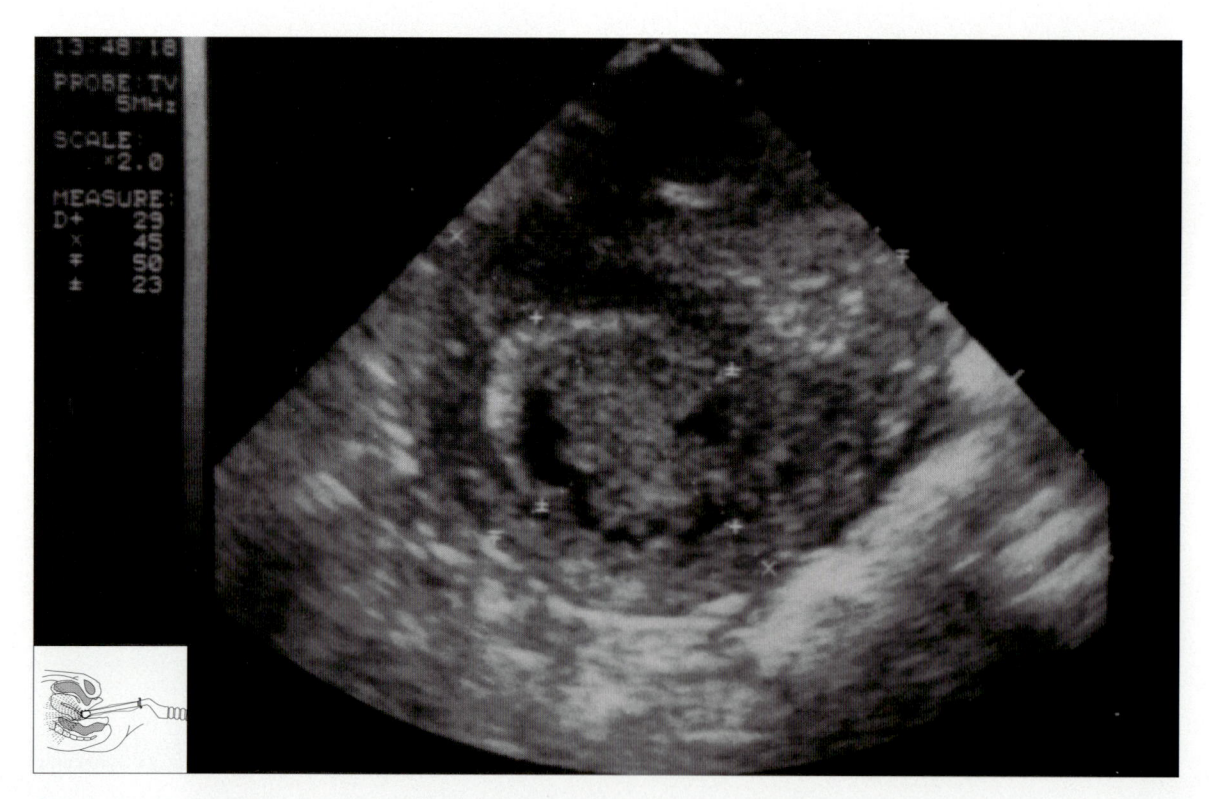

Figure 11-27. Advanced, invasive, necrotic, uterine cancer.

Uterine Cancer

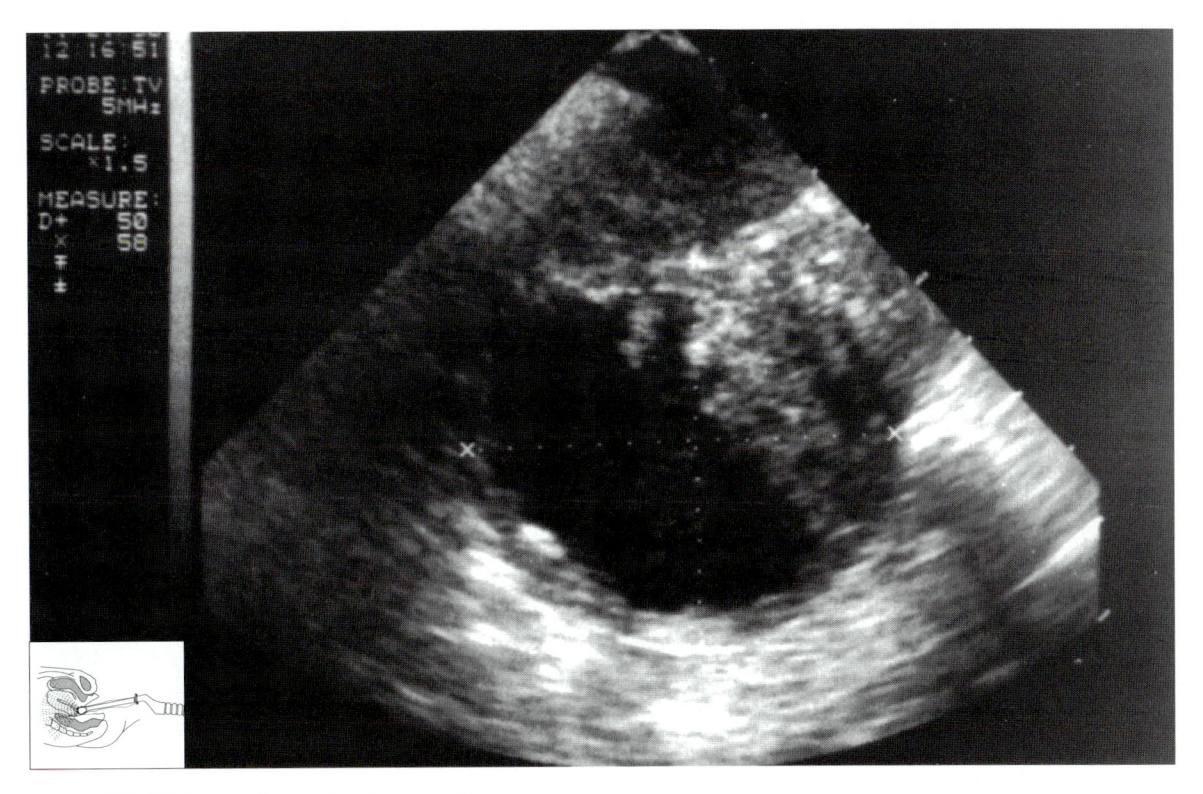

Figure 11-28. Large, hemorrhagic, necrotic corpus cancer.

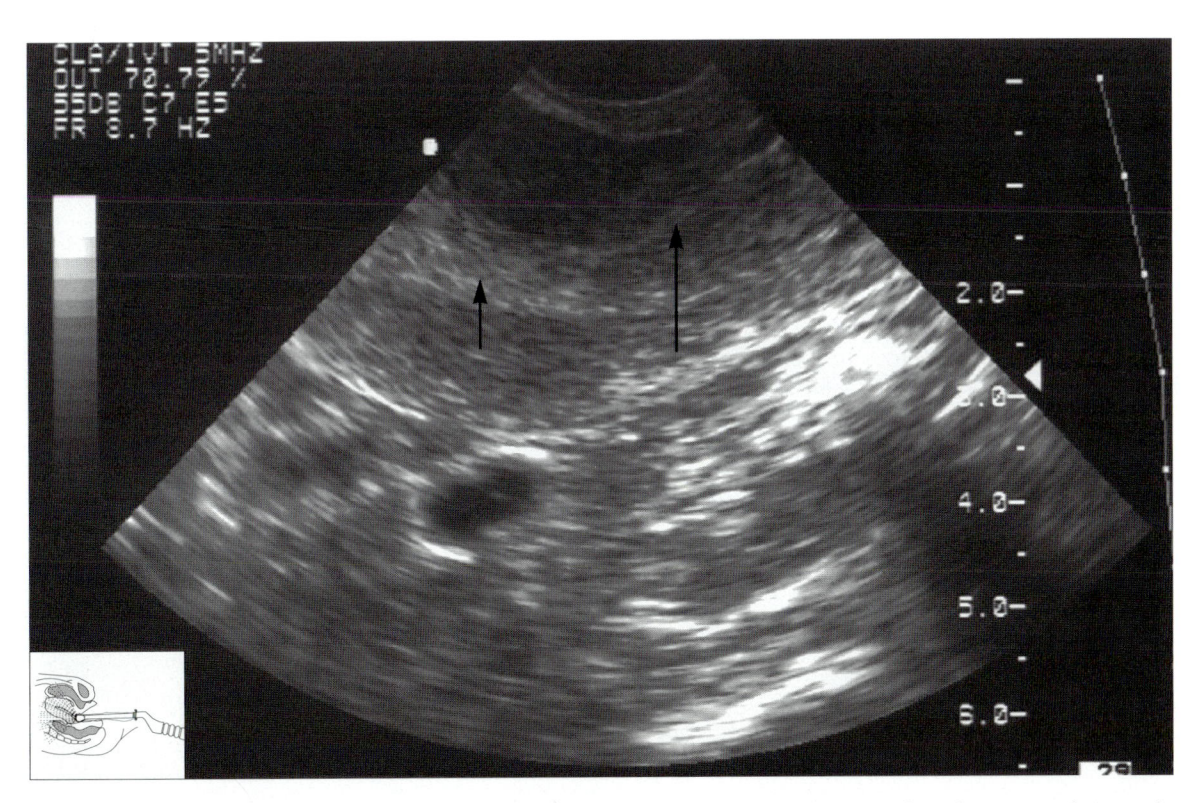

Figure 11-29. Sagittal section through lower uterine segment and upper endocervix. An echogenic endometrial cancer (small arrow) is present as well as an isoechoic prolapsed polyp (large arrow).

An Atlas of Transvaginal Sonography

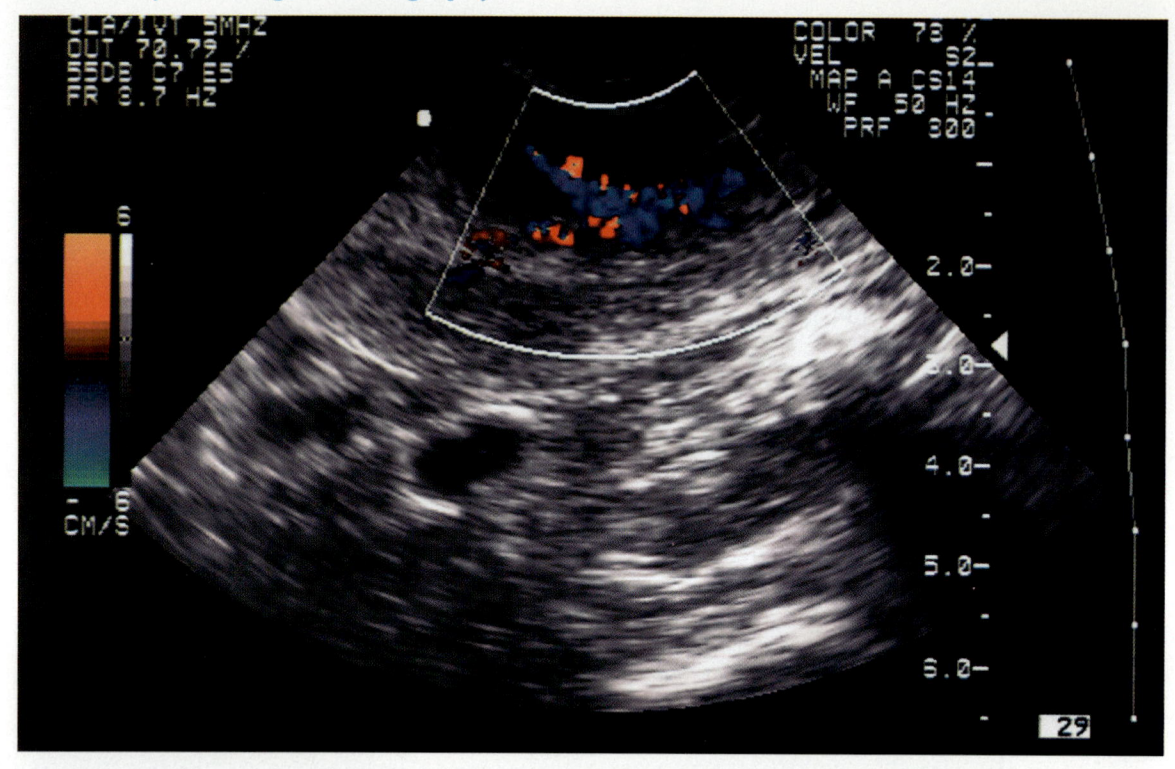

Figure 11-30. Color flow Doppler demonstrates increased flow within the base of the polyp and adjacent myometrium.

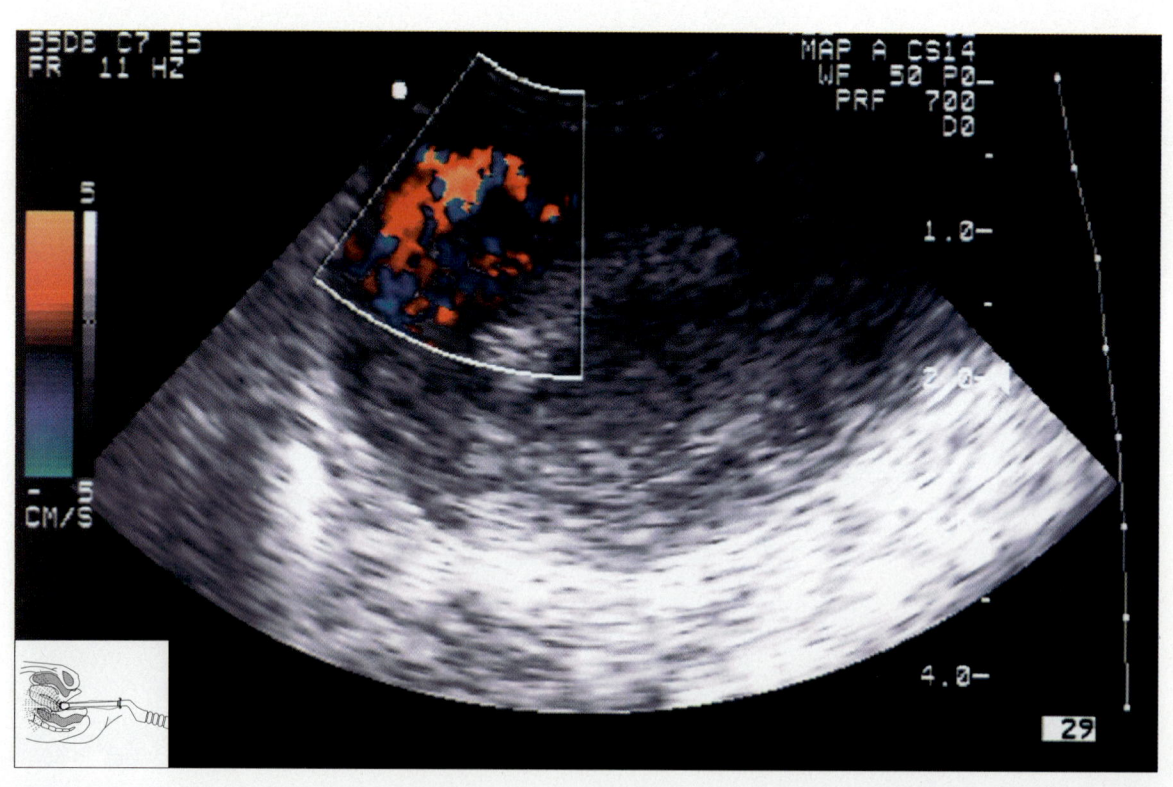

Figure 11-31. Echogenic, invasive, endometrial cancer, with increased myometrial flow demonstrated by color flow Doppler.

Uterine Cancer

Uterine Sarcoma

Uterine sarcomas are rare, accounting for only 1-3% of uterine cancers, but despite their rarity, account for 15% of uterine malignancy deaths. Age at diagnosis varies from the second decade to the eighth decade with a mean age of 55.7 years. Leiomyosarcomas tend to occur at a younger age than the other sarcomas.

As with endometrial cancer, obesity, hypertension, and diabetes are frequently associated with uterine sarcomas, although their etiologic role is not defined. Previous radiation therapy increases the risk of development of uterine sarcoma and unopposed estrogen therapy has rarely been reported with endometrial sarcomas. The malignant transformation of a fibroid is rare, accounting for less than 1% of cases.

Scan Findings

Sonographic features include an enlarged uterus containing either solid or complex echoes. One would expect color flow to be increased in these lesions, but in low-grade, endometrial, stromal sarcoma, blood flow is not increased. Histologically, intratumoral blood vessels are clogged with tumor, perhaps accounting for this finding.

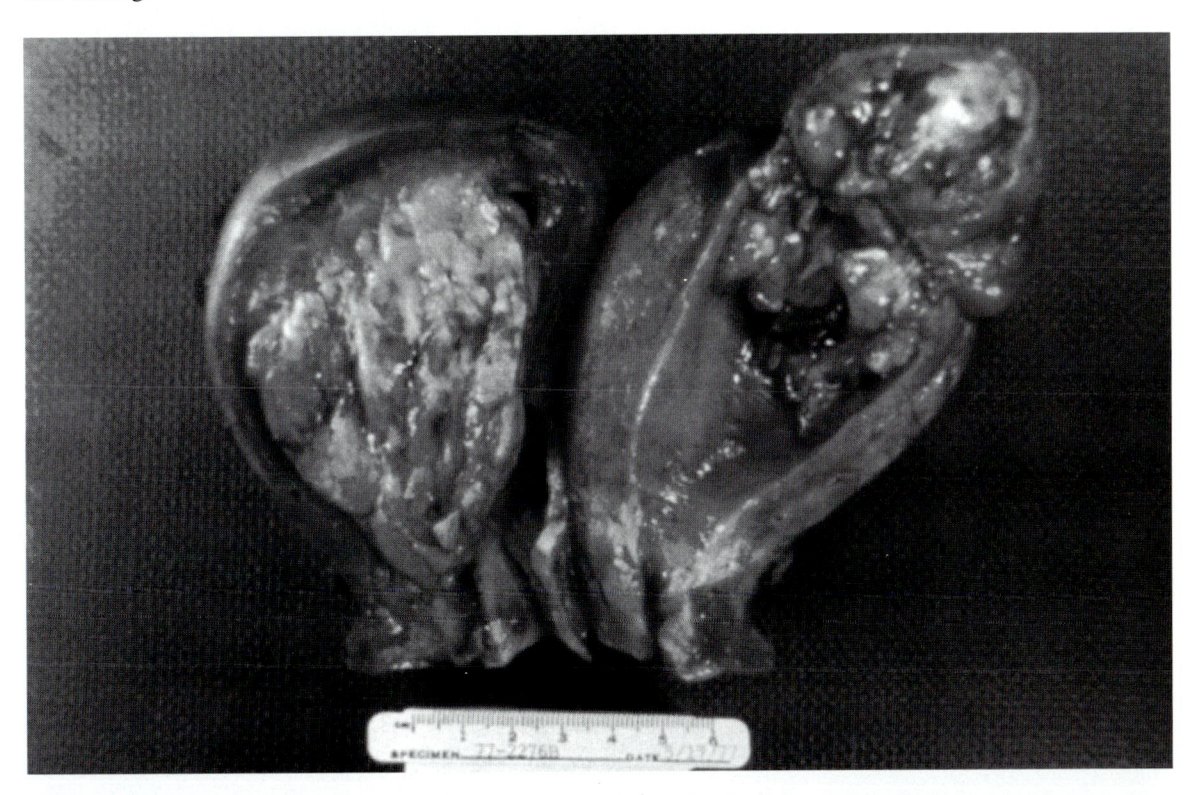

Figure 11-32. Large uterine sarcoma, displaying an intraluminal polypoid tumor distending the uterine cavity, and transmyometrial invasion with exophytic serosal extension.

An Atlas of Transvaginal Sonography

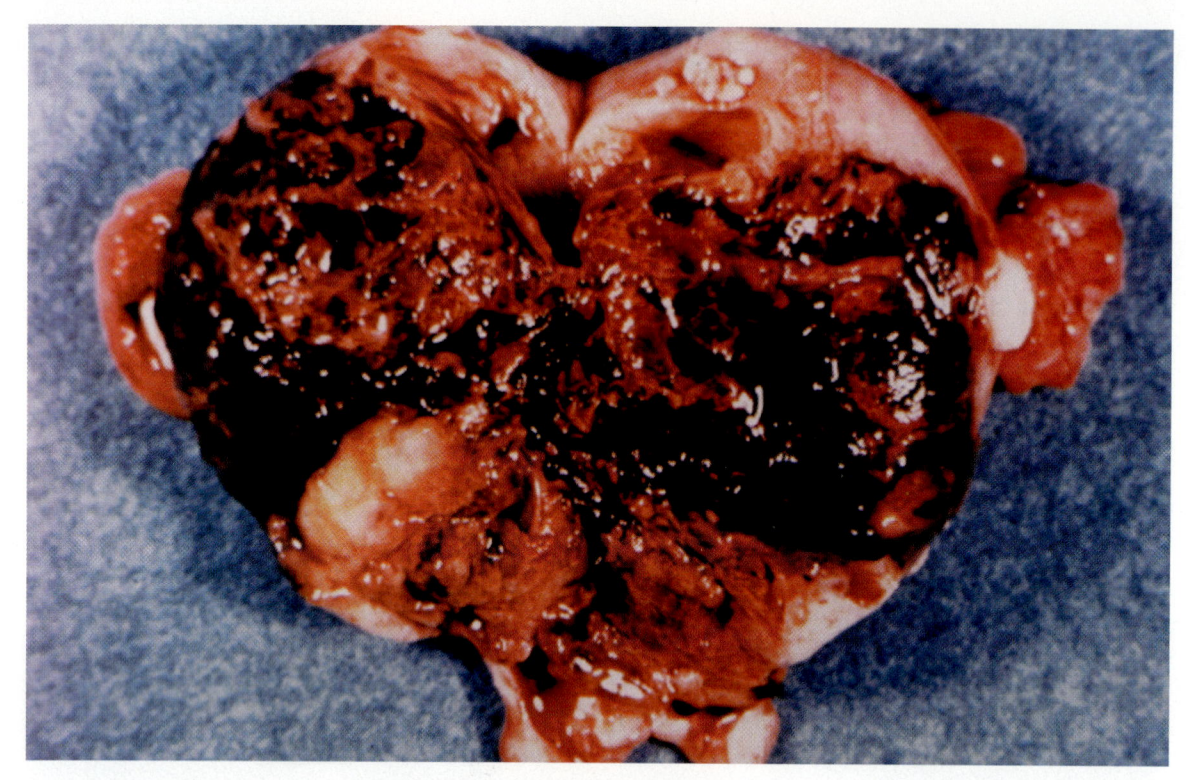

Figure 11-33. Hemorrhagic and necrotic advanced uterine sarcoma.

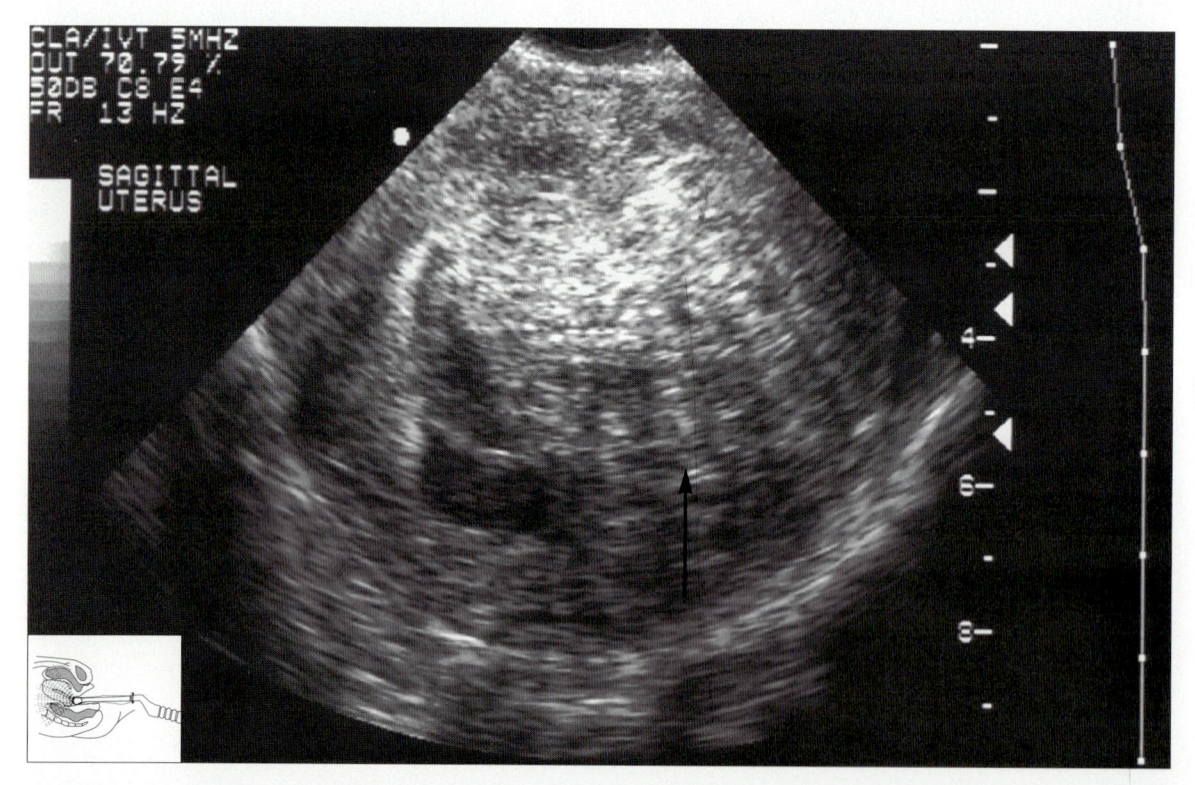

Figure 11-34. An asymmetrically enlarged uterus. The posterior uterine wall is markedly thickened (arrow), but without evidence of a discrete mass, such as a leiomyoma. The endometrium is echoic.

Uterine Cancer

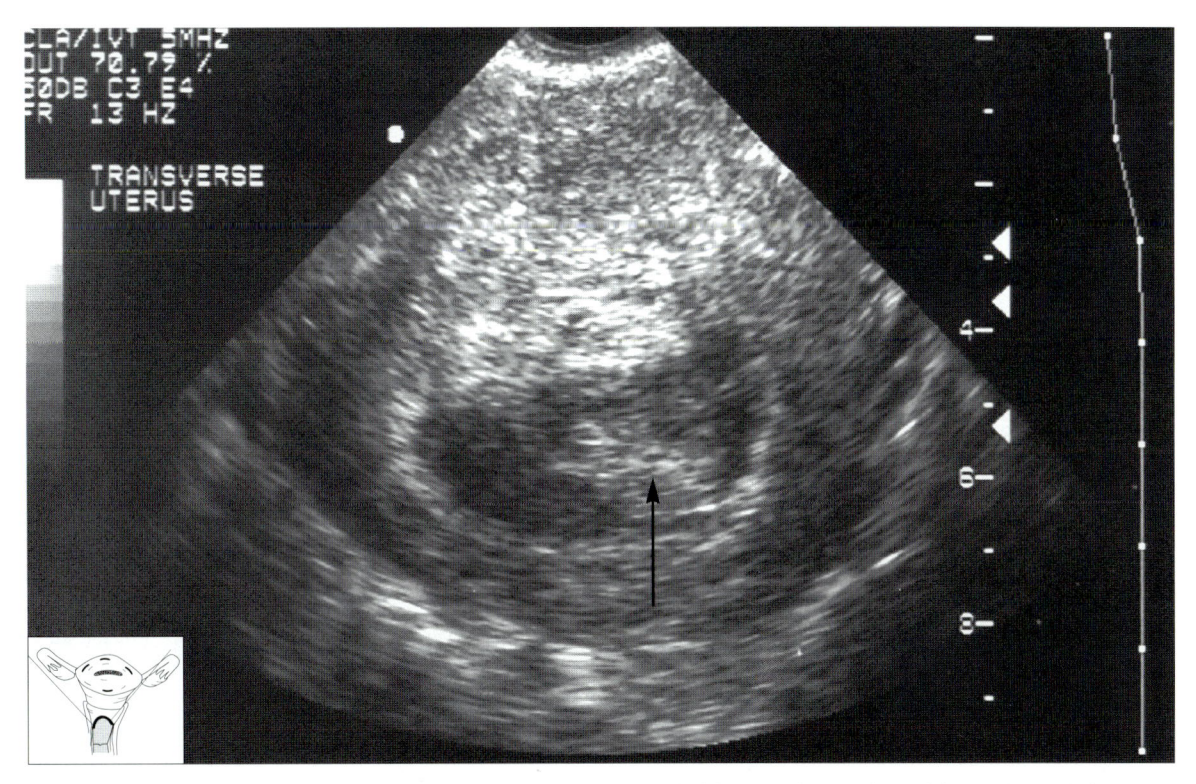

Figure 11-35. Same patient, showing the uterine cavity distended by an echoic polypoid lesion (arrow) that appeared to invade into the myometrium with loss of the subendometrial halo. Pathology confirmed an endometrial stromal sarcoma.

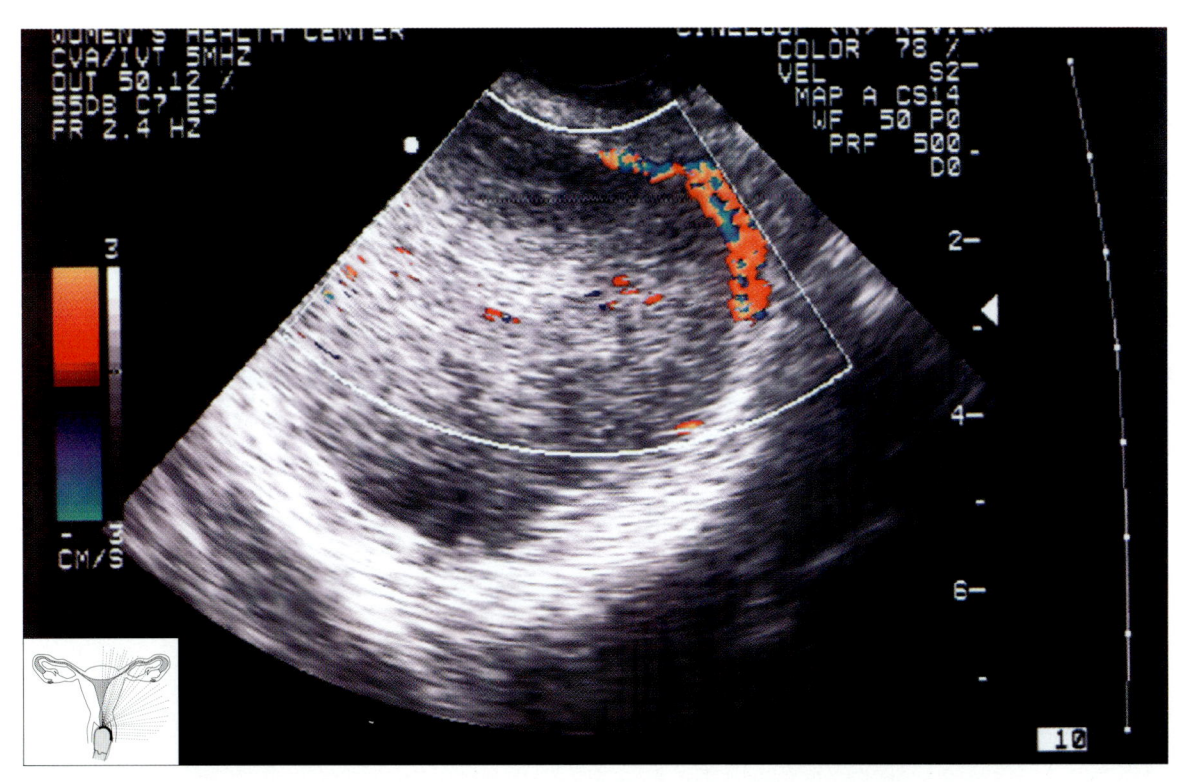

Figure 11-36. Retroperitoneal low-grade, fibrous histiocytoma with peripheral color flow.

An Atlas of Transvaginal Sonography

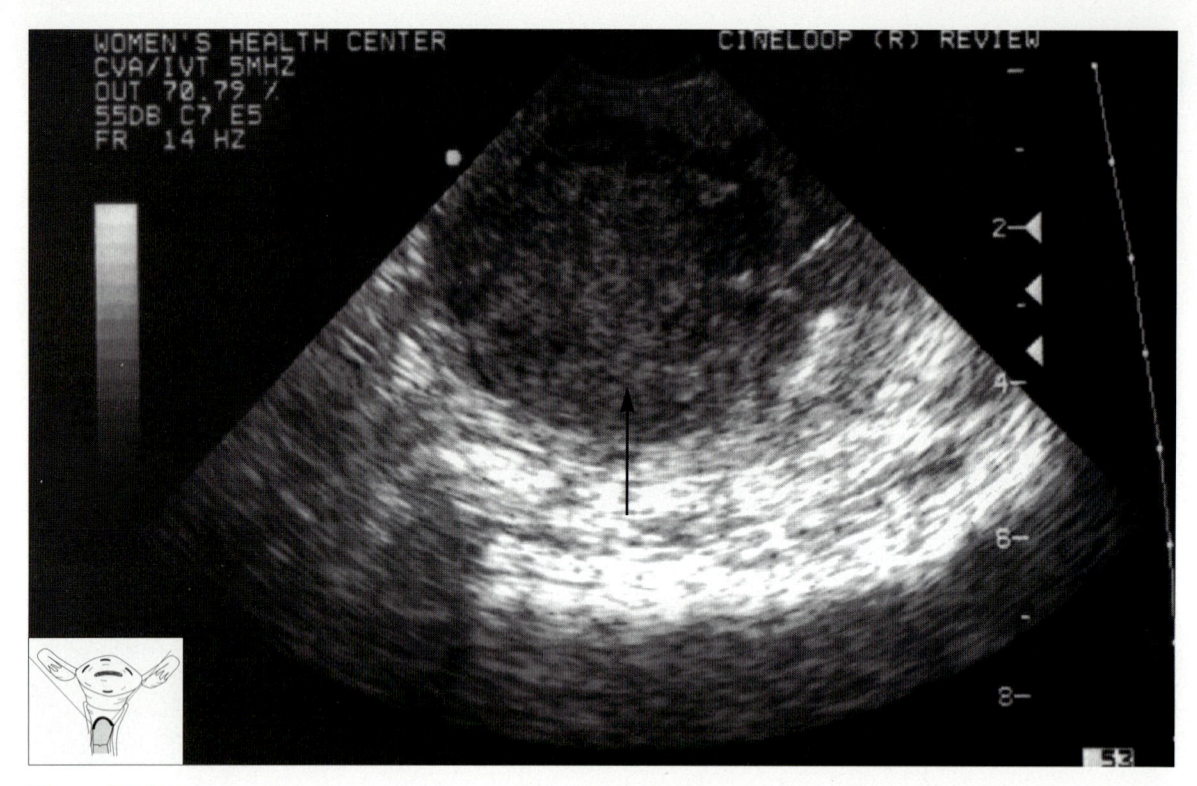

Figure 11-37. *Metastatic melanoma to uterus. TVS demonstrates an isoechoic homogenous lesion (arrow) in the uterine fundus.*

12 Cervical Cancer

Cervical cancer remains a significant cause of morbidity and mortality in the USA. Seven-thousand women are expected to die yearly from cervical cancer. Diagnosis and staging is made clinically, with therapy determined after clinical examination. Early cancer confined to the cervix is best managed by radical hysterectomy, which by definition includes a parametrectomy, and pelvic and para-aortic lymph node dissection. Once the disease has spread beyond the cervix, radiation therapy becomes the more appropriate method of treatment. Determining if the cancer has spread into the parametria is determined by clinical pelvic examination, and is subject to considerable inaccuracies.

Scan Findings

The majority of cervix cancers are recognized clinically as exophytic or ulcerating lesions expanding the cervix, lower uterine segment and parametria. Sonographically, they are solid, hypo- or isoechoic tumors, often producing considerable acoustic shadowing. Except in very early lesions, clear images with distinct anatomic borders are unable to be obtained. Color flow can be variable. In most cases there is increased intratumoral vascularity with dilated abnormal vessels with low resistance. Surprisingly, not all cervix tumors display these color flow changes.

Transvaginal sonography is able to assess parametrial infiltration. Instead of the normal smooth tapering parametria, parametria with carcinomatous infiltration become shortened and blunted, often resulting in deviation of the cervix away from the midline. Color flow confirms dilated abnormal vessels with increased flow and low resistance.

Cervical tumor size correlates well with the frequency of pelvic lymph node metastasis, and hence, survival. Cervical tumor size can be more accurately estimated by TVS than by pelvic examination. Response to therapy, in those patients having chemo or radiotherapy, can be monitored by TVS by regularly assessing tumor size and color flow. The response to therapy is more accurately monitored by TVS than by pelvic exam. Positive pelvic nodes will reduce the survival by one-half. Although an entire survey of the pelvic lymph nodes is not possible, enlarged carcinomatous nodes are able to be identified.

An Atlas of Transvaginal Sonography

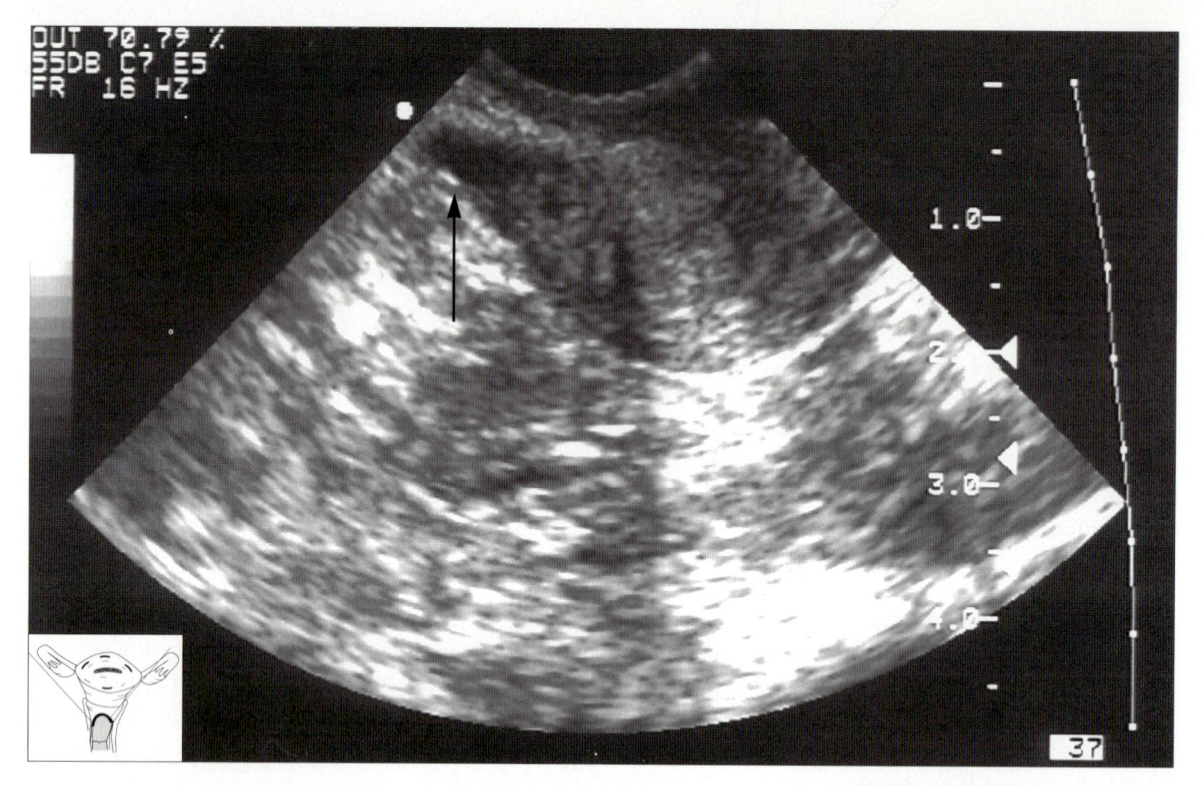

Figure 12-1. Coronal view through cervix and normal parametria (arrow), extending in a fine tapering fashion laterally.

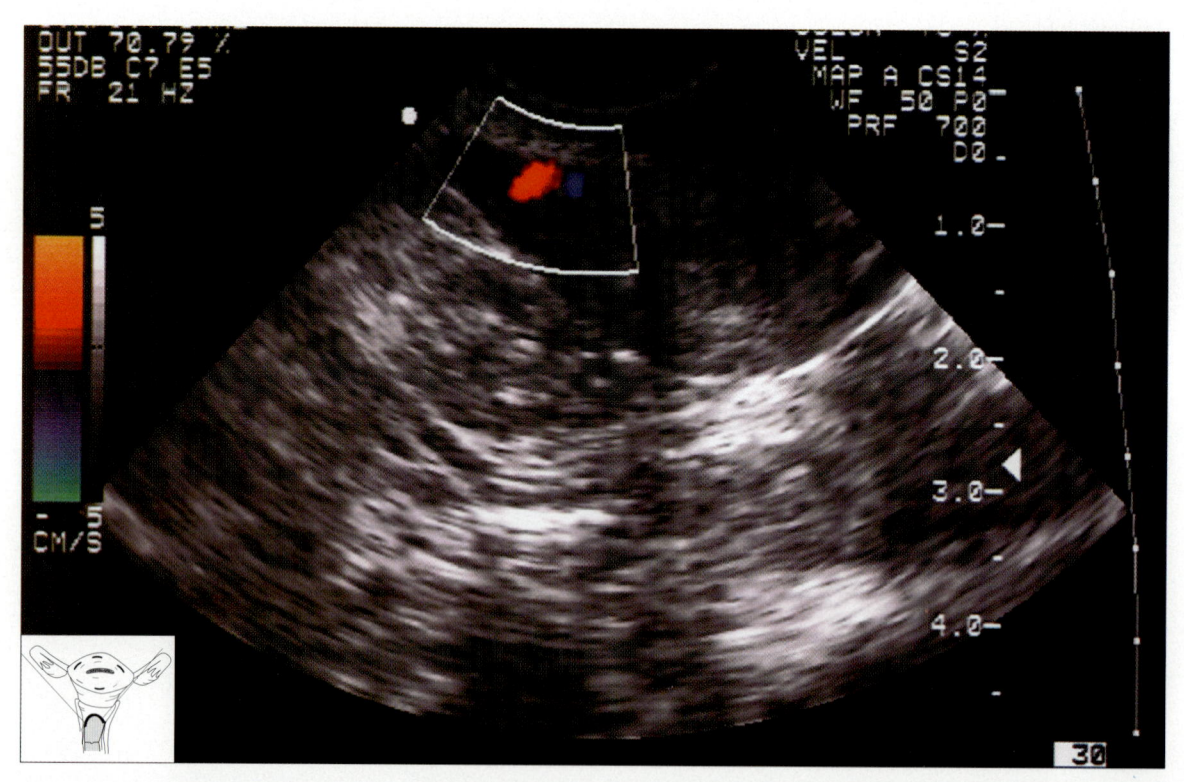

Figure 12-2. Color flow Doppler demonstrating the uterine vessels within the parametrial tissue, lateral to the cervix.

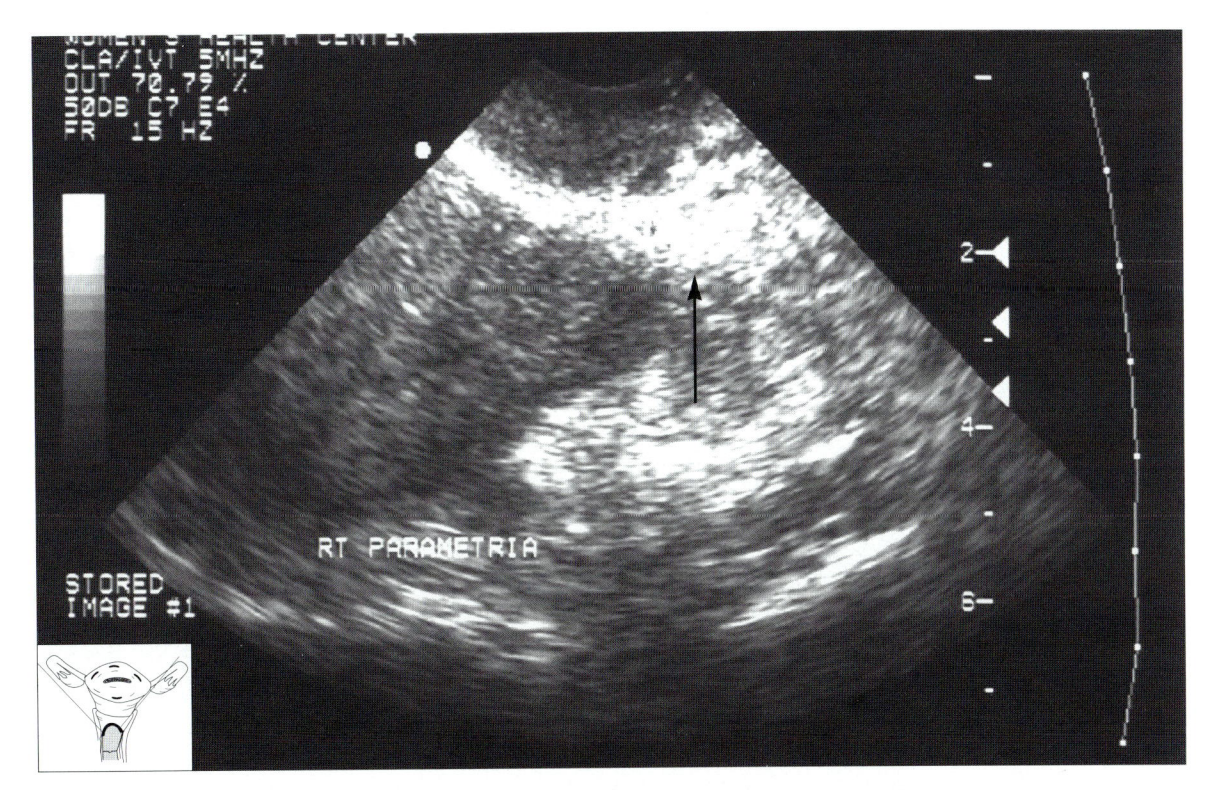

Figure 12-3. Short, blunted, thickened parametria (arrow) in a patient with stage IIB cervix cancer.

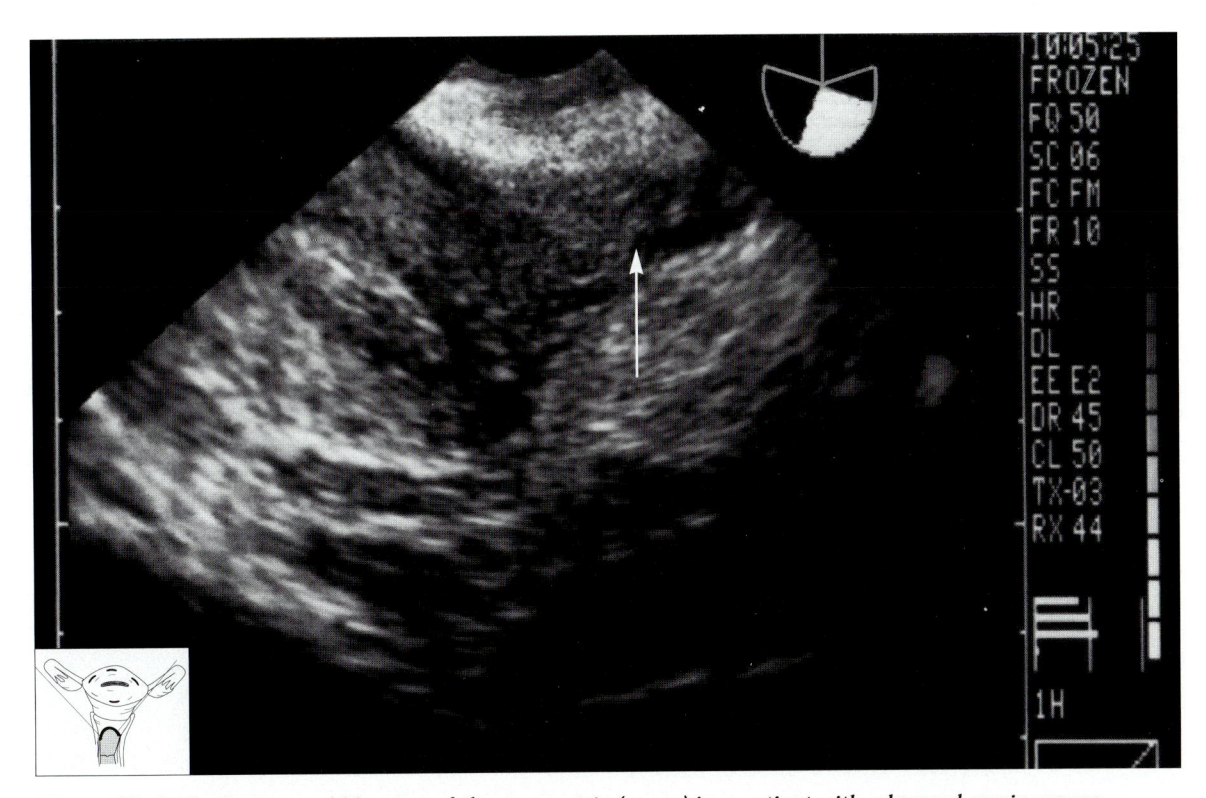

Figure 12-4. Thickening and blunting of the parametria (arrow) in a patient with advanced cervix cancer.

An Atlas of Transvaginal Sonography

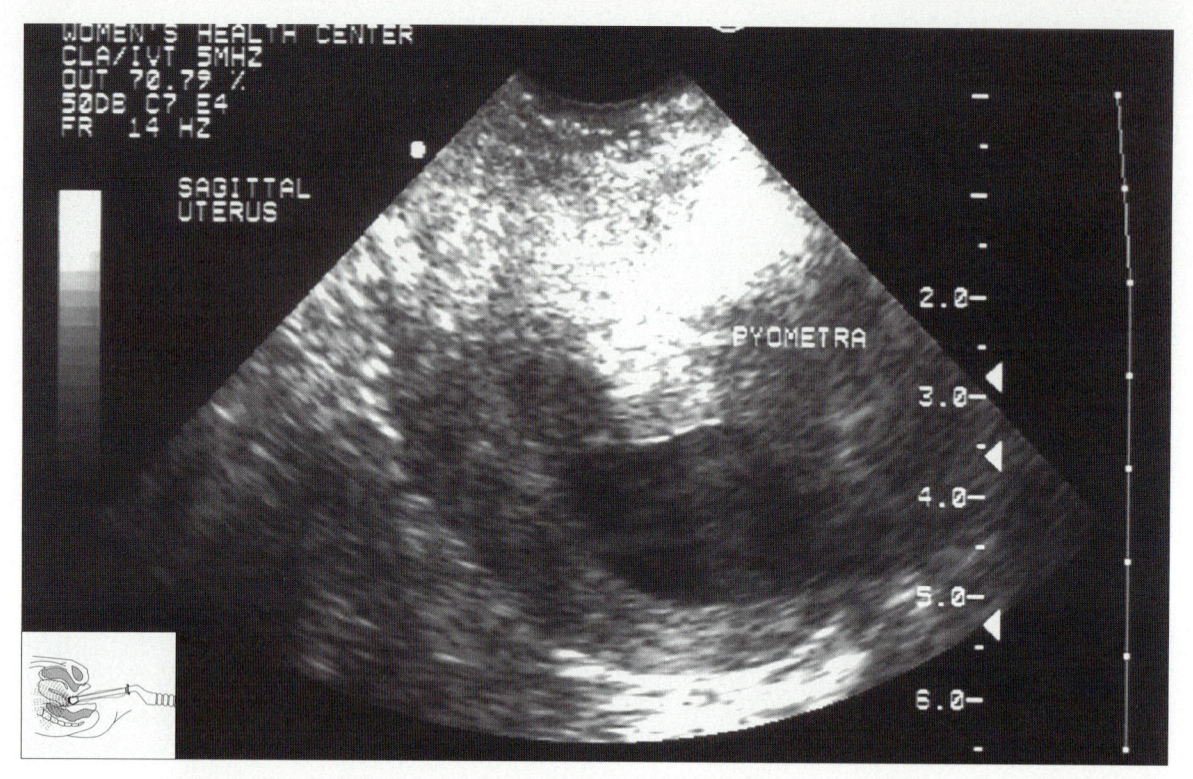

Figure 12-5. *Isoechoic early cervix cancer causing an associated pyometra.*

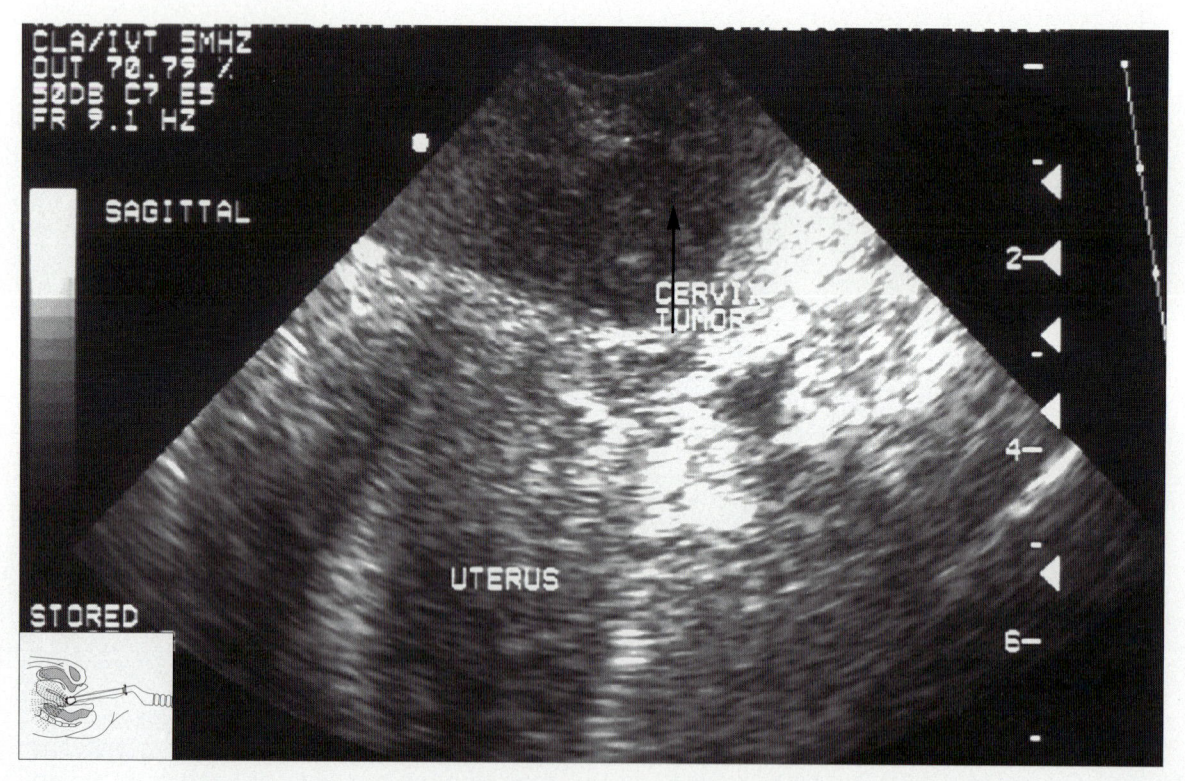

Figure 12-6. *Clearly hypodense cervix cancer (arrow).*

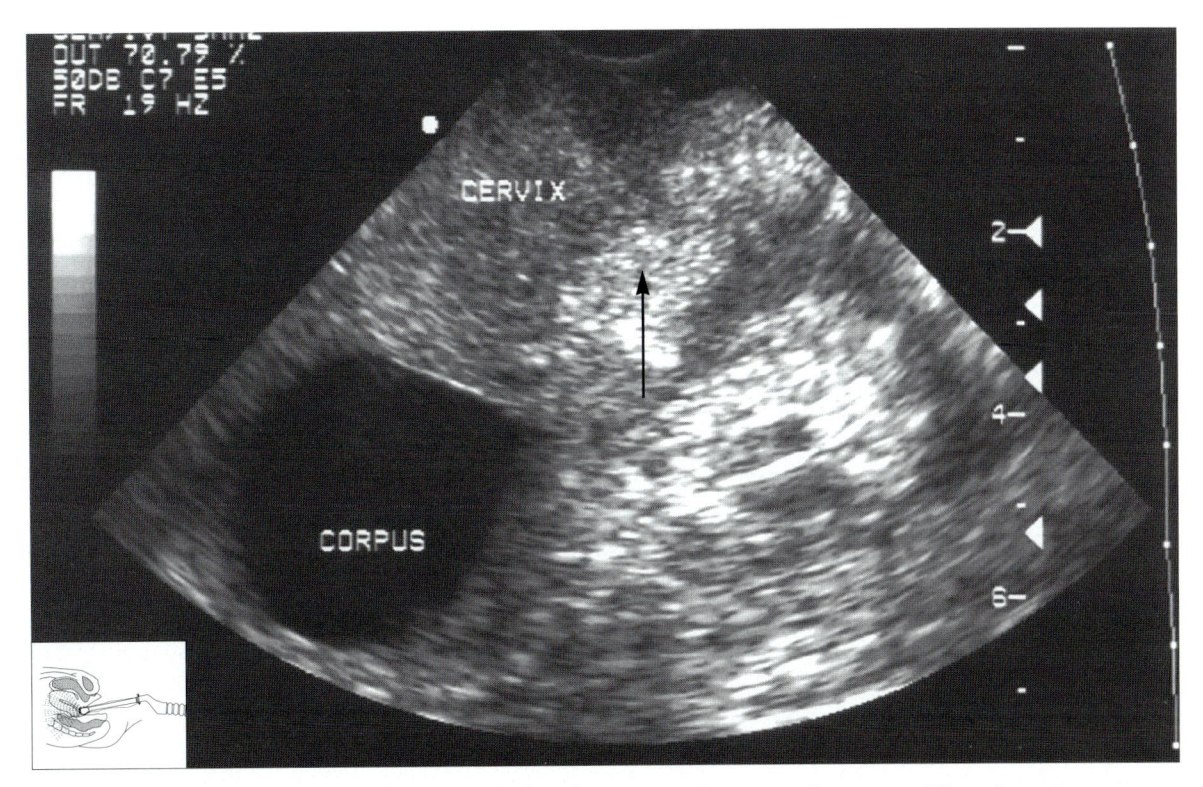

Figure 12-7. Mixed, echogenic, barrel-shaped cervical cancer and associated pyometra. The echogenic area (arrow) in the posterior cervix represents hemorrhage.

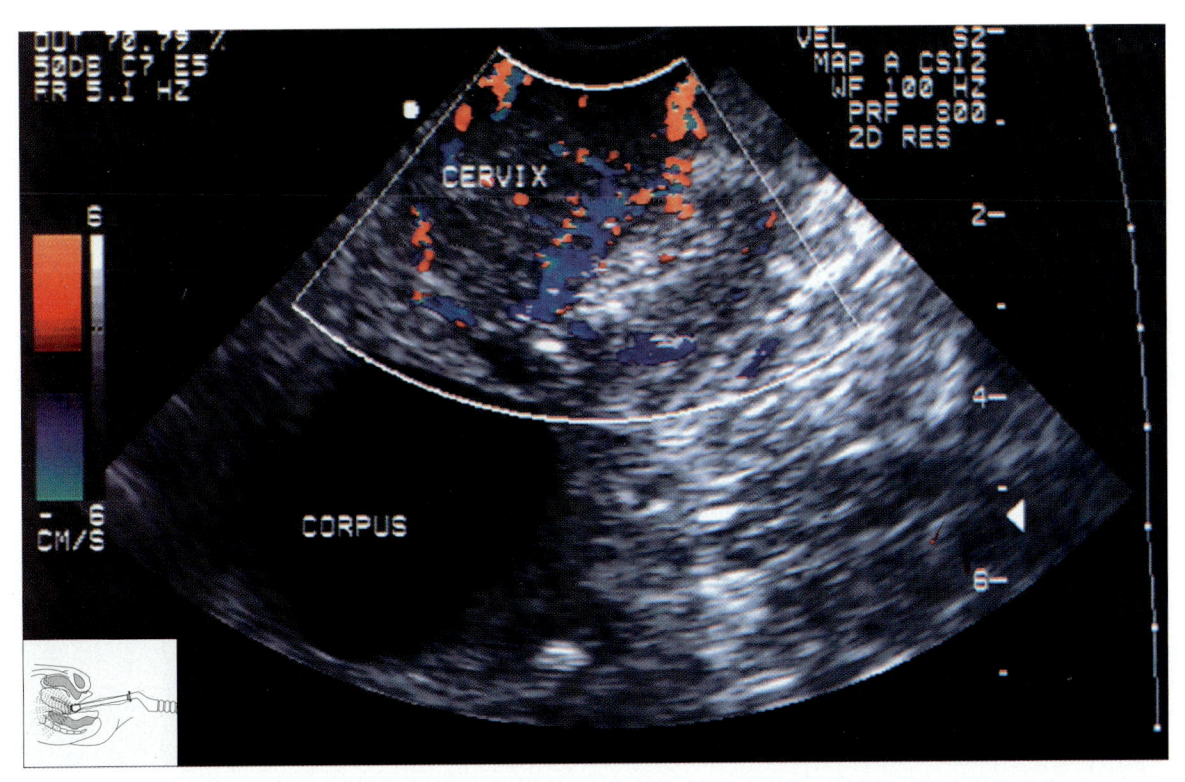

Figure 12-8. Color flow Doppler confirming increased flow.

An Atlas of Transvaginal Sonography

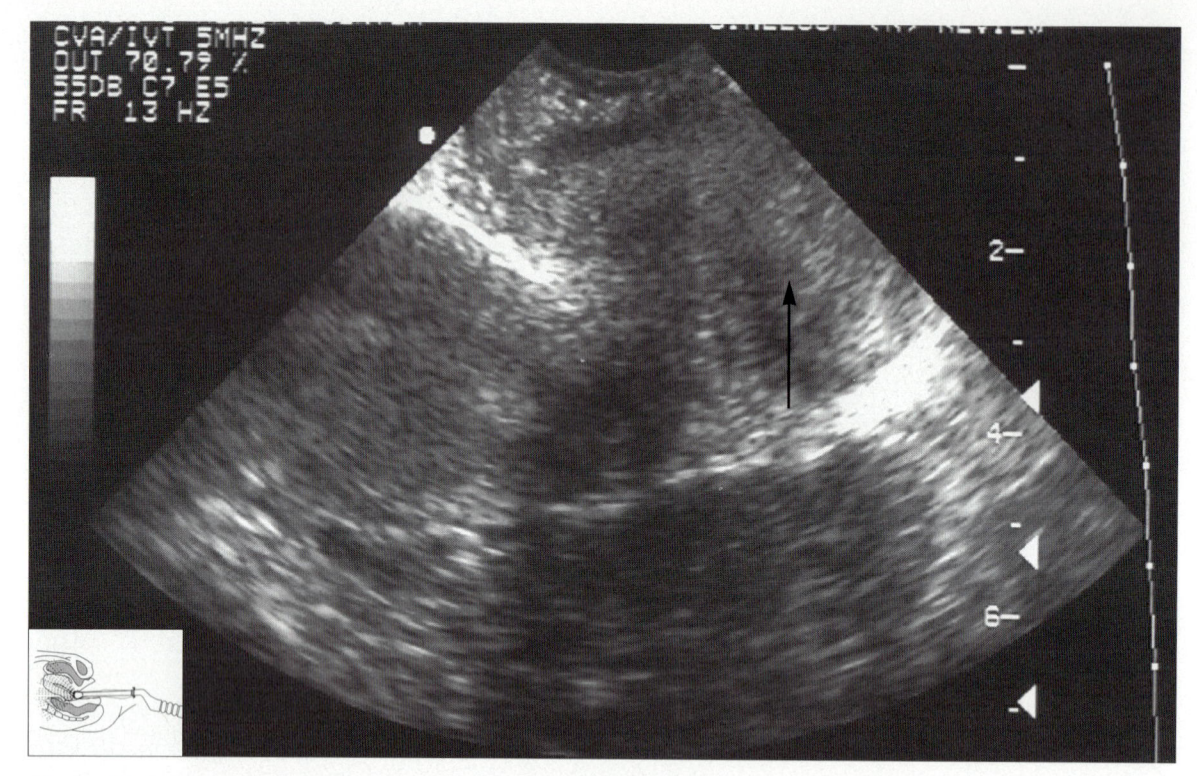

Figure 12-9. Large, isoechoic, barrel-shaped cervix cancer (arrow).

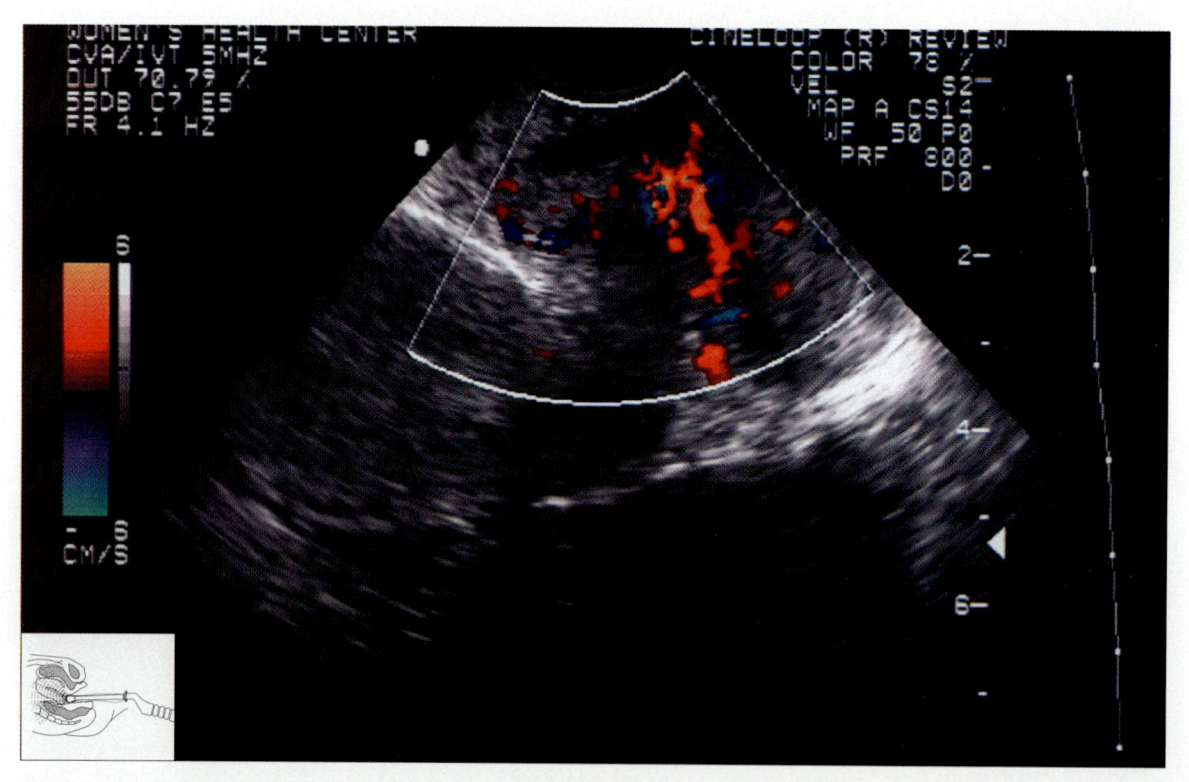

Figure 12-10. Color flow Doppler confirming increased flow.

Cervical Cancer

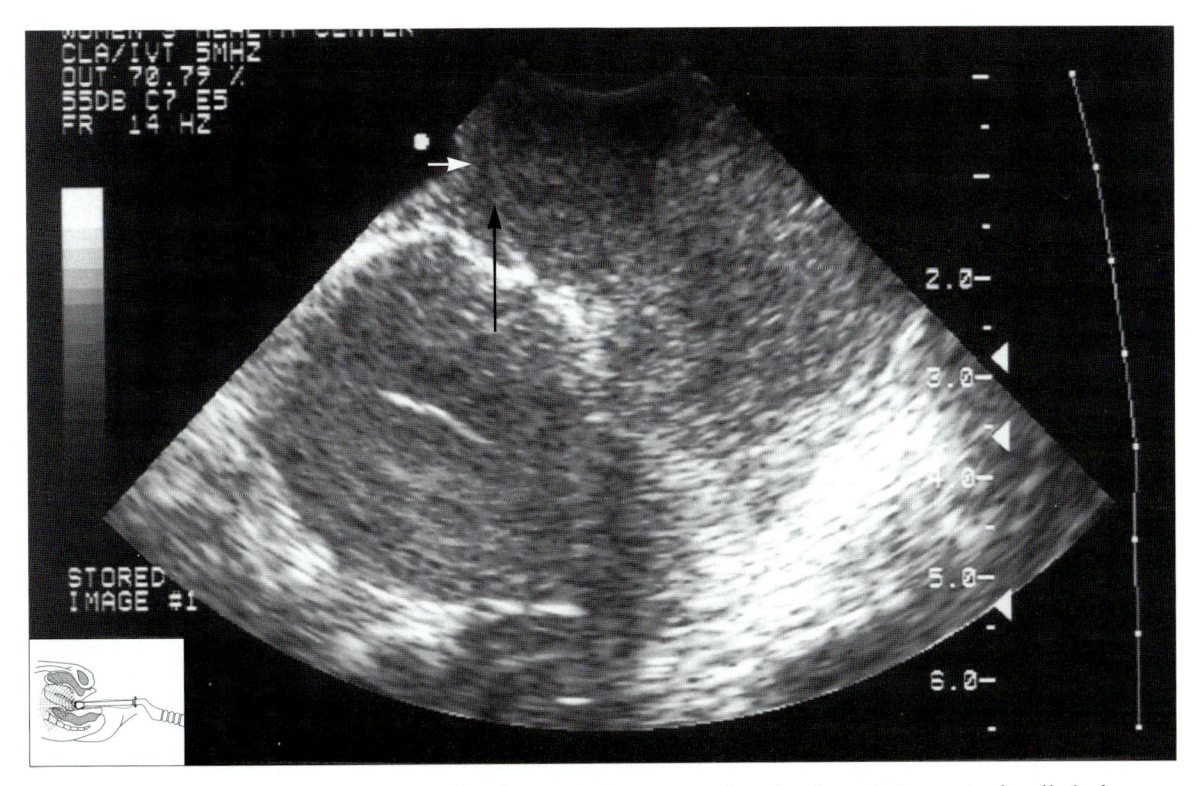

Figure 12-11. Stage IIA cervical cancer. This large isoechoic tumor invades the anterior vaginal wall. A clear plane of normal tissue (arrow) separates the tumor from the bladder.

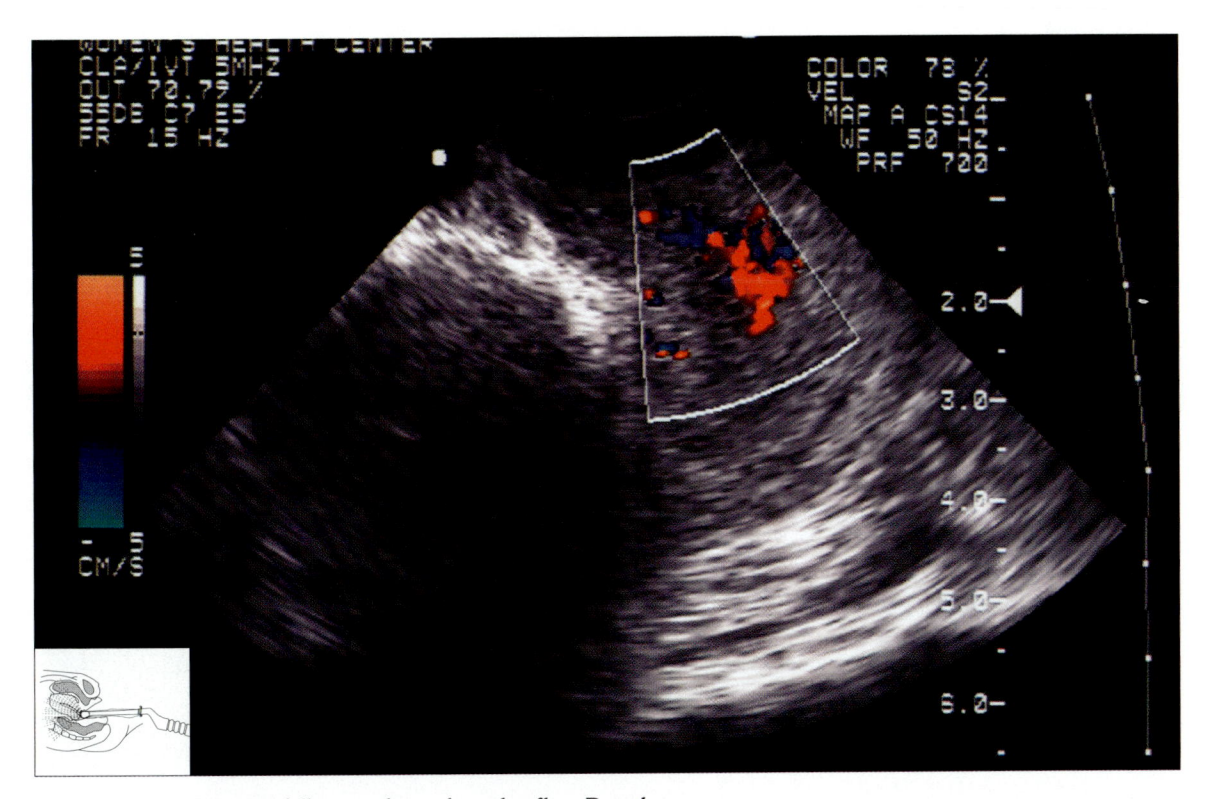

Figure 12-12. Increased flow as shown by color flow Doppler.

An Atlas of Transvaginal Sonography

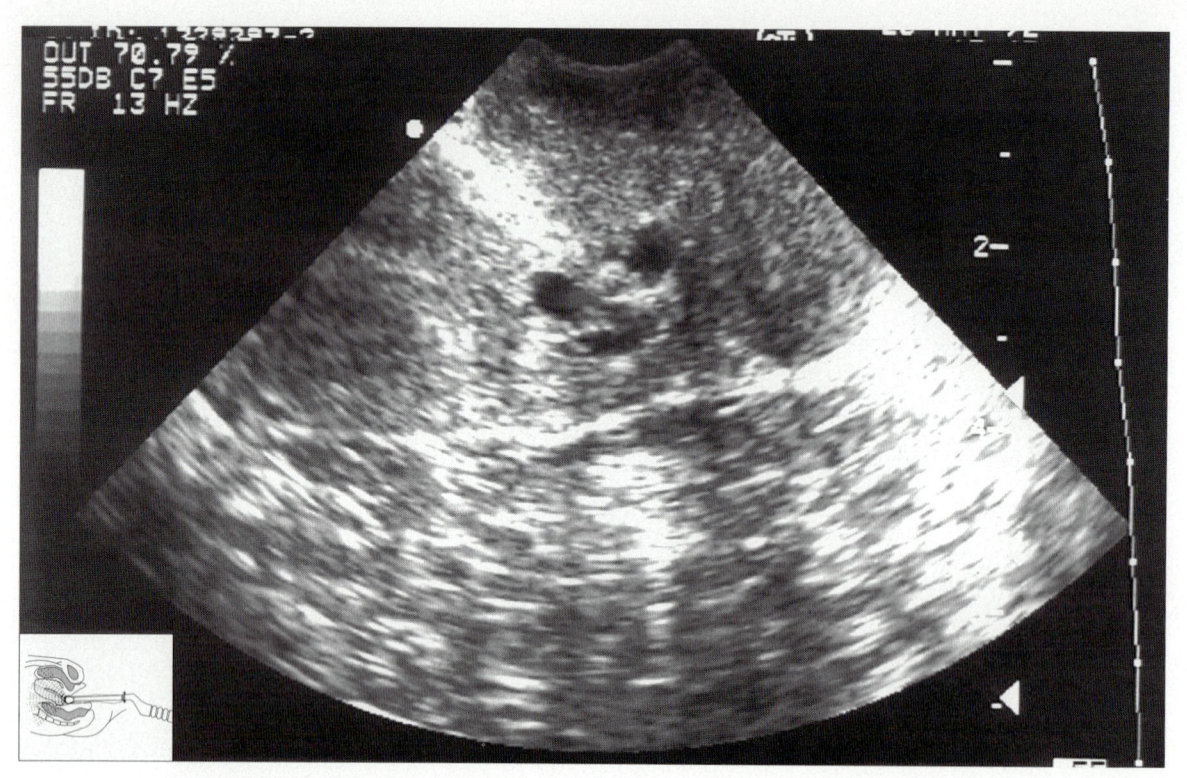

Figure 12-13. Cystic-glandular formation in this adenosquamous cancer of the cervix.

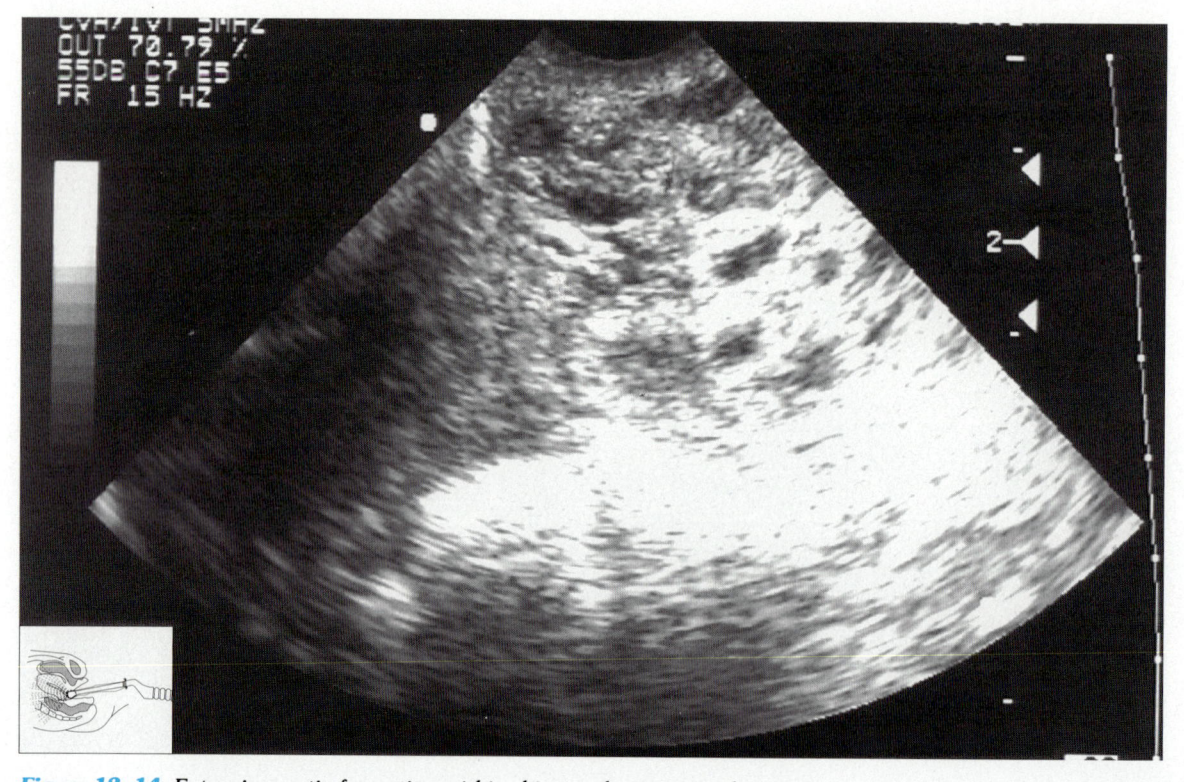

Figure 12-14. Extensive cystic formation within this exophytic cervical cancer.

Cervical Cancer

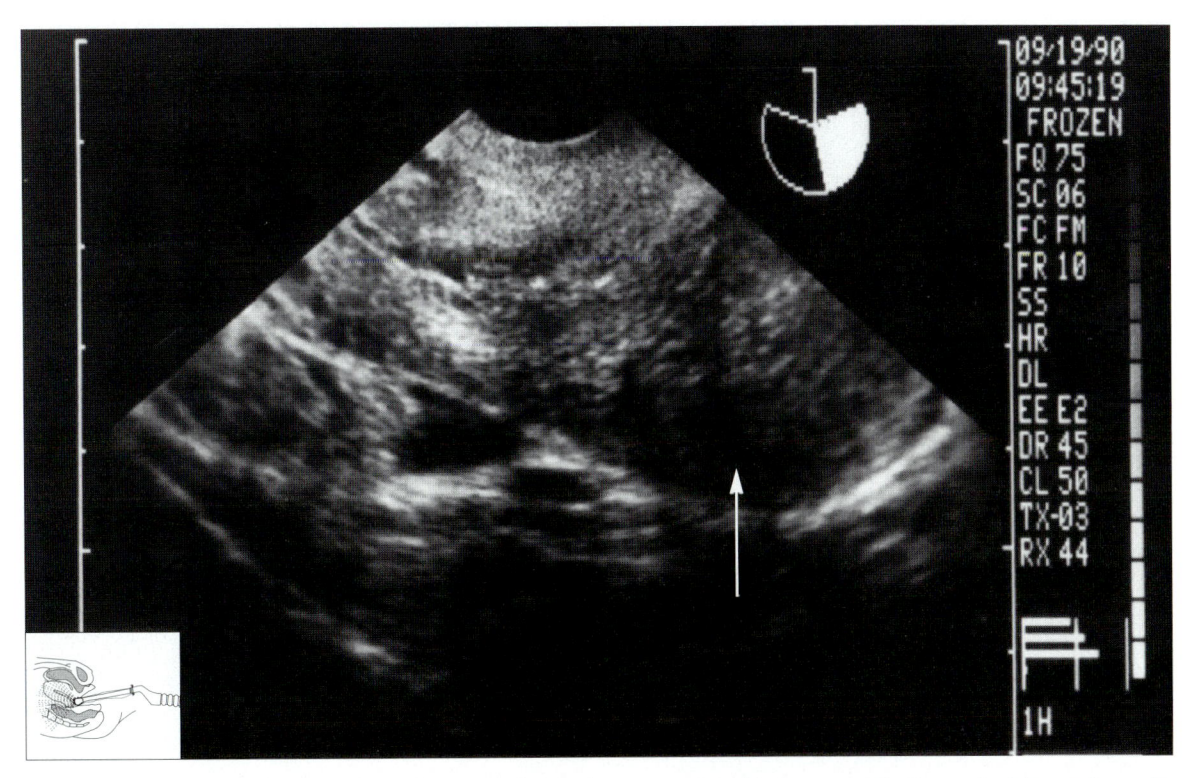

Figure 12-15. Sagittal section through cervix, clearly demonstrating this large exophytic cervical tumor (arrow).

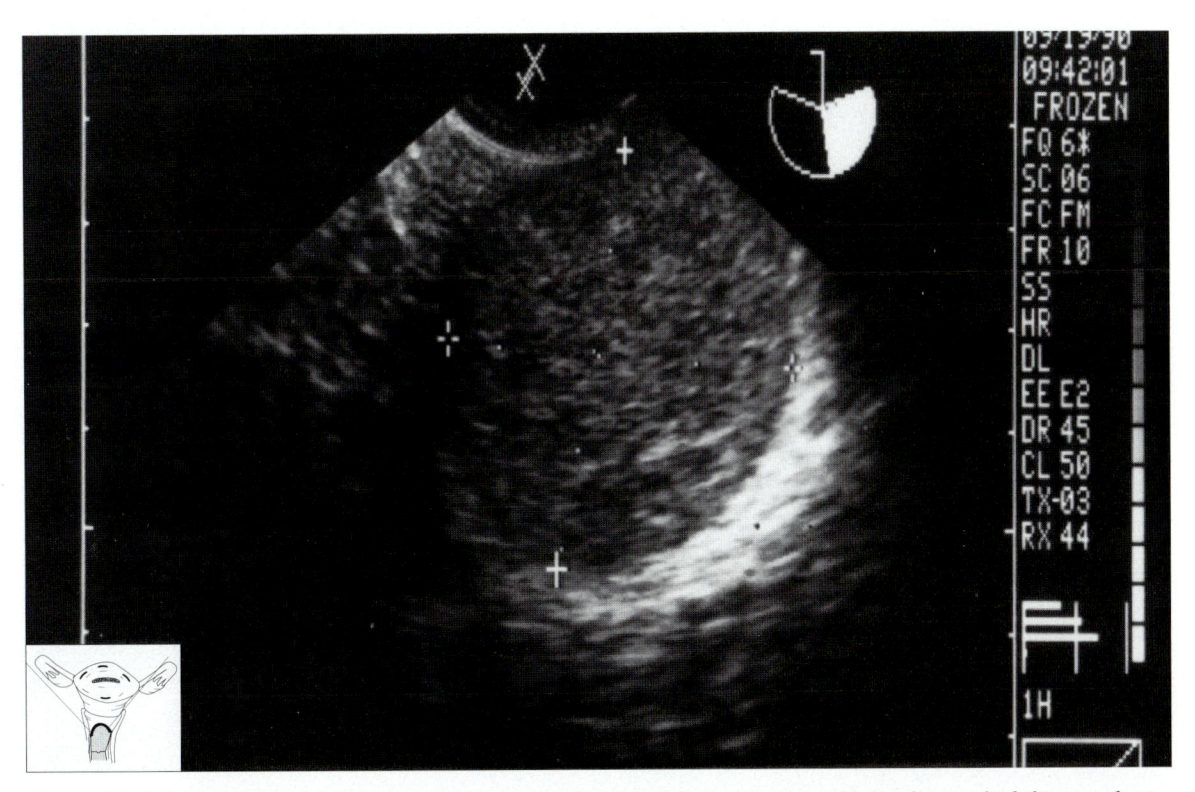

Figure 12-16. Coronal view allows accurate measurement and determination of lateral spread of this exophytic tumor. The patient underwent definitive radiation therapy, and tumor volume regression was accurately determined by TVS.

An Atlas of Transvaginal Sonography

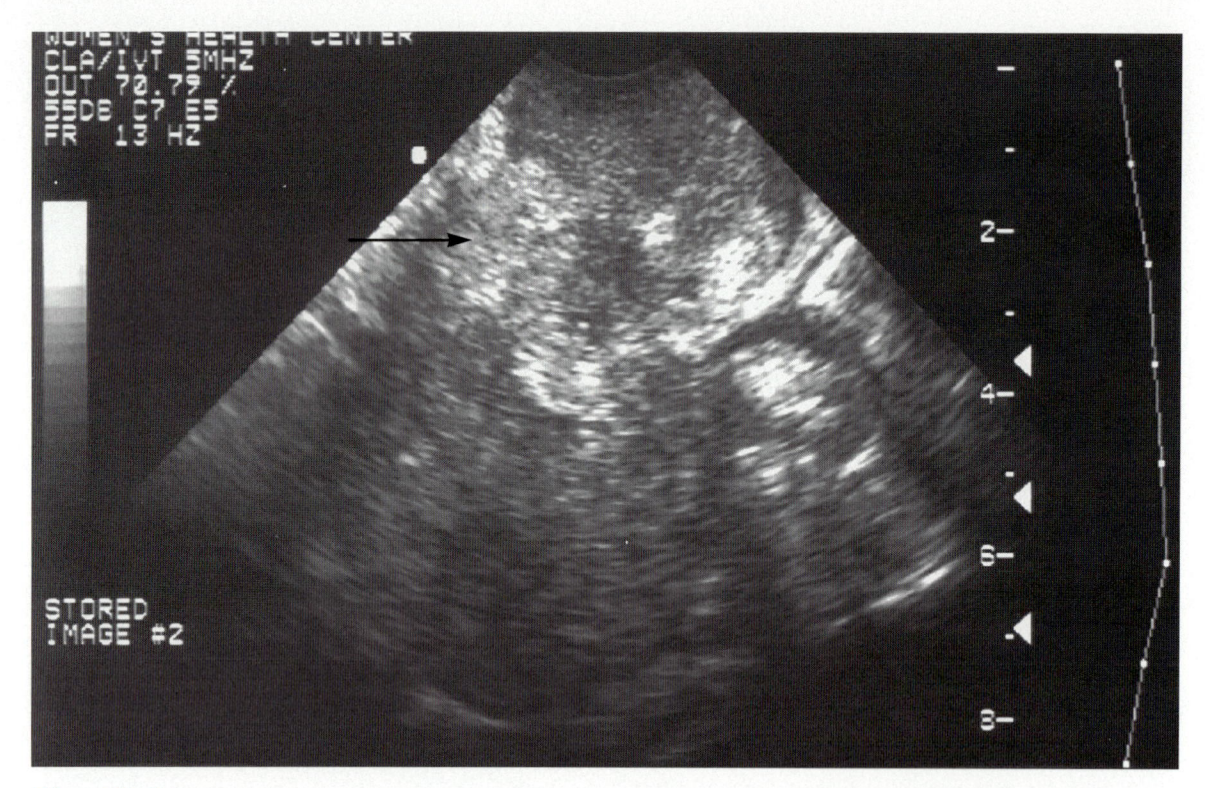

Figure 12-17. Barrel-shaped, echogenic, endocervical cancer (arrow). The ectocervix is isoechoic, and was normal to inspection. Fractional curettage confirmed an invasive endocervical adenocarcinoma.

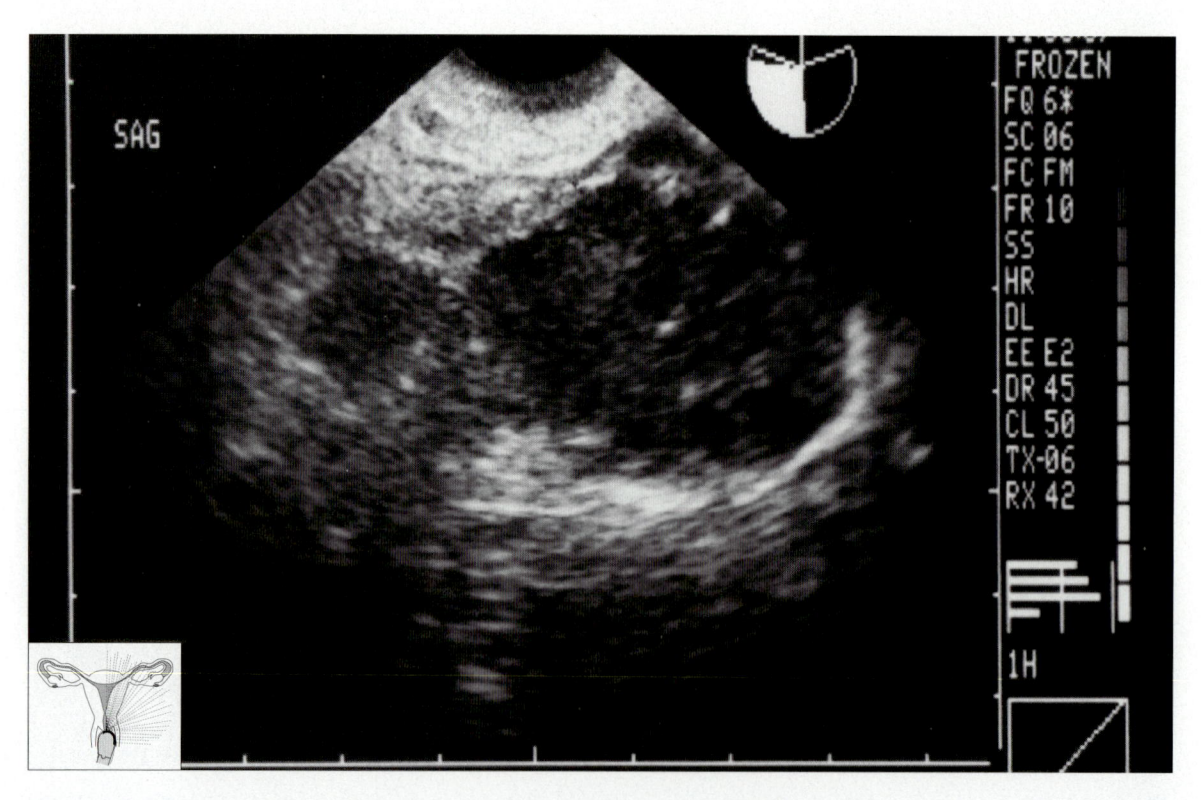

Figure 12-18. Enlarged iliac lymph node in a patient with advanced cervical cancer.

Cervical Cancer

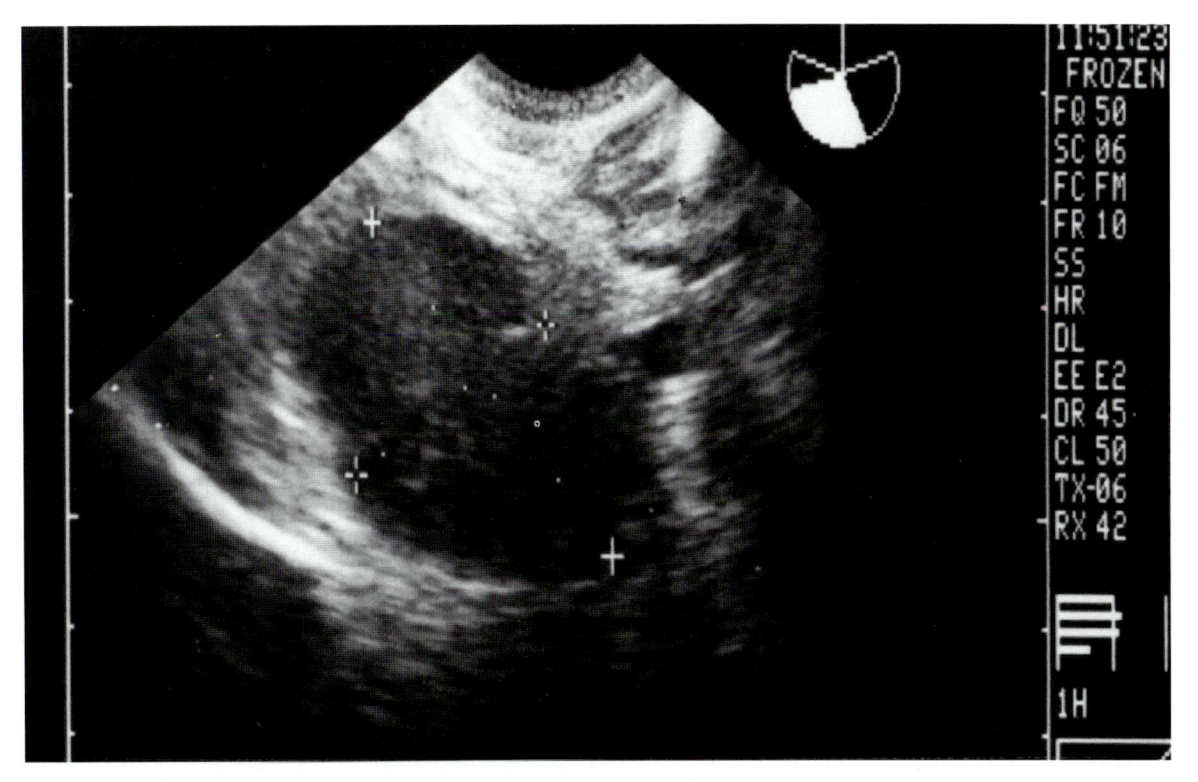

Figure 12-19. Enlarged pelvic lymph node on the pelvic side wall.

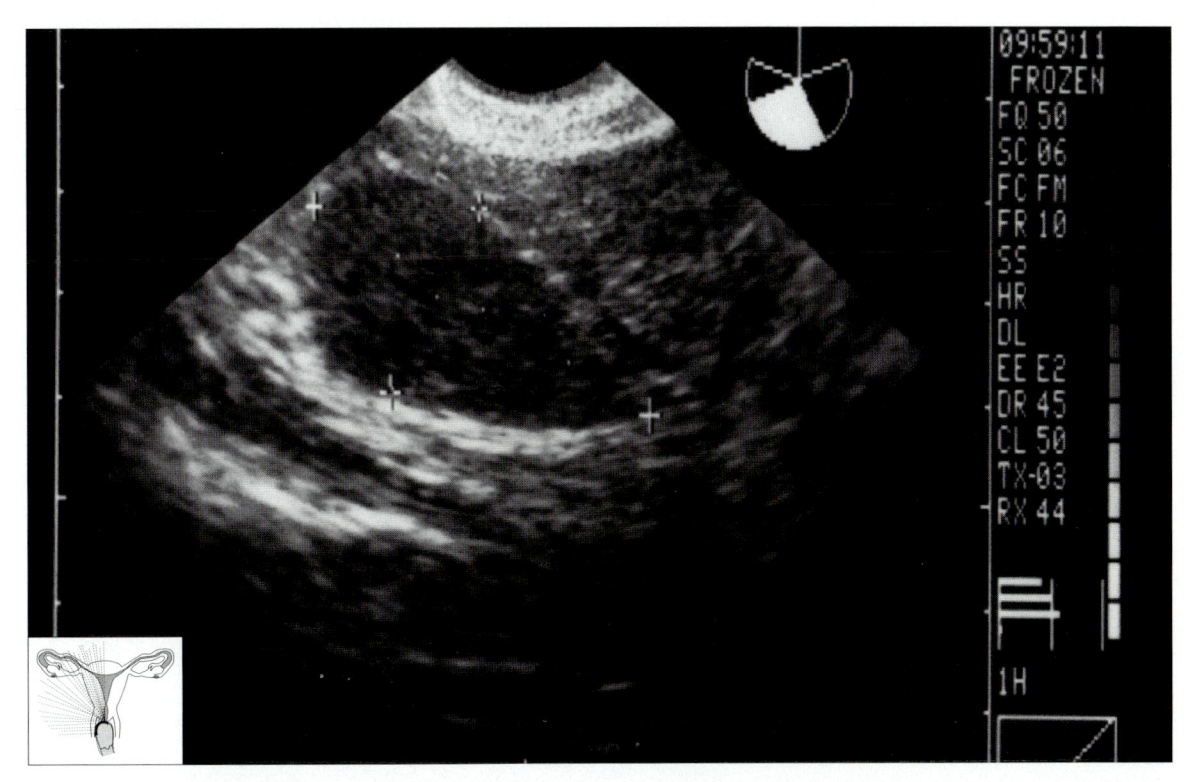

Figure 12-20. Enlarged pelvic lymph node that morphologically looks like an ovary.

13   *Ovarian Cancer*

Ovarian cancer comprises the common epithelial ovarian tumors and the less common germ cell and sex cord stromal tumors. The epithelial variety comprises borderline and malignant types. Serous histology is the predominant histological type, while other less common histologies include mucinous, endometrioid, clear cell, Brenner, and mixed lesions.

Ovarian cancer is a disease of middle and upper socioeconomic classes and occurs most frequently in industrialized countries. It occurs in 1:70 women (1.5%) and 1 in every 100 will die from the disease. Twenty-two-thousand new cases are diagnosed yearly, accounting for 4% of all female cancers. It is the leading cause of death from gynecologic malignancy, causing 12,000 deaths yearly, accounting for more than half of all deaths due to gynecologic malignancies. Without regular screening, early ovarian cancer remains an uncommonly diagnosed entity.

Scan Findings

Sonographic features indicative of a malignant lesion relate to its size, shape, morphology, and persistence. Masses larger than 5-6 cm that are multilocular, complex or solid, which have external excrescences or nodularity or internal papillary excrescences or persist for longer than five weeks in association with increased peritoneal fluid, are highly suspicious for malignancy and should be further evaluated. Depending on the clinical context, this could mean an attempt at hormonal suppression, determination of serum CA-125 level, or color flow Doppler determination of the pulsatility and/or resistance index (PI or RI). If doubt exits, then surgical exploration is warranted.

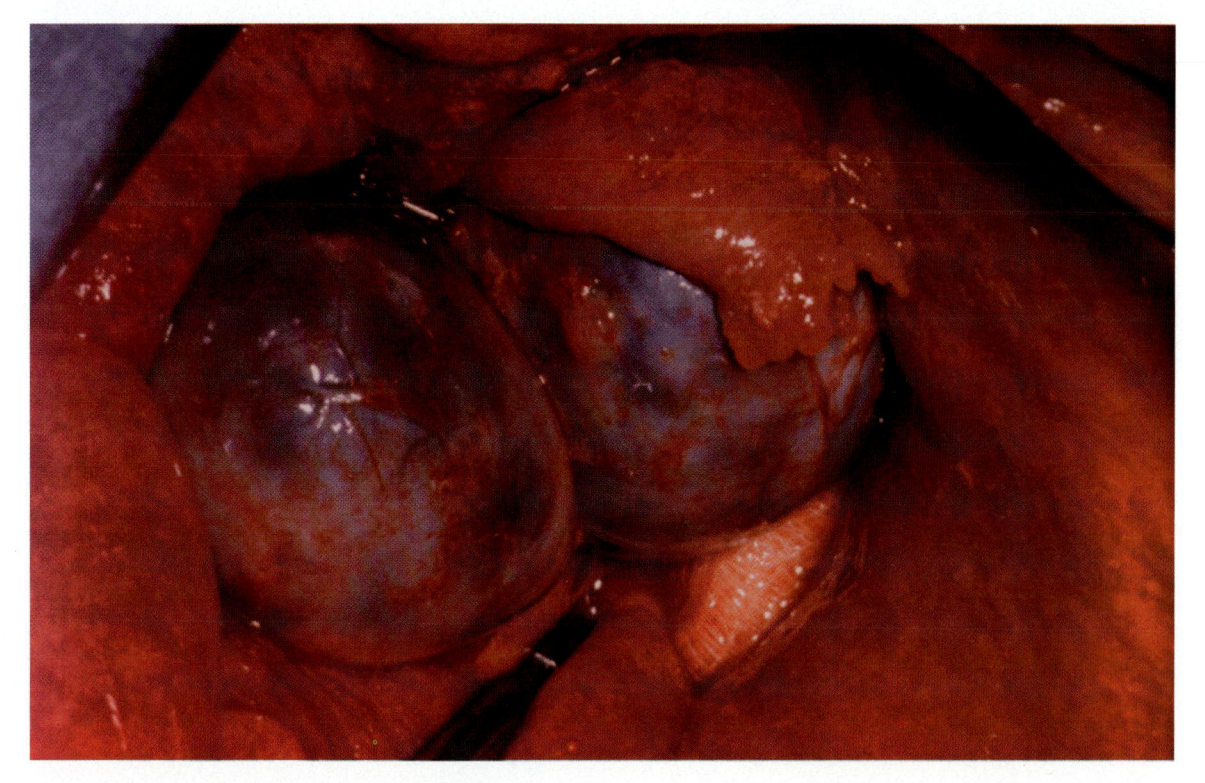

Figure 13-1. Bilateral early ovarian cancers.

An Atlas of Transvaginal Sonography

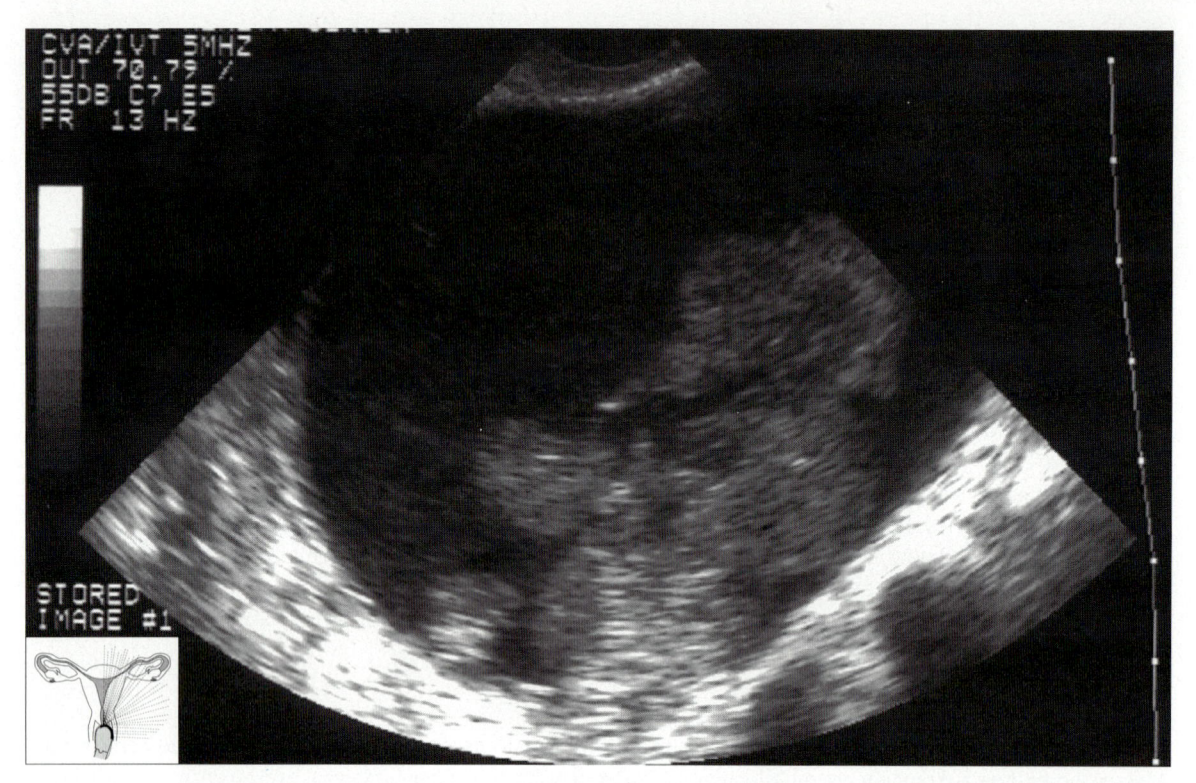

Figure 13-2. *Large complex ovarian cancer with prominent internal papillary excrescences. Disease was localized to the ovaries.*

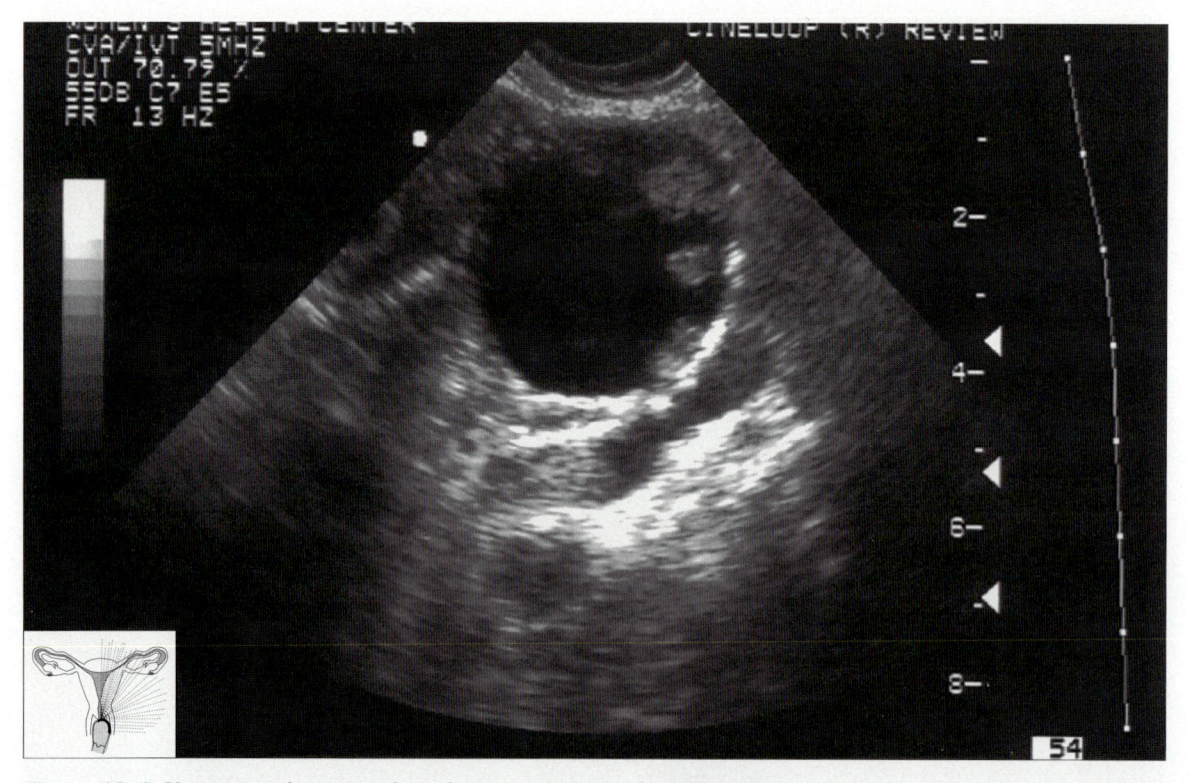

Figure 13-3. *Unsuspected, cystic, adnexal mass with internal papillations.*

Ovarian Cancer

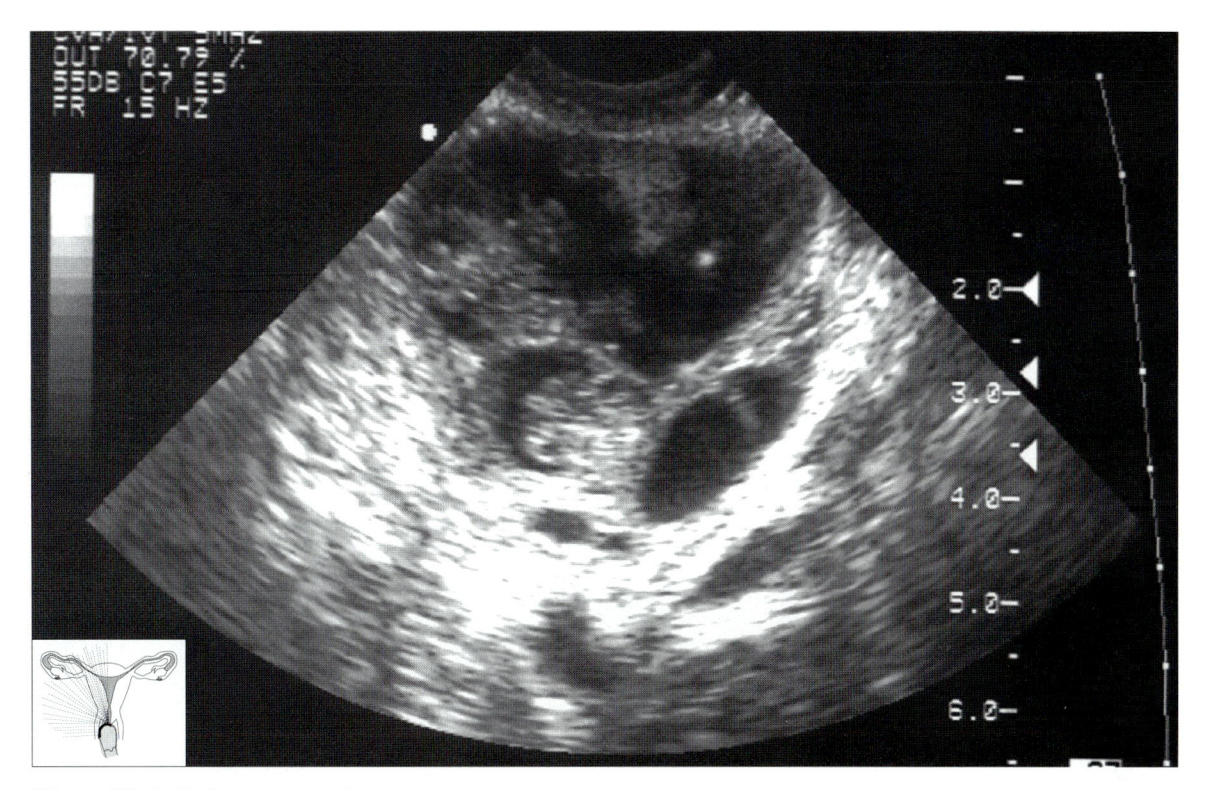

Figure 13-4. Multicystic complex ovary.

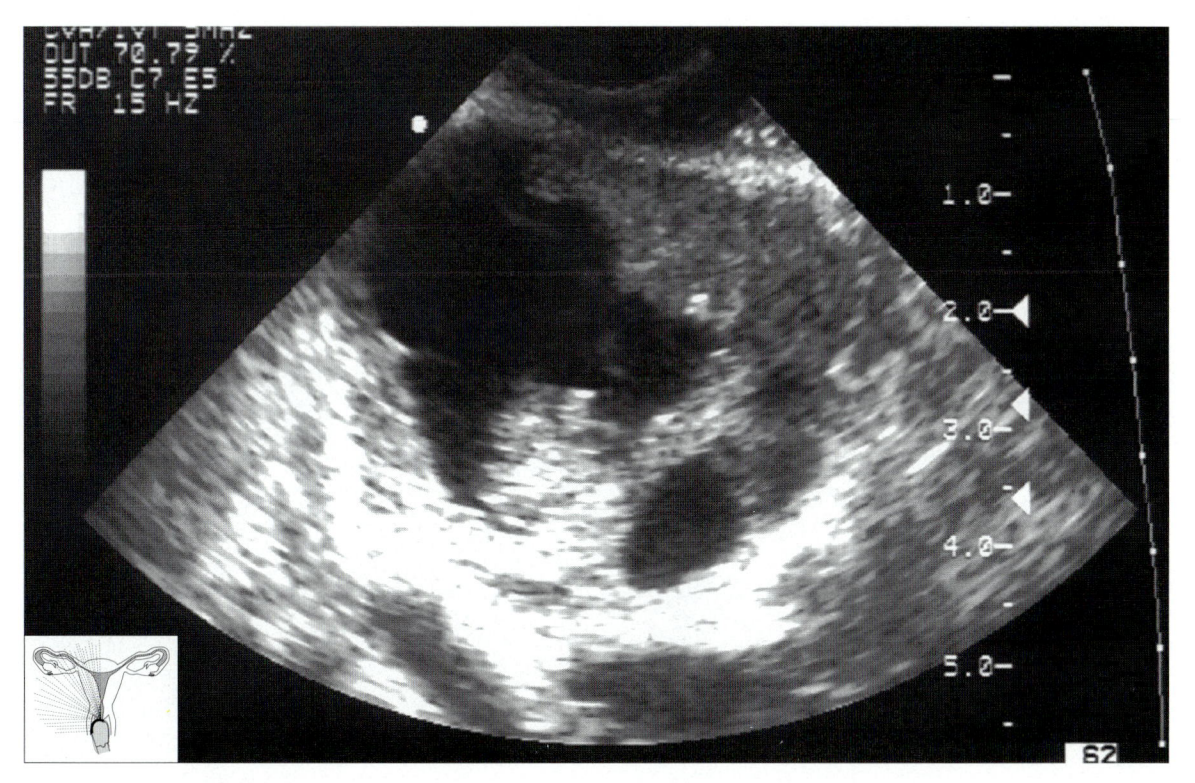

Figure 13-5. Multicystic complex ovarian cancer, FIGO stage IA.

An Atlas of Transvaginal Sonography

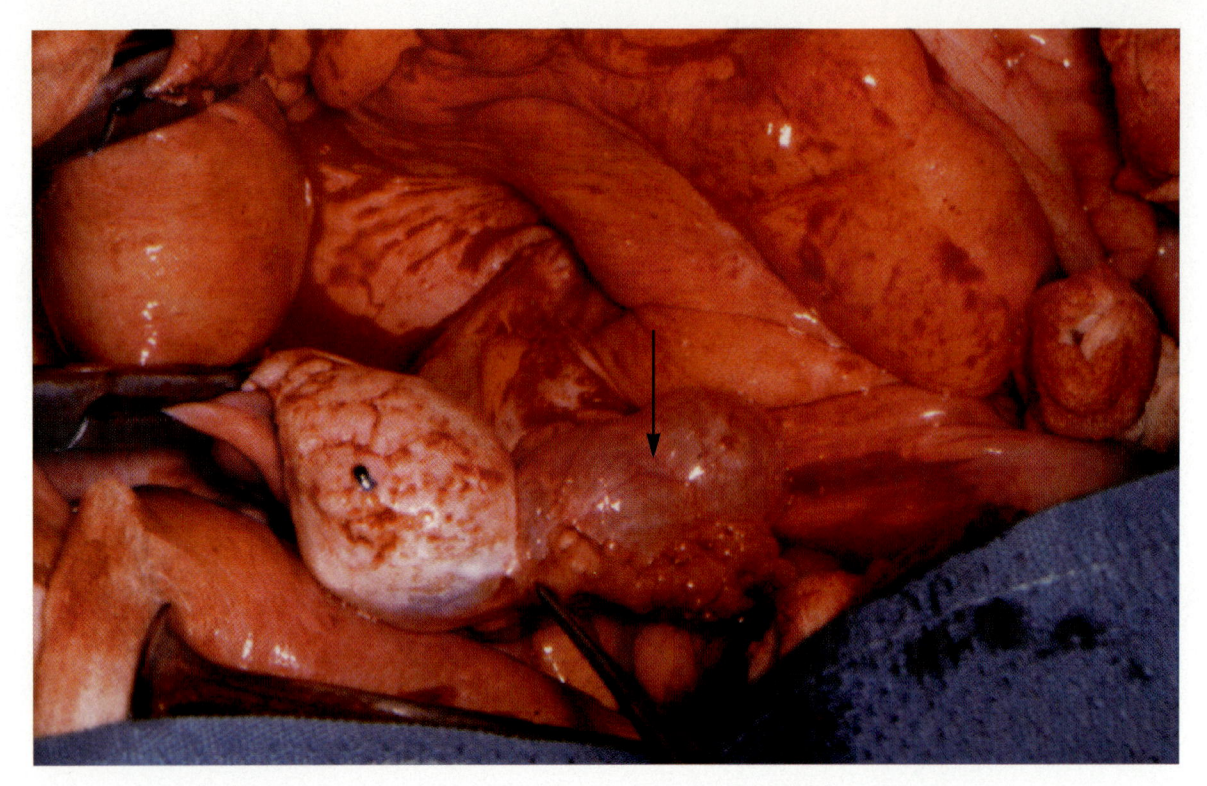

Figure 13-6. Tumor growth arising in the ovary and extending into the fallopian tube (arrow).

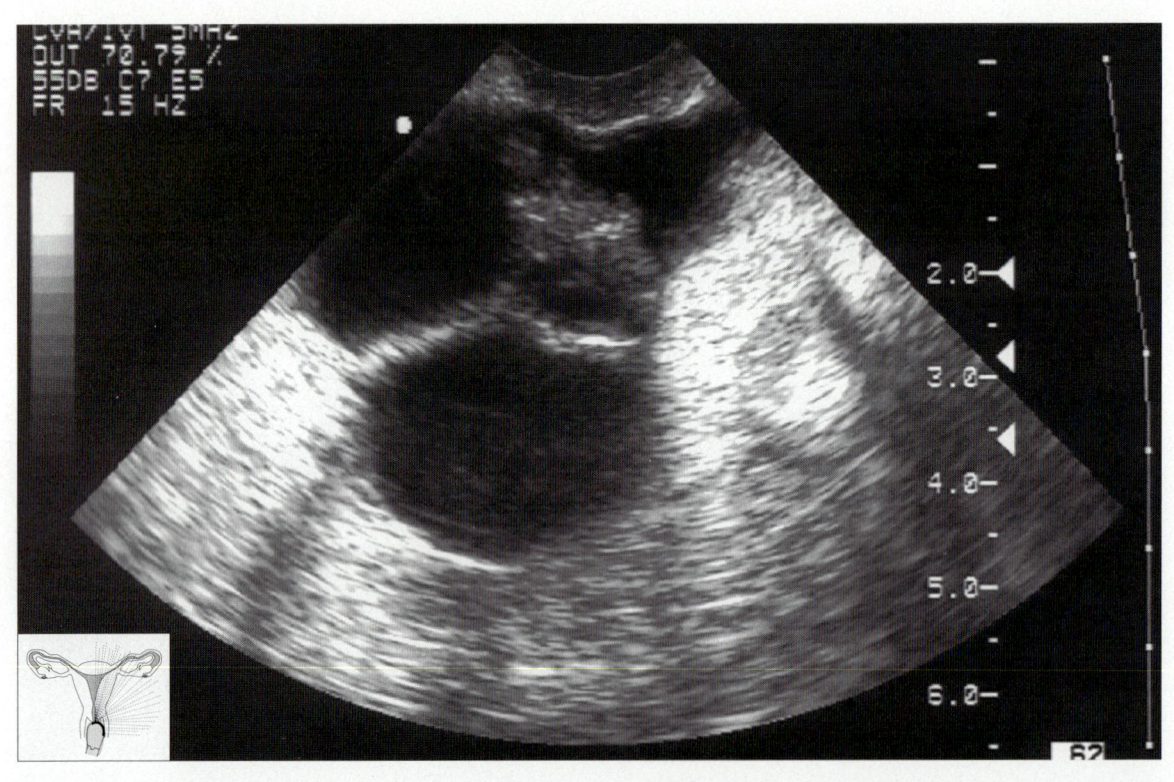

Figure 13-7. Multicystic, early, ovarian cancer, with thickened septae and small solid component.

Ovarian Cancer

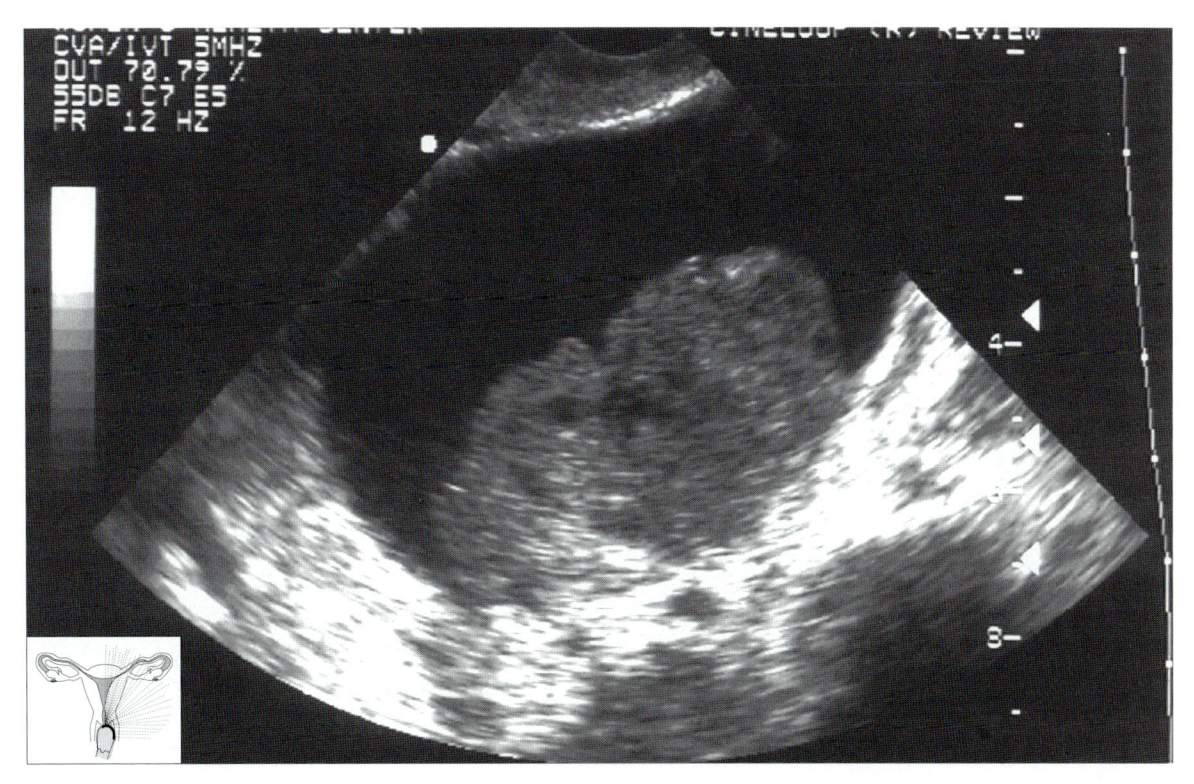

Figure 13-8. Large solid component to the cystic ovarian cancer. On superficial inspection, this may be confused with hemorrhage within a corpus luteum. Color flow Doppler is invaluable.

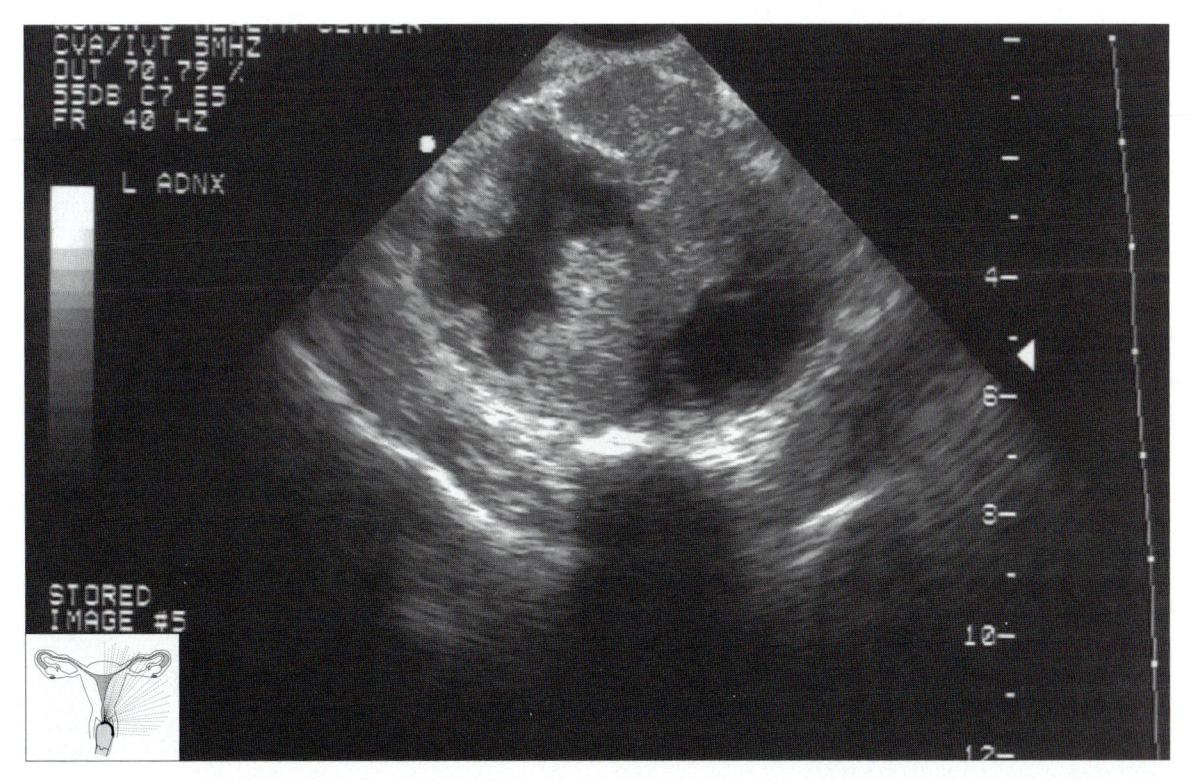

Figure 13-9. Complex Stage IA ovarian cancer.

An Atlas of Transvaginal Sonography

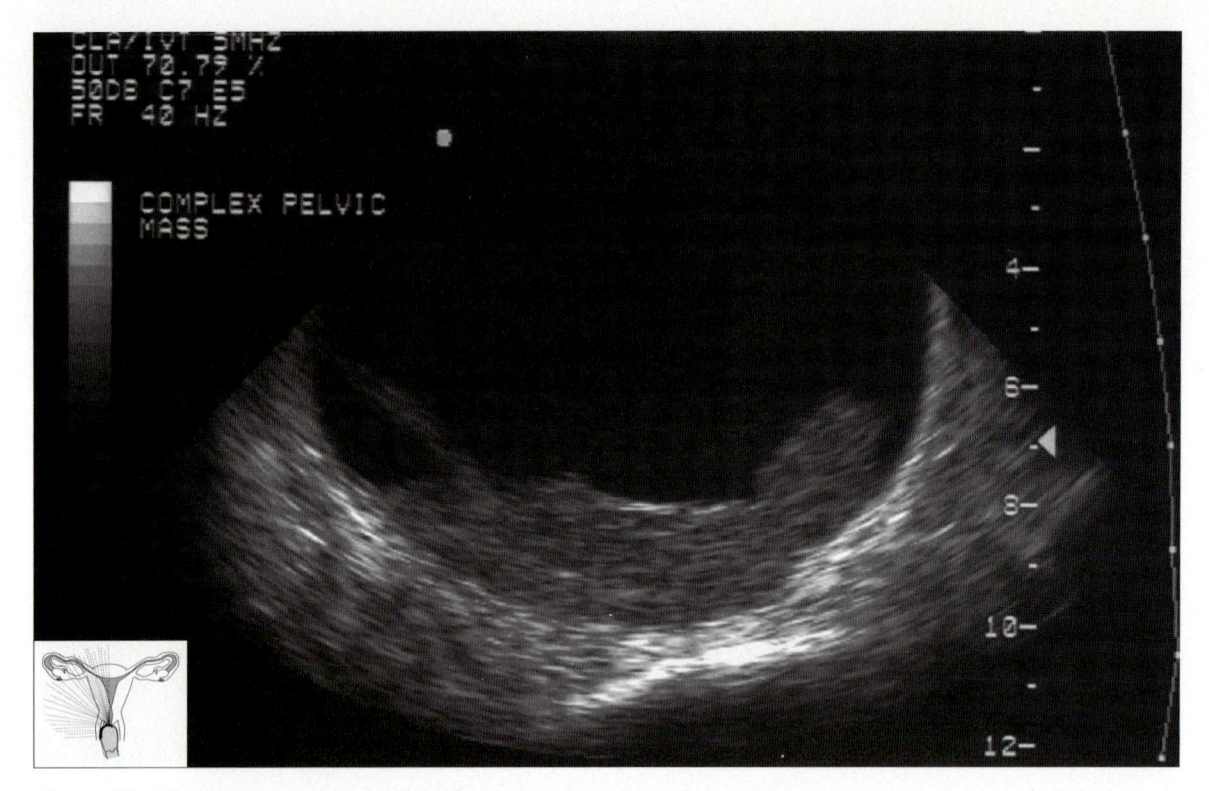

Figure 13-10. Solid component with thick septa in this early ovarian cancer.

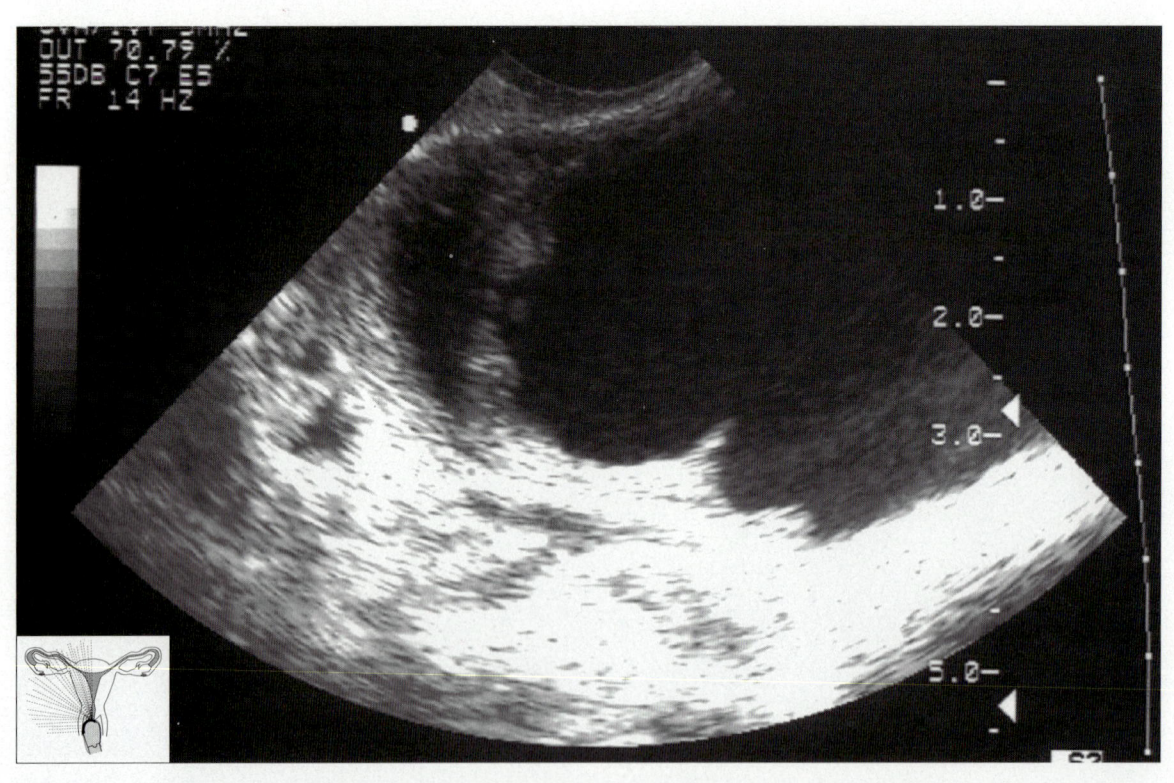

Figure 13-11. Thickened irregular septation and small, solid, papillary projections in this early ovarian cancer.

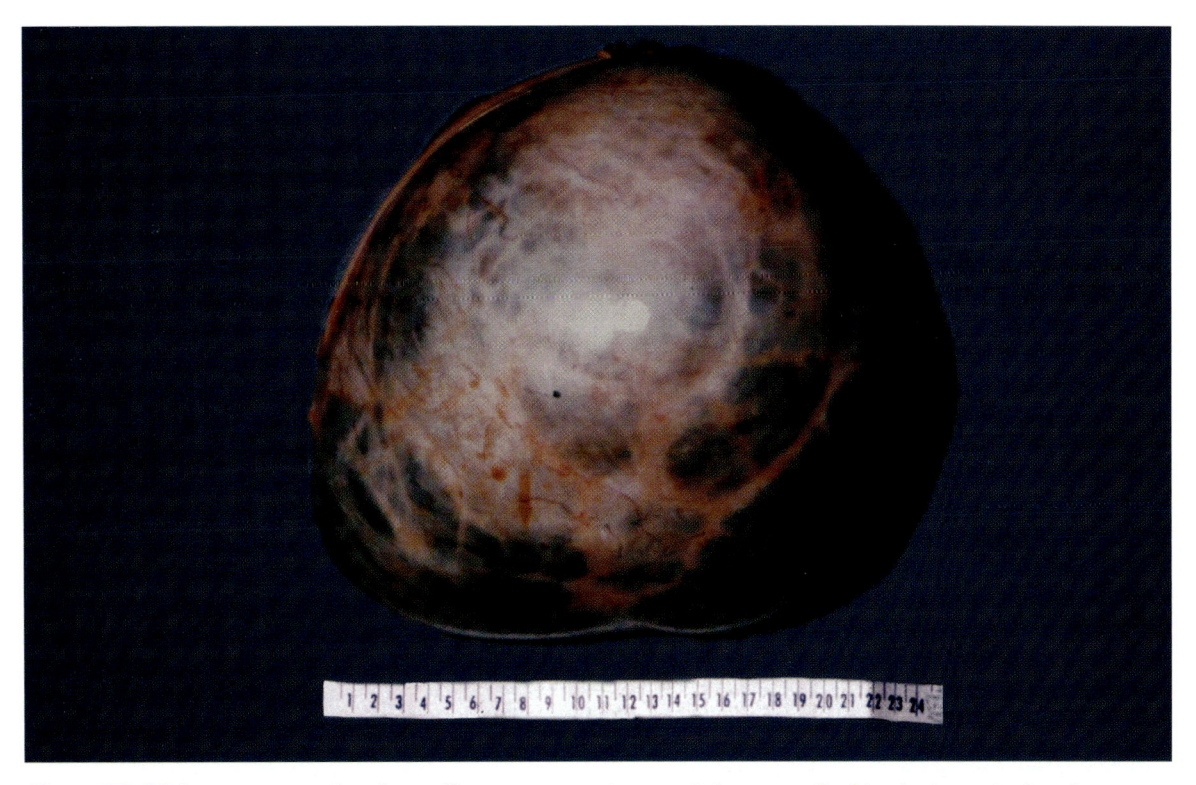

Figure 13-12. Large, encapsulated, papillary serous carcinoma of the ovary. On histologie sectioning there were prominent internal papillations.

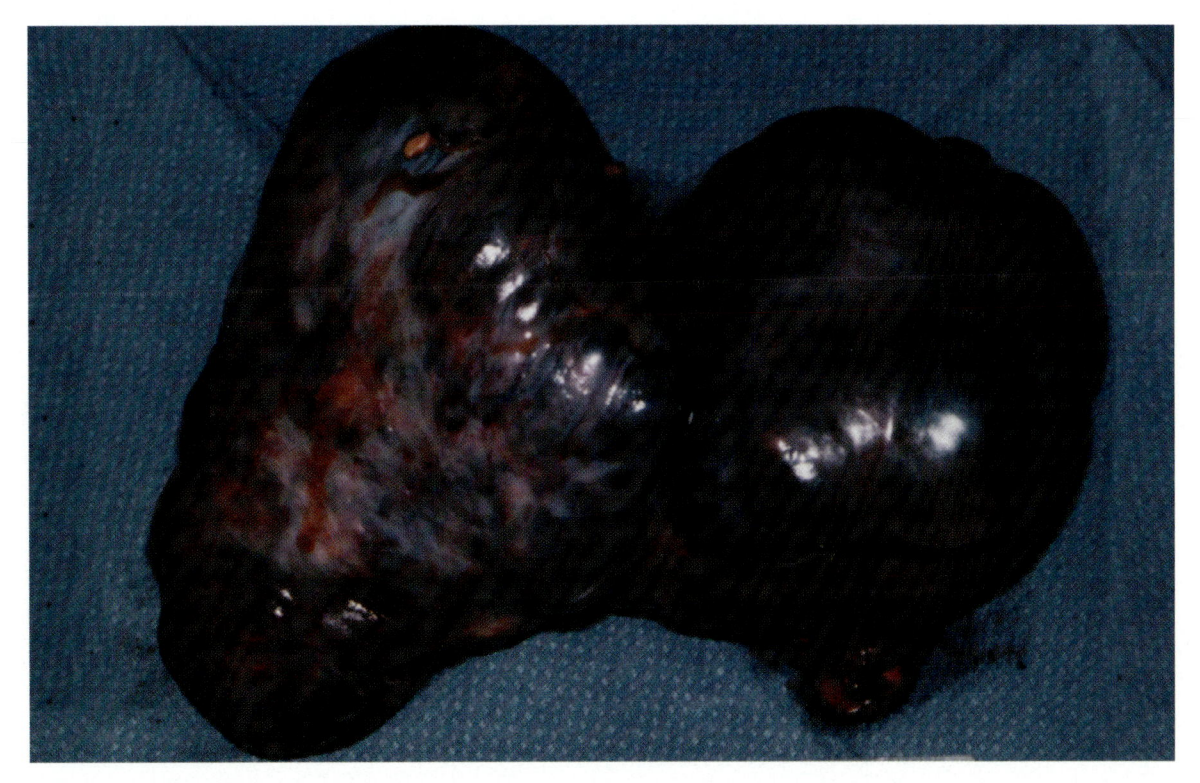

Figure 13-13. Multicystic complex ovarian cancer.

An Atlas of Transvaginal Sonography

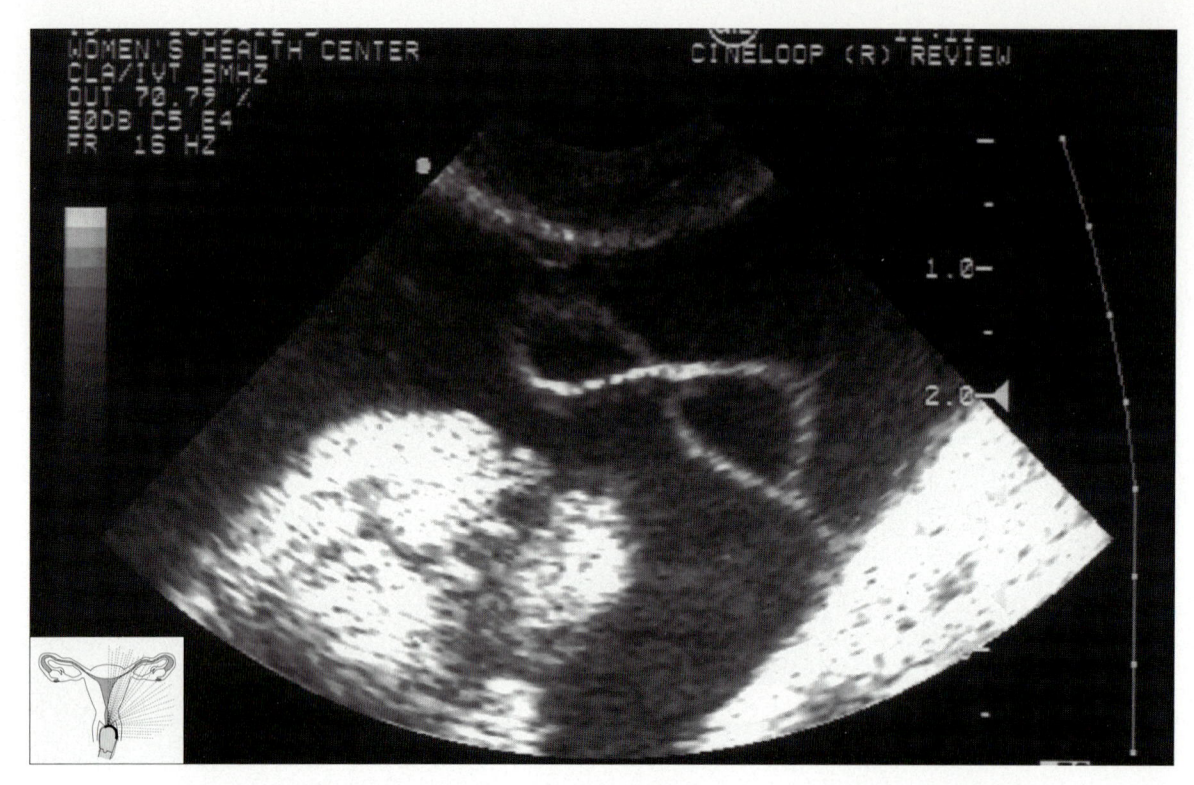

Figure 13-14. Convoluted thin septa adjacent to a large solid component in a complex ovarian cancer.

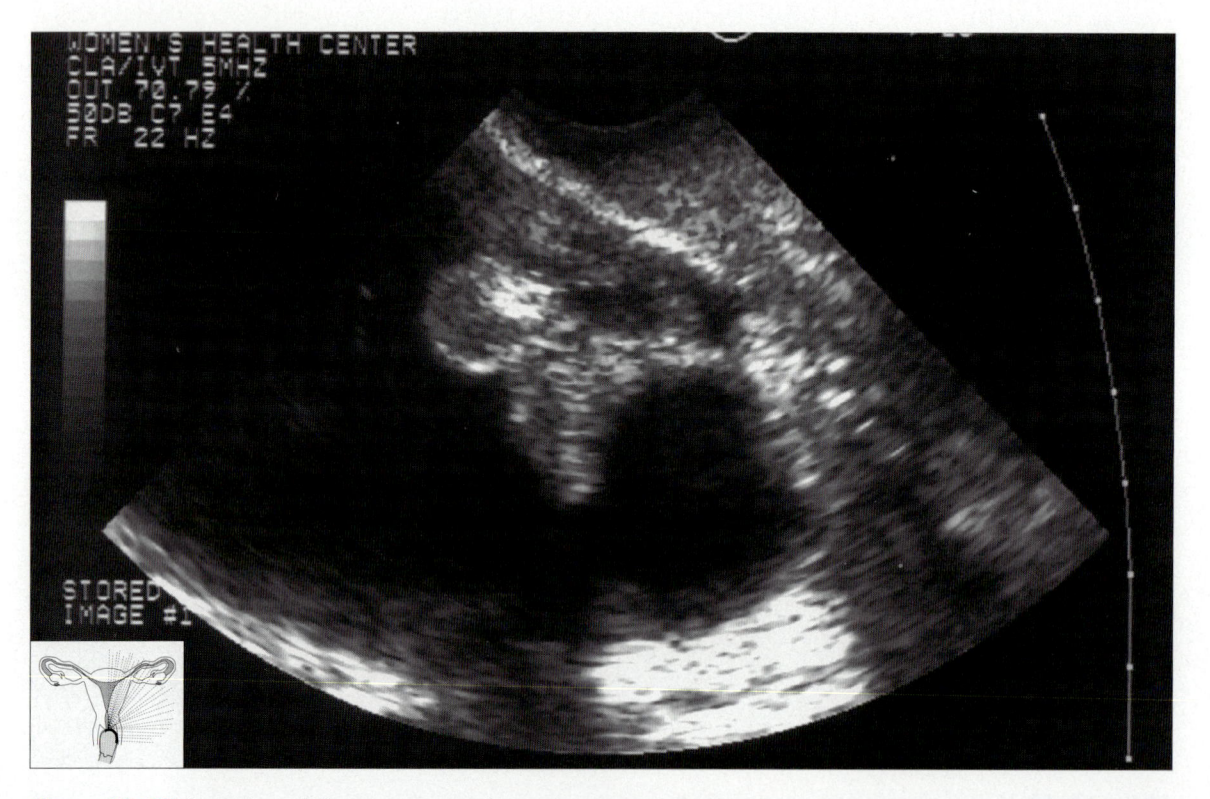

Figure 13-15. Irregular solid component to this early ovarian cancer.

Ovarian Cancer

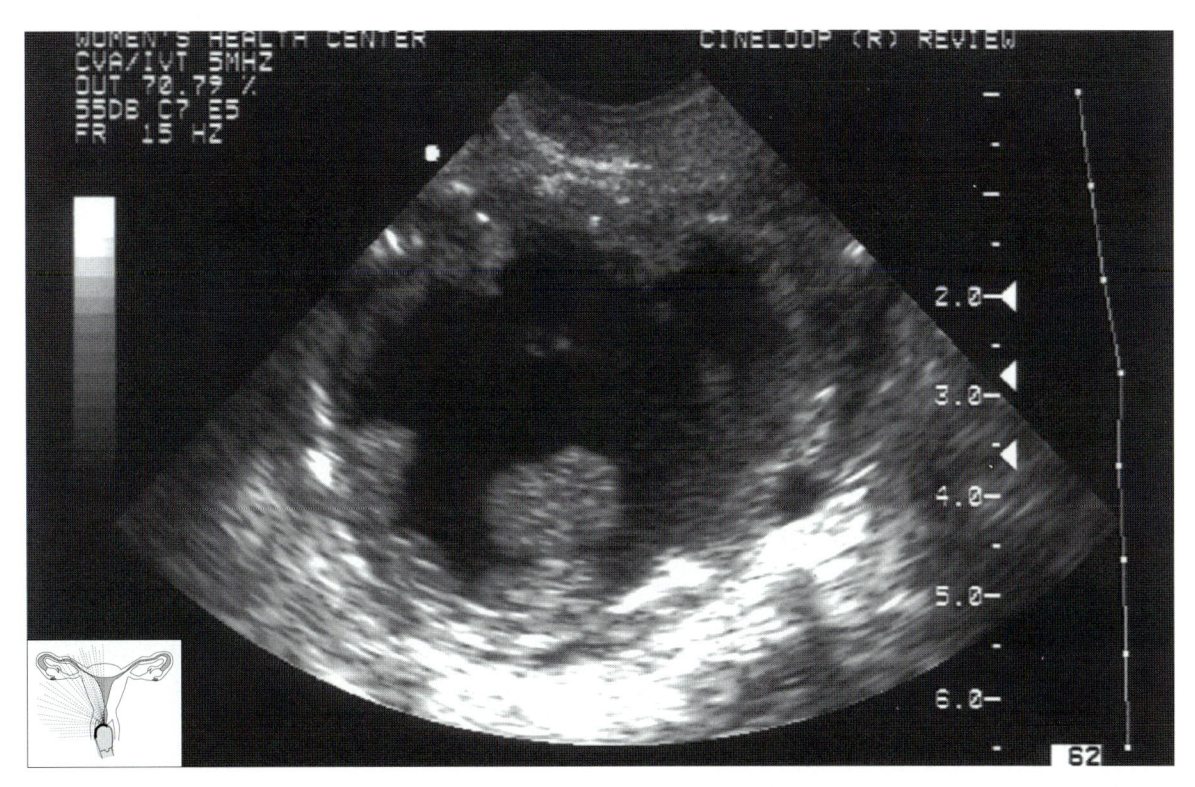

Figure 13-16. Stage IC ovarian cancer with internal and external excrescences.

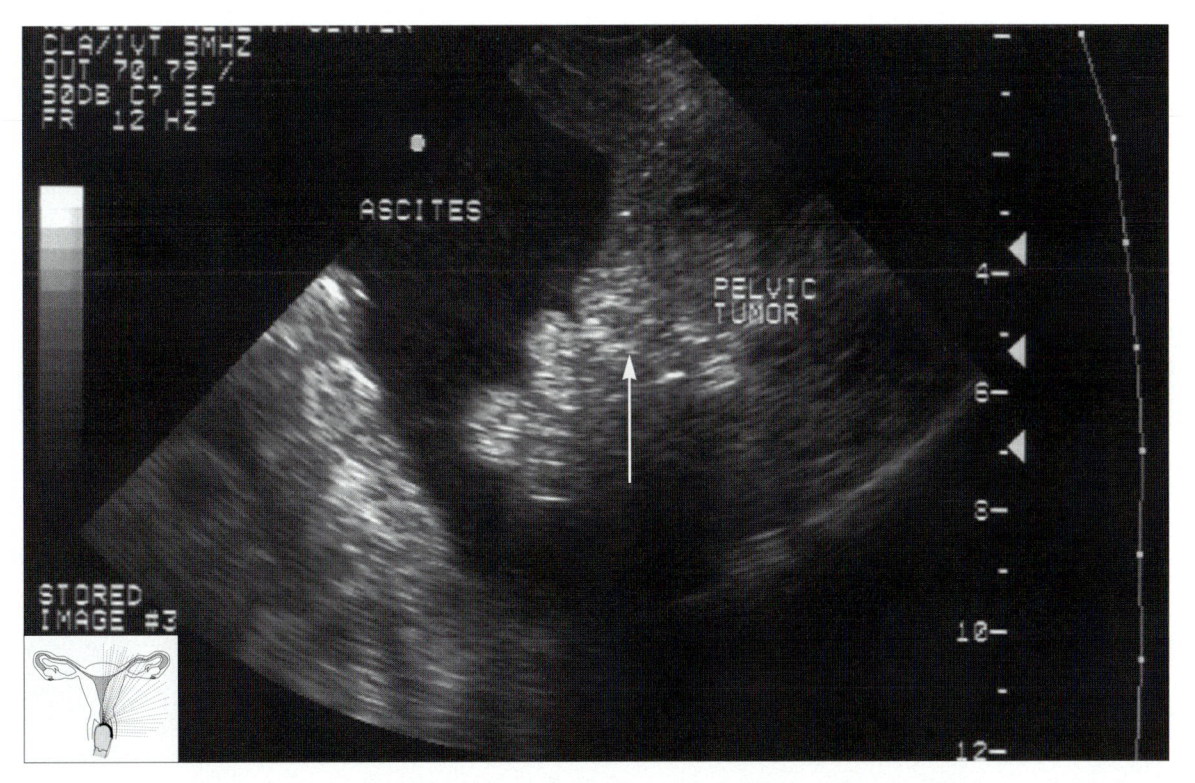

Figure 13-17. Advanced solid pelvic side wall tumor (arrow) surrounded by malignant ascites.

An Atlas of Transvaginal Sonography

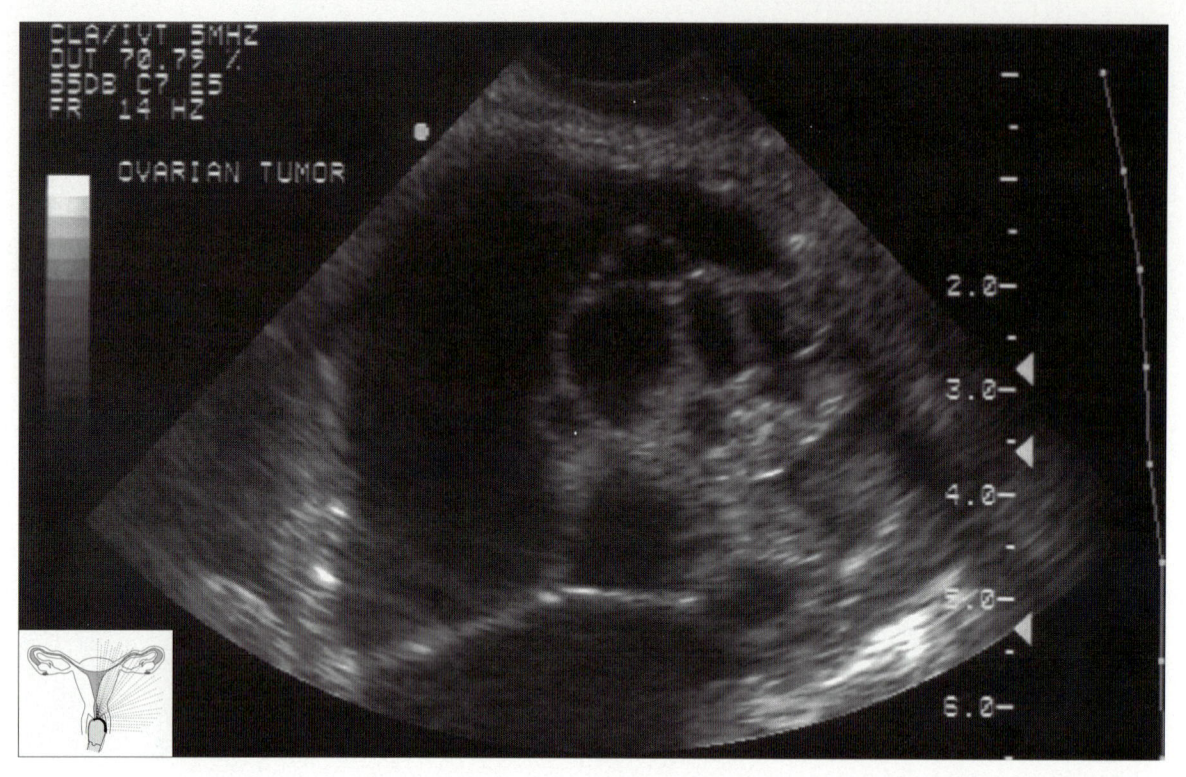

Figure 13-18. Large, advanced, complex ovarian tumor with solid areas, large cystic regions and daughter cysts.

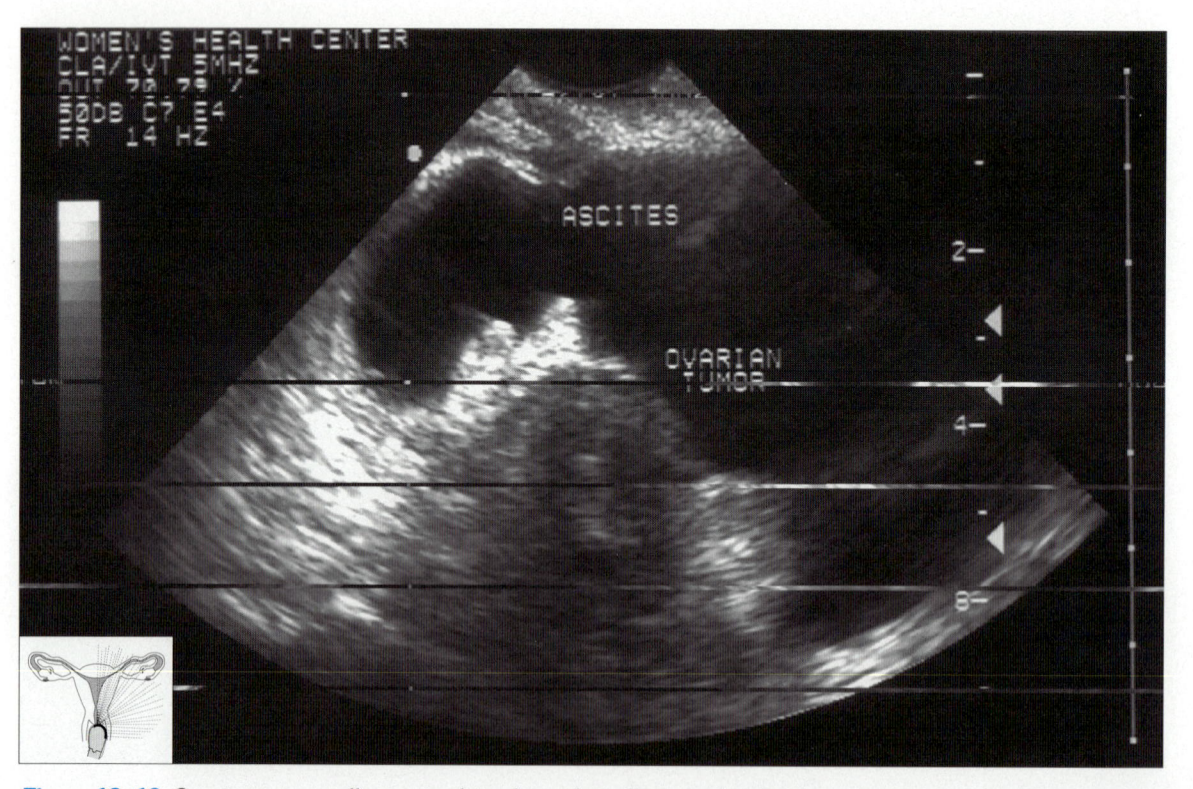

Figure 13-19. Ovarian cancer adherent to the pelvic side wall covered with echoic excrescences and surrounded by malignant ascites.

Ovarian Cancer

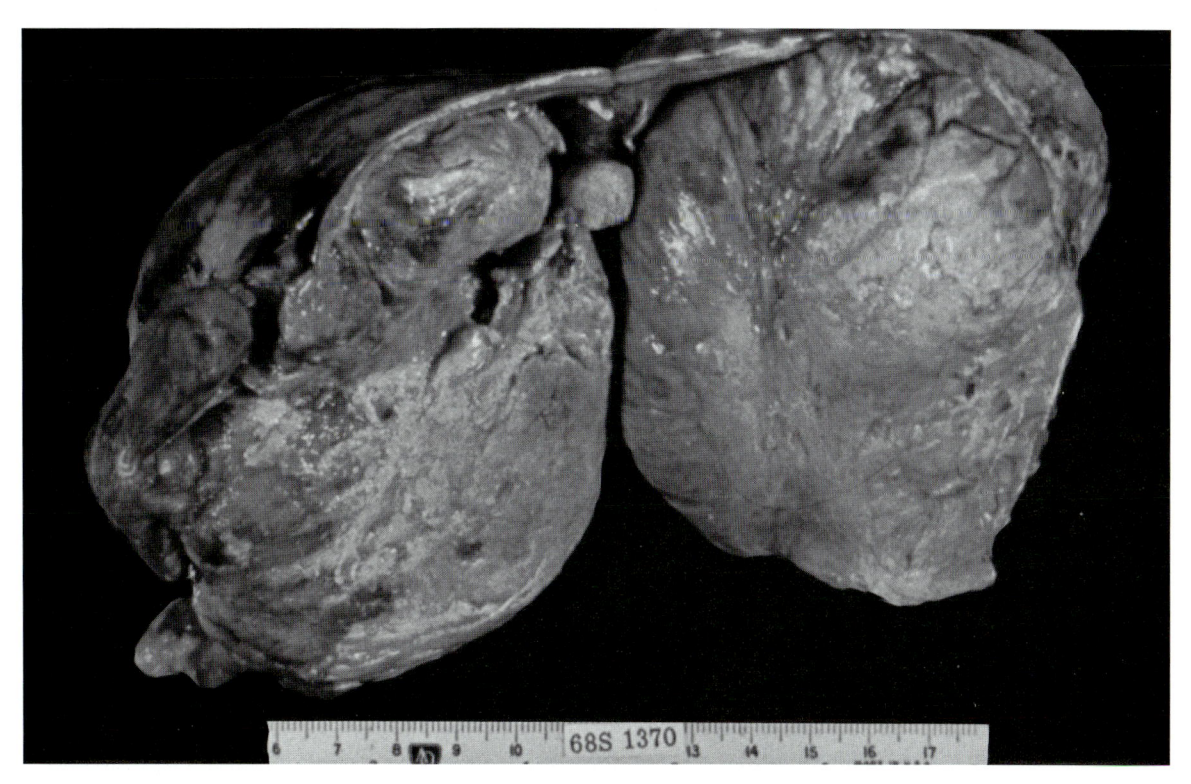

Figure 13-20. Complex endometrioid carcinoma of the ovary.

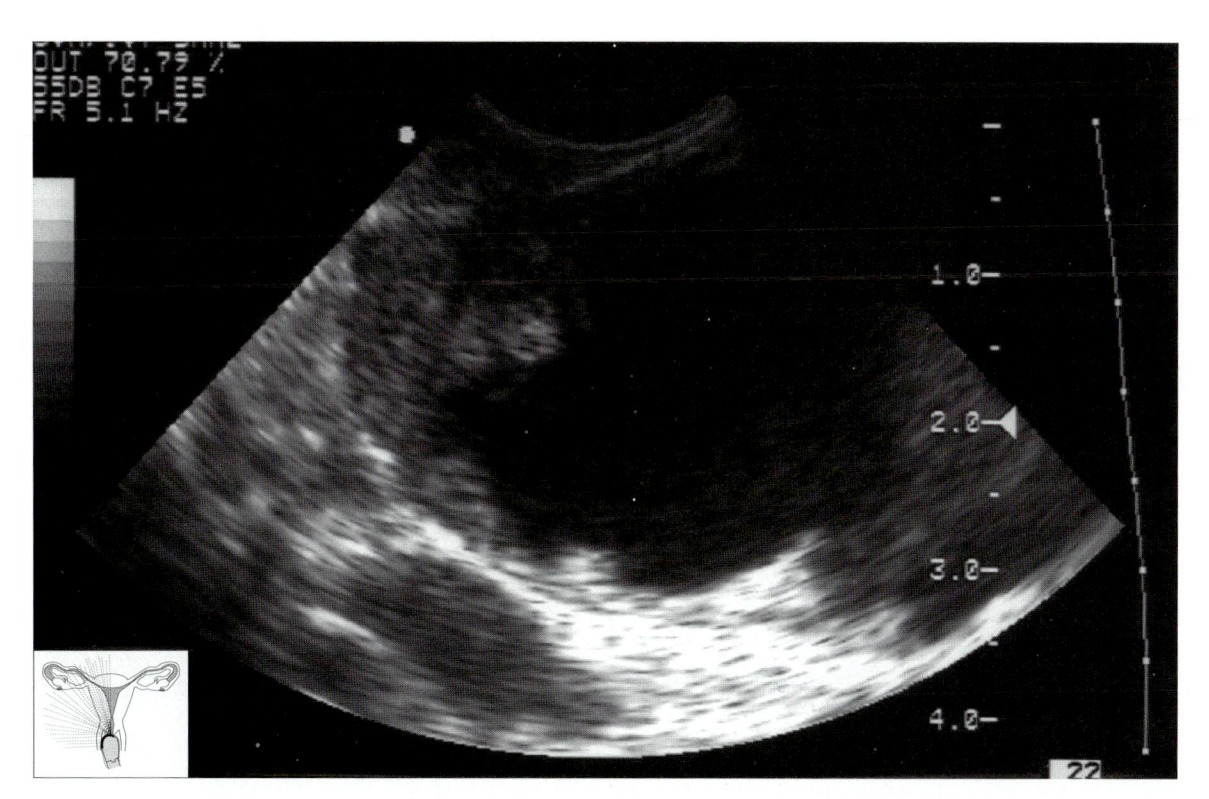

Figure 13-21. Complex ovarian tumor, with solid component and small, internal, papillary projections.

An Atlas of Transvaginal Sonography

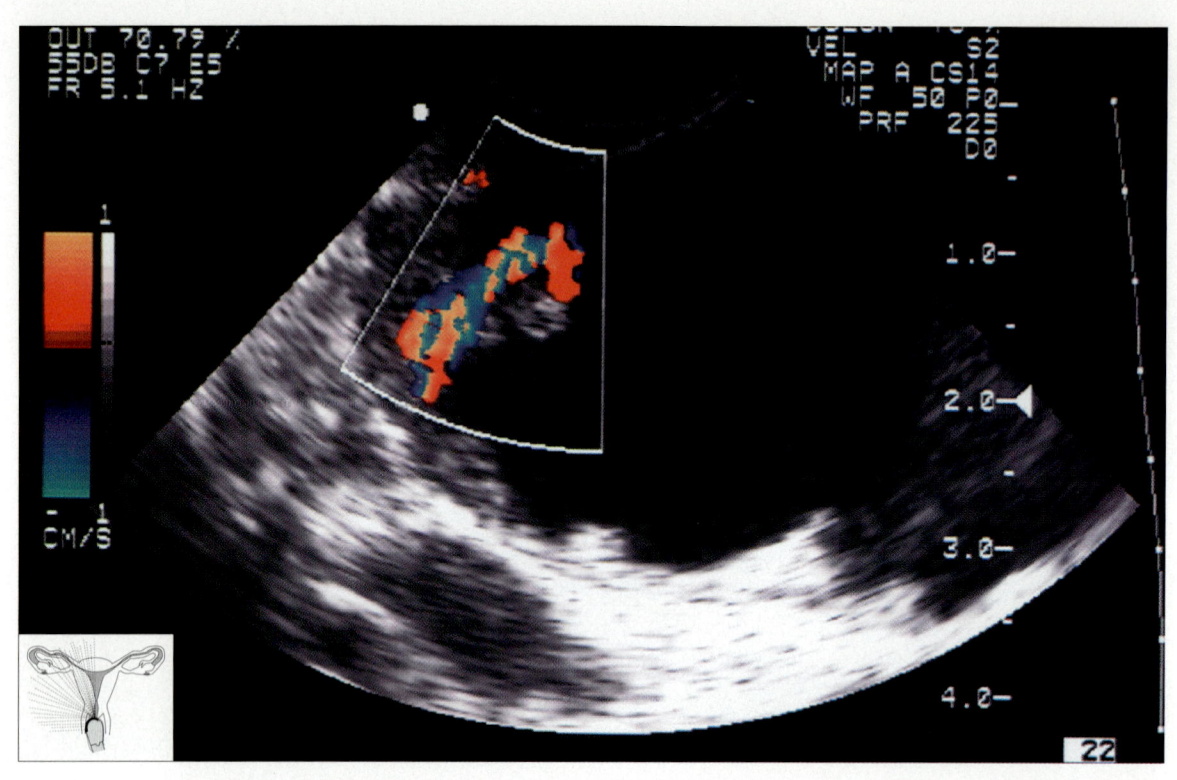

Figure 13-22. Color flow Doppler demonstrates increased flow through the solid component of the cancer.

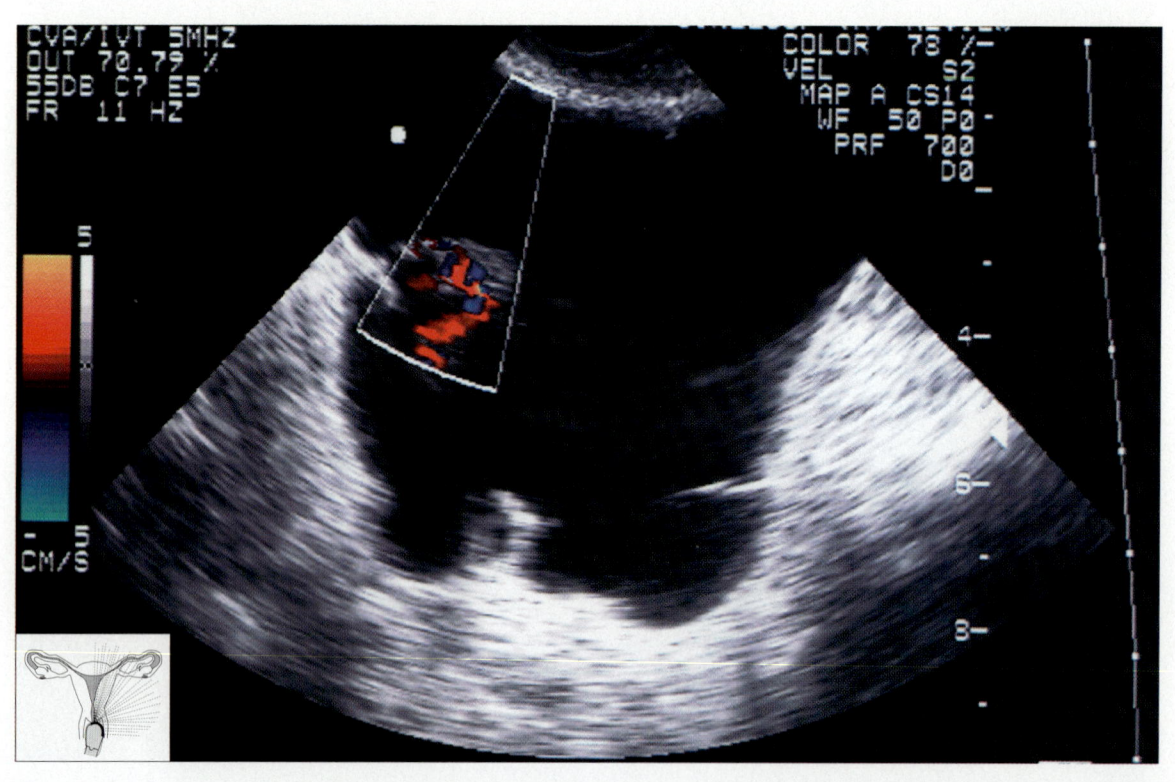

Figure 13-23. Increased color flow through the solid component of this mainly cystic ovarian cancer.

172

Ovarian Cancer

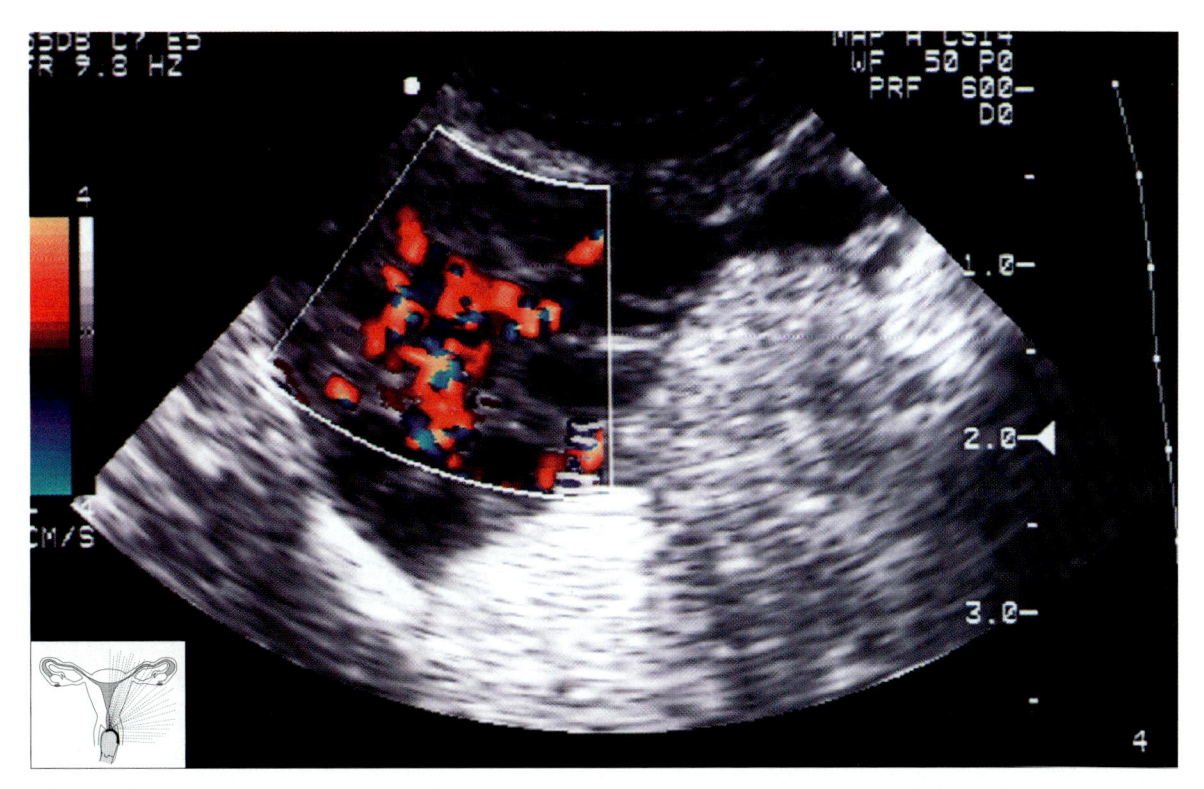

Figure 13-24. Increased color flow in this cystic but otherwise morphologically normal ovary. An early ovarian cancer was confirmed at laparotomy.

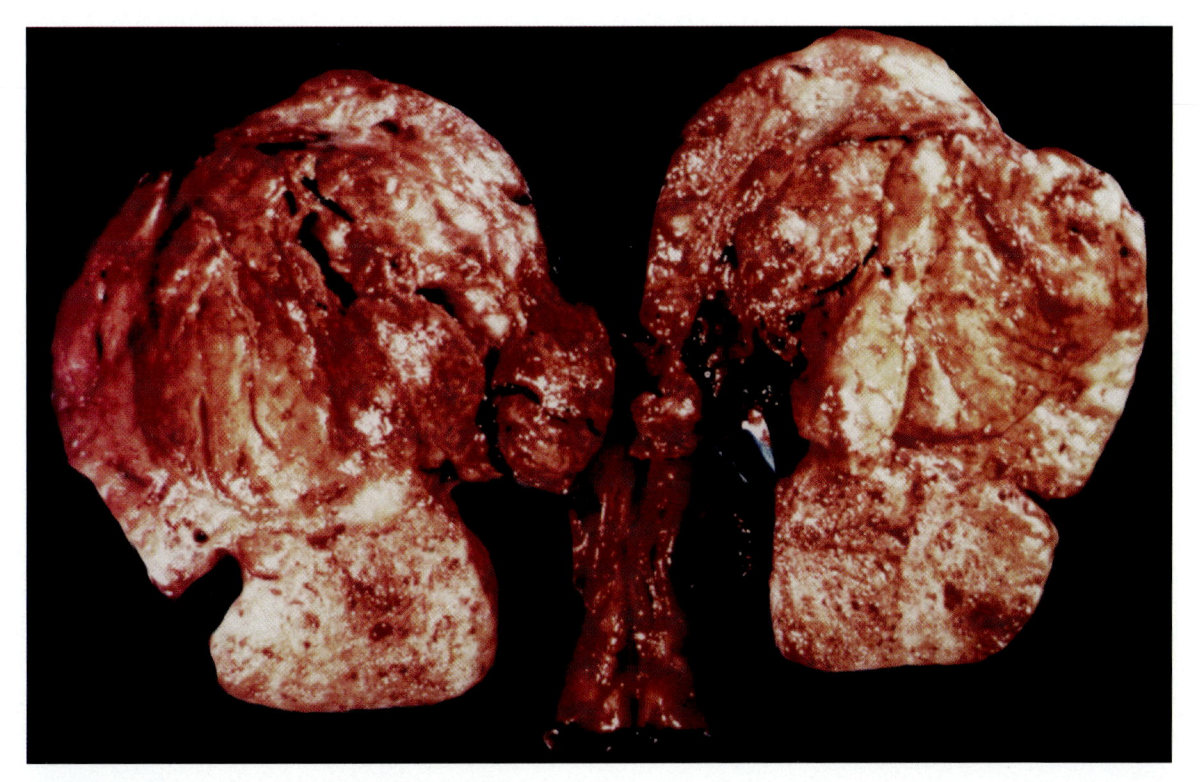

Figure 13-25. Large, solid, ovarian carcinoma.

An Atlas of Transvaginal Sonography

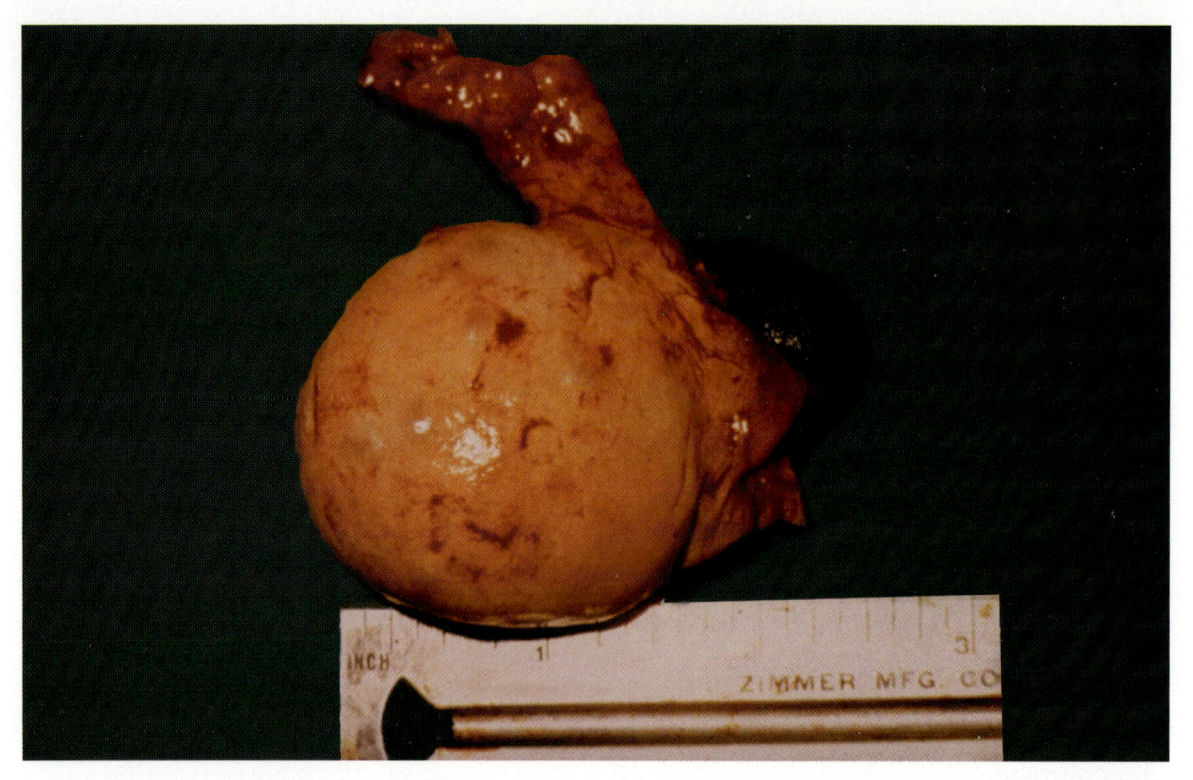

Figure 13-26. This solid, yellowish, ovarian tumor is an endocrinologically functioning Sertoli-Leydig cell tumor.

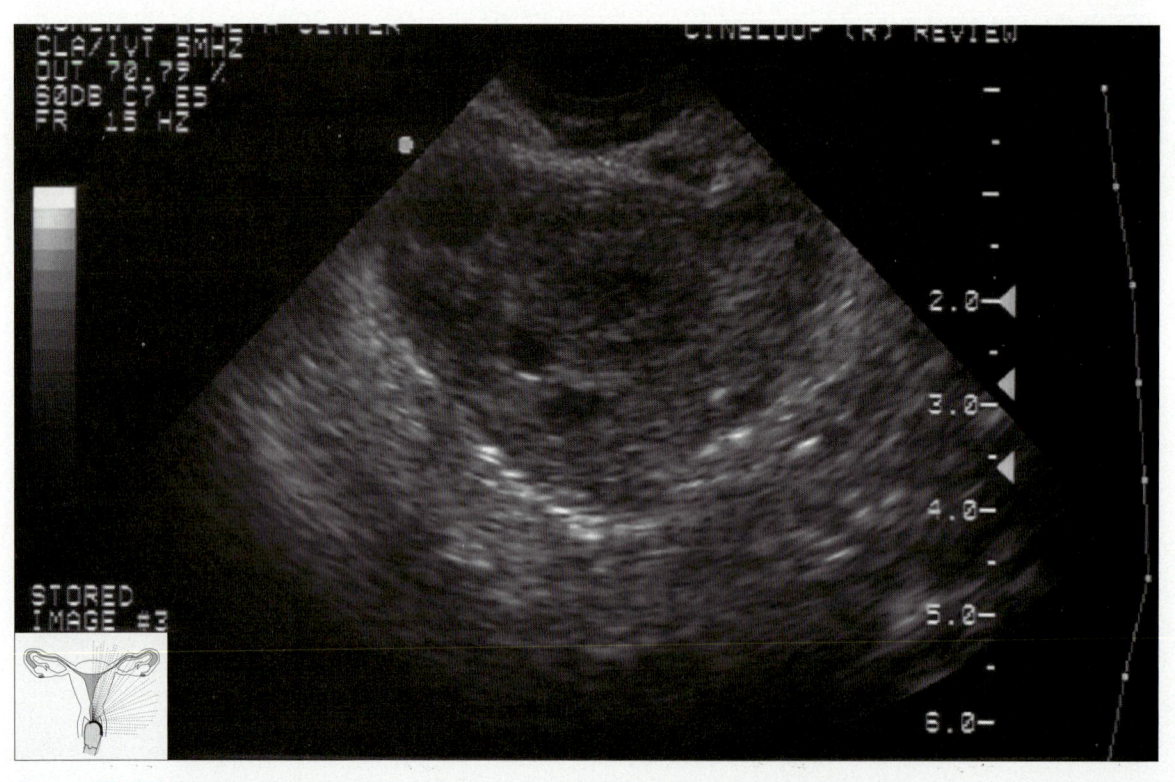

Figure 13-27. Ovarian dysgerminoma. A solid, enlarged, isoechoic, ovarian tumor suggests a germ cell tumor.

Ovarian Cancer

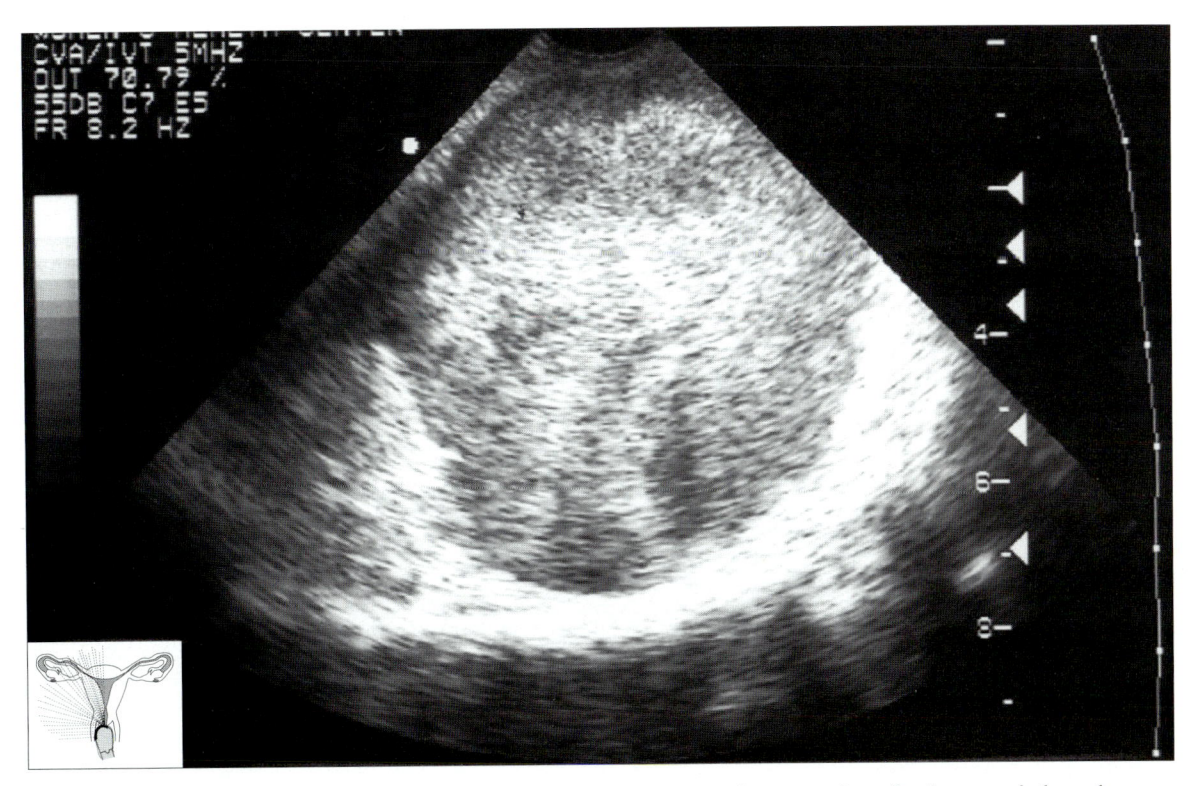

Figure 13-28. Rapidly growing, solid, ovarian tumor in a young woman. It was confirmed to be an endodermal sinus tumor.

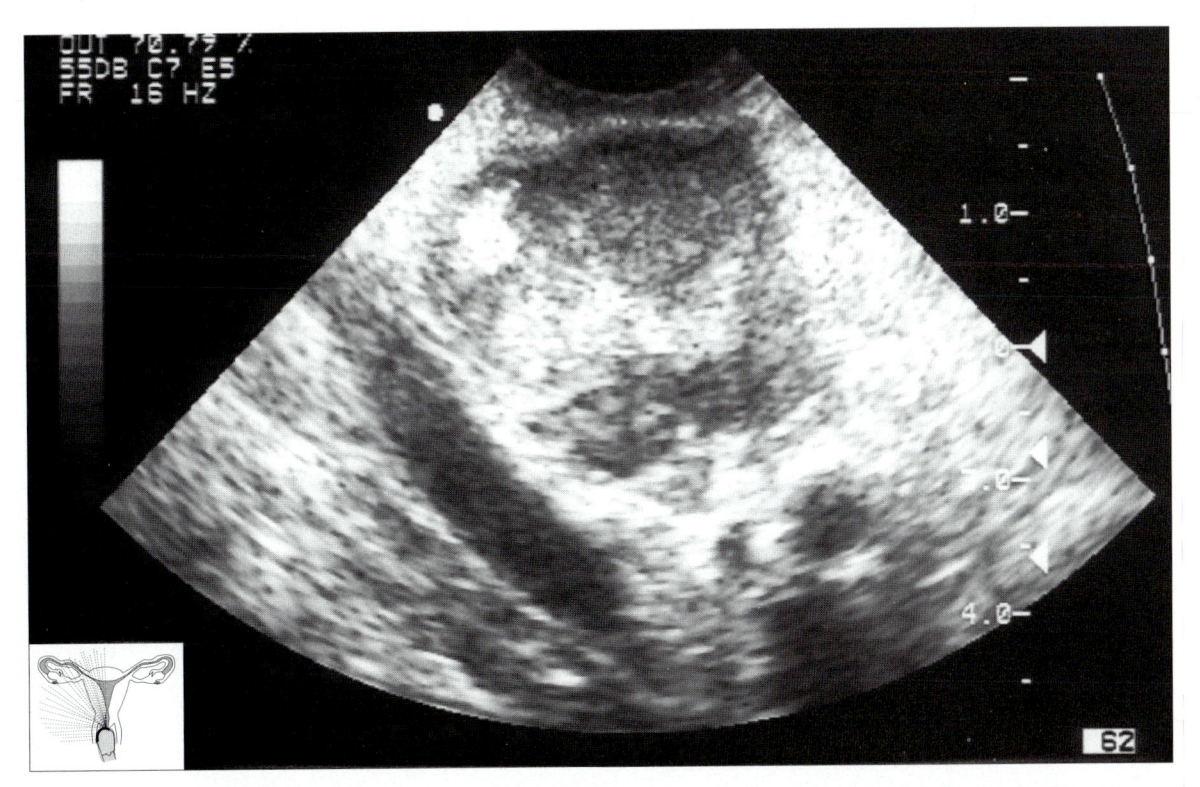

Figure 13-29. This patient had a previous history of colon cancer. Both ovaries were solid, mixed echogenic tumors, confirmed to be metastatic or Krukenberg tumors.

An Atlas of Transvaginal Sonography

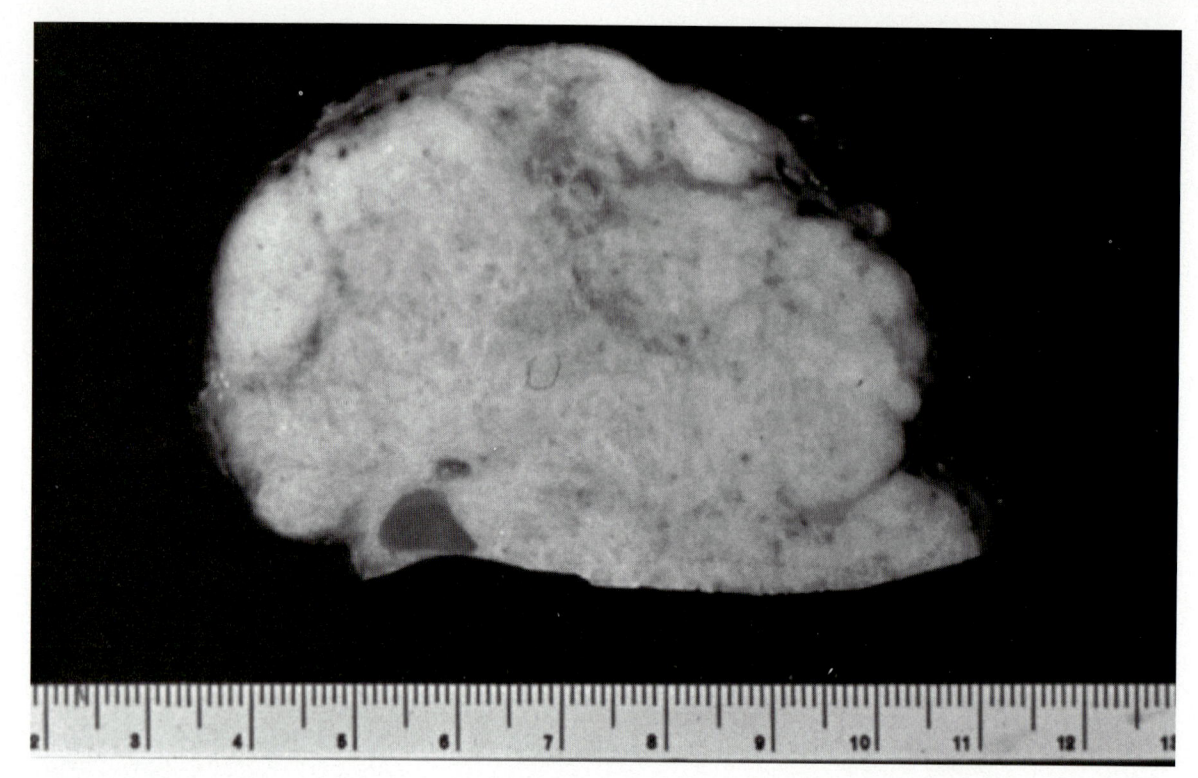

Figure 13-30. Brenner tumor, a solid ovarian tumor, usually benign or low grade malignancy.

14 Recurrent Gynecologic Cancer

The early detection of recurrent gynecologic cancers is compromised by a number of factors, including: inaccurate vaginal examination; previous therapy resulting in dense pelvic fibrosis; and the poor sensitivity of CT scanning.

Scan Findings

Sonographically, a central recurrence appears as a hypoechoic, usually irregular area on the vaginal stump, whose echo pattern usually resembles that of the primary tumor. Suspicious areas on the pelvic side wall usually have more sharply defined borders, especially when the lesion is a carcinomatous lymph node. Color flow can be variable, but it is usual to find recurrent tumors without demonstrable color flow. This is related to the amount of scar tissue present, previous therapy, and vascularity of the recurrence.

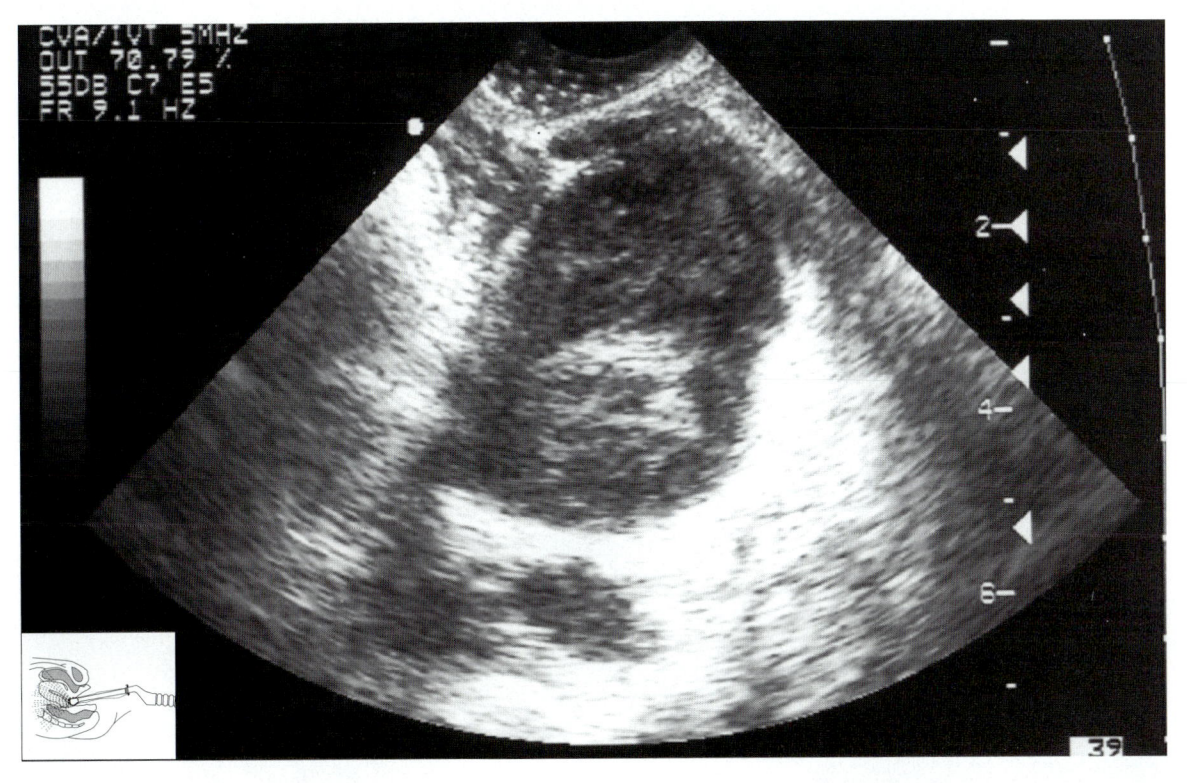

Figure 14-1. Mixed, echogenic, recurrent, mucinous ovarian tumor at the vaginal apex.

An Atlas of Transvaginal Sonography

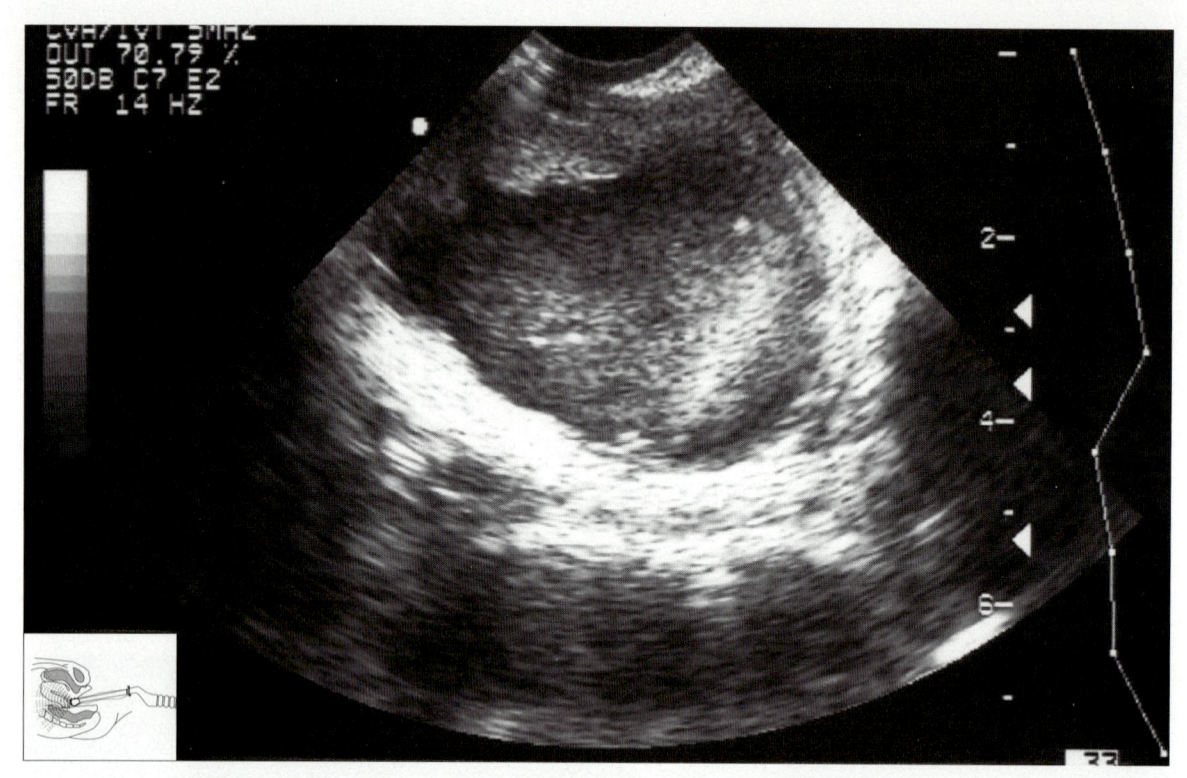

Figure 14-2. Vaginal recurrence of serous ovarian cancer.

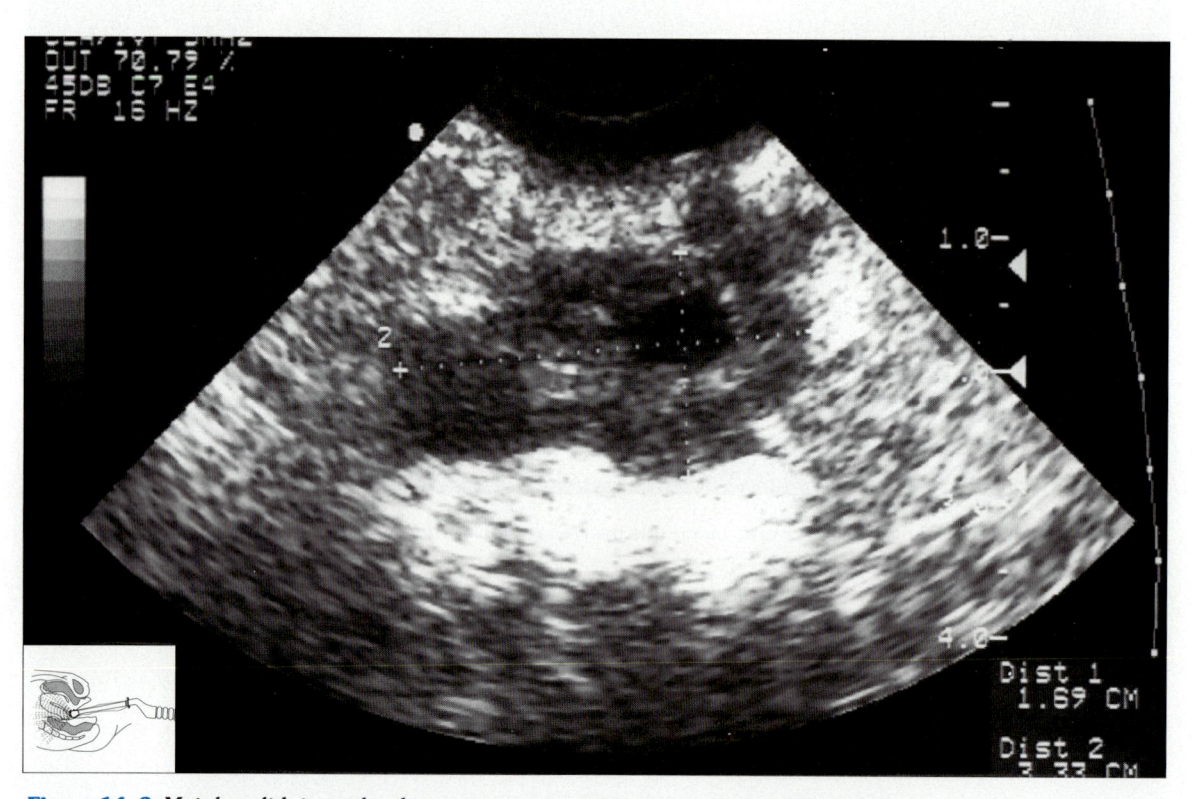

Figure 14-3. Mainly solid, irregular, homogenous, recurrent tumor at the vaginal apex.

Recurrent Gynecologic Cancer

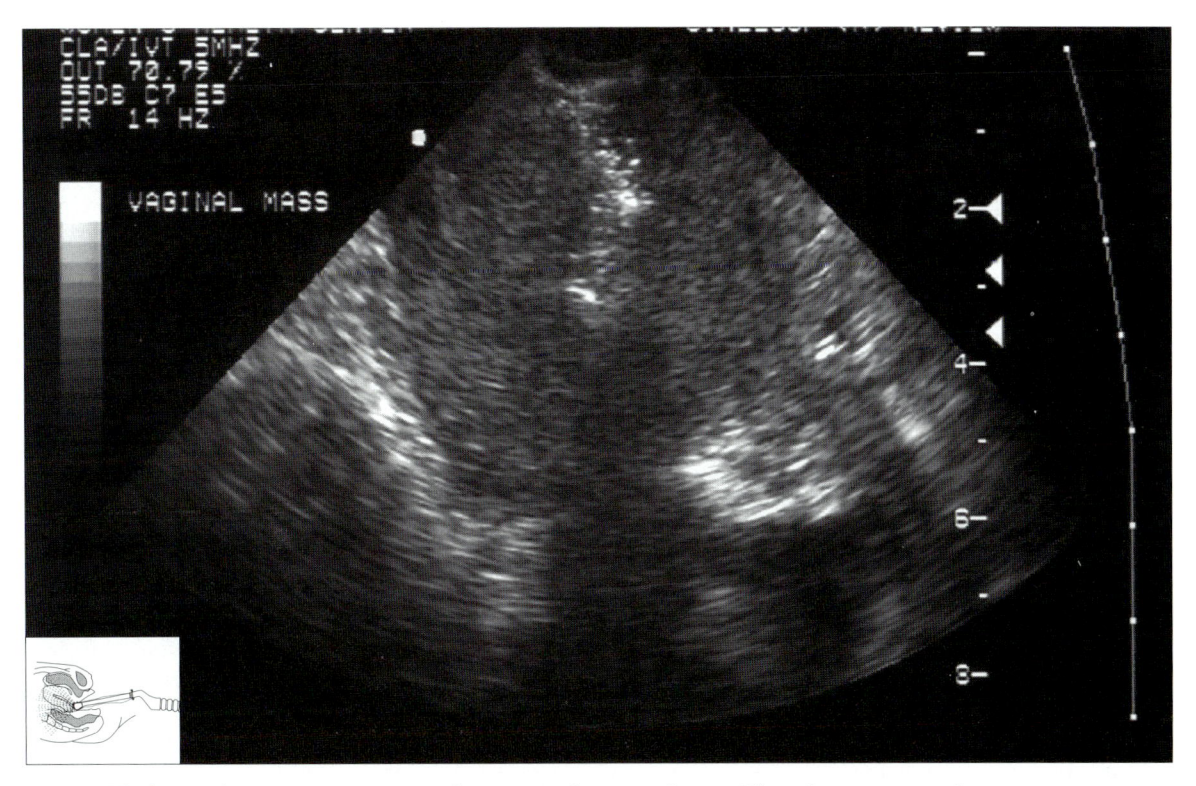

Figure 14-4. Isoechoic, recurrent, cervical tumor at the vaginal apex. The echogenic central portion represents blood. The patient was cured by a total pelvic exenteration.

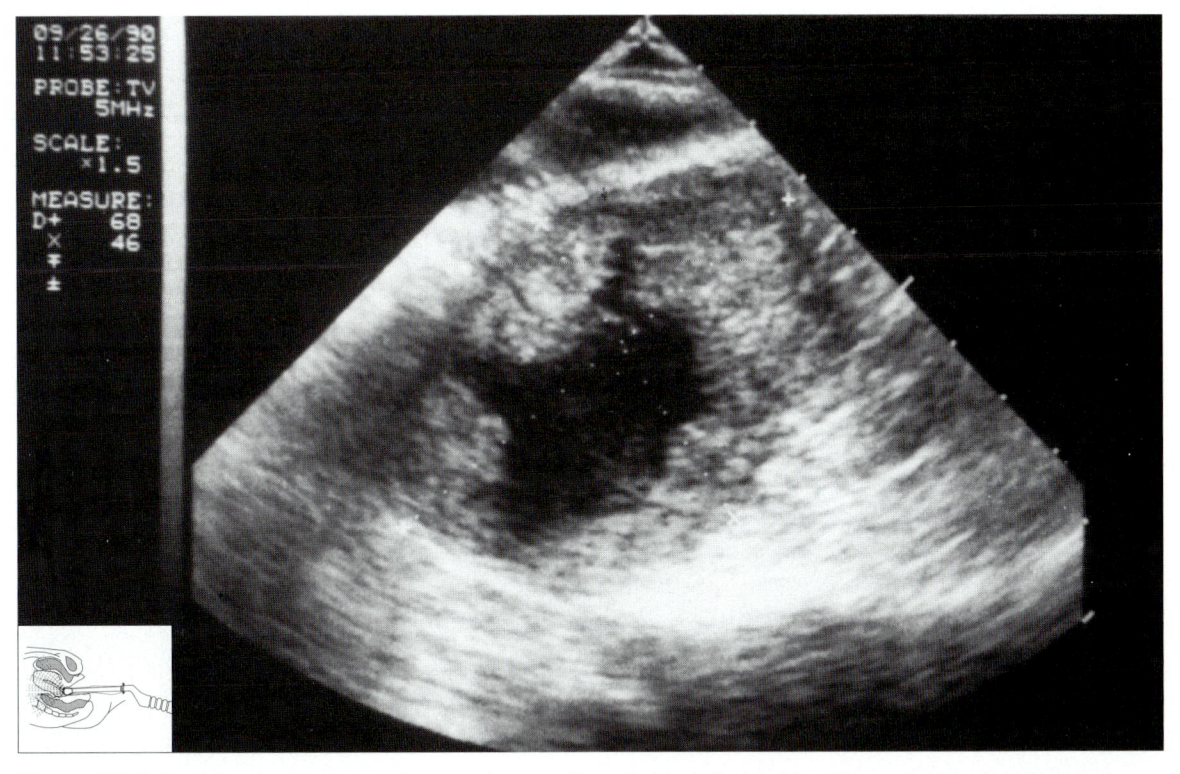

Figure 14-5. Recurrent, necrotic, endometrial cancer lying behind the bladder. The patient had widespread disease at exploratory laparotomy.

An Atlas of Transvaginal Sonography

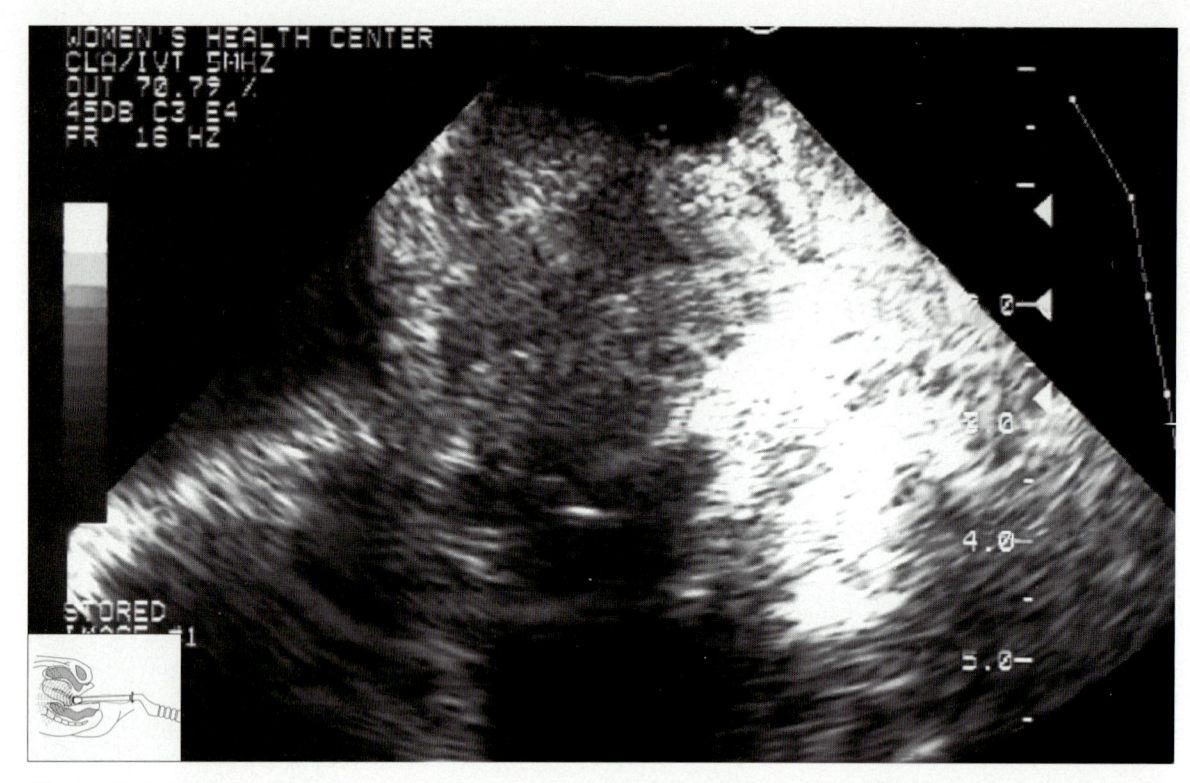

Figure 14-6. Patient with a history of a hysterectomy was referred with a central pelvic mass. TVS confirmed a remnant cervix and no cancer. A review of the records confirms a subtotal hysterectomy was performed.

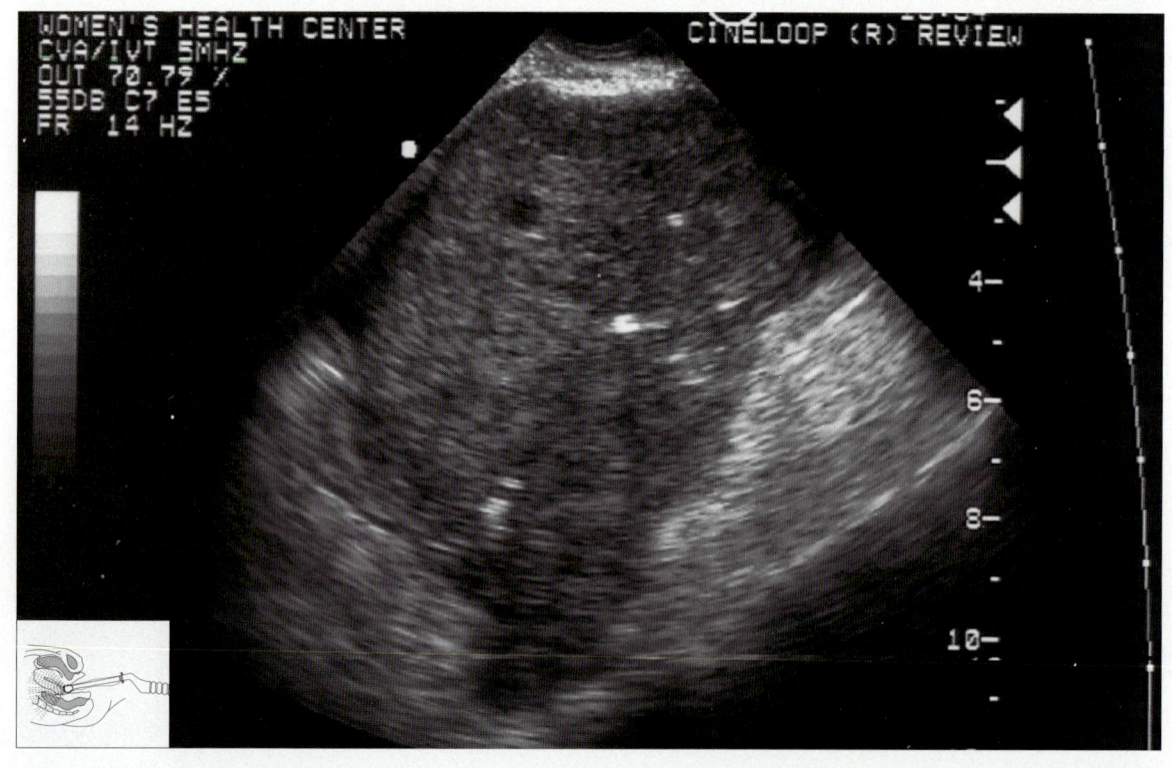

Figure 14-7. Large, homogenous isoechoic, recurrent pelvic cancer with extension to the pelvic side walls, and thus not an operative candidate.

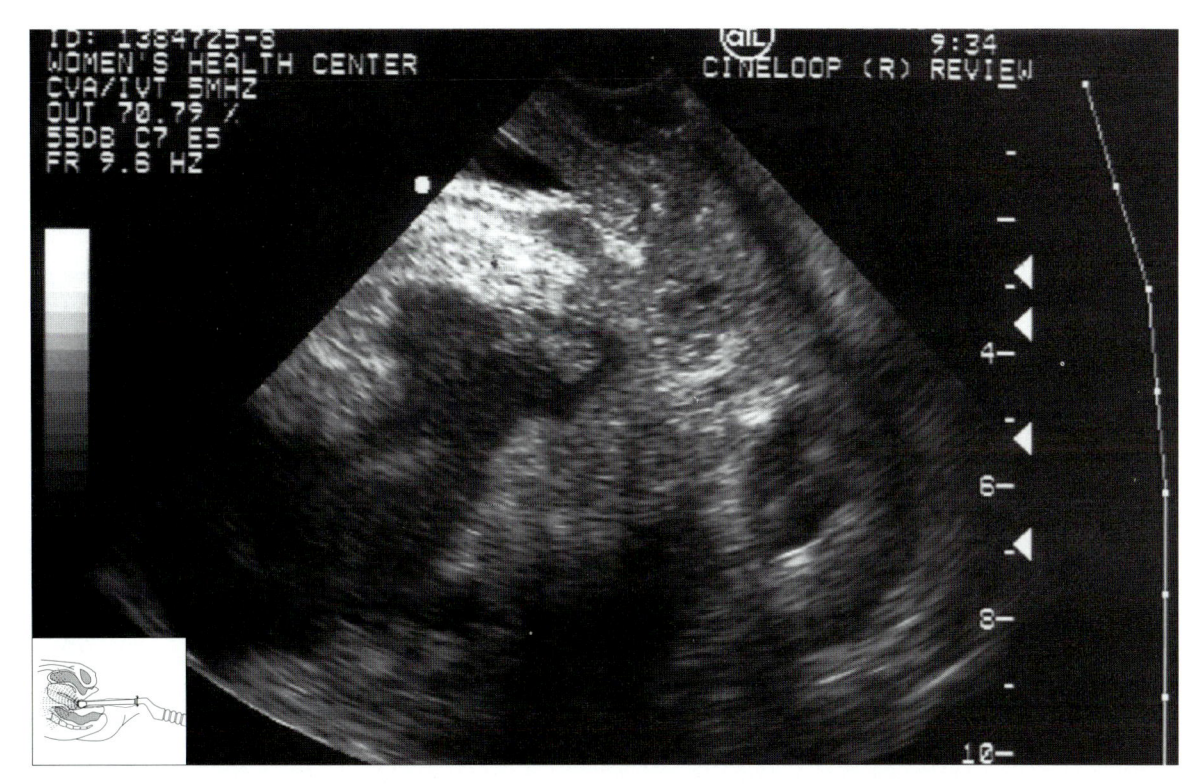

Figure 14-8. Large, necrotic, complex, corpus cancer, in a patient previously irradiated for cervix cancer.

15 Infertility

Transvaginal sonography has established itself as a vital component of the reproductive endocrinologists armamentarium. It is utilized to monitor follicular development in spontaneous and induced cycles, aid in oocyte retrieval, and confirmation of pregnancy.

Scan Findings

Mature follicles typically measure 17-25 mm in diameter. They may contain intrafollicular echoes, originating from clusters of granulosa cells that are torn off the follicle wall at ovulation. After ovulation, the follicular wall becomes irregular, as the follicle becomes "deflated." The corpus luteum appears as a hypoechoic structure with an irregular wall and often contains internal echoes corresponding to blood. As the luteal phase progresses, the wall of the corpus luteum becomes thickened by the process of luteinization.

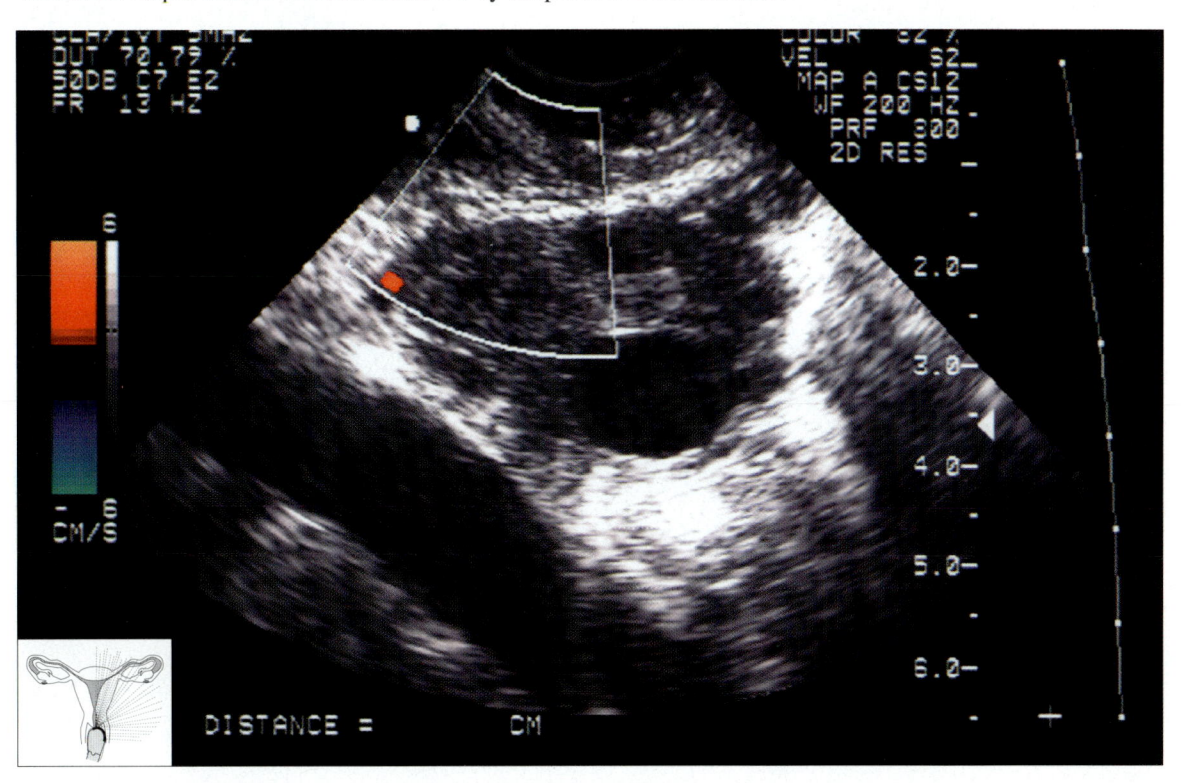

Figure 15-1. Developing follicular cyst appearing as a distinct, "punched out," anechoic cyst.

An Atlas of Transvaginal Sonography

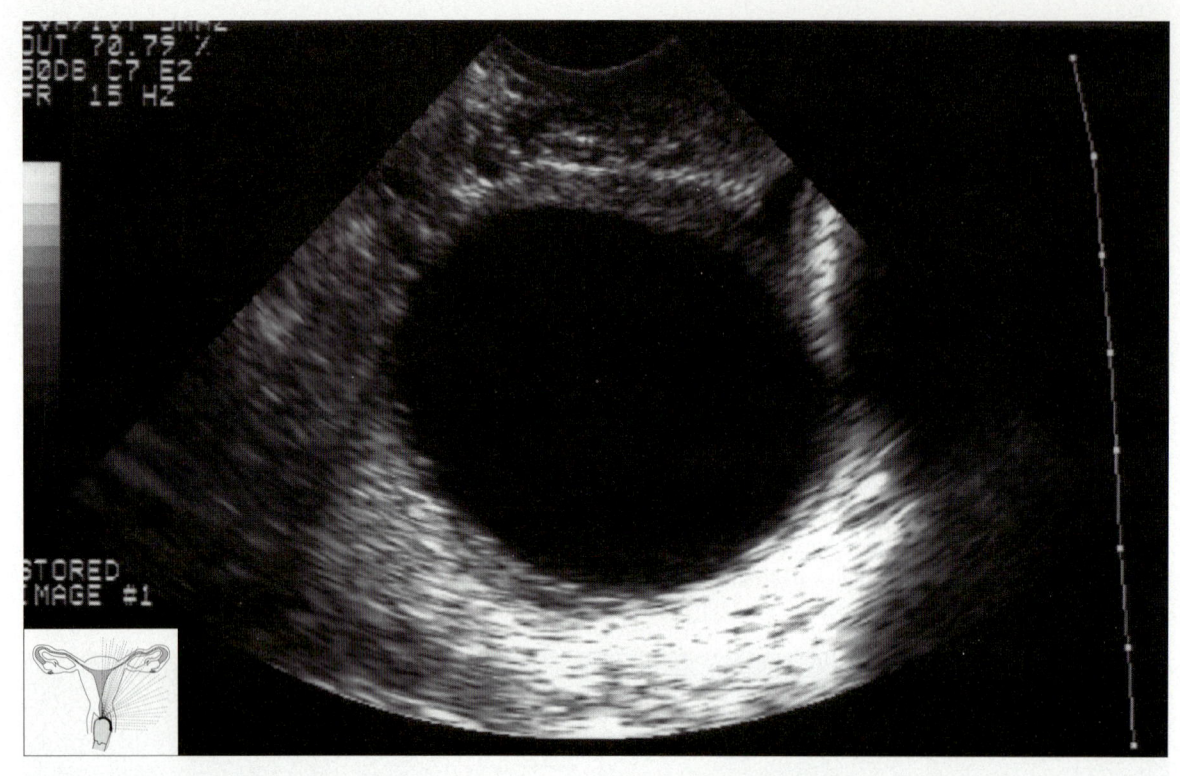

Figure 15-2. Mature follicular cyst. Normal ovarian cortex is seen around the cyst.

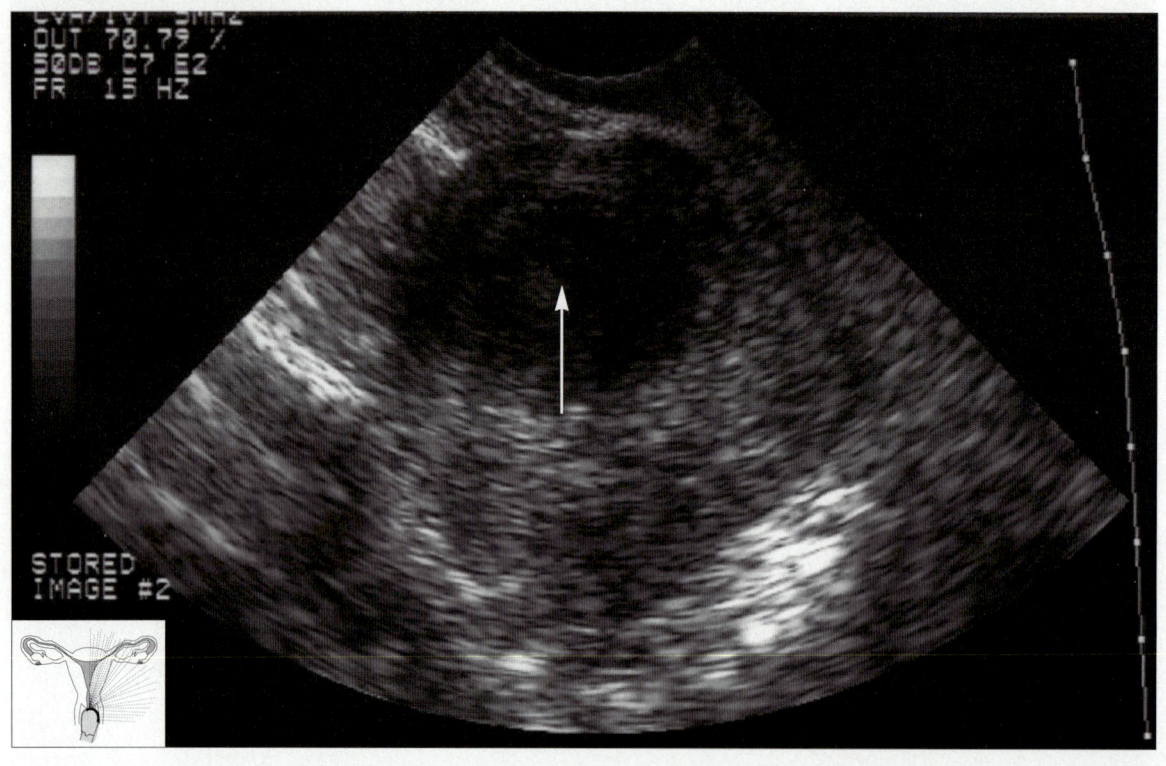

Figure 15-3. Corpus luteum cyst, with irregular, indistinct borders and intracyst echoes (arrow) corresponding to blood.

Infertility

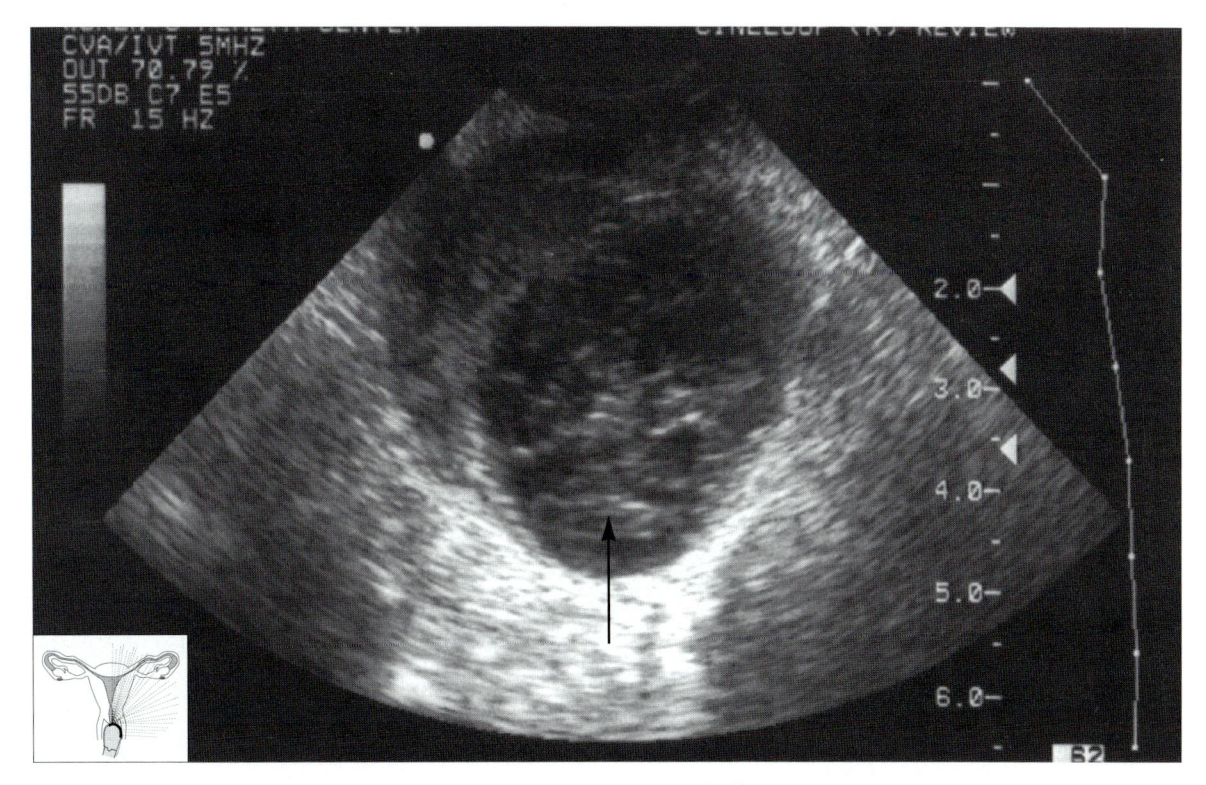

Figure 15-4. Hemorrhagic corpus luteum with prominent internal echoes (arrow) consistent with clotting blood.

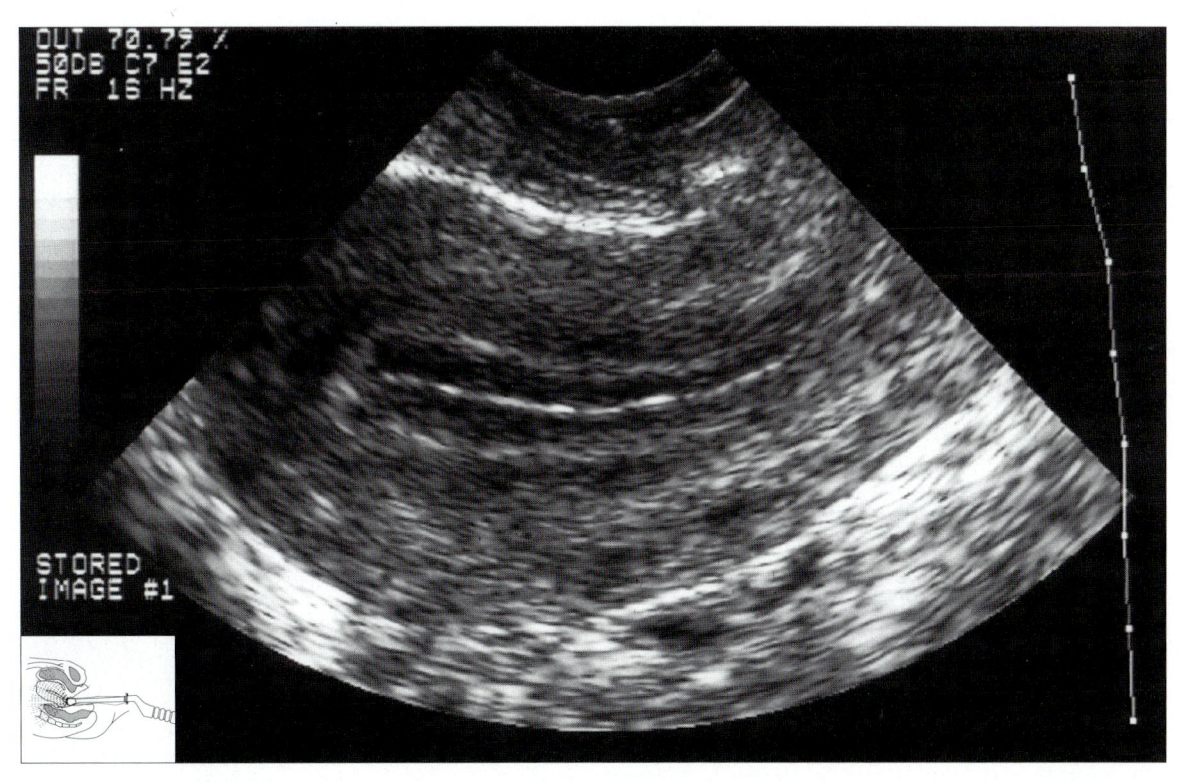

Figure 15-5. Midcycle-stimulated endometrium, with the characteristic "three line sign."

An Atlas of Transvaginal Sonography

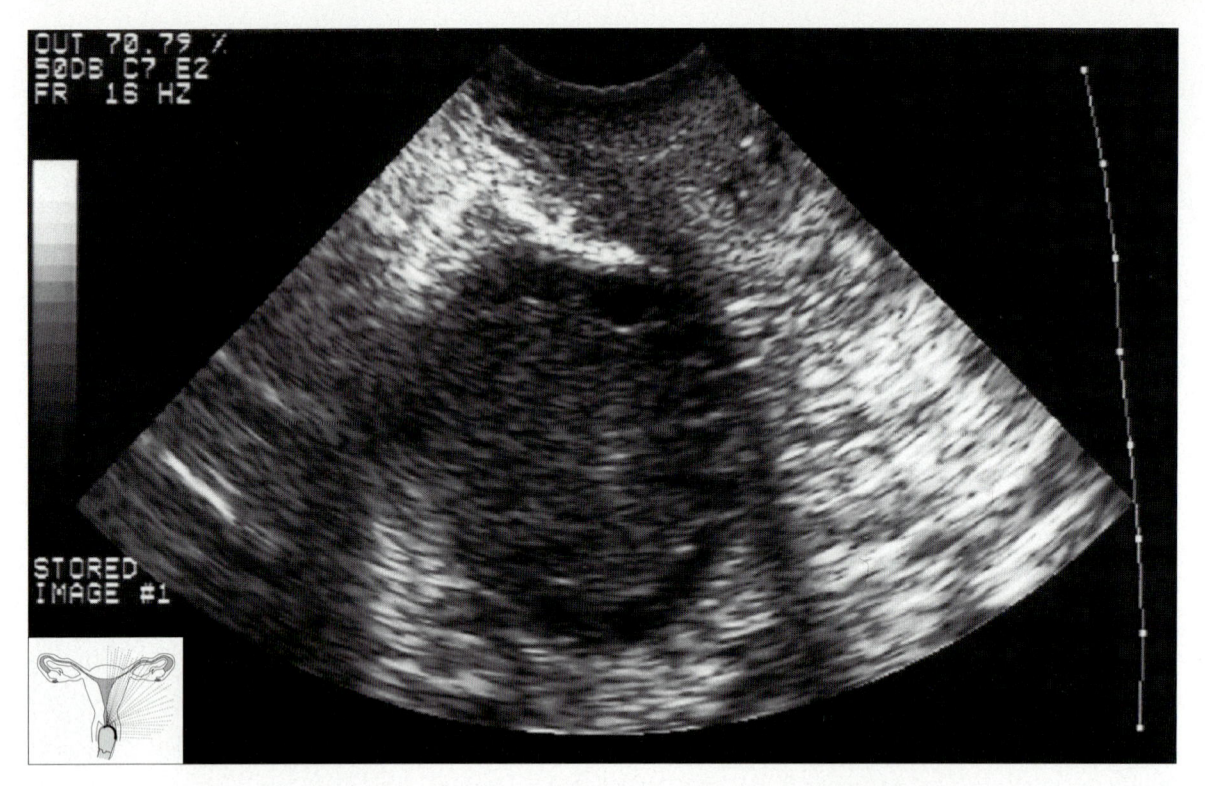

Figure 15-6. Small, subcortical, ovarian cysts, typically seen in polycystic ovary syndrome.

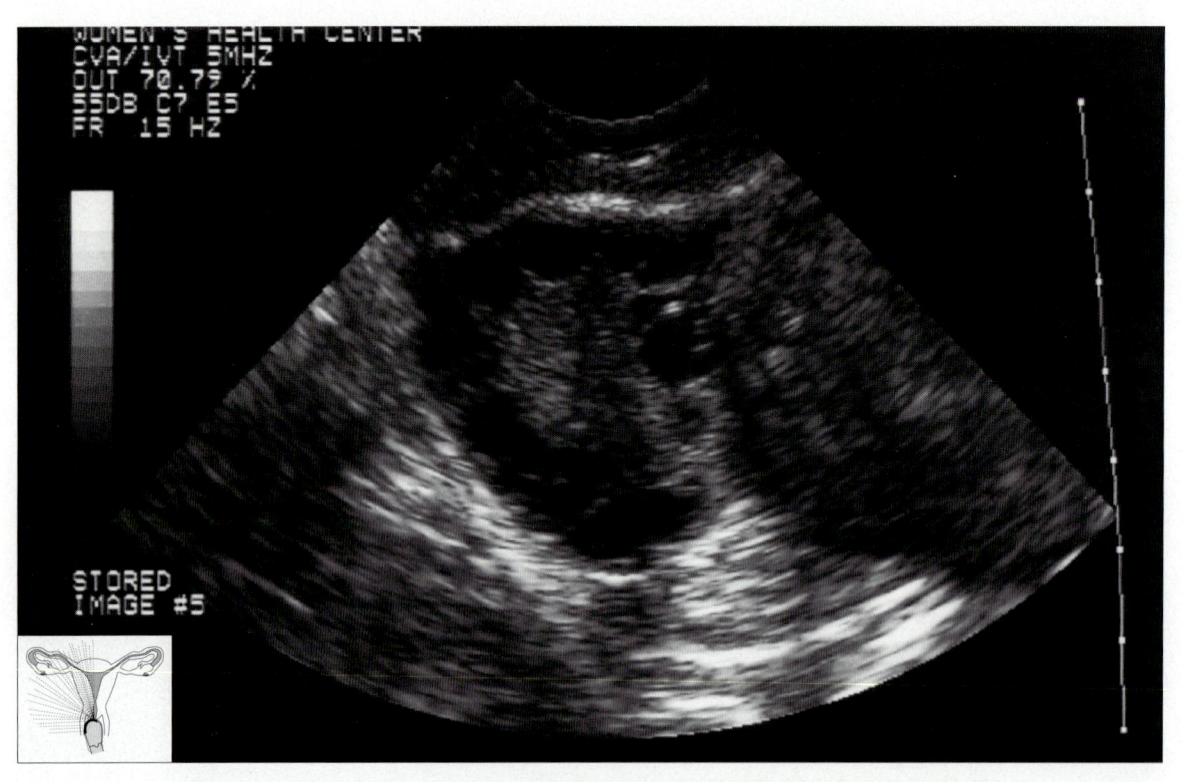

Figure 15-7. Larger, subcortical, ovarian cysts, typically seen in polycystic ovary syndrome.

Infertility

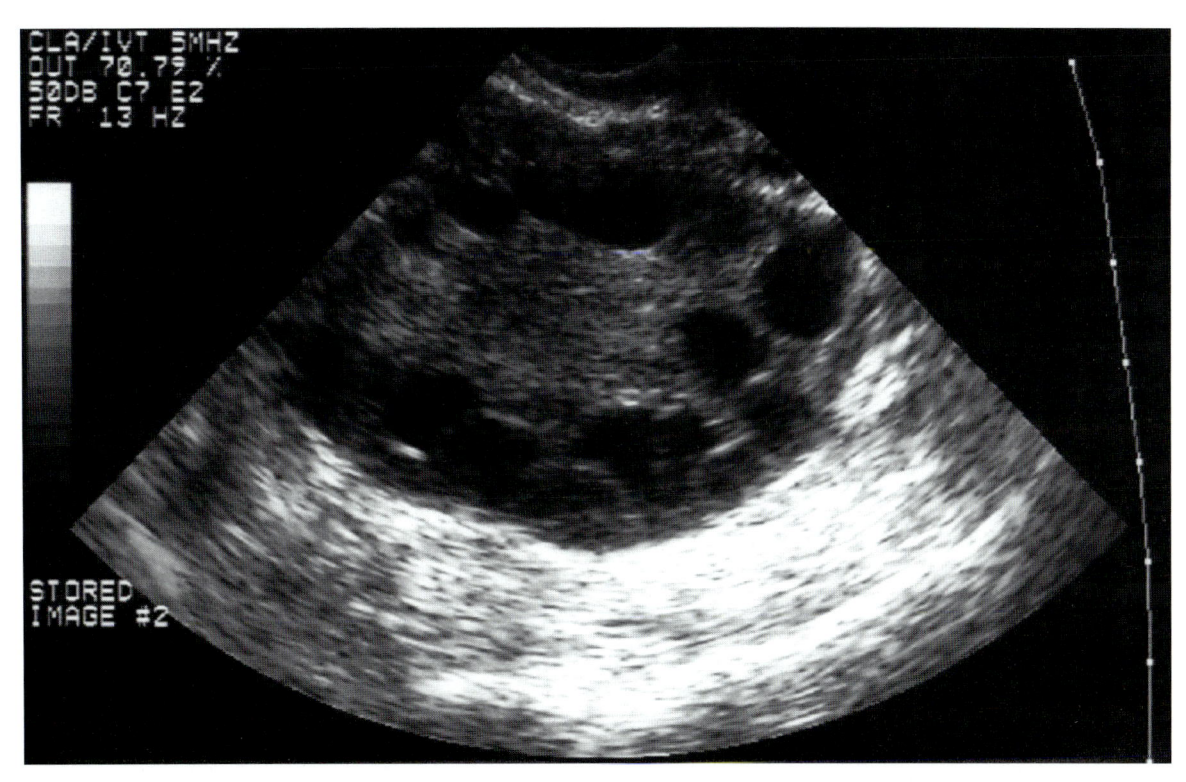

Figure 15-8. Large, subcortical, ovarian cysts, typically seen in polycystic ovary syndrome.

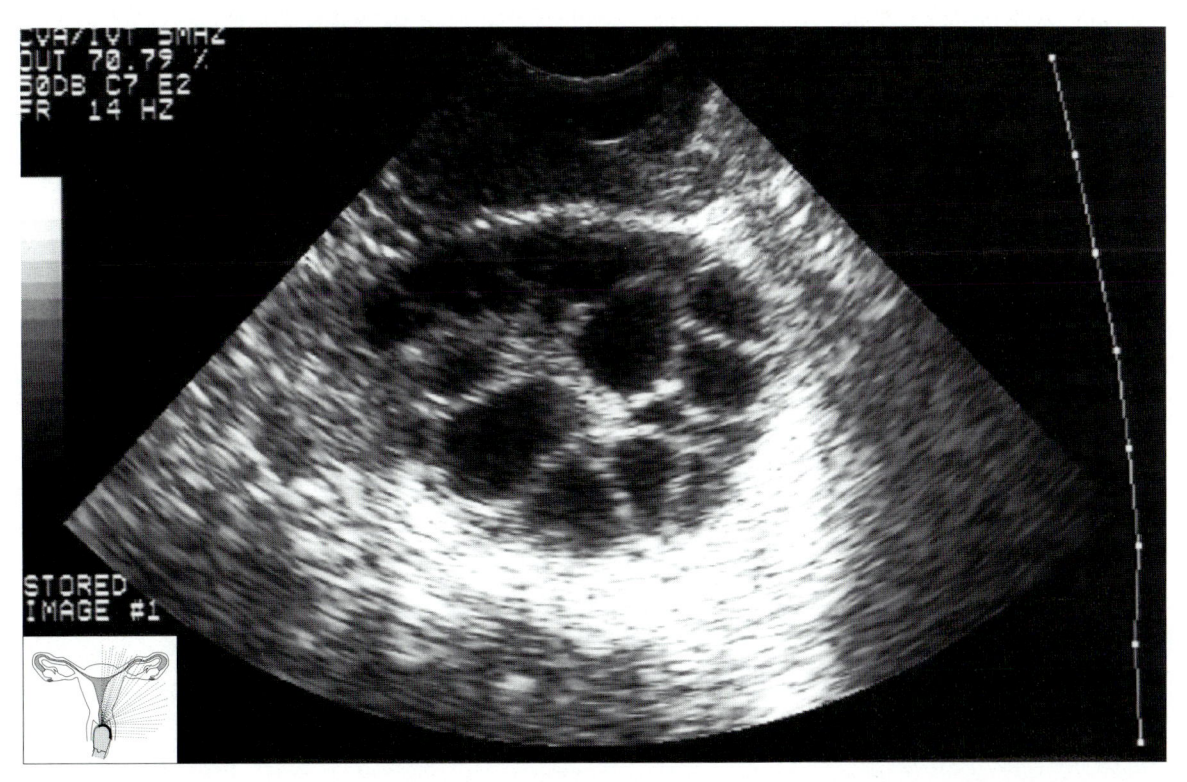

Figure 15-9. Pergonal-stimulated polycystic ovary (early).

An Atlas of Transvaginal Sonography

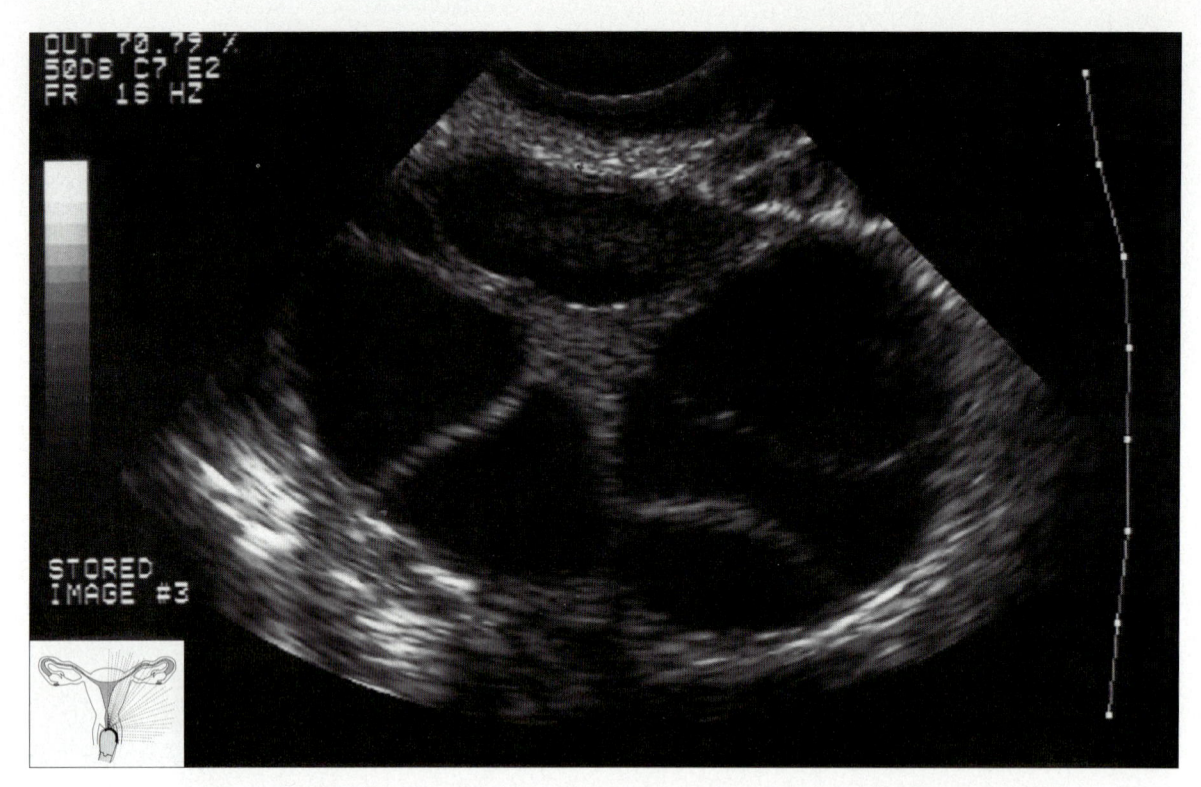

Figure 15-10. Pergonal-stimulated polycystic ovary (mid-cycle).

Hyperstimulation Syndrome

A potential risk of stimulated cycles is the ovarian hyperstimulation syndrome. Presentations vary in severity from mild, with minor abdominal discomfort, to severe with pleural effusion, ascites, and circulatory collapse.

Scan Findings

The sonographic appearance in the more severe cases is classic. The ovaries are bilaterally enlarged and tender and may contain several hypoechoic areas. The pelvic contents are seen floating in a sea of ascitic fluid.

Infertility

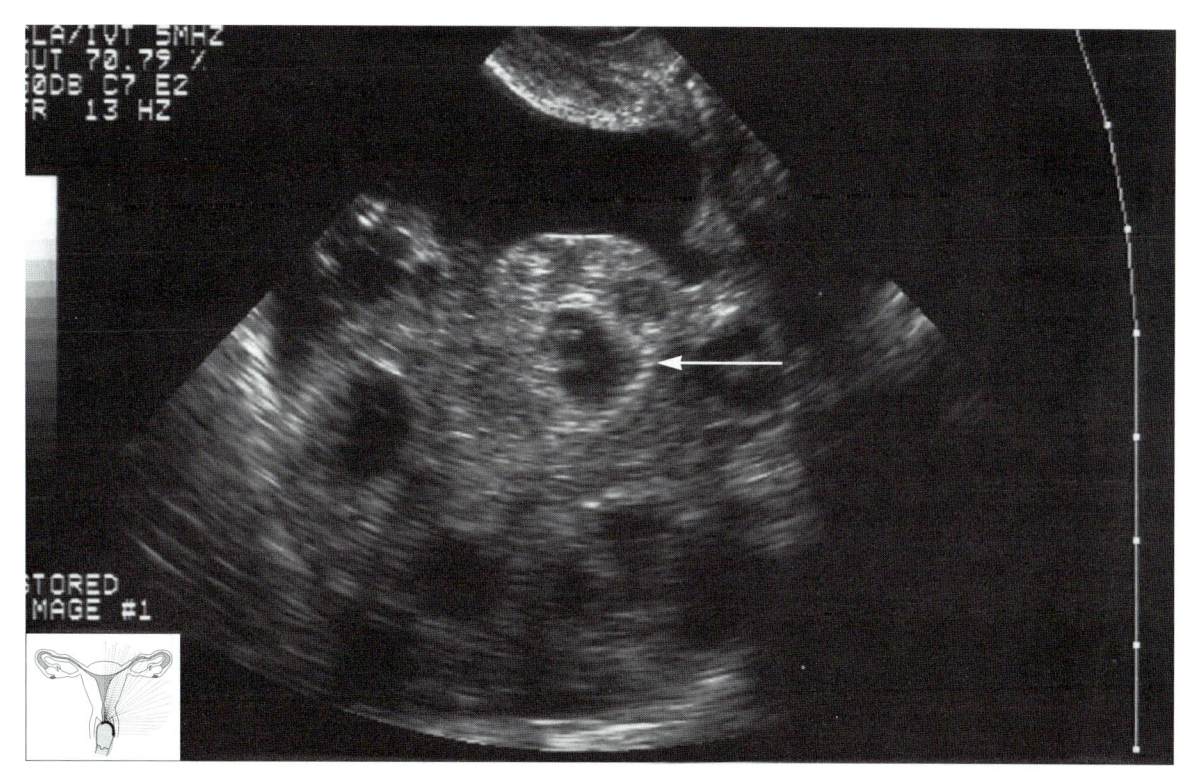

Figure 15-11. *Hyperstimulated ovary post-retrieval. Numerous collapsed cysts (arrow) are clearly seen.*

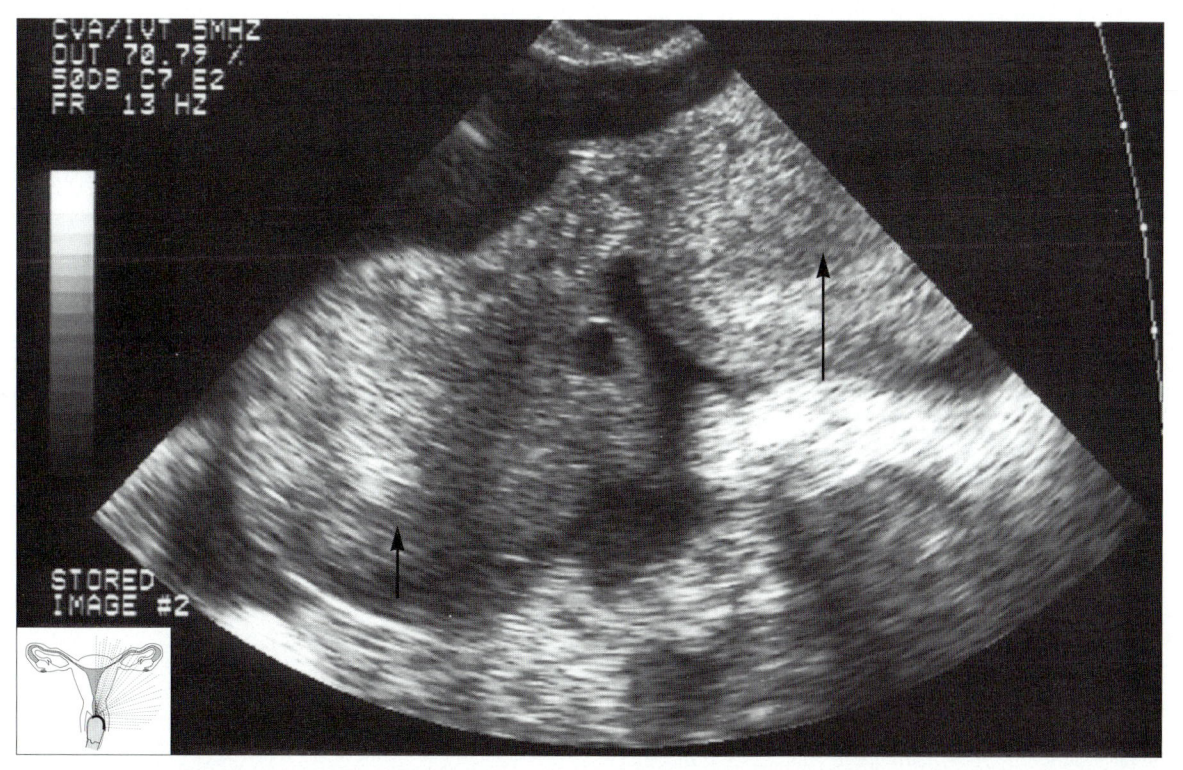

Figure 15-12. *Significant ascites surround the ovary (small arrow) on the left and the uterus (large arrow). The patient had severe hyperstimulation syndrome.*

An Atlas of Transvaginal Sonography

Congenital Uterine Abnormalities

It beyond the scope of this *Atlas* to discuss the classification of Mullerian fusion defects. They are usually characterized by a history of infertility, recurrent abortion, and prematurity. They are classified as vaginal atresia, unicornuate uterus, uterine didelphys, bicornuate uterus, septate uterus, and the DES-exposed T-bar uterus.

Scan Findings

Retention of vaginal or uterine blood or secretions (hematocolpos or hematometra) due to vaginal atresia is easily recognized by transvaginal sonography. The upper vagina and uterus are distended by echogenic fluid. The other fusion defects are best identified in the luteal phase of the menstrual cycle, when the echogenic endometrium is most prominent. A fusion defect may be suspected by the identification of an abnormal uterine contour and the finding of a duplicated endometrial stripe.

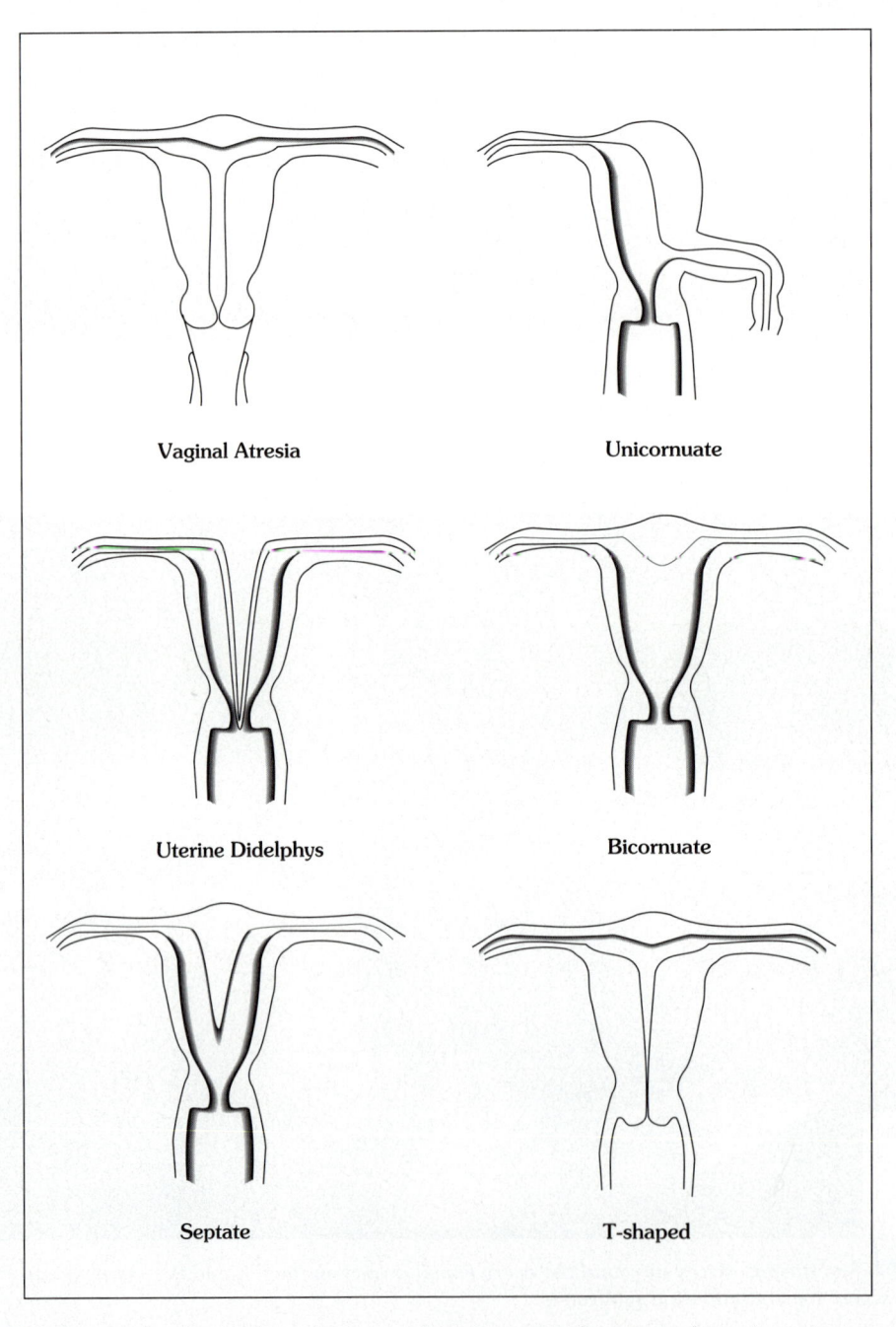

Figure 15-13. Diagram illustrating the major types of uterine anomalies: *vaginal atresia, unicornuate uterus, uterine didelphys, bicornuate uterus, septate uterus, and T-shaped uterus.*

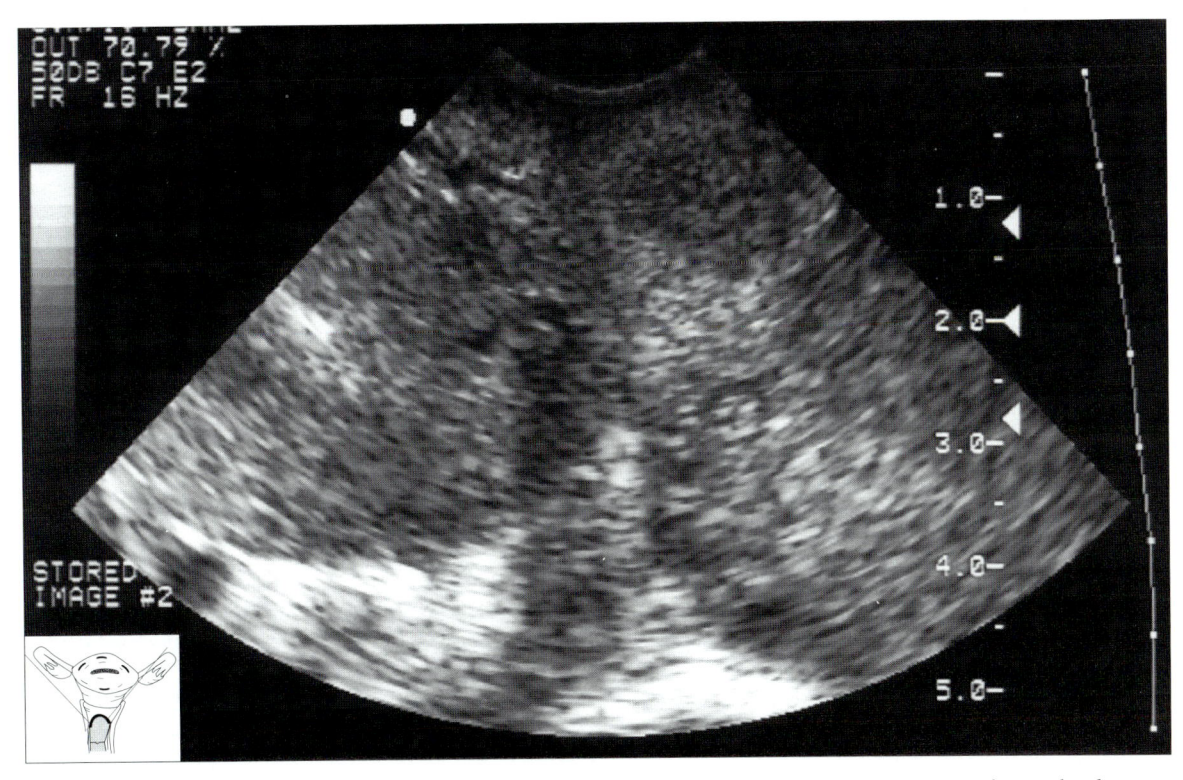

Figure 15-14. Bicornuate uterus. In the early proliferative phase the endometrial linings are not always clearly seen.

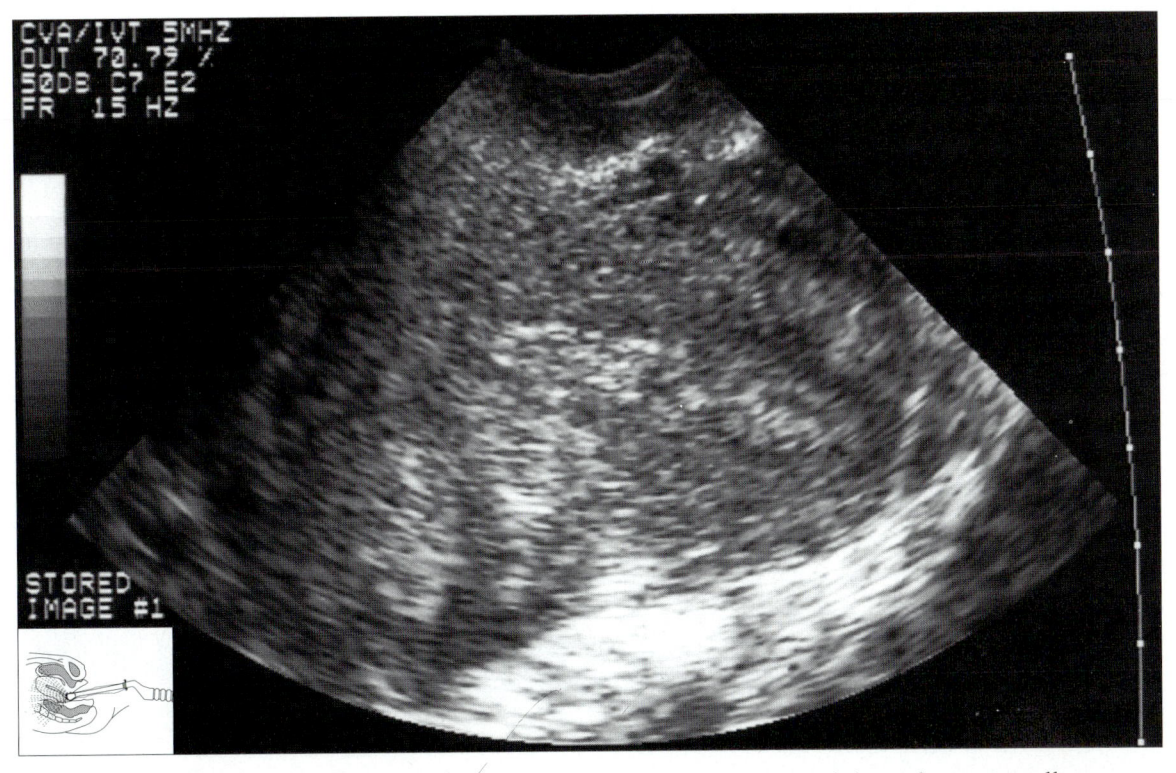

Figure 15-15. Bicornuate uterus in midcycle. The increasing echogenicity of the endometrium allows easier identification.

An Atlas of Transvaginal Sonography

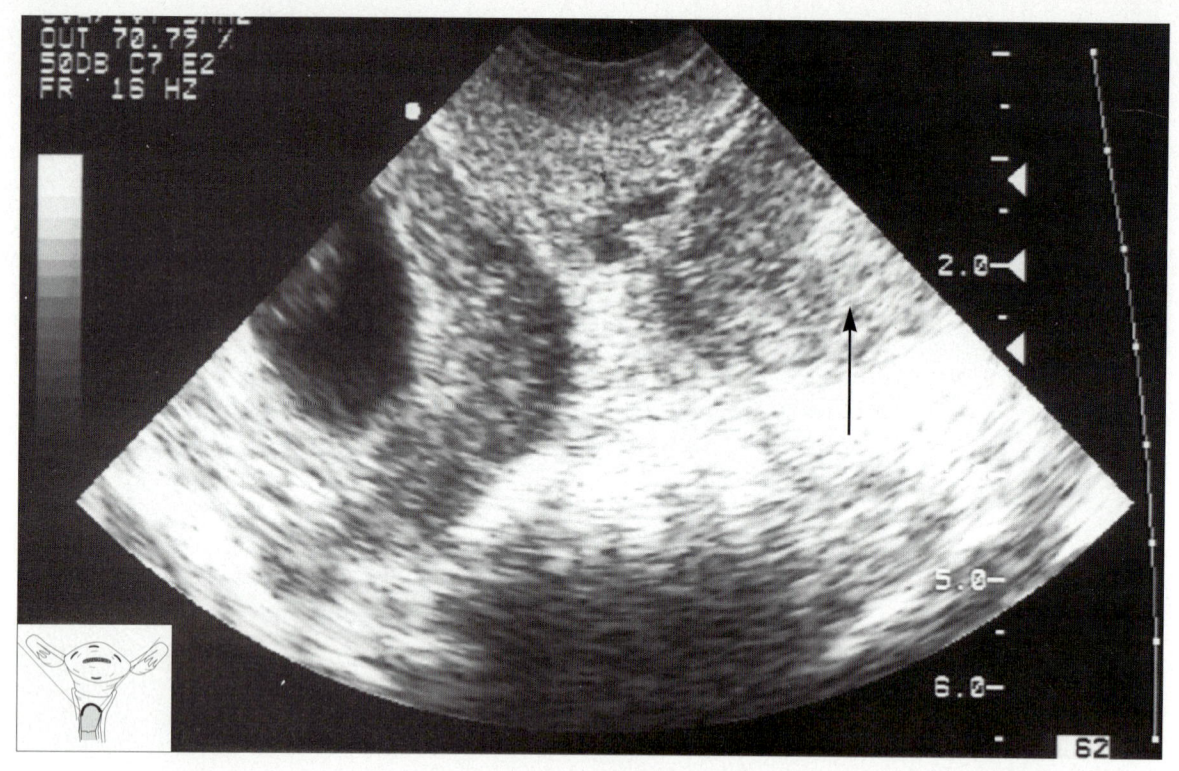

Figure 15-16. Bicornuate uterus with pregnancy in the left horn and rudimentary right horn (arrow).

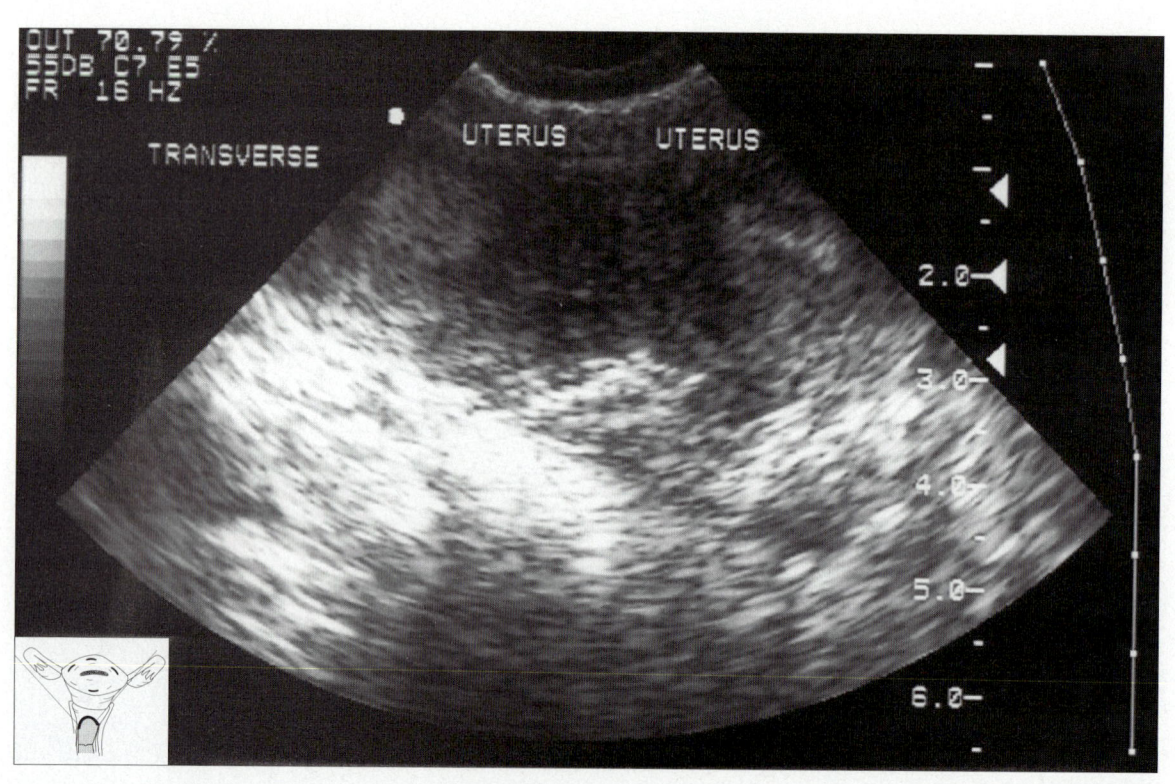

Figure 15-17. Bicornuate uterus in the early luteal phase.

192

Infertility

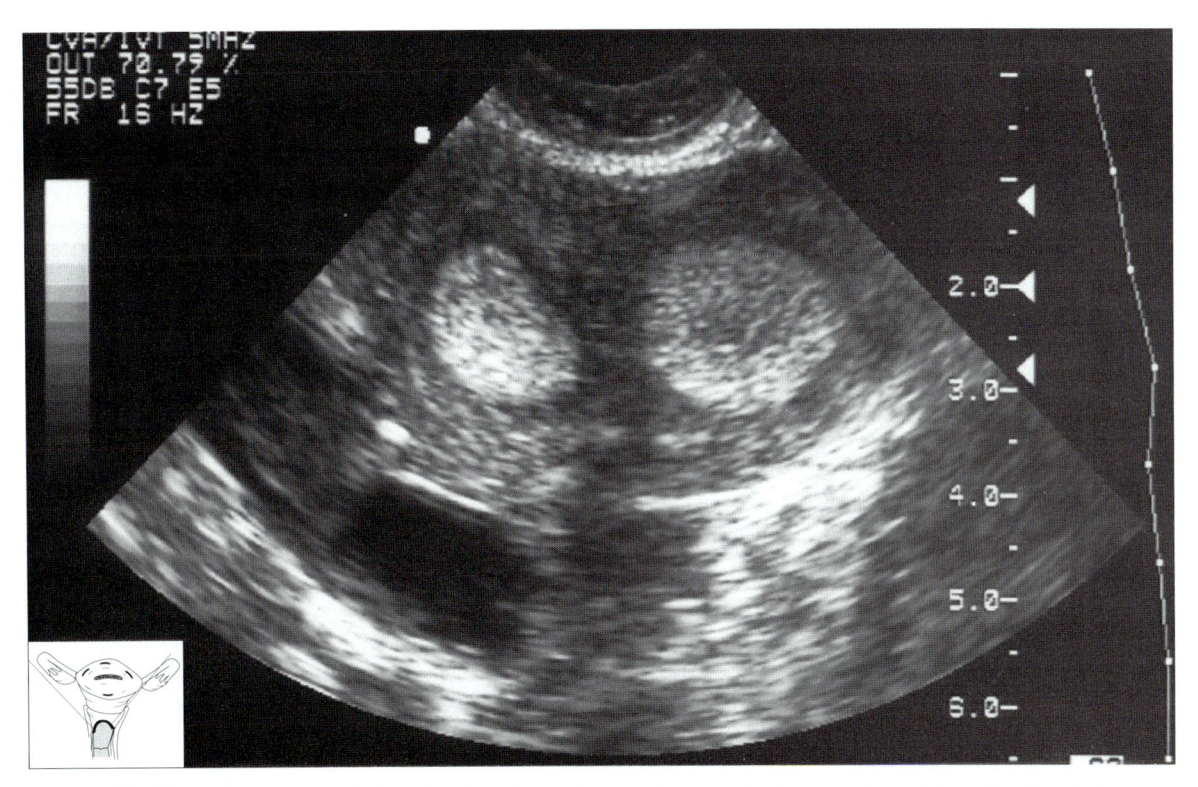

Figure 15-18. In the late luteal phase both endometrial cavities are clearly seen. A septate and subseptate uterus needs to be excluded.

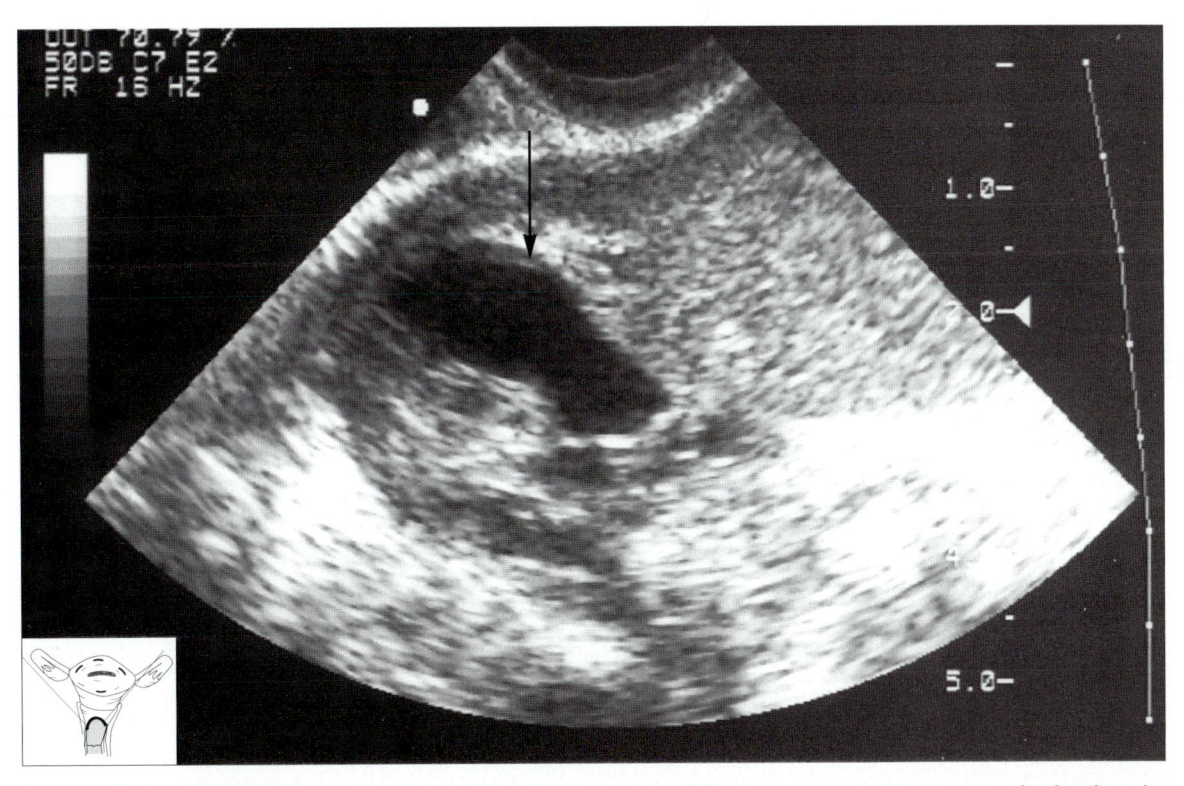

Figure 15-19. Hydrosalpinx and its associated tubal damage and blockage are a common cause of infertility. A sausage-shaped cystic mass (arrow) is draped over the ovary, and lies adjacent to the uterus.

An Atlas of Transvaginal Sonography

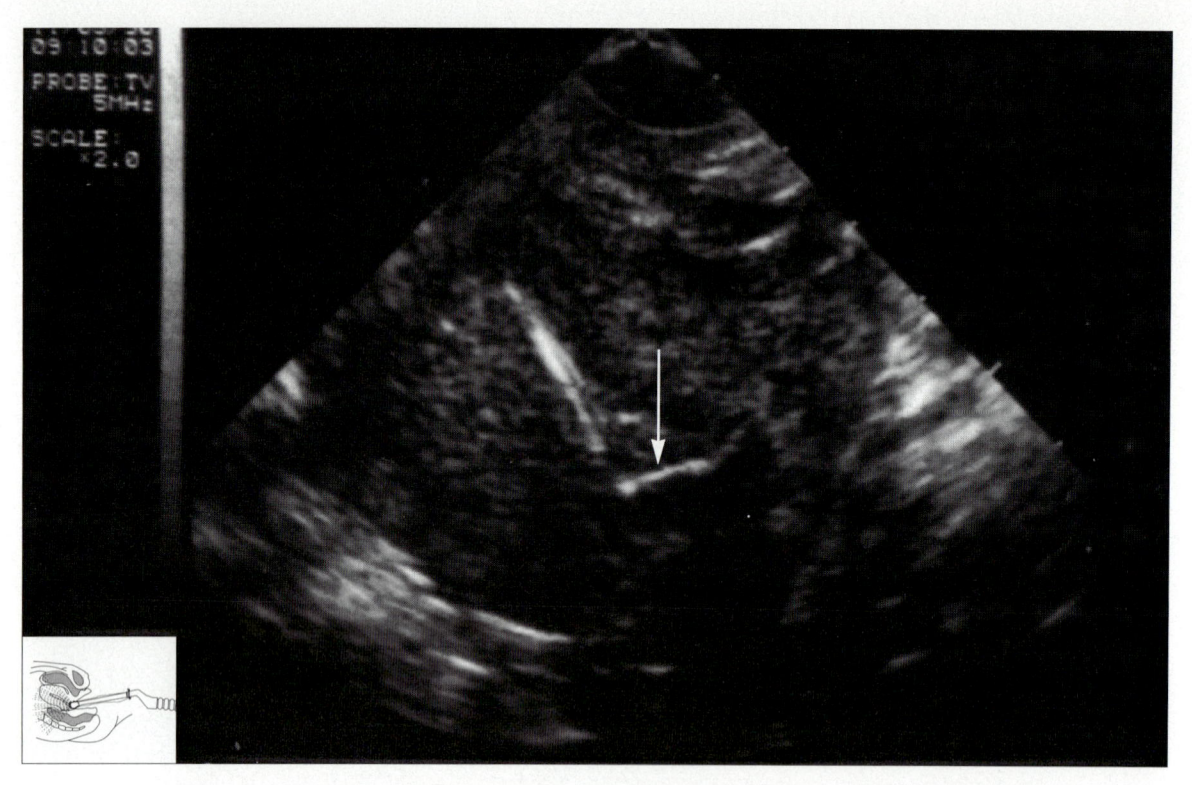

Figure 15-20. Intrauterine contraceptive device (Copper T). One arm of the T is clearly visible (arrow).

16   Urinary Tract

The urinary tract comprises the upper (kidney and abdominal ureter) and lower tracts (pelvic ureter, bladder, and urethra). While the upper tract is out of the sonographic range of the vaginal transducer, useful clinical information can be obtained from careful assessment of the lower urinary tract.

The size, shape, position, and relations of the urinary bladder vary with the amount of urine it contains and age of the patient. The empty bladder is somewhat rounded and lies completely within the pelvic cavity. As it distends with urine, it rises up into the abdomen and may reach the level of the umbilicus. The bladder wall is composed of a mucous membrane, a submucosa, a muscular coat of smooth detrusor muscle, and is covered by serosal peritoneum. The urethra is a 4 cm fibromuscular tube that serves as a passage of urine from the bladder to the exterior. It extends downward and forward from the neck of the bladder.

Scan Findings

Although often ignored sonographically, the bladder should be imaged during every examination. The sonographic appearance of the lower urinary tract is dependent upon the differing acoustic impedances of the different structures. After inserting the probe into the vagina, the symphysis and pubic rami are first visualized. The symphysis appears as a dense, uniform, hyperechoic, midline structure that can be distinguished from surrounding connective tissue by the shape of the inferior half of the pubis and its immobility during coughing or straining. The pubis is lateral to the symphysis, and as it is composed of trabecular bone, with a dense cortex, sonographically appears as a hypoechoic body with a hyperechoic inferior border. Immediately posterior are the bladder and urethra.

The bladder appears as a hypoechoic structure because of its stored urine. The course of the urethra is indicated by the acoustic characteristics of the adjacent tissues. The sonographic appearance of the bladder wall varies with its degree of distention. When empty or only partially distended, the wall should be less than 6 mm in thickness. The bladder mucosal pattern is prominent with slight irregularity and tufting. When the bladder is distended, its wall appears as a thin echogenic line. A pathologically thickened bladder wall is thus more easily appreciated when the bladder is distended.

The ureters are fibromuscular tubes connecting the kidney to the bladder. They are closely related to the cervix and vagina and enter the base of the bladder at the trigone. Under normal circumstances, the ureters are unable to be visualized by sonography. Occasionally, the "ureteric jet phenomenon" can be seen. This is an echogenic spurt of urine passing from the ureter into the bladder.

An Atlas of Transvaginal Sonography

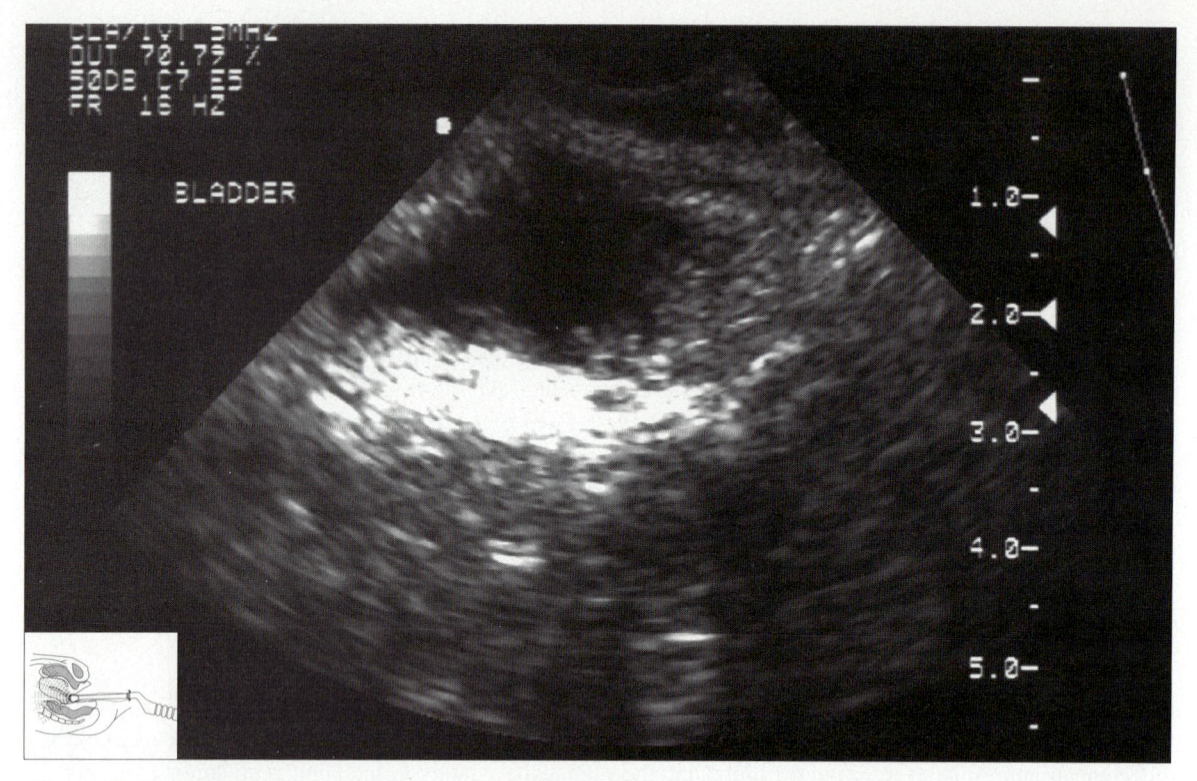

Figure 16-1. Normal bladder wall. When only partially distended, the walls appear thickened and with prominent mucosal irregularity.

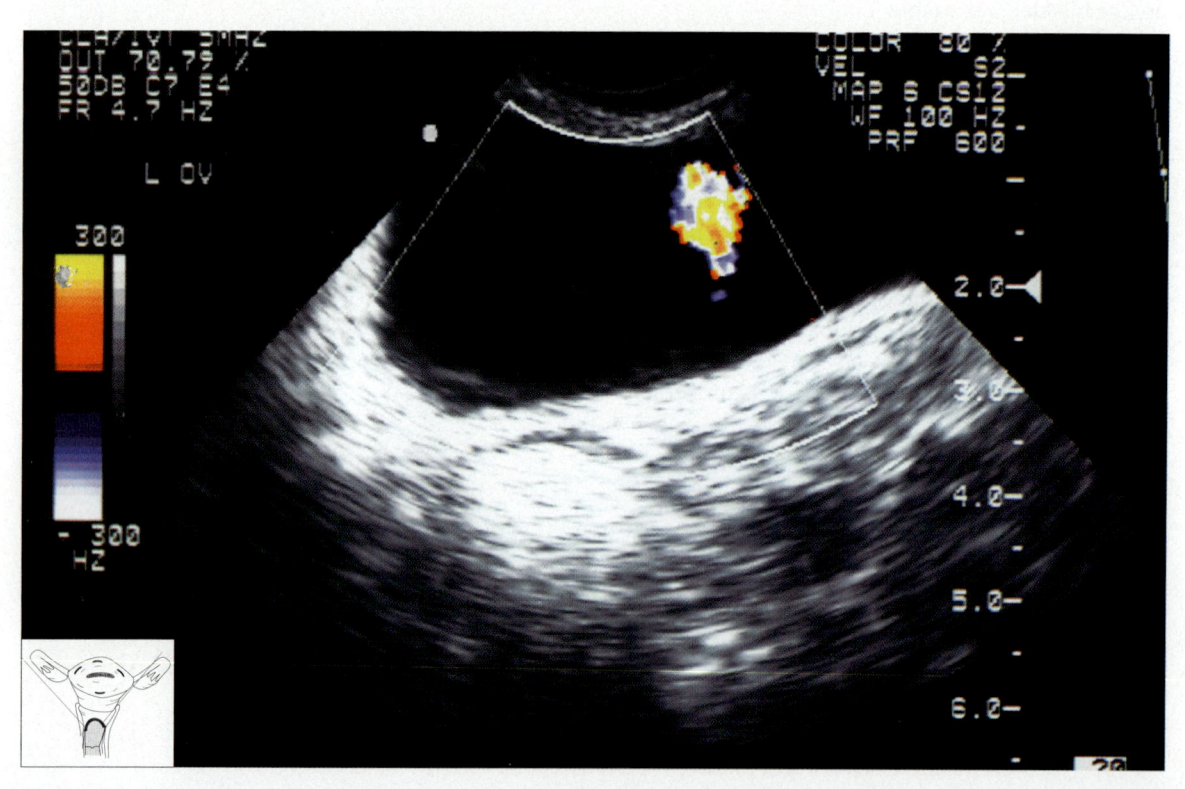

Figure 16-2. With increasing bladder distention, its walls become thin and echoic. The ureters are usually not visible but color flow Doppler demonstrates the "ureteric jet phenomenon."

196

Urinary Tract

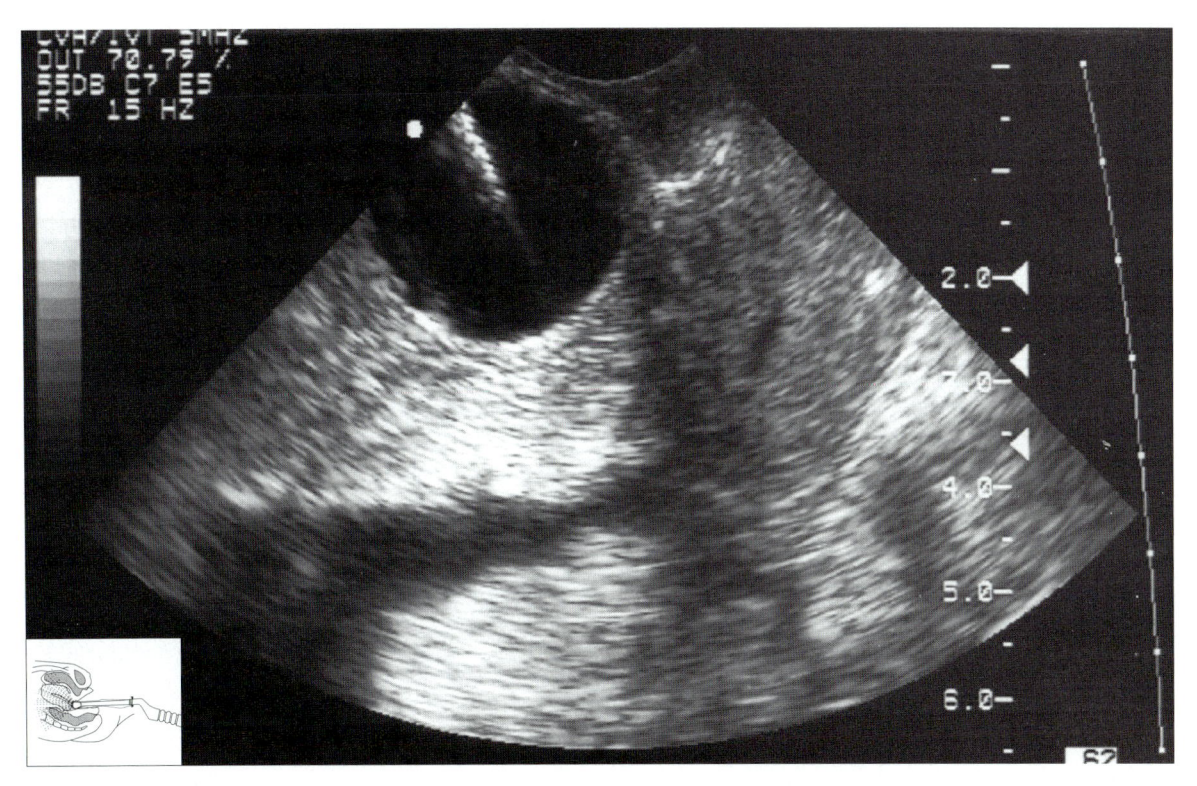

Figure 16-3. Foley catheter, anterior to the uterus.

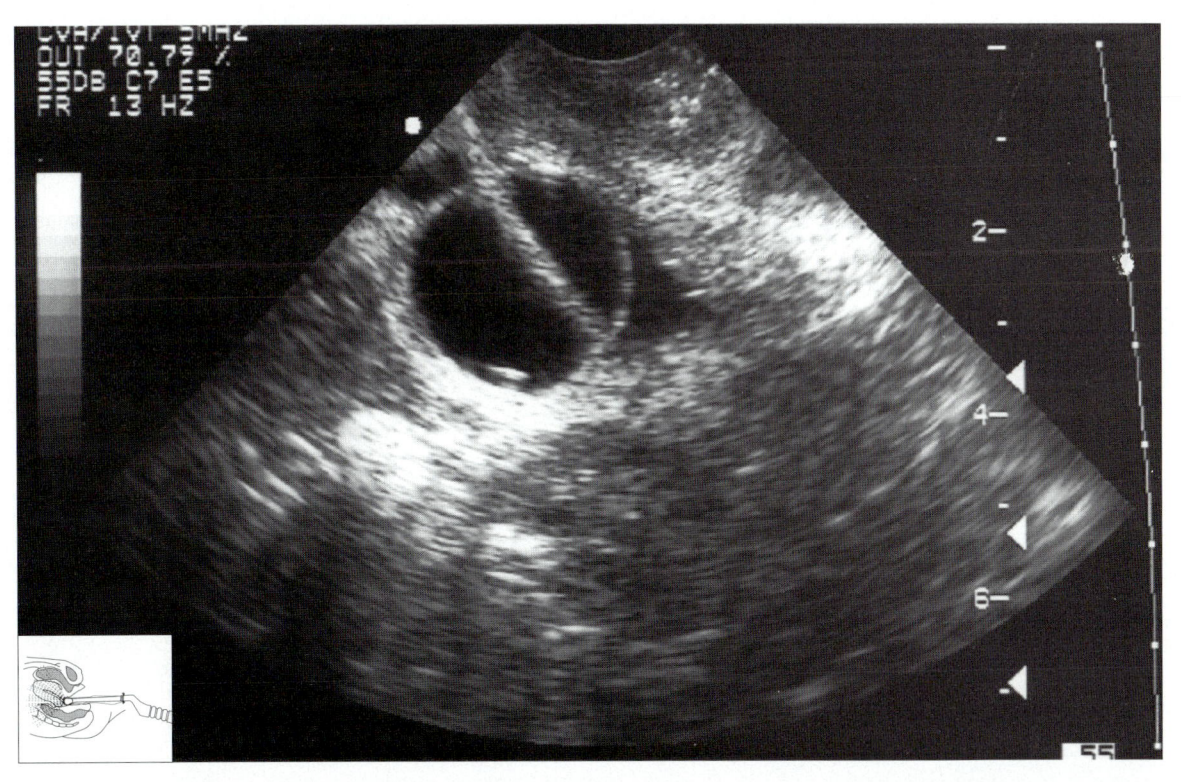

Figure 16-4. Clear view of Foley balloon, catheter, and small amount of surrounding urine within the bladder.

An Atlas of Transvaginal Sonography

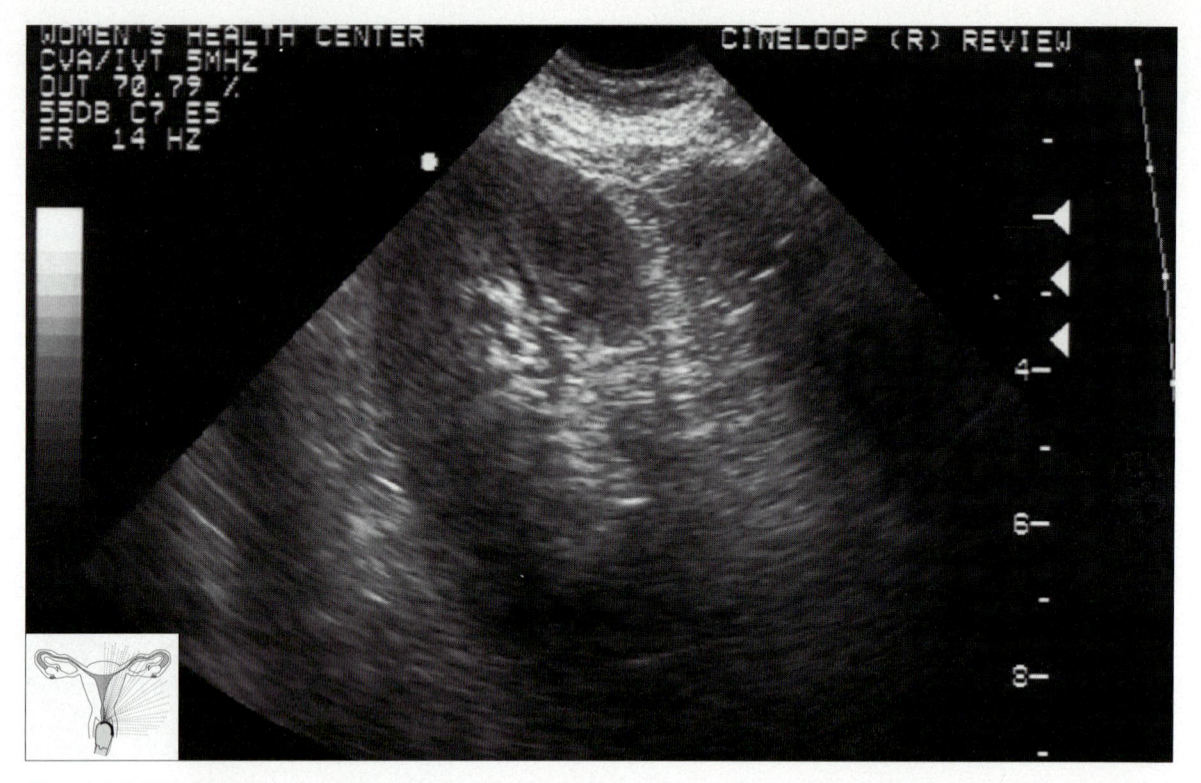

Figure 16-5. Pelvic kidney, with its echoic collecting system and isoechoic cortex, once seen, should never be forgotten, as inadvertent removal has disastrous results.

Benign Urinary Tract Pathology
Ureteric Obstruction

Ureteric obstruction, either partial or complete from either benign or malignant causes, results in a distended urine-filled ureter. This distended ureter, or hydroureter, is seen depending on the site of the obstruction. In low ureteric obstruction the distended ureter is seen lateral to the cervix, and can be traced up the pelvic side wall to the iliac vessels.

Scan Findings

Due to limitations in the depth of view, high ureteric obstructions may not be seen by TVS. Where doubt exists as to the nature of the tubular structure, vascular structures can be excluded by color flow Doppler. Low ureter obstruction can be diagnosed by TVS. The ureter is seen as a distended tubular structure on the pelvic side wall, and can be seen crossing the iliac vessels.

Urinary Tract

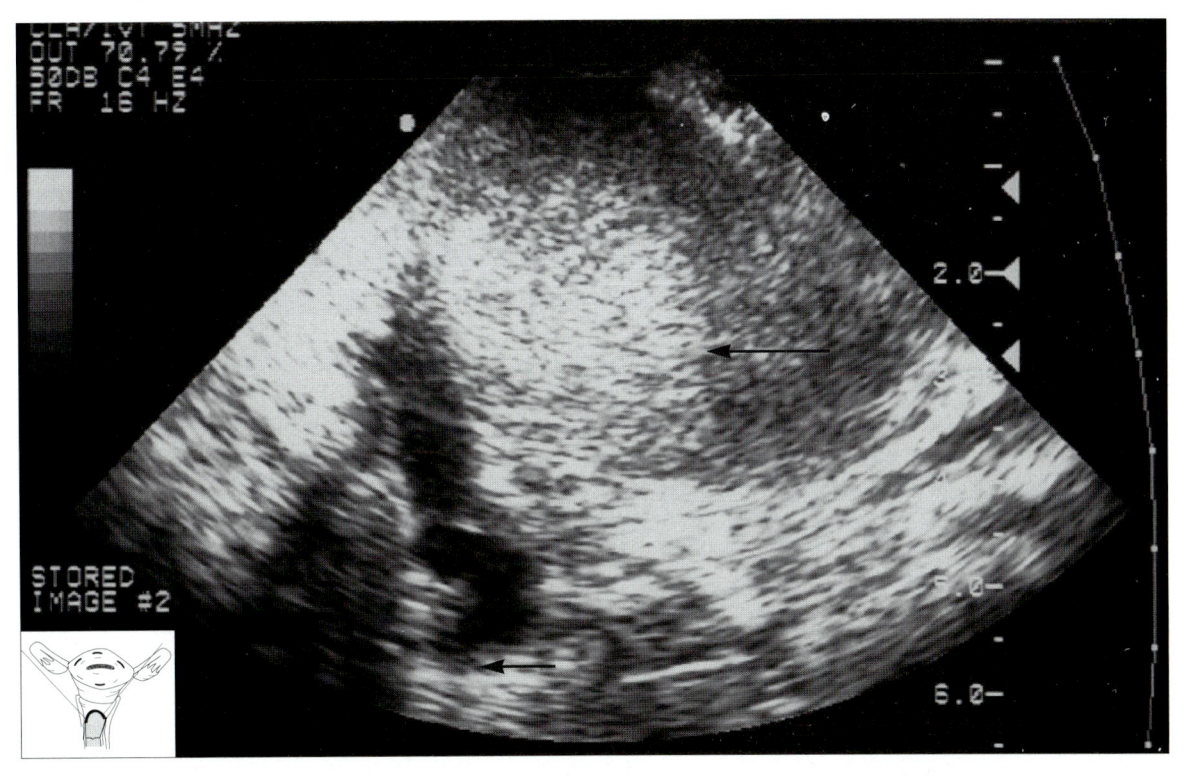

Figure 16-6. Patient with a large Stage IIIB cervix cancer (large arrow), extending to the pelvic side wall, and causing ureteric obstruction (small arrow).

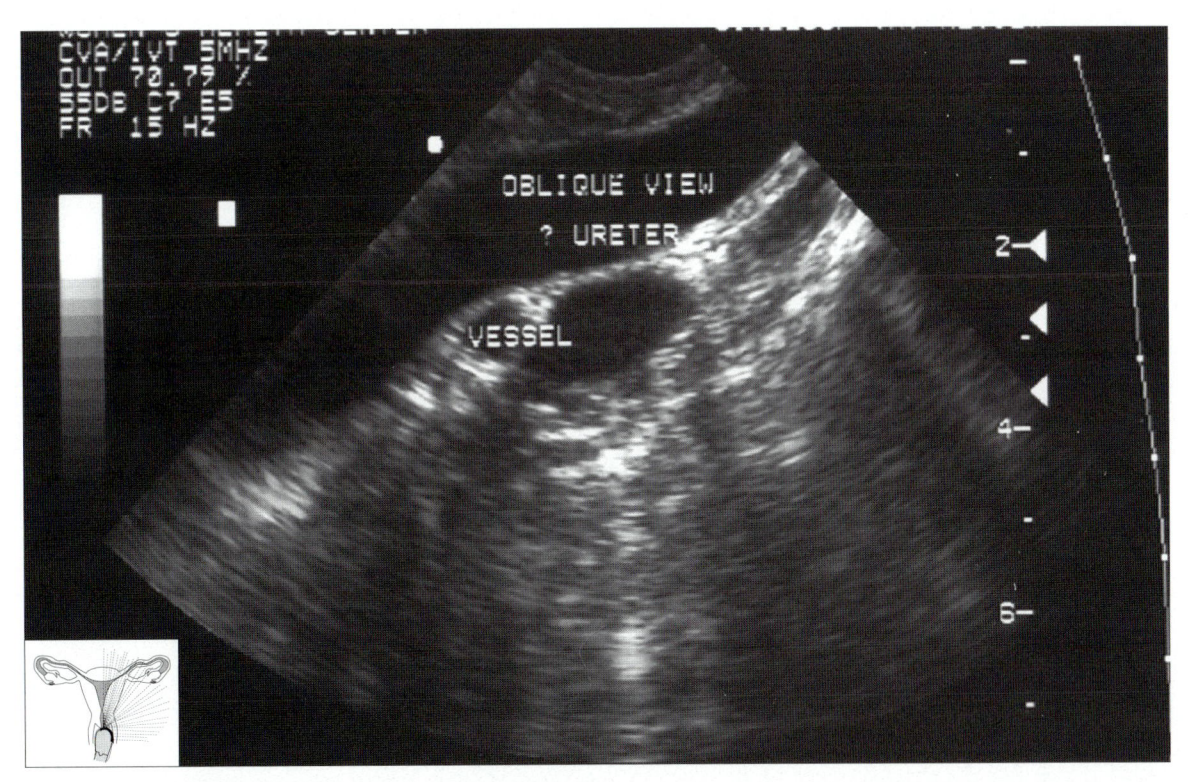

Figure 16-7. Hydroureter seen crossing the iliac vessels.

17   Bowel

The bowel extends from the stomach to the anus, and comprises the small or upper bowel and the large or lower bowel. Shadowing from intraluminal gas may be reduced by fasting the patient prior to the scan. Unwanted bowel loops may also be pushed away by the abdominal hand to provide a clear view of pelvic structures.

The small intestine, composed of the duodenum, jejunum, and ileum is the major site of digestion. The ileum is the only clinically relevant portion of the small bowel to the transvaginal sonographer. Although attached to the posterior abdominal wall by its mesentery, the ileum is the most mobile portion of the alimentary tract. Likewise, the rectum and sigmoid are the only sonographically relevant portions of the large bowel for the transvaginal sonographer. The sigmoid colon may be mobile and seen on either side of the lower pelvis, while the rectum is fixed posterior to the uterus, in the midline.

Scan Findings

Isolated loops of small bowel are rarely visualized sonographically, unless loops are full of fluid, in which case the wall is thin and its mucosal pattern unremarkable. More commonly the small bowel appears sonographically as a peristatic, ground glass-appearing mass-like structure. Air within the small bowel produces posterior acoustic shadowing.

The sonographic appearance of the sigmoid colon and rectum is dependent upon the amount of gas, fluid, and feces within its lumen. Stool has a mixed echogenicity and may dilate the colon or rectum, while bowel gas may appear hyperechoic and produces characteristic posterior shadowing.

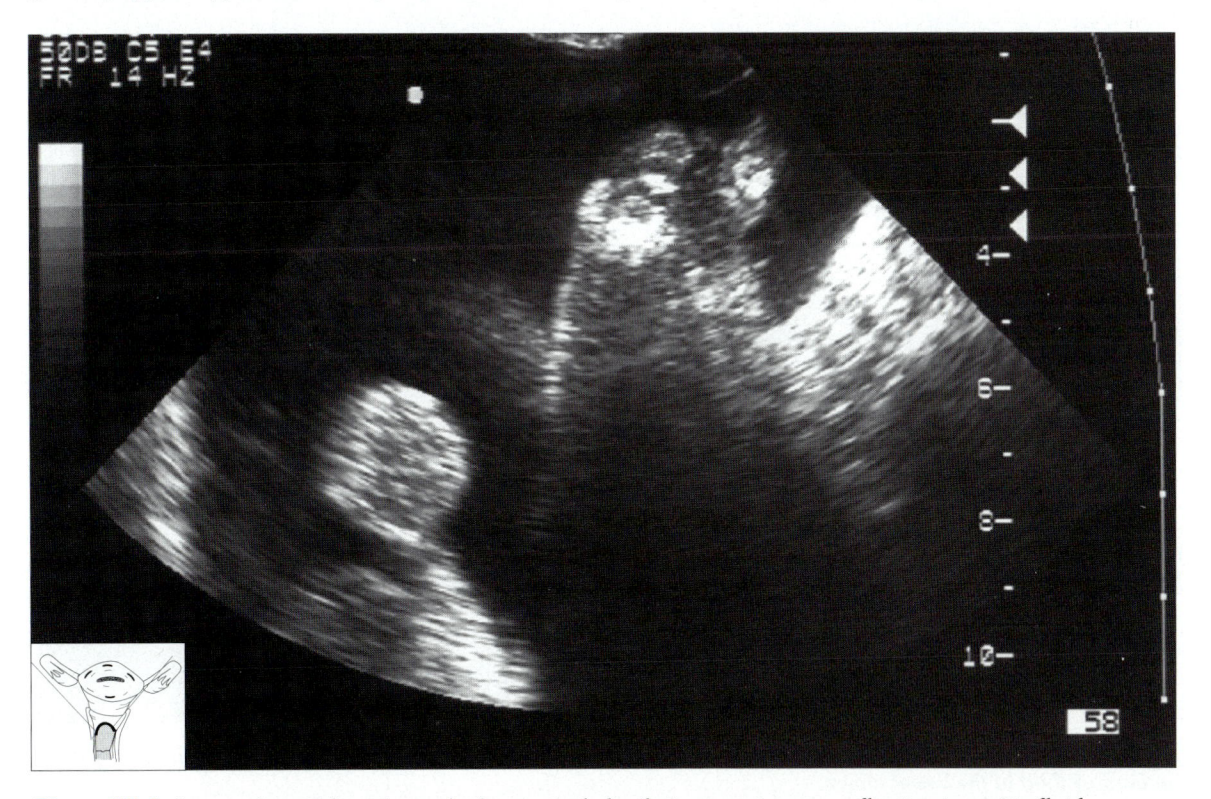

Figure 17-1. Loops of small bowel attached posteriorly by their mesentery, seen floating in ascitic fluid.

An Atlas of Transvaginal Sonography

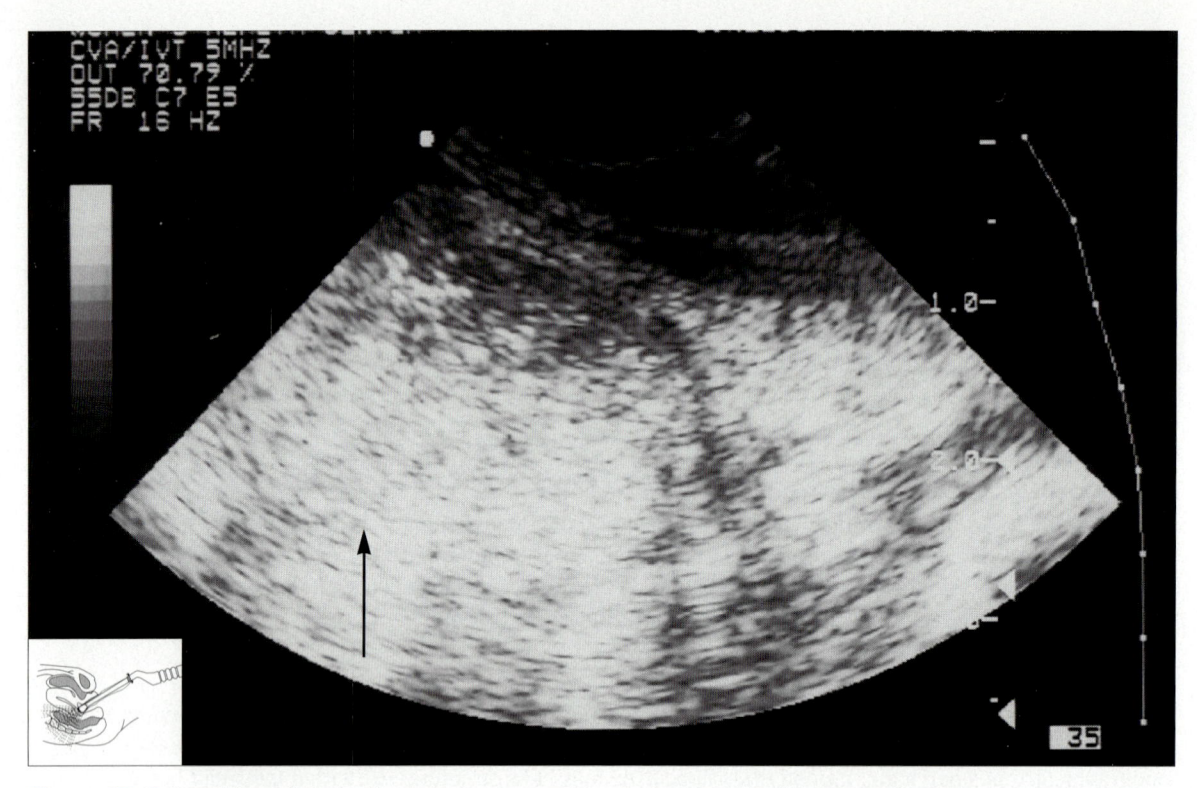

Figure 17-2. Small bowel is usually seen as a peristaltic mass of mixed echogenicity (arrow).

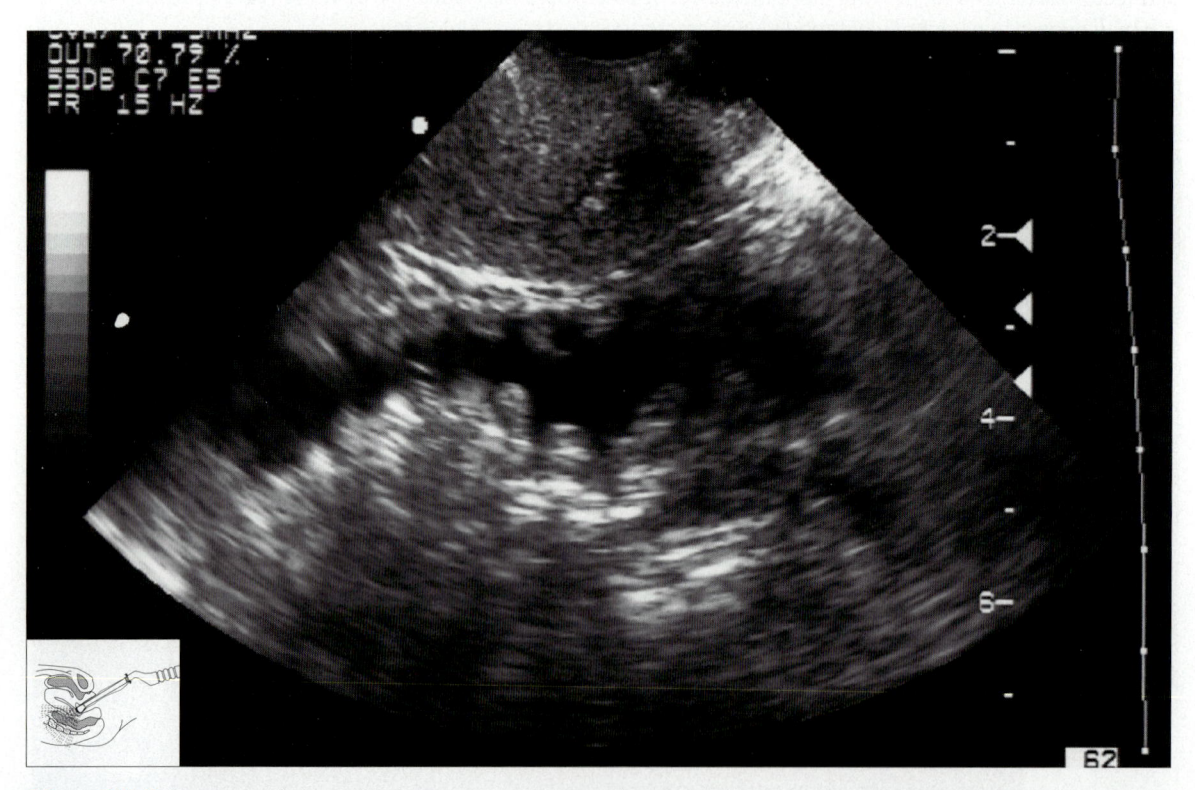

Figure 17-3. Segment of sigmoid colon seen posterior to the cervix. Normal mucosal pattern is seen due to the amount of fluid in the bowel lumen.

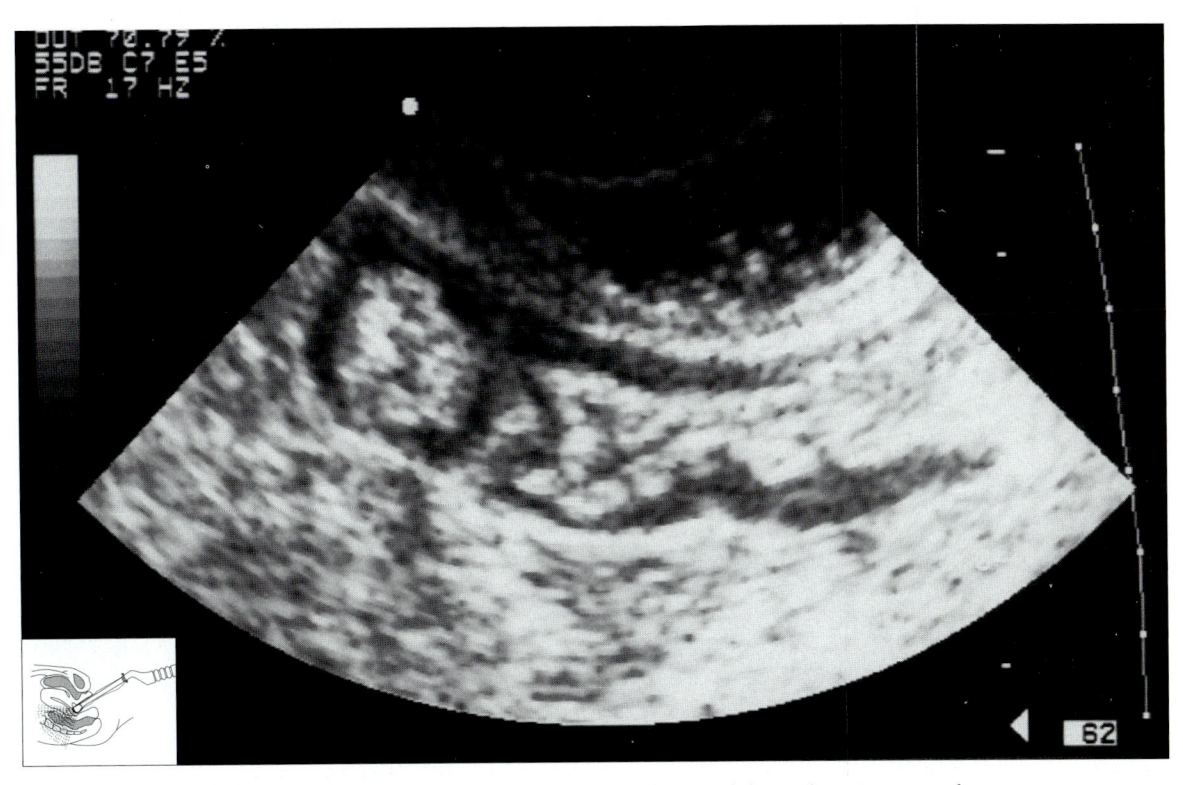

Figure 17-4. The mucosa in this segment of rectosigmoid is flattened, but otherwise normal.

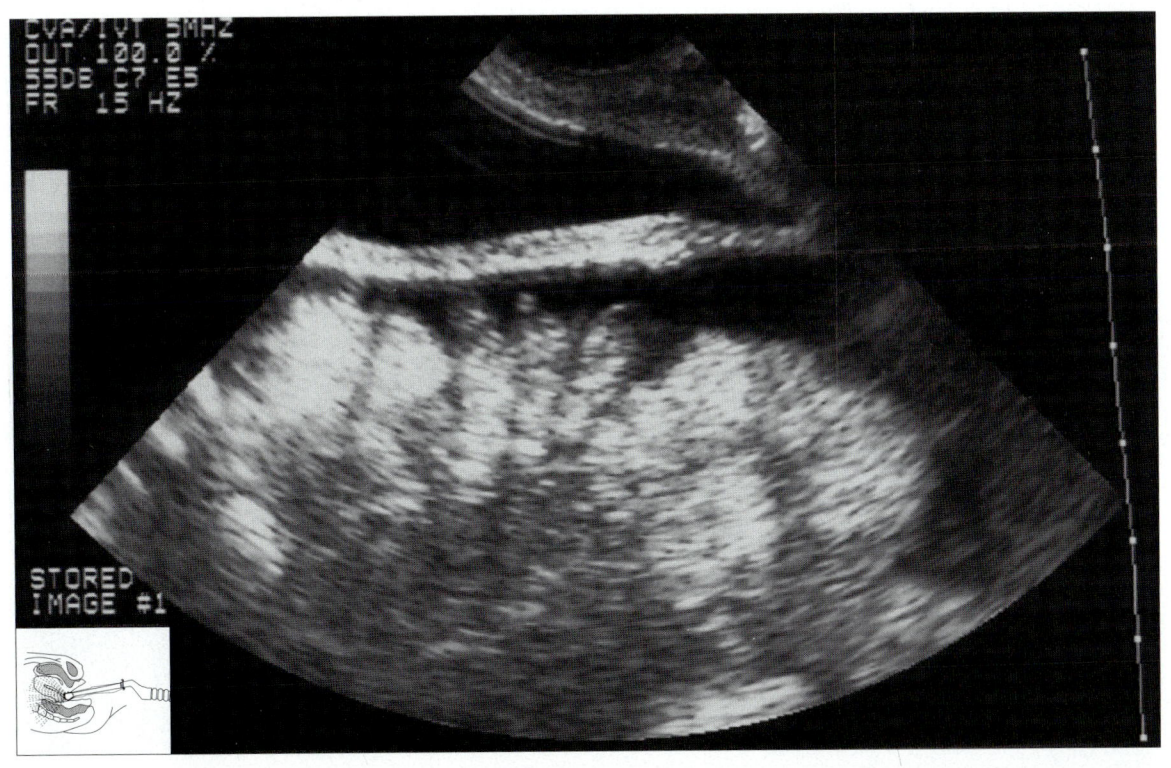

Figure 17-5. A segment of sigmoid colon is seen posterior to the bladder. Ascitic fluid allows recognition of the large bowel haustrations. Fecal content is echogenic.

An Atlas of Transvaginal Sonography

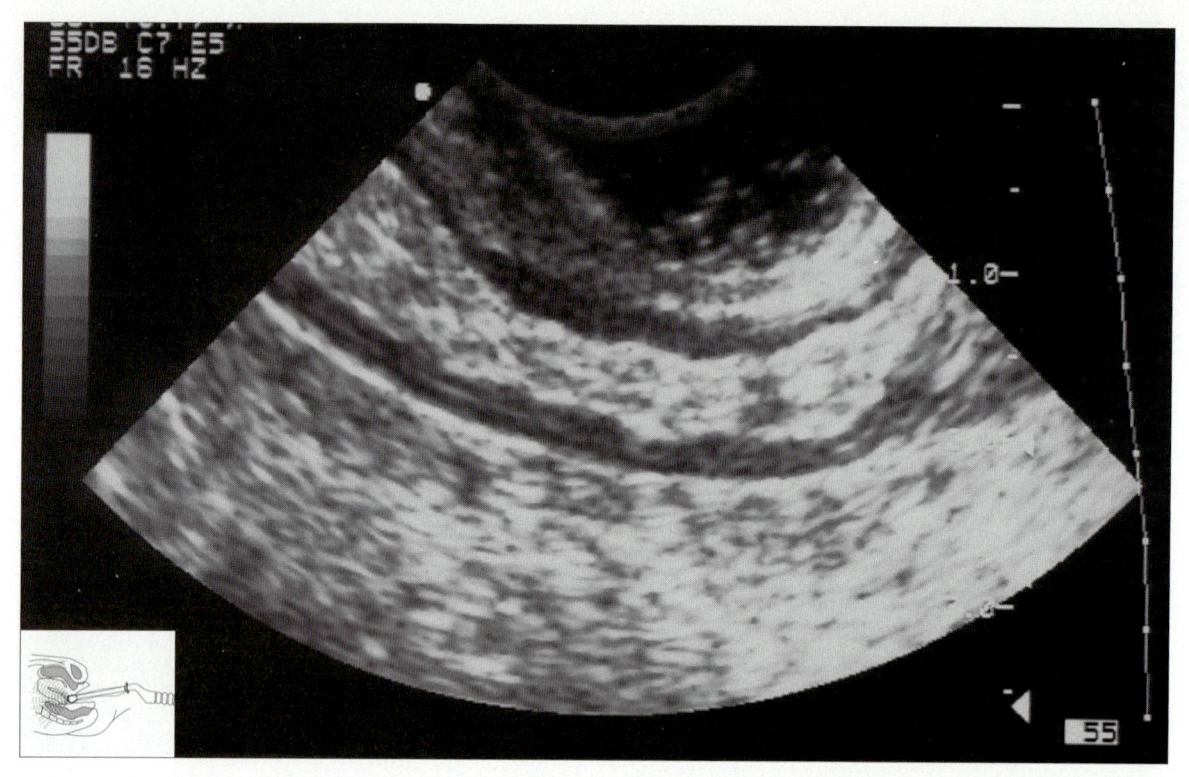

Figure 17-6. A water enema can enhance visualization of the colonic mucosa, by increasing through transmission of the ultrasound beam. Fecal content is echogenic.

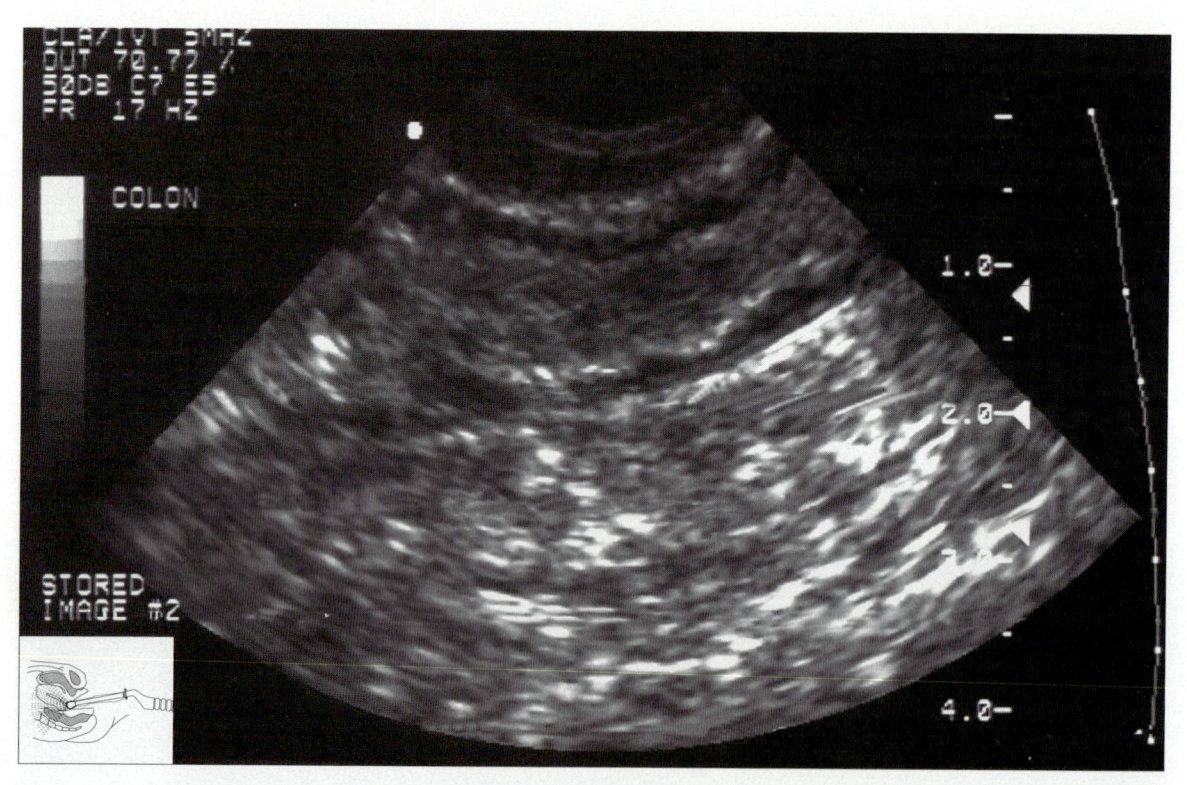

Figure 17-7. The fecal stream can take on different sonographic appearances depending on its consistency, and the amount of fluid and gas present. This fecal stream is isoechoic.

Bowel

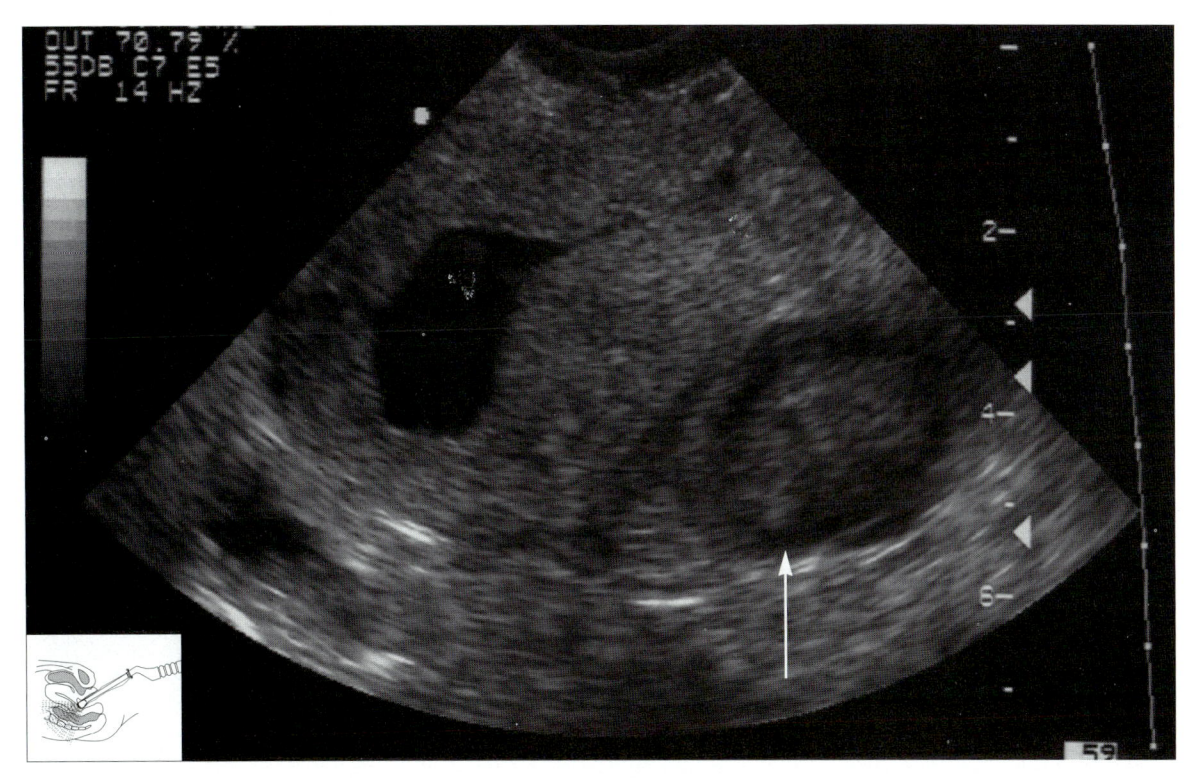

Figure 17-8. Sagittal section of an anteverted uterus with hydrometra. In the cul-de-sac is a section of large bowel (arrow) that could be easily mistaken for an adnexal mass.

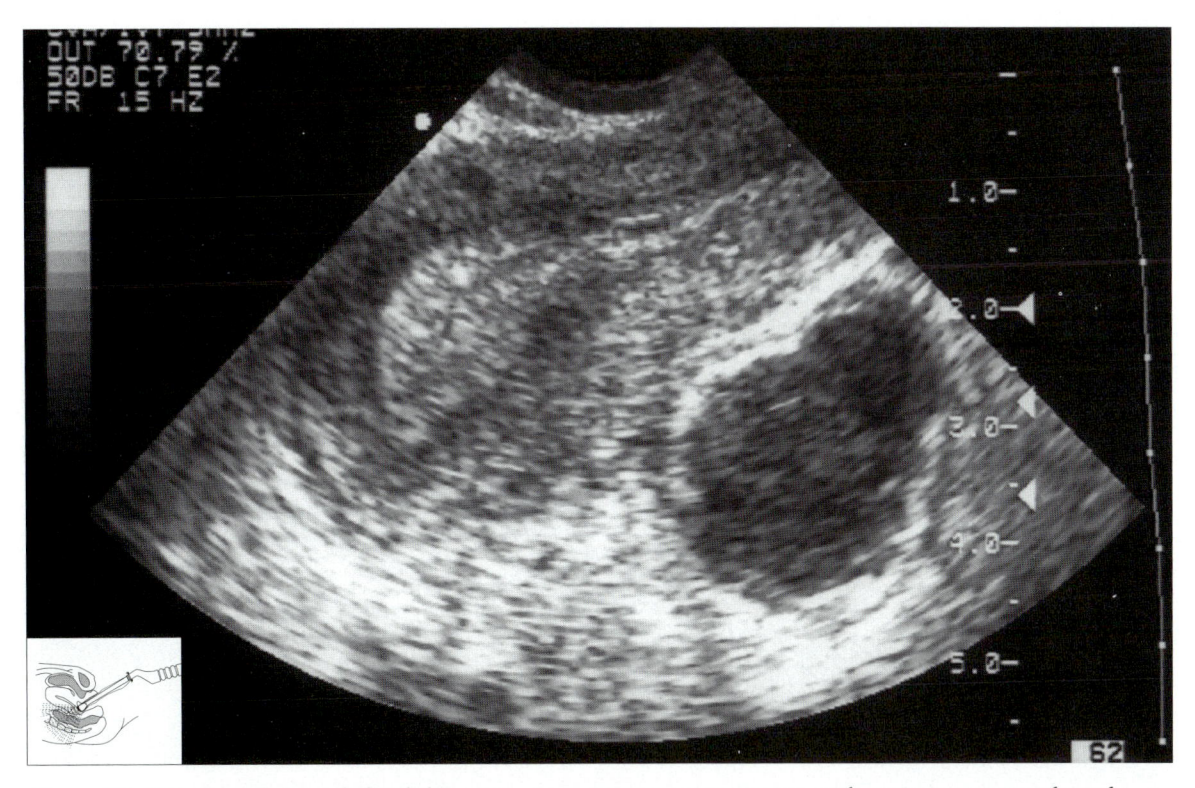

Figure 17-9. In the cul-de-sac behind this uterus is an apparent tumor mass, with an apparent capsule and echogenic contents. Continued observation confirmed peristaltic activity.

205

An Atlas of Transvaginal Sonography

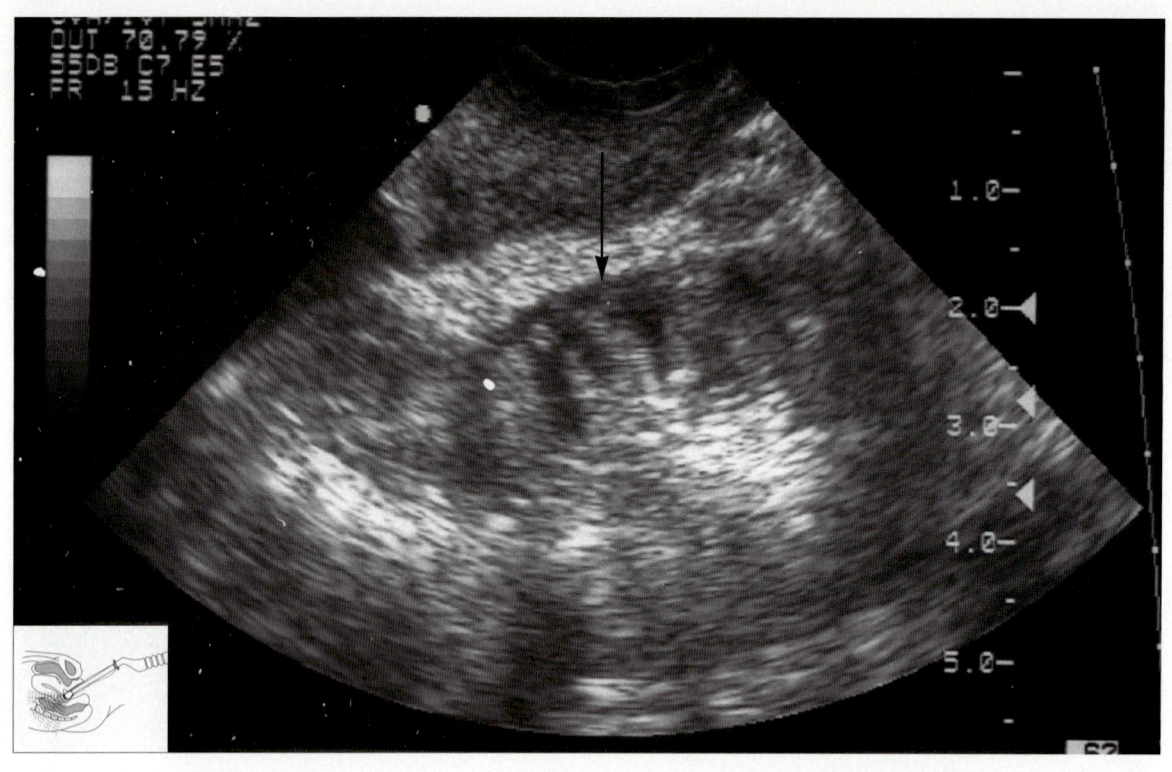

Figure 17-10. Echoic thickened bowel wall (arrow) in a patient with pseudomembranous colitis.

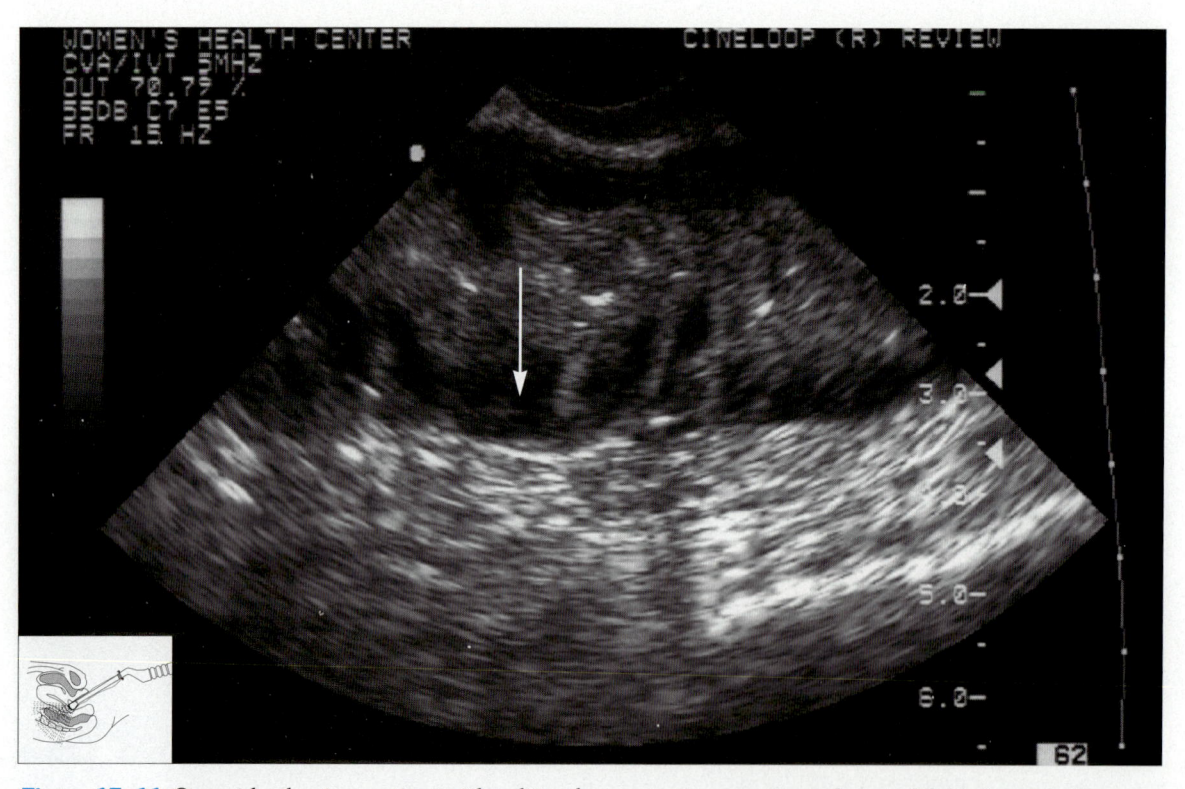

Figure 17-11. Sigmoid colon in a patient with colitis, demonstrating prominent haustral folds (arrow), the so-called "thumbprint" effect.

Bowel

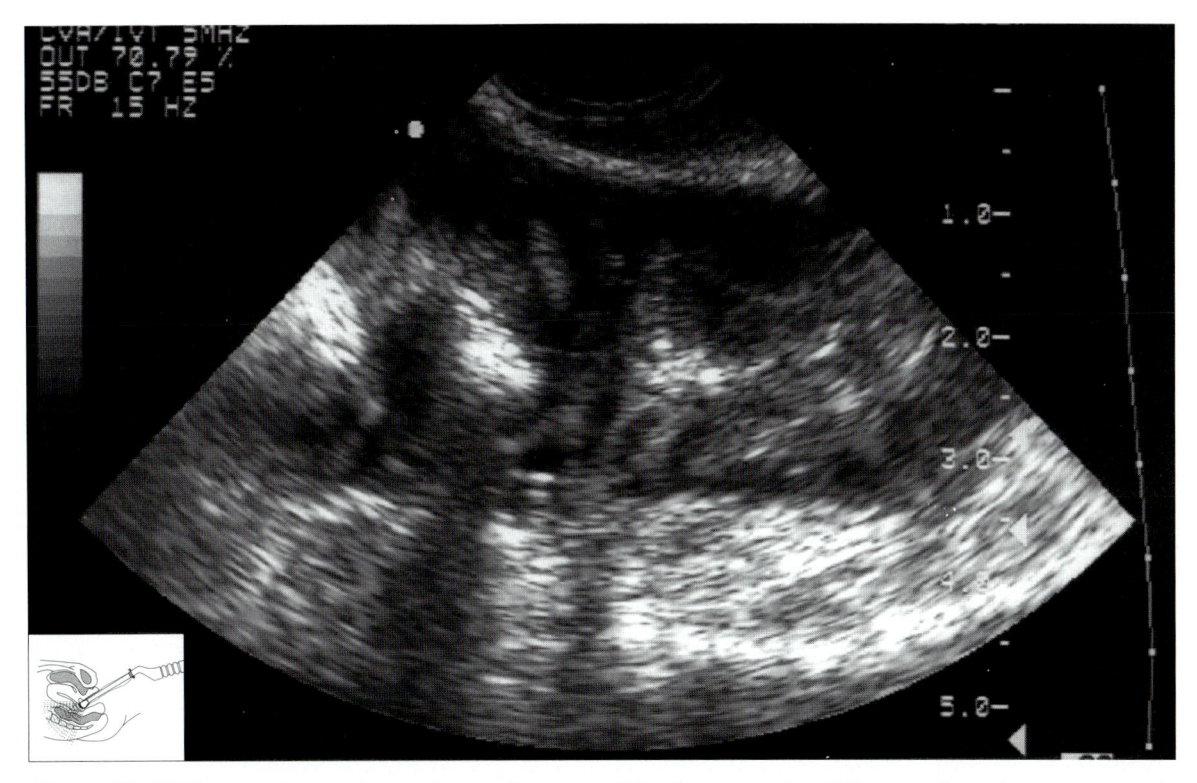

Figure 17-12. *Same patient with pseudo membranous colitis, demonstrating different echogenic appearance of the fecal stream with echoic areas interspersed among the isoechoic fecal stream.*

18   Miscellaneous Lesions

A variety of non-gynecologic or miscellaneous lesions which can cause considerable diagnostic dilemma, may be visualized by transvaginal sonography. These include pelvic varicosities, the presence of free fluid or ascites, pelvic hematoma, enlarged pelvic lymph nodes, and lymphocysts.

Pelvic Lymph Nodes

Pelvic lymph nodes drain the lower extremities and pelvic organs. They are small structures surrounding the pelvic vessels.

Scan Findings

Under normal conditions, pelvic lymph nodes are not seen by TVS. Conditions causing lymph node enlargement include infectious and metastatic spread from cancers. When enlarged, pelvic lymph nodes are seen as isoechoic masses of variable size on the pelvic side wall. On superficial inspection they can be mistaken for an ovary. Color flow tends not to be increased in enlarged lymph nodes.

Lymphocysts

Lymphocysts are collections of lymphatic fluid commonly seen after radical pelvic surgery.

Scan Findings

Lymphocysts have a variable appearance. They can assume any size, and their internal morphology can be cystic, multicystic or complex. On color flow Doppler, low-volume blood flow can be seen through the septae within the cysts.

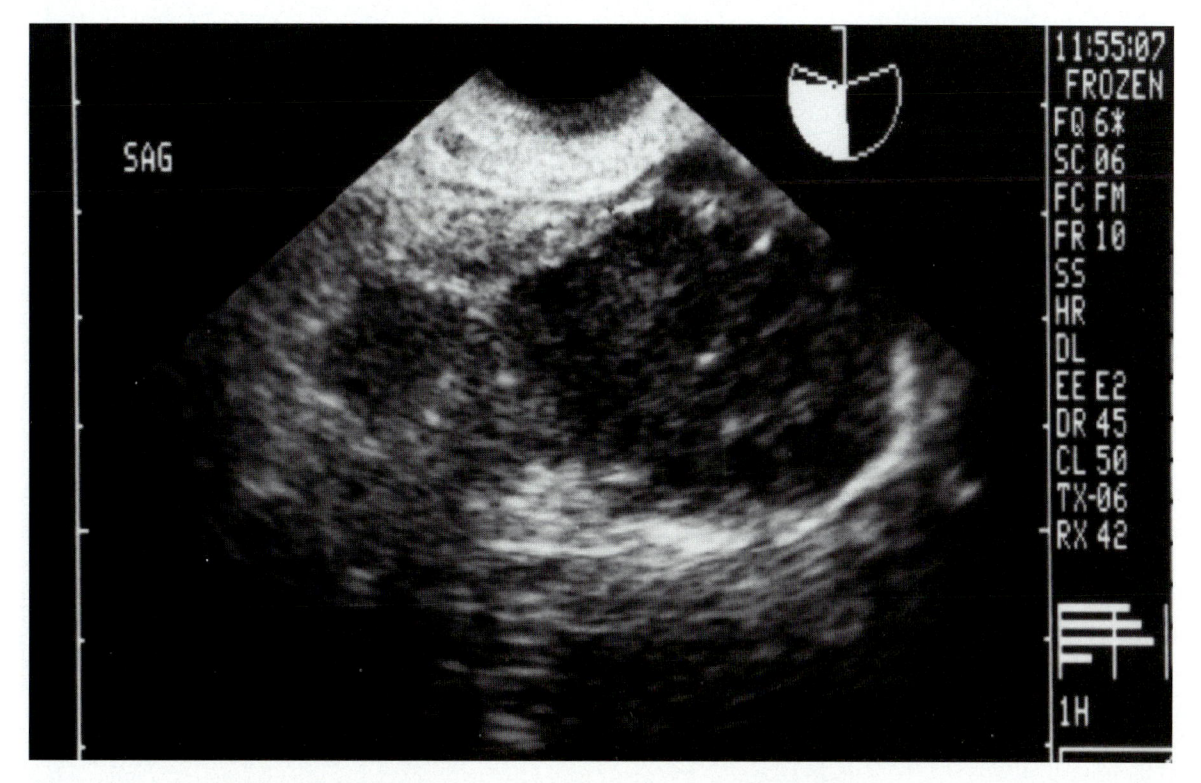

Figure 18-1. Enlarged iliac lymph node in a patient with advanced cervical cancer.

An Atlas of Transvaginal Sonography

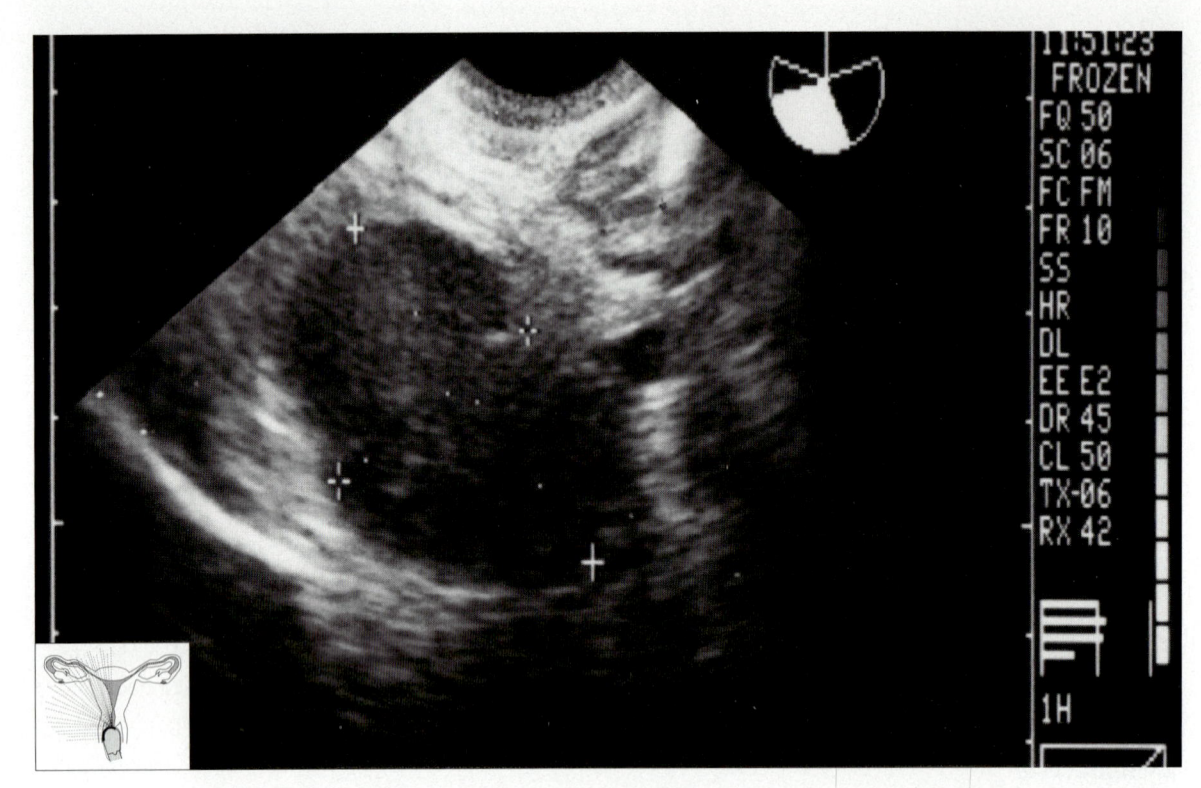

Figure 18-2. Enlarged pelvic lymph node on the pelvic side wall.

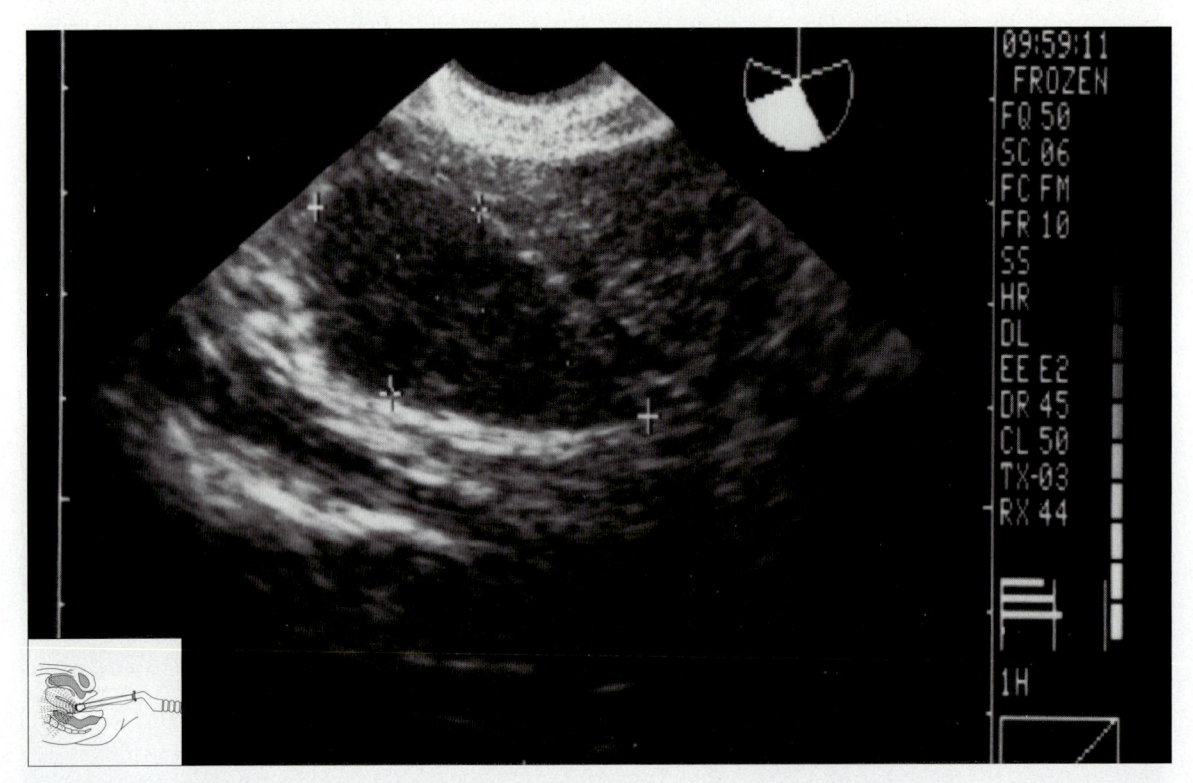

Figure 18-3. Enlarged pelvic lymph node, that morphologically looks like an ovary.

Miscellaneous Lesions

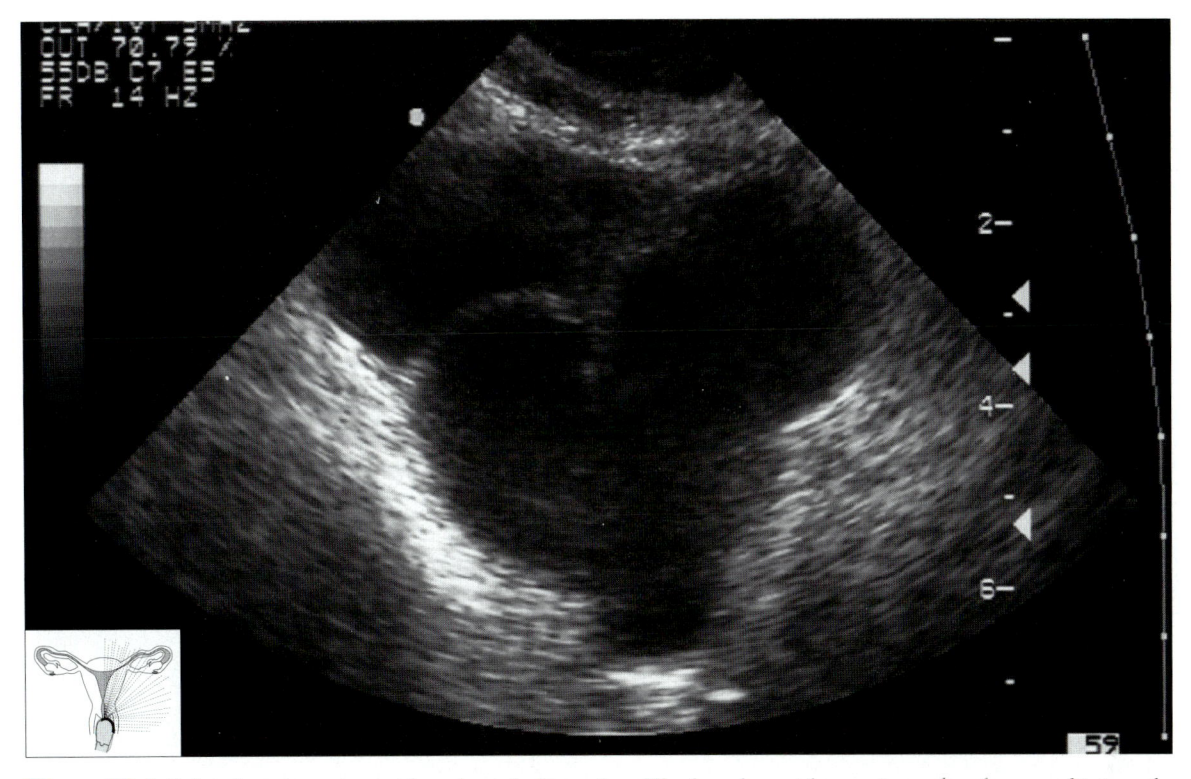

Figure 18-4. Pelvic lymphocyst, post-lymph node dissection. The lymphocyst has an irregular shape and internal septations that superficially could be confused with an ovarian tumor.

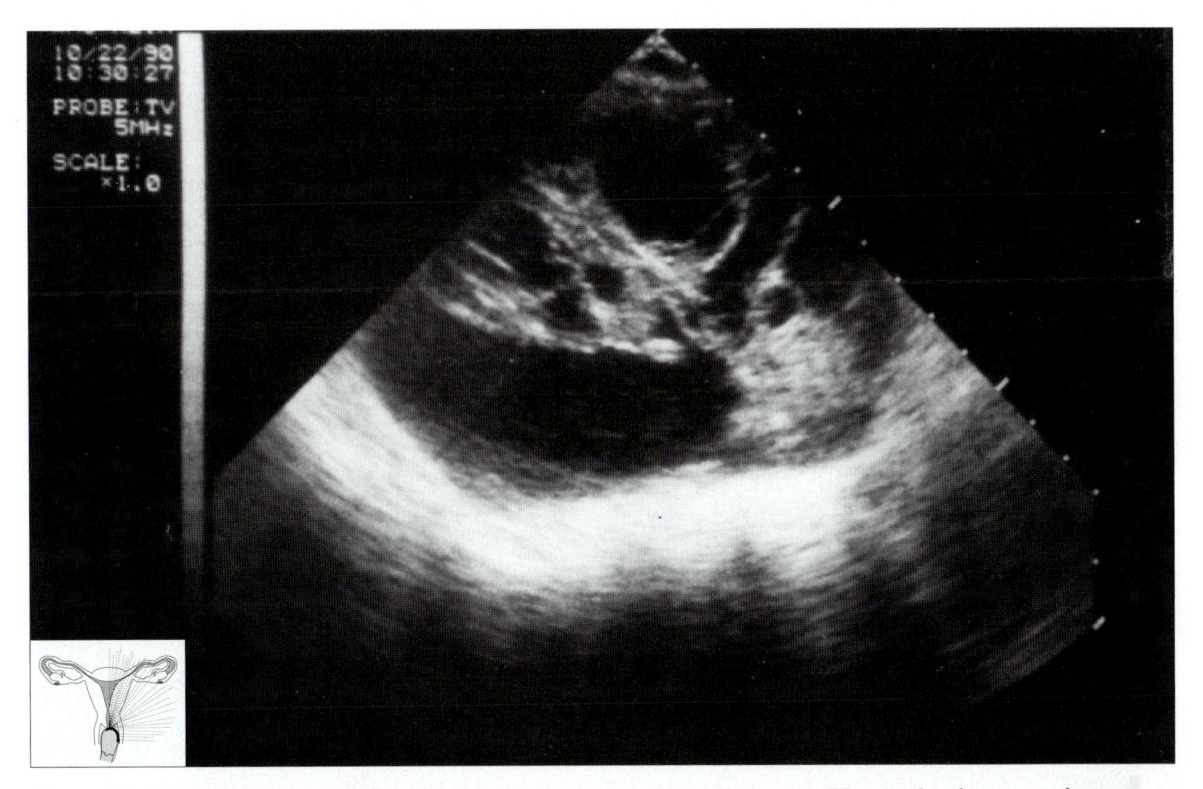

Figure 18-5. Chronic pelvic lymphocyst, appearing as a complex pelvic mass. The cyst borders are indistinct, which is one of its differentiating features.

An Atlas of Transvaginal Sonography

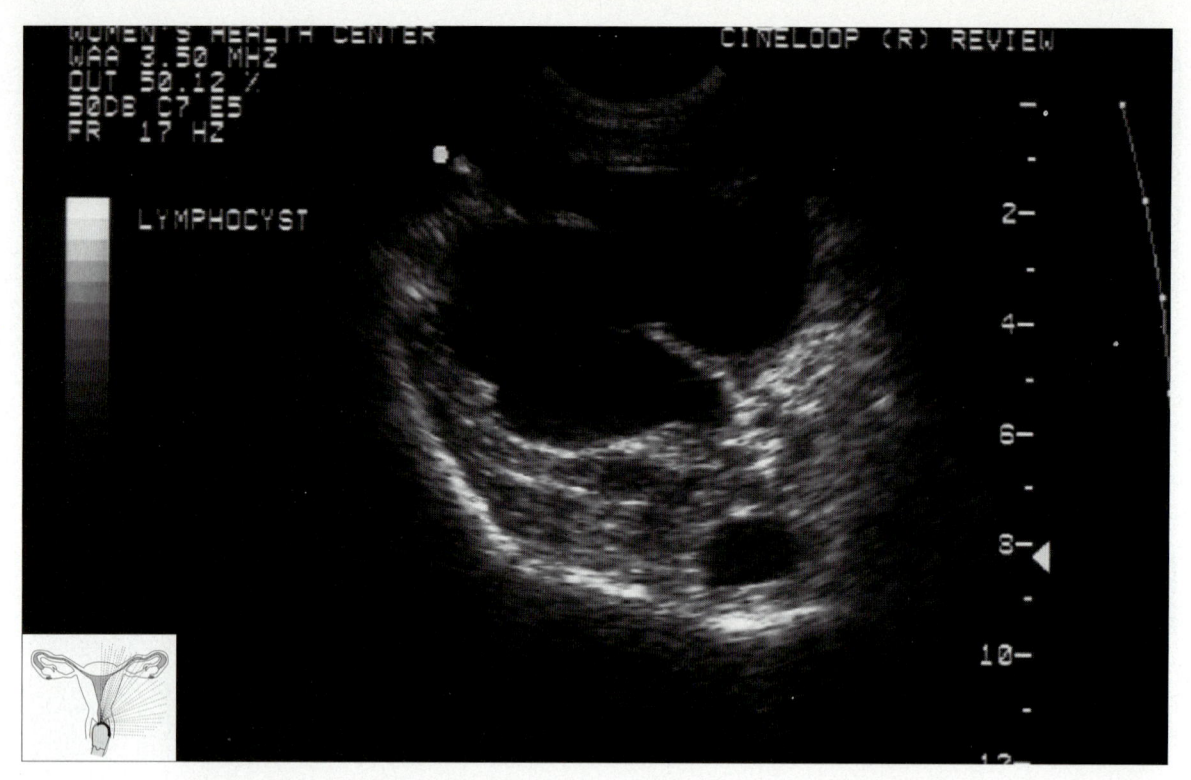

Figure 18-6. Pelvic side wall lymphocyst with large solid component and pseudo septa.

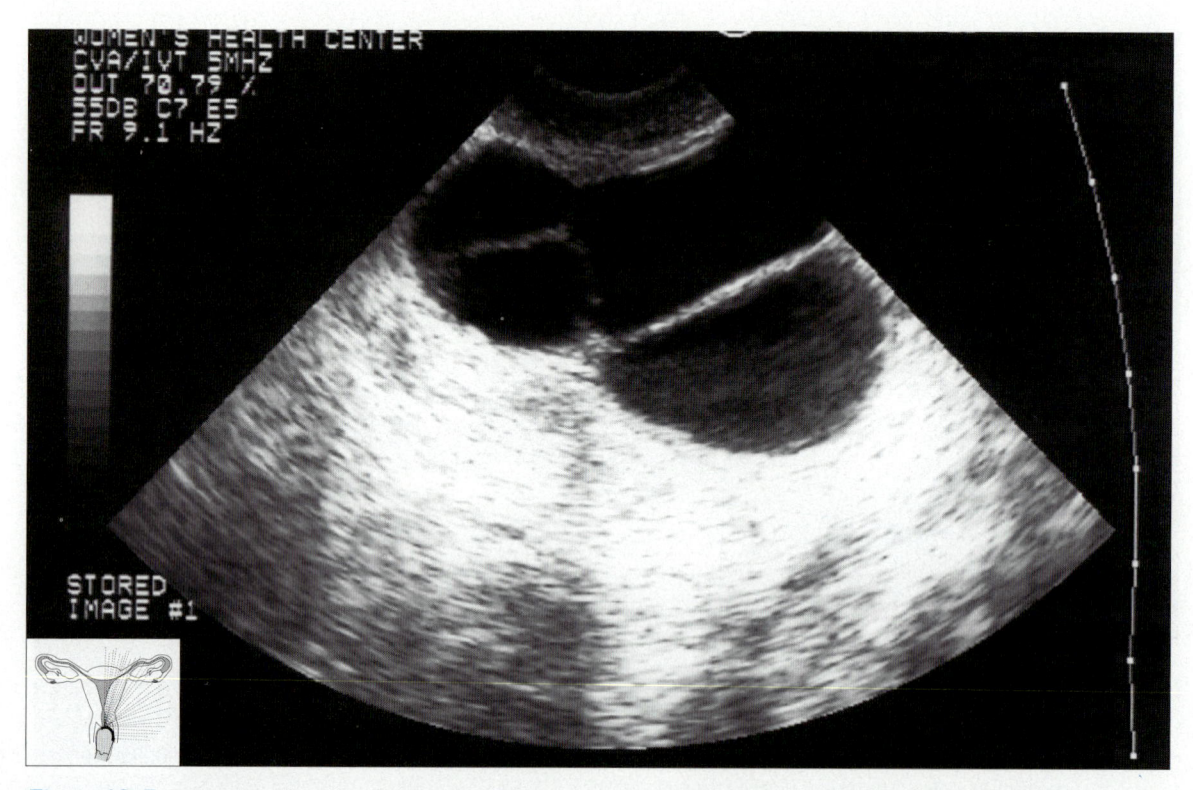

Figure 18-7. Pelvic lymphocyst with daughter cysts in a patient's status post-lymph node dissection for endometrial cancer.

Miscellaneous Lesions

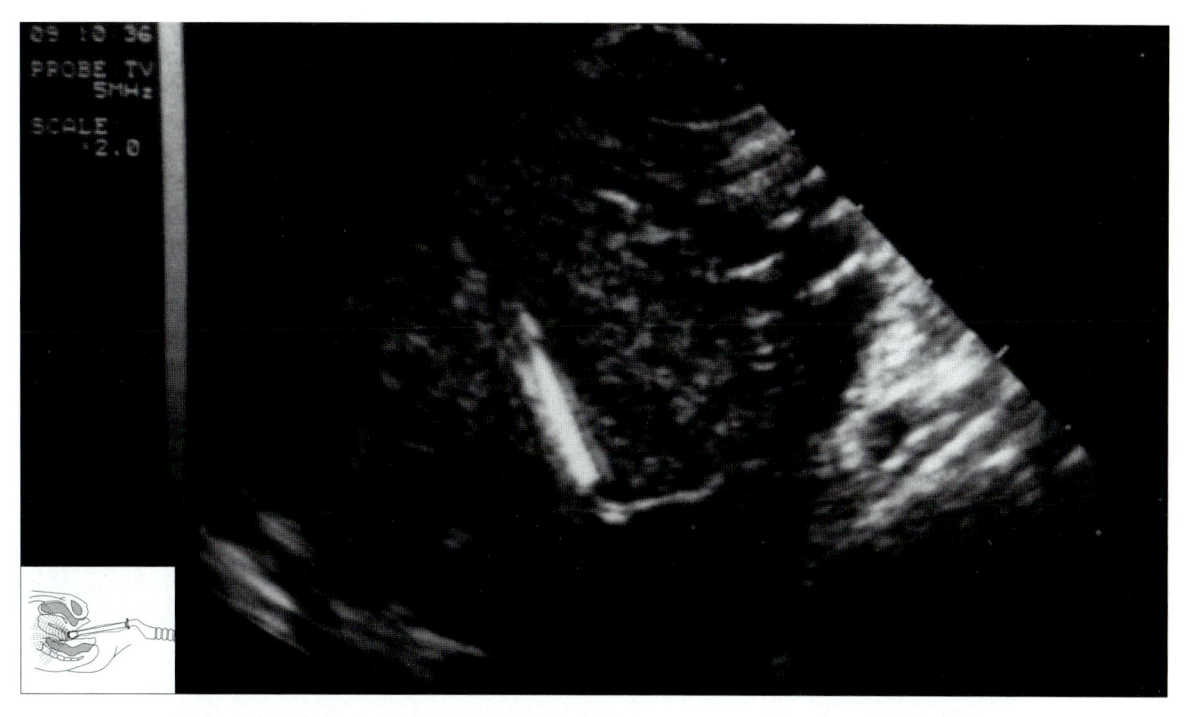

Figure 18-8. Copper T, intrauterine contraceptive device.

Pelvic Varicosities

Pelvic varicosities are dilated and congested veins arising from either the ovarian or uterine vessels. Patients can be asymptomatic or complain of pelvic pain and pelvic congestion.

Scan Findings

Dilated pelvic veins can be identified by gray-scale sonography as distended tubular structures, which need to be distinguished from distended fallopian tubes, multilocular ovarian cysts, or fluid-filled bowel loops. They are often found in the broad ligament just lateral to the cervix but can also be seen adjacent to the ovary in the infundibulopelvic ligament. Color flow imaging easily confirms the vascular nature of these structures.

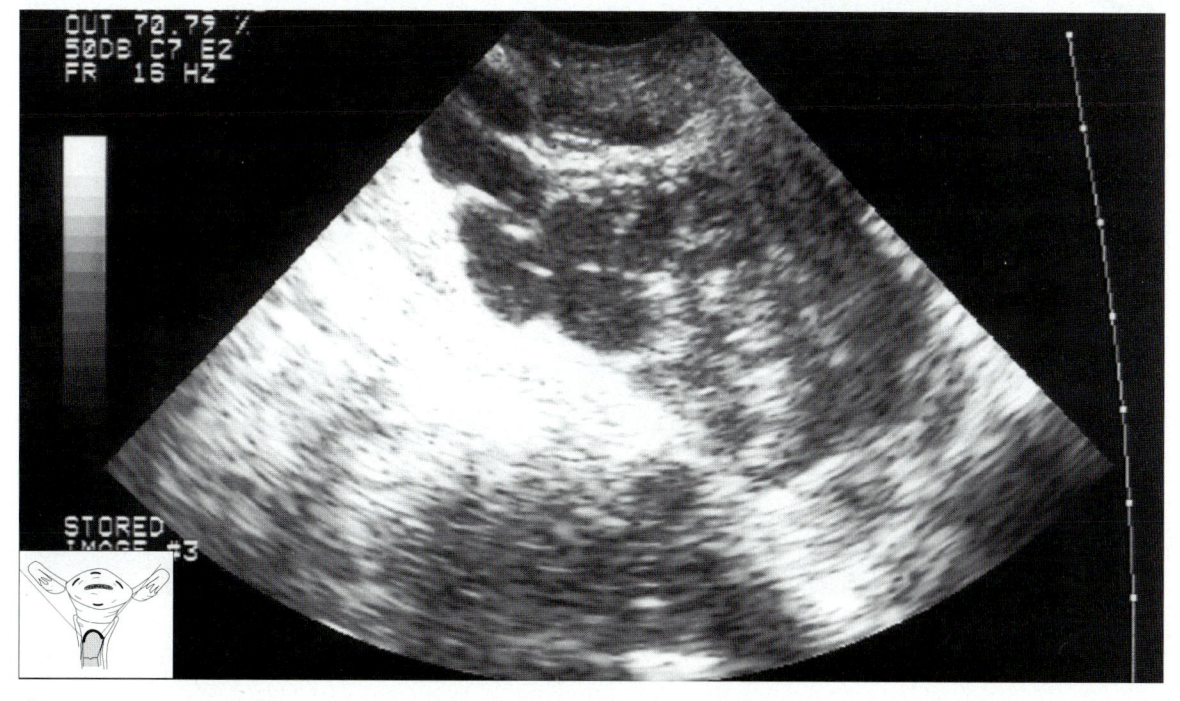

Figure 18-9. Cysts, hydrosalpinx or vessels?

An Atlas of Transvaginal Sonography

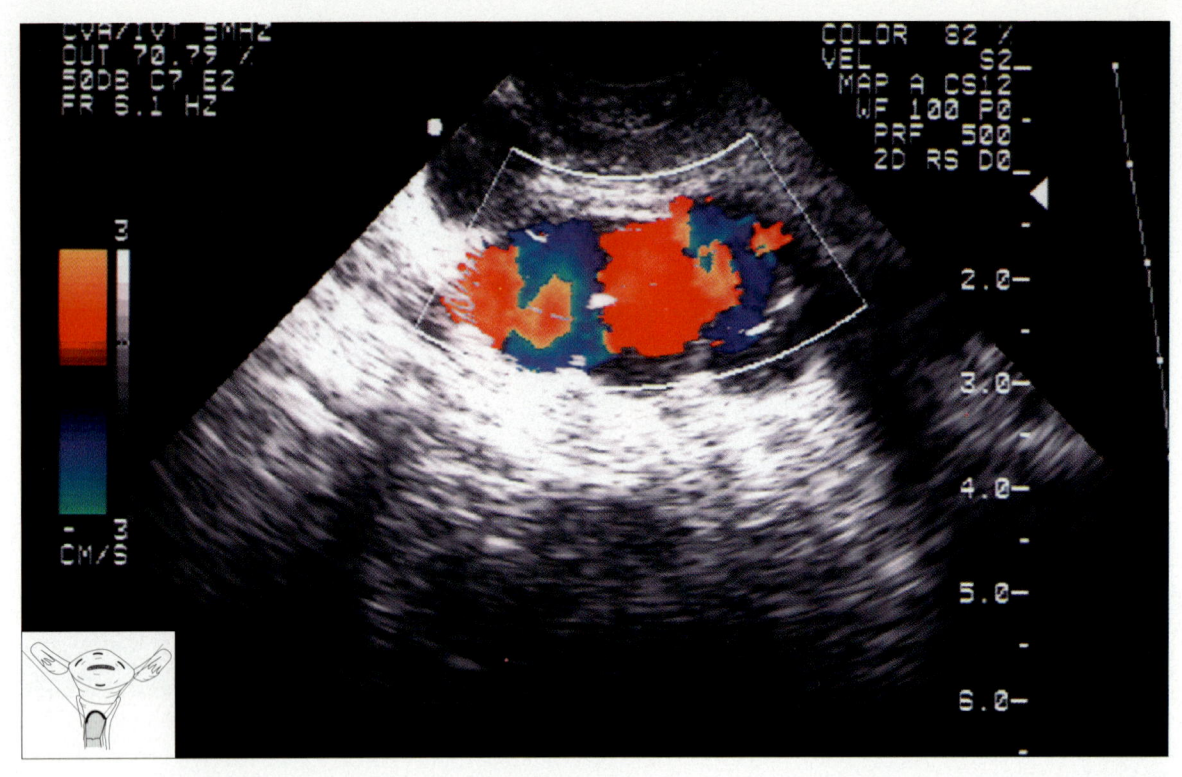

Figure 18-10. Color flow Doppler confirms pelvic varicosities.

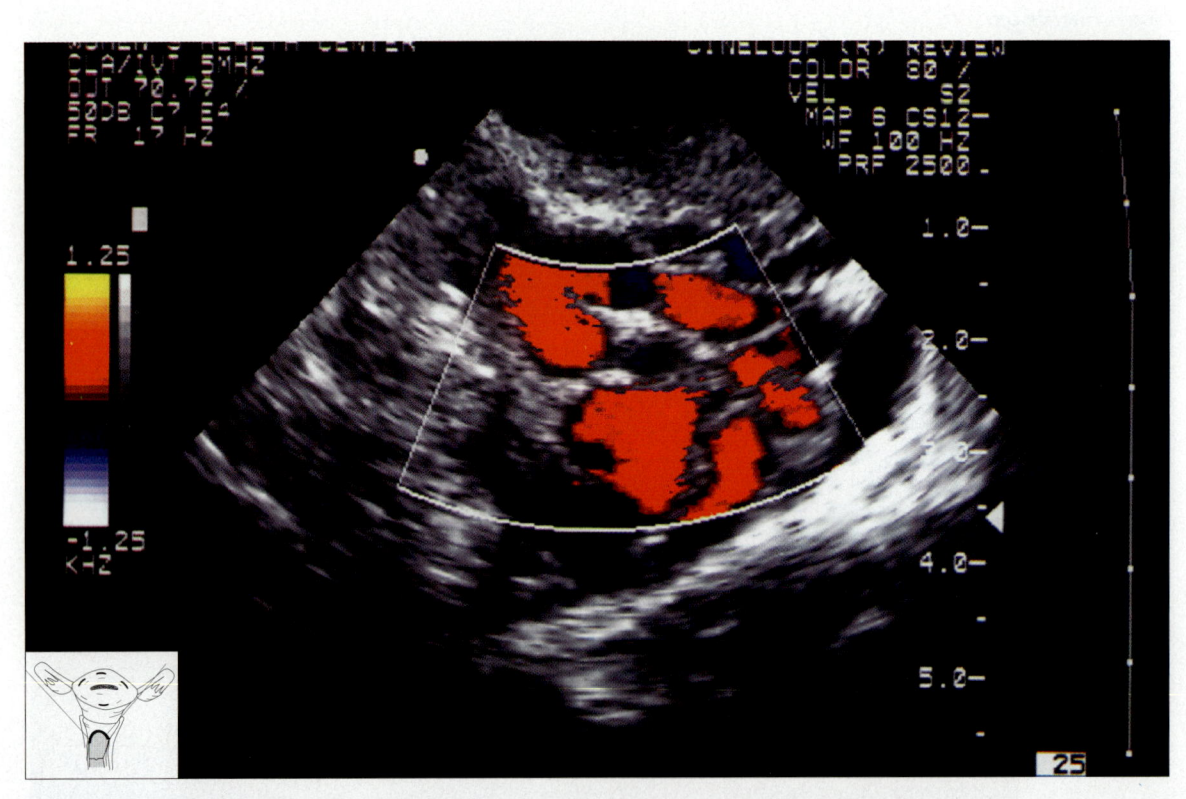

Figure 18-11. Pelvic varicosities confirmed by color flow Doppler in a patient with pelvic pain.

Miscellaneous Lesions

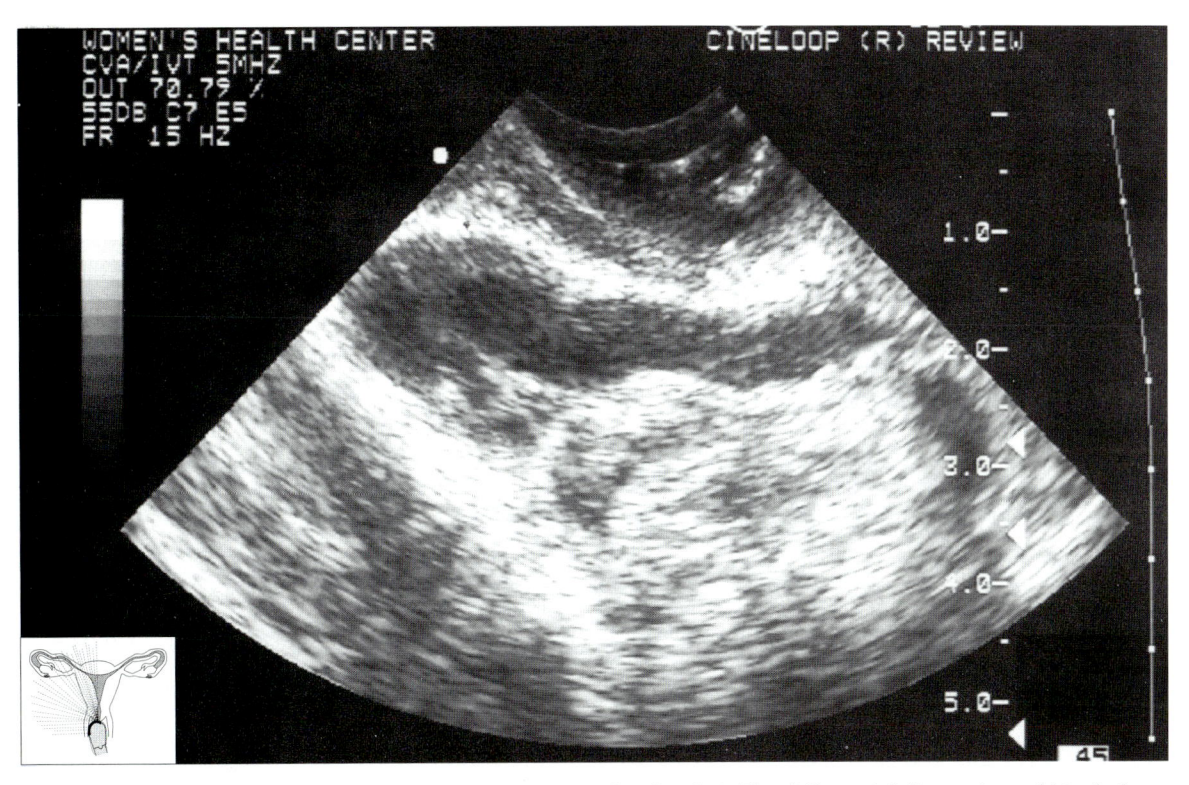

Figure 18-12. Tubular adnexal structure in a patient with infertility. The differential diagnosis could include hydrosalpinx.

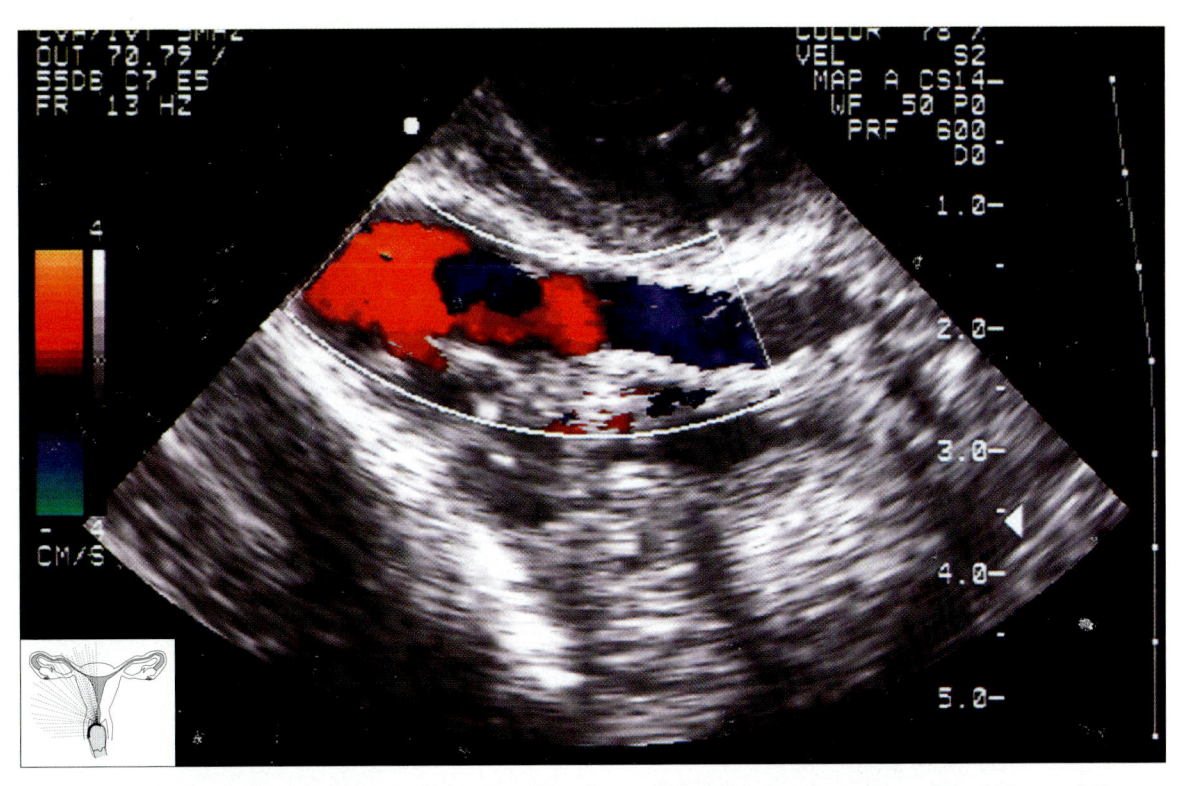

Figure 18-13. Same patient as above. Color flow Doppler confirms the vascular nature of the lesion and the diagnosis of pelvic varicosities.

An Atlas of Transvaginal Sonography

Free Fluid and Ascites

A small amount of peritoneal fluid is normally seen throughout the menstrual cycle. Around ovulation, periovarian fluid is seen, while up to 5 ml of free fluid may be seen in the cul-de-sac under normal conditions.

Scan Findings

An increase in the amount of free peritoneal fluid is easily demonstrated by TVS. The uterus and bowel are outlined by anechoic fluid if a transudate is present, whereas exudates or blood may contain echoes.

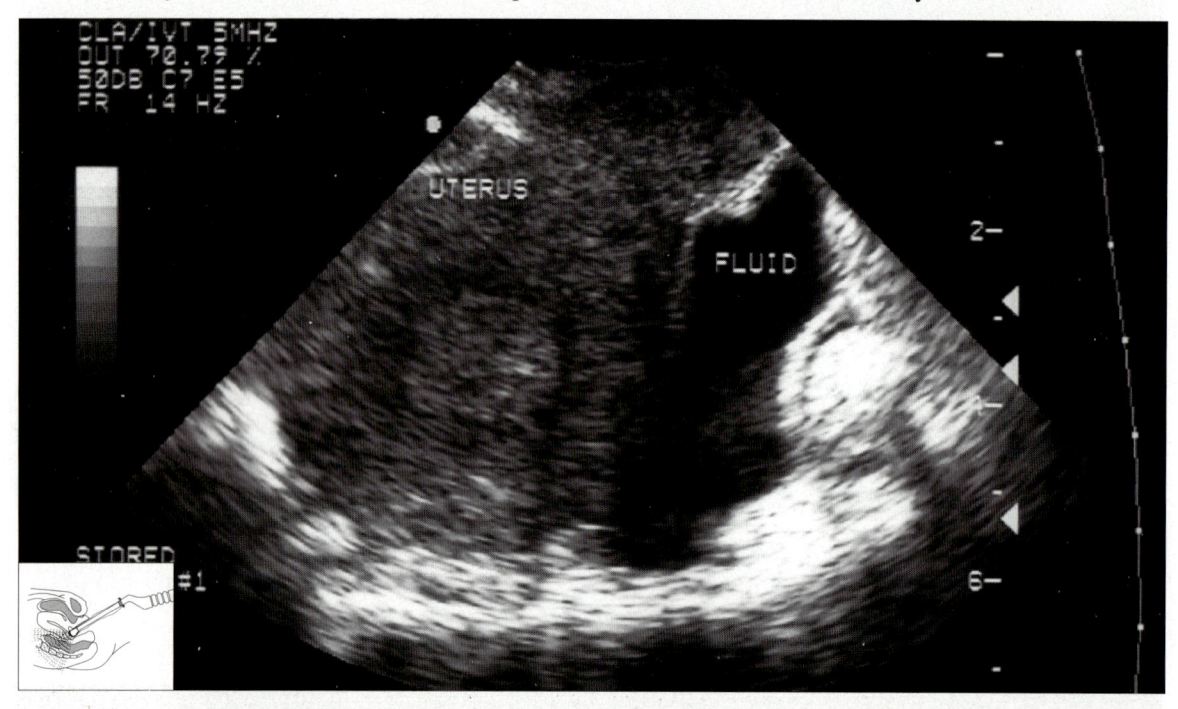

Figure 18-14. Ascitic fluid in the cul-de-sac easily demonstrated by TVS.

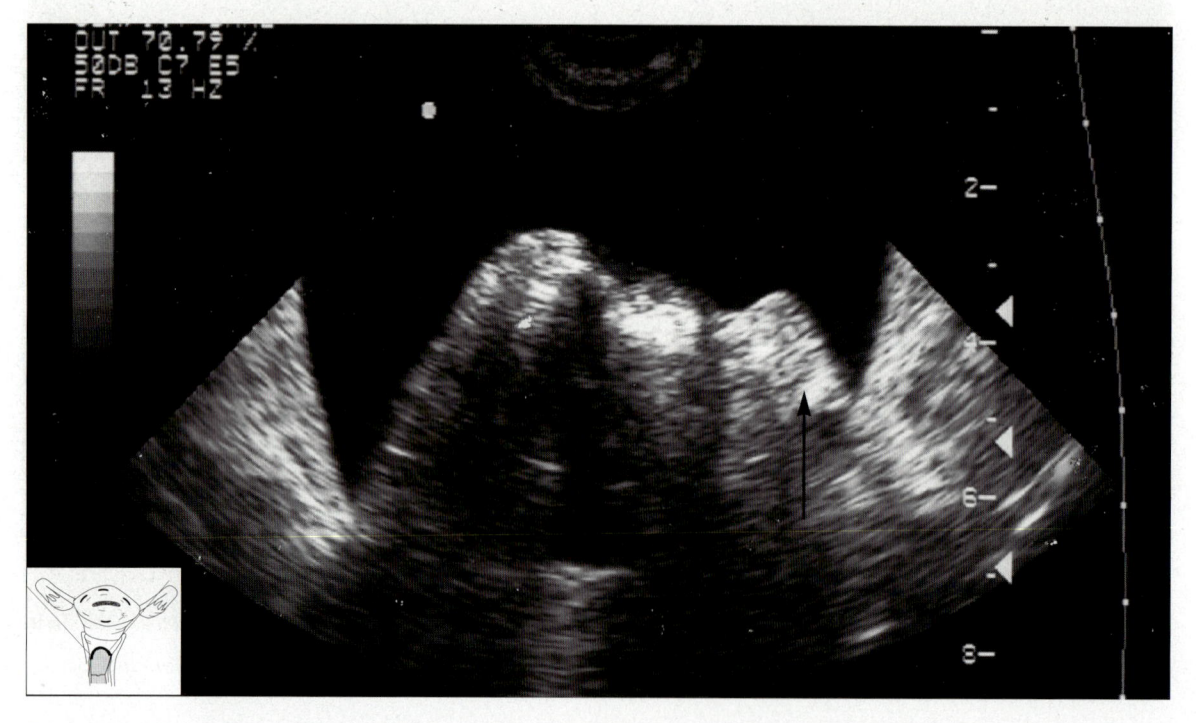

Figure 18-15. Large ovarian cyst. Bowel loops tend to float on ascitic fluid, whereas large serous ovarian tumors compress the bowel posteriorly (arrow).

Miscellaneous Lesions

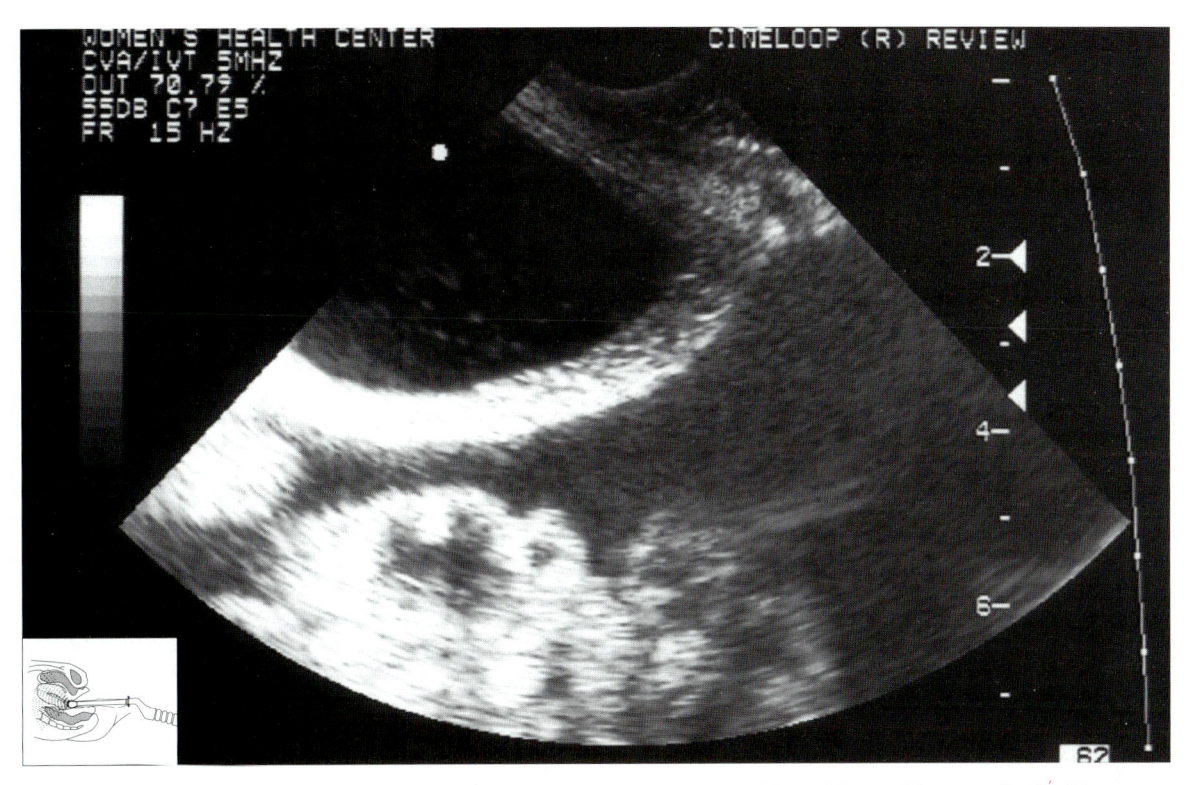

Figure 18-16. Blood-stained malignant ascites outlines the bladder and bowel loops. Urine in the bladder is anechoic, whereas blood in the malignant ascites produces low-grade echoes.

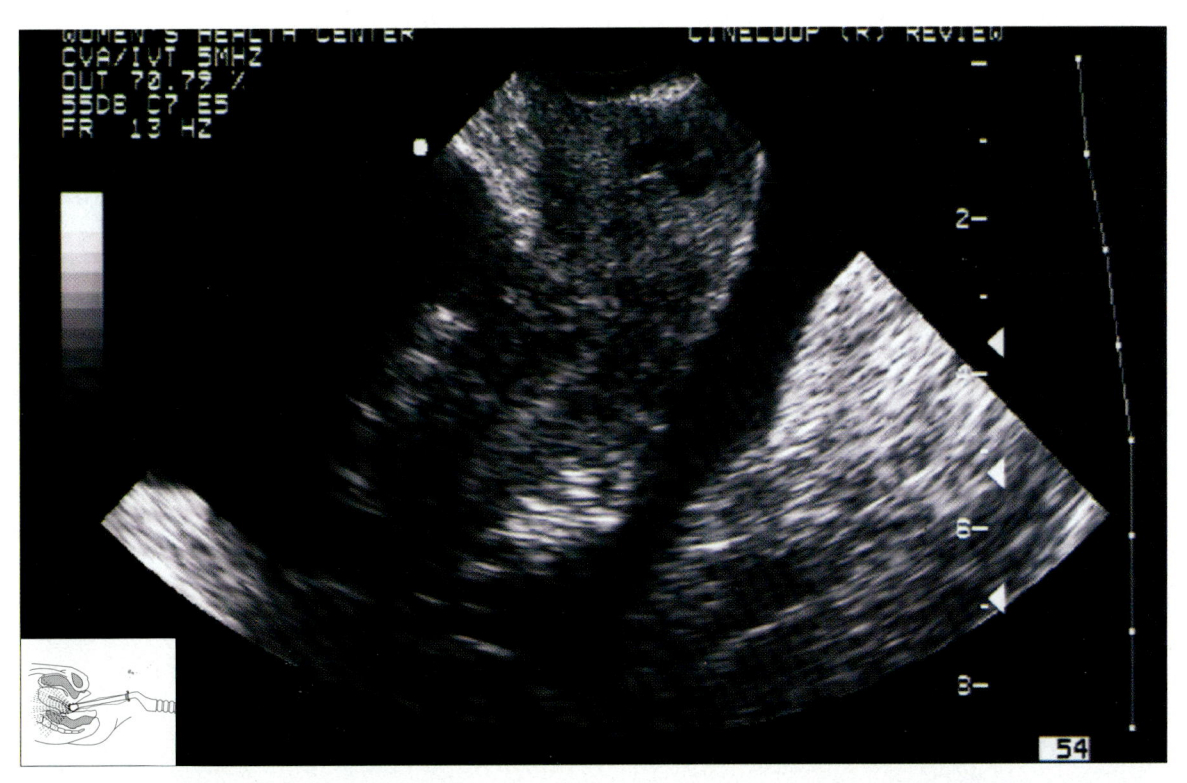

Figure 18-17. Ascites from liver disease. The uterus with calcified arcuate vessels is suspended within ascitic fluid.

217

An Atlas of Transvaginal Sonography

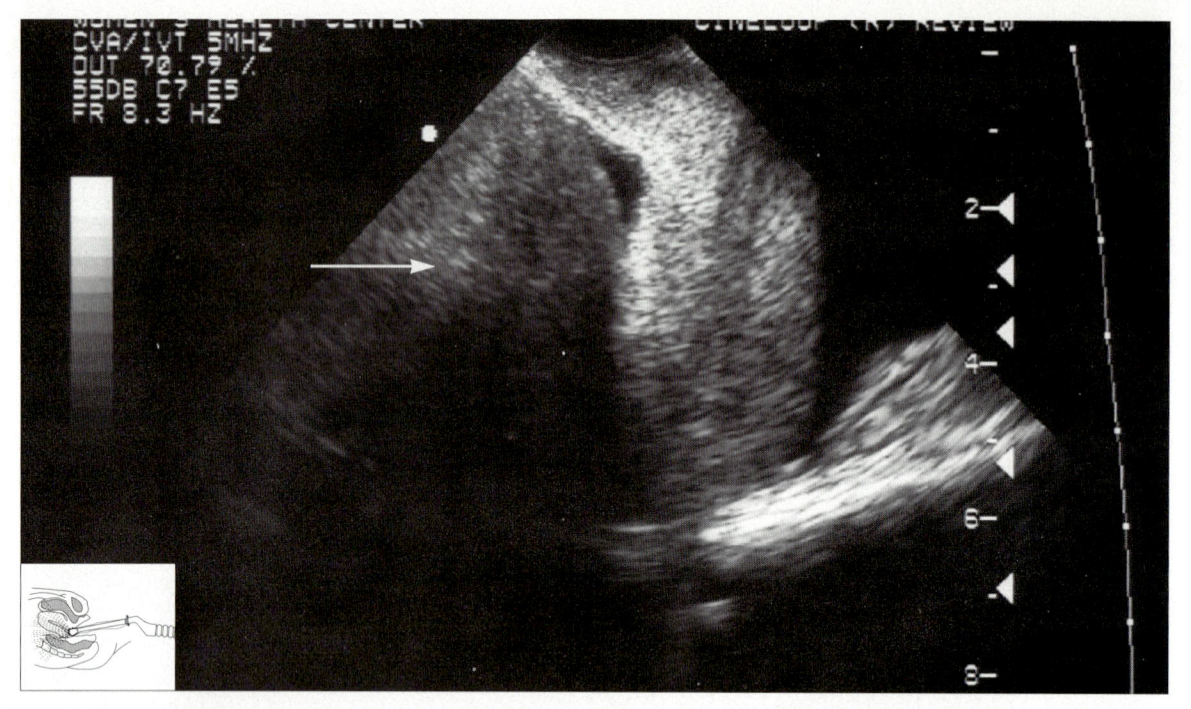

Figure 18-18. Meigs' syndrome: ascites, pleural effusion in association with a benign ovarian fibrothecoma (arrow).

Pelvic Hematoma

Pelvic hematomas or collections are usually seen in the postoperative period, usually after a hysterectomy, but by its dependent nature, any intraabdominal fluid may potentially accumulate within the cul-de-sac.

Scan Findings

Typically what is seen in a pelvic hematoma is an ill-defined, mixed echogenic mass situated at the apex of the vagina or cul-de-sac. If large enough the hematoma can displace adjacent structures, especially the vagina and bowel. Color flow is characteristically absent. A decision can be made at this stage as to the best route of drainage, whether through the vaginal apex, via a posterior colpotomy or through the rectum.

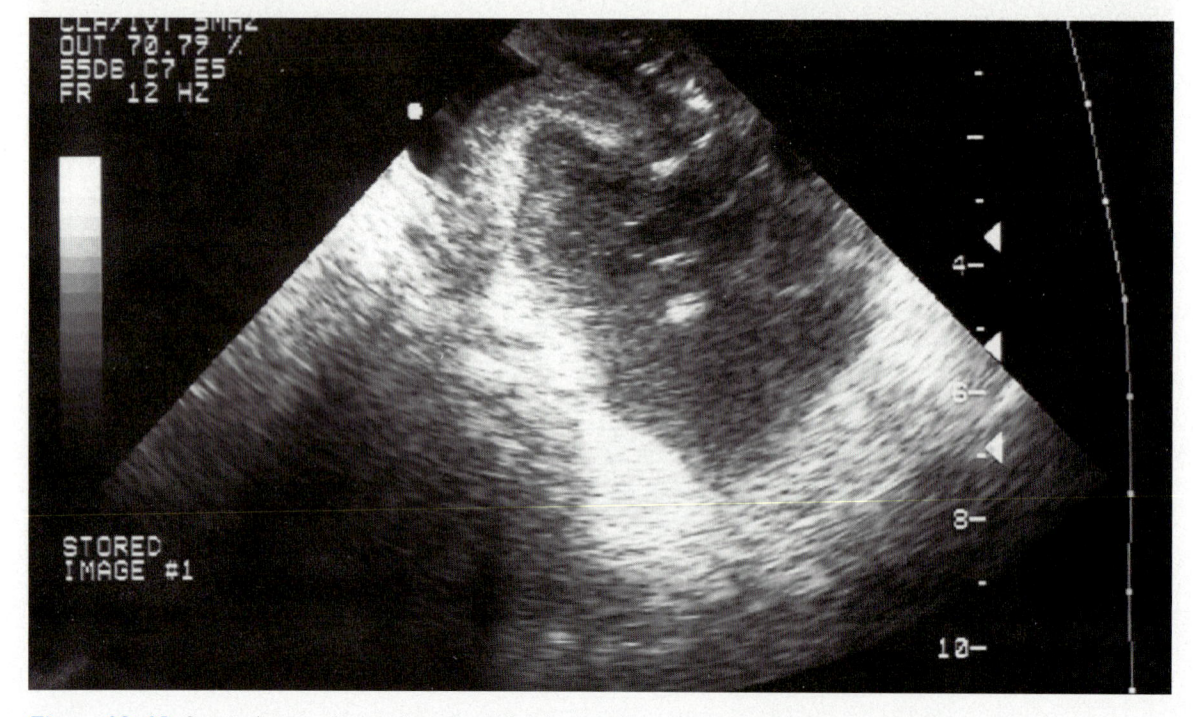

Figure 18-19. Sagittal view of a moderate-sized pelvic abscess after a radical hysterectomy.

Miscellaneous Lesions

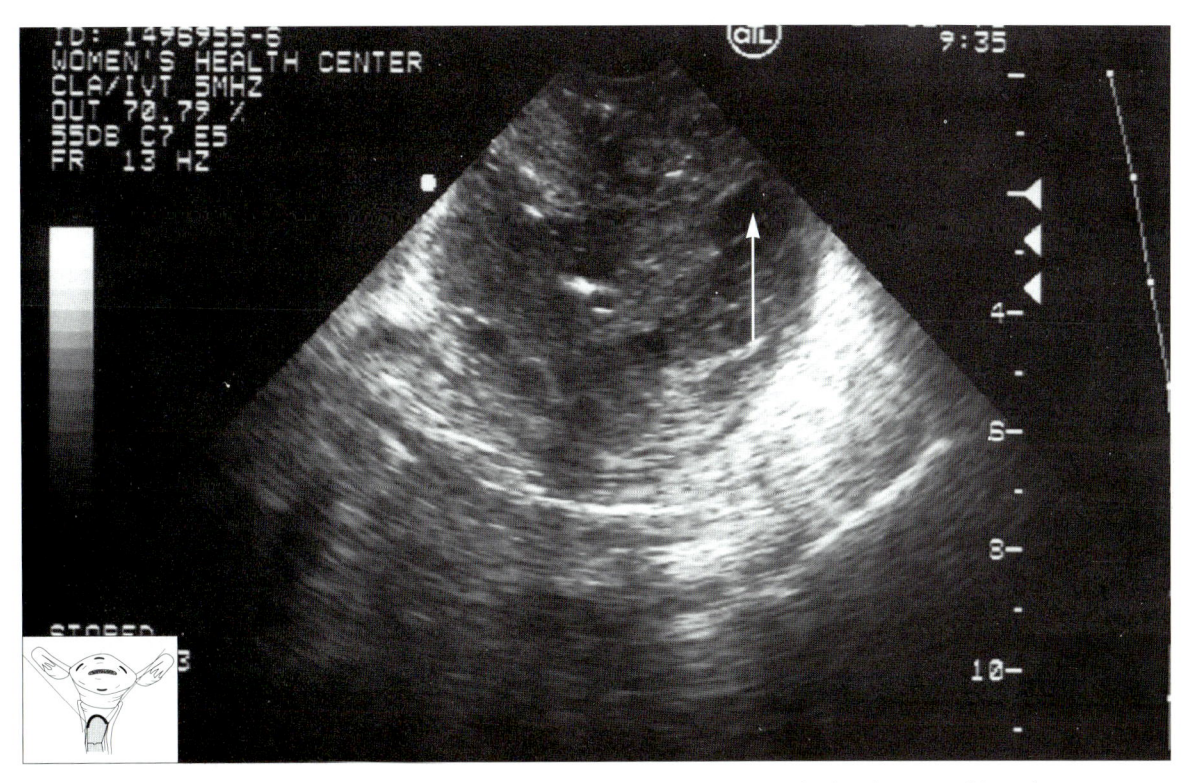

Figure 18-20. Coronal view demonstrates the abscess to be well-circumscribed with areas of liquefactive necrosis (arrow).

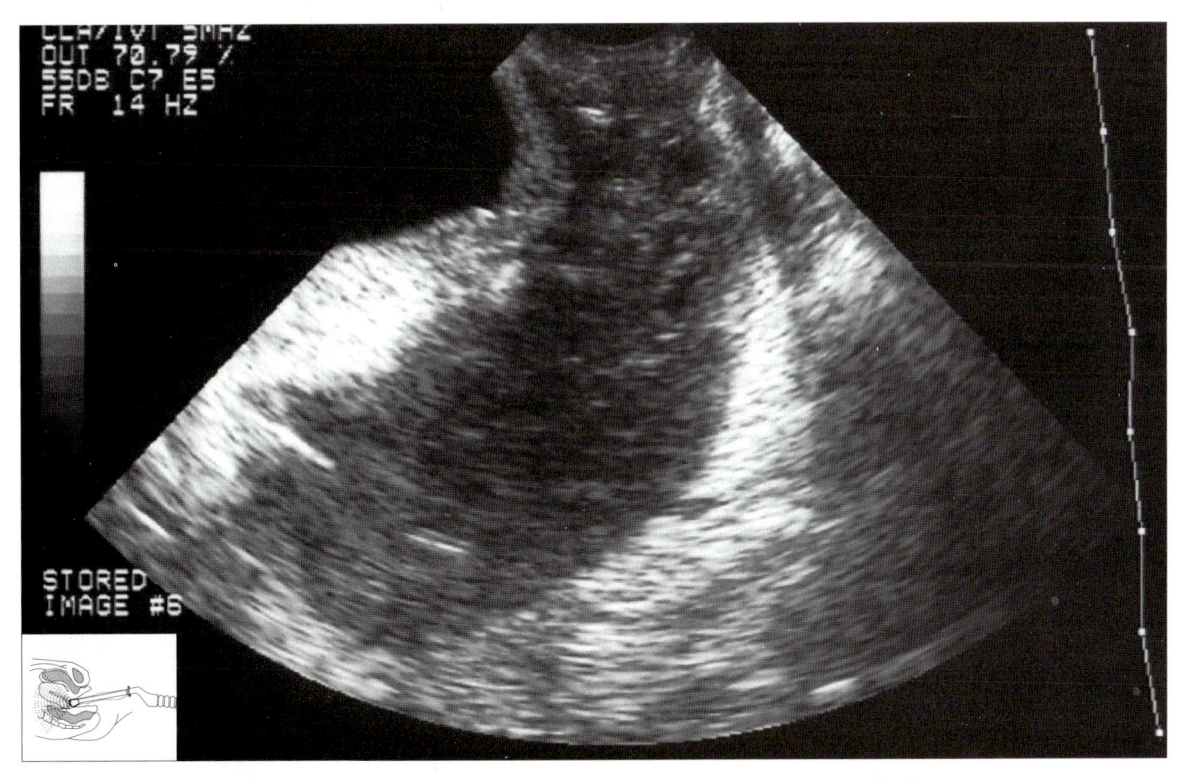

Figure 18-21. Follow-up scan confirms dramatic increase in size, prompting surgical evacuation.

An Atlas of Transvaginal Sonography

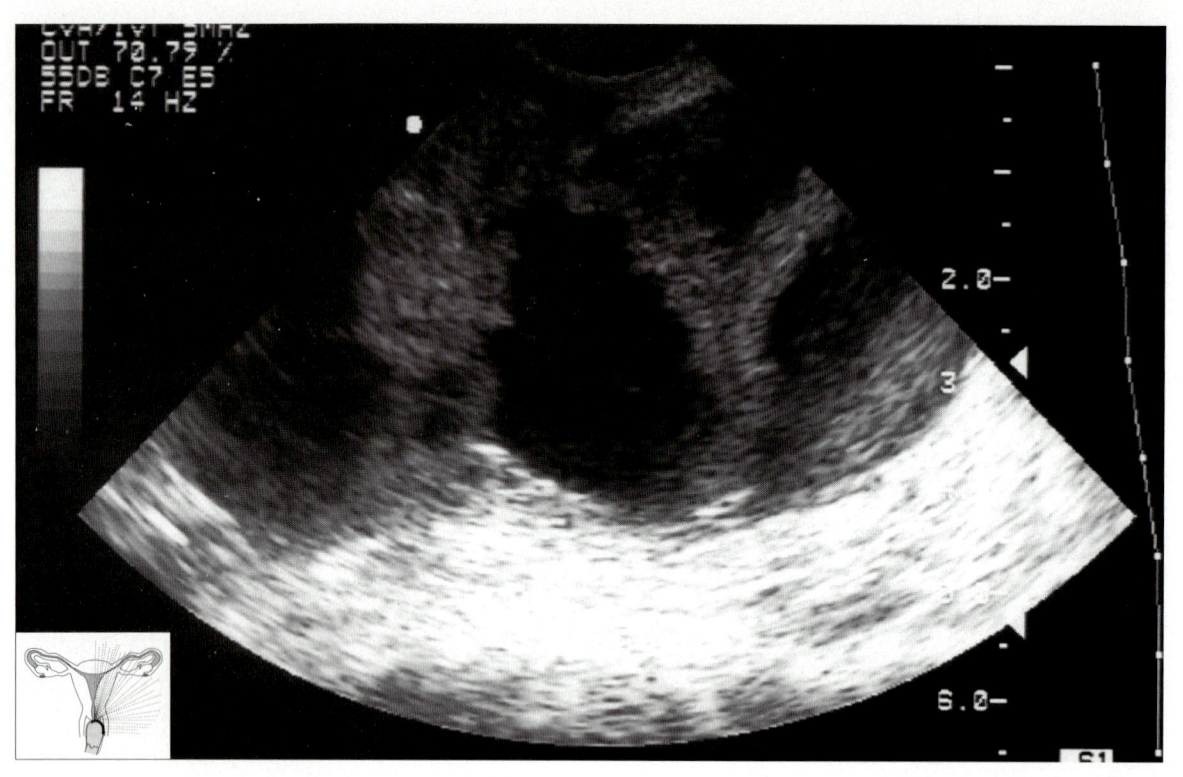

Figure 18-22. Retroperitoneal pelvic hematoma, post-radical pelvic surgery.

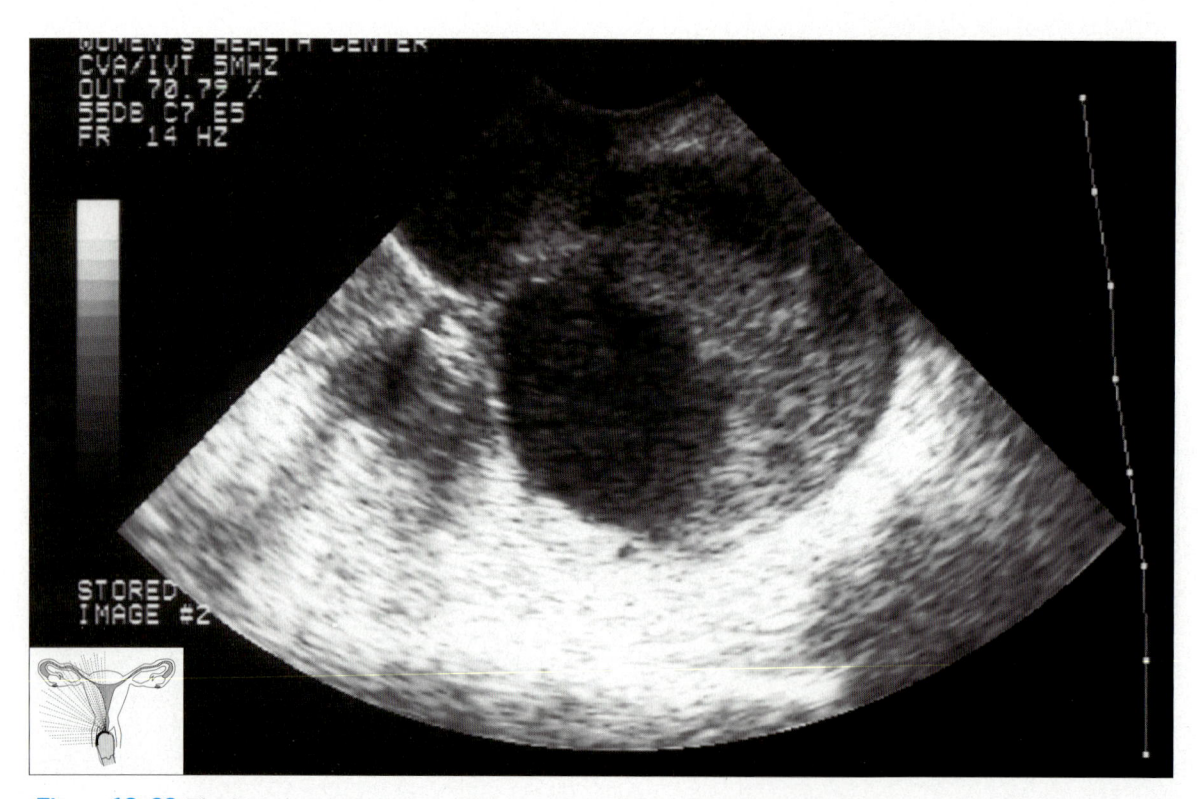

Figure 18-23. The hematoma is similar in appearance to hemorrhagic ovarian cysts.

Miscellaneous Lesions

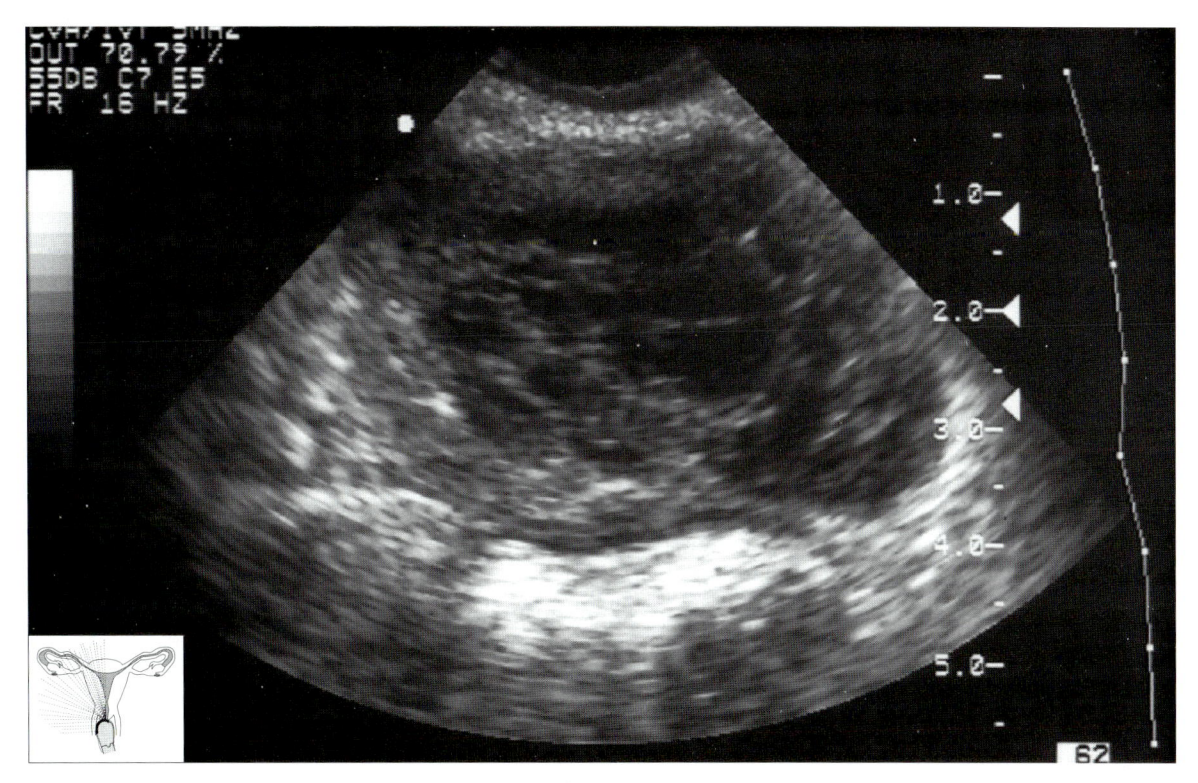

Figure 18-24. Pelvic hematoma: with the passage of time the internal clot solidifies, producing "pseudo septa" and "pseudocysts."

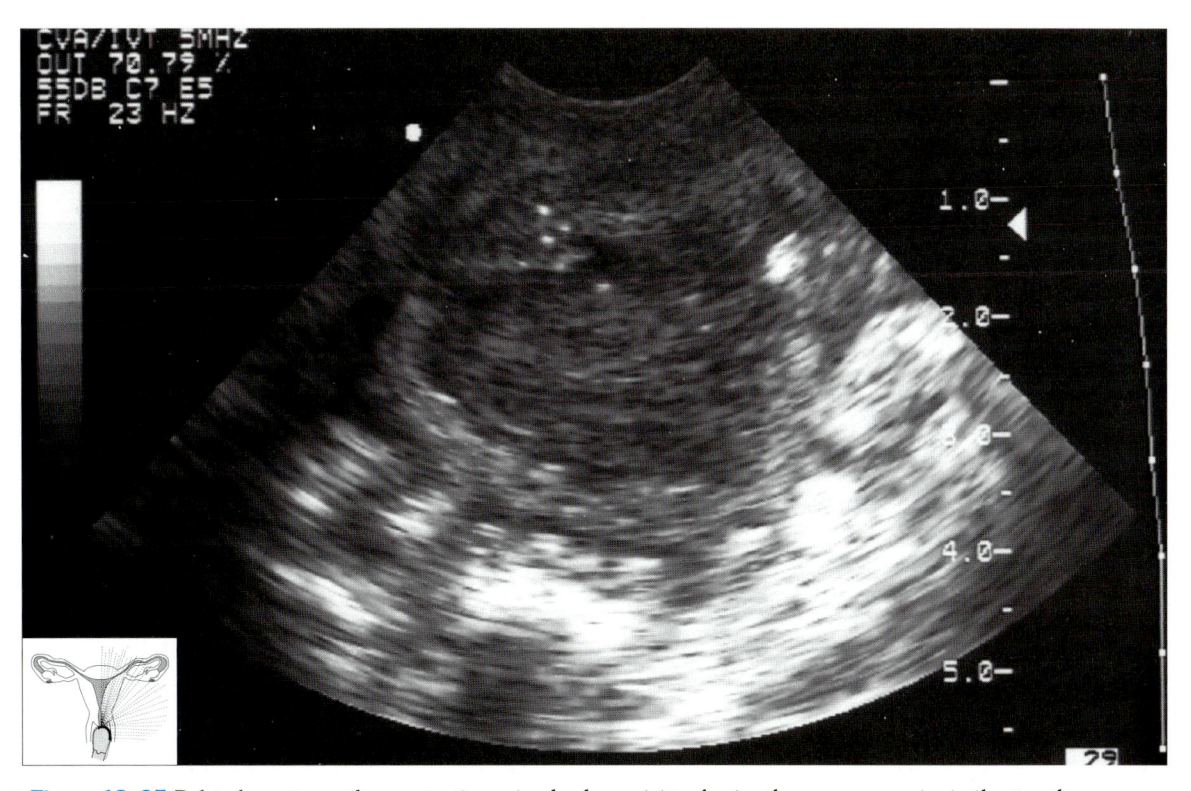

Figure 18-25. Pelvic hematoma demonstrating mixed echogenicity. Again, the appearance is similar to a hemorrhagic ovarian cyst.

Bibliography

Andolf E, Jorgensen C. A prospective comparison of clinical ultrasound and operative examination of the female pelvis. J Ultrasound Med 1988; 7: 617-620.

Andolf E, Svalenius E, Astedt B. Ultrasonography for early detection of ovarian carcinoma. Br J Obstet Gynaecol 1986; 93: 1286-1289.

Averette HE, Dudan RC, Ford JH. Exploratory celiotomy for surgical staging of cervical cancer. Am J Obstet Gynecol 1972; 113: 1090-1096.

Bagshawe KD. Trophoblastic disease. In Advances in Obstetrics and Gynecology, edited by RM Caplan and WJ Sweeney. Williams and Wilkins, Baltimore, 1978, p 225.

Baltzer J, Goepcke W. Tumor size and lymph node metastases in squamous cell carcinoma of the uterine cervix. Arch Gynakologe 1981; 227: 271-278

Bast RC, Klug TL, St John E et al. A radioimmunoassay using a monoclonal antibody to monitor the course of epithelial ovarian cancer. N Eng J Med 1983; 309: 883-887.

Bernaschek G, Deutinger J, Kratochwil A. Endosonography in Obstetrics and Gynecology. Springer-Verlag Berlin Heidelberg: 97-122; 1990.

Bernaschek G, Janisch H. Ene Methode zur Objektivierung des Parametrienbefundes beim Zervixkarzinom. Gevburtshilfe Frauenheilkd 1983; 43: 498-500.

Bourne T, Campbell S, Steer C, Whitehead MI and Collins WP. Transvaginal colour flow imaging: a possible new screening technique of ovarian cancer. Br Med J 1989; 68: 131-135.

Bourne TH, Campbell S, Whitehead MI, Royston P, Steer CV, Collins WP. Detection of endometrial cancer in postmenopausal women by transvaginal ultrasonography and colour flow imaging. Br Med J 1990; 301: 369

Breckenridge JW, Kurtz AB, Ritchie WGM, Macht EL. Postmenopausal uterine fluid collection: indicator of carcinoma. AJR 1982; 139: 529-534.

Buttram VC, Gibbons WE. Mullerian anomalies: a proposed classification (an analysis of 144 cases). Fertil Steril 1979; 3: 397-344.

Campbell S, Bhan V, Royston P, Whitehead MI, Collins WP. Transabdominal ultrasound screening for early ovarian cancer. Br Med J. 299; 1363-1367, 1989.

Carter J and Twiggs LB. The role of transvaginal sonography in gynaecologic oncology. In: Progress in Obstetrics and Gynaecology, Volume 10, Chapter 19. (John Studd, ed), Churchill Livingstone Press, pp 341-357 (1993).

Carter J, Atkinson K, Coppleson M, Elliott P, Solomon J et al. Proliferating and invasive epithelial ovarian tumours in young women. Aust NZ J Obstet Gynaecol 1989; 29: 3(1): 245-249

Carter J, Carson LF and Twiggs L.B.. An update on gestational trophoblastic disease. Postgraduate Obstet Gynecol 1991; 11(8): 1-8.

Carter J, Carson LF and Twiggs LB. Gynecologic Oncology. In: Transvaginal Ultrasound, (David Nyberg, Lyndom Hill, Marcela Bohm-Velez and Ellen Mendelson eds), St. Louis, Mosby Year Book Publishers, pp 241-265 (1992).

Carter J, Carson LF, Byers L, Moradi MM, Elg SA, Adcock LL, Prem KA and Twiggs LB. Transvaginal ultrasound in gynecologic oncology. Obstet Gynecol Surv 1991; 46(10): 687-696.

Carter J, Elg S, Moradi M, Byers L, Adcock L, Prem K, Carson LF and Twiggs LB. Transvaginal sonography as an adjunct to the clinical staging of cervical cancer. J Clin Ultrasound 1992; 20: 283-287.

Carter J, Fowler J, Carlson J, Carson L and Twiggs LB. Just how accurate is the pelvic examination? A prospective comparative study. J Repro Med 1993. (In press).

Carter J, Fowler J, Carlson J, Carson L and Twiggs LB. Prediction of malignancy using transvaginal color flow Doppler in patients with gynecologic tumors. Int J Gynecol Cancer. 1993; 3:279-284.

Carter J, Perrone T, Carson LF, Carlson JW and Twiggs LB. Uterine malignancy predicted by transvaginal sonography and color flow Doppler Ultrasonography. J Clin Ultrasound 1993; 21:405-408

Carter J. Early detection of ovarian cancer by transvaginal ultrasound. Clinical Developments in Women's Cancer 1991; 5 (1): 1-4.

Carter JR, Carlson JW, Fowler JM, Carson LF and Twiggs LB. TVS and CFD in assessment of uterine cancer. 1993.

Carter JR, Carlson JW, Fowler JM, Carson LF, Twiggs LB. Persistent Post-Molar GTD: Use of Transvaginal Sonography and Color Flow Doppler to Diagnose Invasive Moles. Aust NZ J Obstet Gynecol 1993; 33: 4-6.

Carter JR, Fowler JM, Carlson JW, Saltzman A, Byers LJ, Hartenbach E, Carson L and Twiggs LB. Flow Characteristics in Benign and Malignant Gynecologic Tumors Using Transvaginal Color Flow Doppler. Obstet Gynecol 1994;83(1): 1-6.

Carter JR, Fowler JM, Carlson JW, Saltzman AK, Byers LJ, Carson LF and Twiggs LB. Transvaginal color flow doppler in the assessment of gestational trophoblastic disease. J Ultrasound Med 1993; 12:595-599.

Carter JR, Ruhr D, Okagaki T, Fowler JM. Uterine lipoleiomyoma: a rare tumor. J Ultrasound Med 1993;12:491-492.

Chambers CB, Unis JS. Ultrasonographic evidence of uterine malignancy in the postmenopausal uterus. Am J Obstet Gynecol 1986; 154: 1194-1199.

Coppleson M, Elliott PM, Ried BL. Puzzling changes in cervical cancer in young women. Med J Aust 1987; 146: 406-408.

DuBose T. Fetal heart tones. J Ultrasound Med 1989; 8: 407-408.

Elliott PM, Tattersall MHN, Coppleson M et al. The changing character of cervical cancer in young women. Br Med J 1989; 298: 288-290.

Evans DH, Barrie WW, Asher MJ, Bentley S and Bell PRF. The relationship between ultrasonic pulsatility index and proximal arterial stenosis in a canine model. Circ Res 1980; 46: 470-475.

Fasoli M, Ratti E, Franceschi S, LaVecchia C, Pecorelli S and Mangioni C. Management of gestational trophoblastic disease: results of a cooperative study. Obstet Gynecol 1982; 60: 205.

Fleischer AC, Dudley BS, Entman SS, Baxter JW, Kalemeris GC and James AE. Myometrial invasion by endometrial carcinoma: sonographic assessment. Radiology 1987; 162: 307-310.

Folkman J, Merler E, Abernathy C, Williams G. Isolation of a tumor factor responsible for angiogenesis. J Exp Med 1971; 33: 275

Gill RW. Accuracy calculations for ultrasonic pulsed Doppler blood flow measurements. Aust Phys Eng Sci Med 1982; 5:51-57.

Goswamy RK, Campbell S, Royston JP et al. Ovarian size in postmenopausal women. Br J Obstet Gyaecol 1988; 95: 795-801.

Goswamy RK, Campbell S, Whitehead MI. Screening for ovarian cancer. Clinics Obstet Gynecol 1983; 10 (3): 621-643.

Granberg S, Wikland M. A comparison between ultrasound and gynecologic examination for detection of enlarged ovaries in a group of women at risk for ovarian carcinoma. J Ultrasound Med 1988; 7: 59-64.

Heintz AP, Hacker NF, Lagasse LD. Epidemiology and etiology of ovarian cancer: A review. Obstet Gynecol 1985; 66: 127-135.

Jacobs I, Bridges J, Reynolds C, Staabile I, Kemsley P, Grudzinskas J, Oram D. Multimodal approach to screening for ovarian cancer. The Lancet 1988; 6: 268-271.

Jain KA, Jeffrey RB, Sommer FG. Gynecologic vascular abnormalities: diagnosis with Doppler US. Radiology 1991; 178: 549-551.

Jellins J, Kossoff G, Boyd J and Reeve TS. The complementary role of Doppler to the B-mode examination of the breast. Proc 28th Meeting AIUM, J Ultrasound Med 1983; 2: 29-37.

Julian C. General concepts and characteristics of ovarian cancer. In Novak's Gynecology. H Jones and G Jones (Eds): Textbook of Gynecology, (10th ed), Baltimore. Williams and Wilkins Publishers, 1978, p 543.

Kurjak A, Predanic M. New scoring system for prediction of ovarian malignancy based on transvaginal color Doppler sonography. J Ultrasound Med 1992; 11: 631-636.

Kurkak A, Jurkovic D, Alfirevic Z and Zalud I. Transvaginal color Doppler imaging. J Clin Ultrasound 1990; 18: 227-234.

Lagasse LD, Ballon SC, Berman MI, Watring WG. Pretreatment lymphangiography and operative evaluation in carcinoma of the cervix. Am J Obstet Gynecol 1979; 134: 219-224.

Lande IM, Hill MC, Cosco FE, Kator NN. Adnexal and cul-de-sac abnormalities: transvaginal sonography. Radiology 1988; 166: 325-332.

Lange P. Clinical and histological studies on cervical carcinoma. Precancerous, early metastasis and tubular structures in the lymph nodes. Acta Pathol Microbiol Scand Suppl 1960; 143: 9-162

Long MG, Boultbee JE, Begent RHJ, Hanson ME, Bagshawe KD. Preliminary Doppler studies on the uterine artery and myometrium in trophoblastic tumours requiring chemotherapy. Br J Obstet Gynecol 1990; 97: 686-689.

Lynch HT, Bewtra C and Lynch JF. Familial ovarian carcinoma. Clinical nuances. Am J Obstet Gynecol 1986; 81: 1073-1076.

Lynch HT, Bowtra C, Wells IC Schuelke GS and Lynch JF. Hereditary ovarian cancer clinical and biomarker studies. Cancer Genetics in Women (HT Lynch and S Kullander, Eds), CRC Press, Boca Raton, FL, p 49-97. 1987

Mittelstaedt CA. Abdominal ultrasound, New York, 1987, Churchill Livingstone, pp230-371.

Nicolini U, Belloti M, Bonazzi B, Zamberletti D et al. Can ultrasound be used to screen for uterine malformations? Fertil Steril 1987; 47: 89-93.

Osmerw R, Volksen M, Schauer A. Vaginosonography for early detection of endometrial carcinoma? Lancet 1990; 335: 1569-1571.

Piver MS, Chung WS. Prognostic significance of cervical lesion size and pelvic node metastasis in cervical carcinoma. Obstet Gynecol 1975; 46: 507-510.

Rubin MC, Preston AL. Adnexal masses in post-menopausal women. Obstet Gynecol 1987; 70: 578-581.

Schildkraut JM, Thompson WD. Relationship of epithelial ovarian cancer to other malignancies within families. Genet Epidemiol 1988; 5:355-367.

Schneider DF, Bukovsky I, Winraub Z, Golan A and Caspi E. Transvaginal ultrasound diagnosis and treatment follow-up of invasive gestational trophoblastic disease. J Clin Ultrasound 1990; 18: 110-113.

Schulman H, Fleischer A, Farmakides G et al. Development of uterine artery compliance in pregnancy as detected by Doppler ultrasound. Am J Obstet Gynecol 1986; 155: 1031-1036.

Scott WW, Rosenshein NB, Siegelmann SS, Sanders RC. The obstructed uterus. Radiology 1981; 141: 767-770.

Steinkampf MP. Transvaginal sonography. J Reprod Med 1988; 33(12): 931-937.

Strickland B. The value of arteriography in the diagnosis of bone tumors. Br J Radiol 1959: 32: 705-713.

Tessler FN, Schiller VL. Perrella RR, Sutherland ML, Grant EG. Transabdominal versus endovaginal pelvic sonography: prospective study. Radiology. 1989; 170: 553-556.

Wei P, Ouyang P. Trophoblastic disease in Taiwan. Am J Obstet Gynecol 1961; 85: 844.

Zander J, Baltzer J, Lohe KJ, Ober KG, Kaufmann C. Carcinoma of the cervix: an attempt to individualize treatment. Am J Obstet Gynecol 1981; 139: 752-759.